Quantitative Estimation and Prediction
of Human Cancer Risks

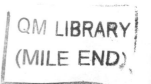

International Agency for Research on Cancer

The International Agency for Research on Cancer (IARC) was established in 1965 by the World Health Assembly, as an independently financed organization within the framework of the World Health Organization. The headquarters of the Agency are at Lyon, France.

The Agency conducts a programme of research concentrating particularly on the epidemiology of cancer and the study of potential carcinogens in the human environment. Its field studies are supplemented by biological and chemical research carried out in the Agency's laboratories in Lyon, and, through collaborative research agreements, in national research institutions in many countries. The Agency also conducts a programme for the education and training of personnel for cancer research.

The publications of the Agency are intended to contribute to the dissemination of authoritative information on different aspects of cancer research. Information about IARC publications and how to order them is available via the Internet at: http://www.iarc.fr/

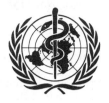

INTERNATIONAL AGENCY FOR RESEARCH ON CANCER
WORLD HEALTH ORGANIZATION

Quantitative Estimation and Prediction of Human Cancer Risks

Edited by
S. Moolgavkar, D. Krewski, L. Zeise,
E. Cardis and H. Møller

IARC Scientific Publications No. 131

International Agency for Research on Cancer
Lyon, France
1999

Published by the International Agency for Research on Cancer,
150 cours Albert Thomas, 69372 Lyon cédex 08, France

Distributed by Oxford University Press, Walton Street, Oxford OX2 6DP, UK
(fax: +44 1865 267782) and in the USA by Oxford University Press, 2001 Evans Road, Carey,
NC 27513 (fax: +1 919 677 1303). All IARC publications can also be ordered directly from IARC*Press*
(fax: +33 04 72 73 83 02; E-mail: press@iarc.fr).

IARC Library Cataloguing in Publication Data

Quantitative estimation and prediction of human cancer risks /
editors, S. Moolgavkar ... [et al.]

(IARC scientific publications ; 131)

1. Neoplasms – epidemiology
2. Risk Assessment I. Moolgavkar, Suresh H
II. Series

ISBN 92 832 2131 1   (NLM Classification W1)
ISSN 0300-5085

Printed in France

Contents

E. Cardis, L. Zeise, M. Schwarz and S. Moolgavkar

Foreword

Modern societies are constantly striving to balance the health risks of exposures to products and byproducts of industrial processes against the economic benefits that accrue from such activity. There is no unified approach to regulation of toxic agents. Regulatory agencies in industrialized countries have adopted different approaches to regulation. A common problem, however, is that regulation must most often be based on incomplete scientific knowledge. In particular, human data on exposure to the agent of interest are often not available, and regulation must be based on information from experimental studies. Even when epidemiological data are available, exposures are typically regulated at levels far below the observed levels in order to assure an adequate margin of safety.

This volume provides a review of current practice at various regulatory agencies and a broad survey of the principles underlying the quantitative estimation and prediction of cancer risks. A large part of the book is devoted to a discussion of state-of-the-art biology based quantitative models that are increasingly being used for analyses of experimental and epidemiological data. This volume should be of interest to all professionals interested in cancer risk assessment.

Paul Kleihues
Director

Contributors

B. Armstrong
Cancer Control Information Centre
NSW Cancer Council
P.O.Box 572
Kings Cross NSW 2011
Australia

P. Boffetta
Unit of Environmental Cancer Epidemiology
International Agency for Research on Cancer
150 cours Albert Thomas
69372 Lyon Cedex 08
France

E. Cardis
Unit of Radiation and Cancer
International Agency for Research on Cancer
150 Cours Albert-Thomas
69372 Lyon Cedex 08
France

V.J. Feron
Toxicology Division
TNO Nutrition & Food Research Institute
P.O.Box 360
3700 AJ Zeist
The Netherlands

K. Hemminki
Center for Nutrition and Toxicology
Karolinska Institute
Novum
141 57 Huddinge
Sweden

D. Krewski
University of Ottawa, Department of Medicine &
Department of Epidemiology & Community
Medicine
451 Smyth Rd.
Ottawa, Ontario K1H 8M5
Canada

A.J. McMichael
London School of Hygiene
Keppel Street
London WC1H OBT
UK

H. Møller
Centre for Research in Health & Social Statistics
The Danish National Research Foundation
Sejrogade 11
2100 Copenhagen Ø
Denmark

S. Moolgavkar
Fred Hutchinson Cancer Research Center
1100 Fairview Avenue N
MP-665
Seattle, WA 98109
USA

M. Schwarz
Institute of Toxicology
University of Tübingen
Wilhelmstrasse 56
72074 Tübingen
Germany

A. Woodward
Wellington School of Medicine
University of Otago
P.O.Box 7343
Wellington South
New Zealand

L. Zeise
Reproductive and Cancer Hazard Assessment
Section
Office of Environmental Health Hazard
Assessment
1515 Clay Street, 16th Floor
Oakland, CA 94612
USA

Acknowledgements

The editors thank Dr C. Wild for his extensive contributions to previous drafts of this book, Drs D. Bell, G.G. Chabot, U. Meyer, R. Montesano, G. Romeo, R. Saracci and E. Taioli for help in reviewing the contributions to this volume, and Mrs O. Drutel, Mrs M. Geesink and M. Garroni-Pichelingat for secretarial help.

Quantitative Estimation and Prediction of Human Cancer Risks
S. Moolgavkar, D. Krewski, L. Zeise, E. Cardis and H. Møller
IARC Scientific Publications No. 131
International Agency for Research on Cancer, Lyon, 1999

1: Quantitative Estimation and Prediction of Human Cancer Risk: Its History and Role in Cancer Prevention

Anthony J. McMichael and Alistair Woodward

1.1 Introduction

As cancer research advances, we accumulate epidemiological data, measure carcinogenic exposures more precisely, understand better the relationship of animal and cell-assay test data to human cancer risks, and learn more about the mechanisms of carcinogenesis. By definition, qualitative evaluation of the weight of evidence from human, animal and other studies does not make full use of this range of knowledge; it assesses whether there is a hazard, but not how great the risk is. Many groups in society, including scientists, want to know more than simply whether cancer risks exist, and are pressing for information about the magnitude of these risks. For example, regulators want such information to guide them when they set priorities for the control of cancer-causing agents in the environment. Consumer organizations press for full disclosure of the harmful effects of new appliances and drugs. Industrial groups want to quantify risks in order to estimate the benefits (and costs) of changing current work practices. Courts of law seek quantitative estimates of cancer risks to assist decisions on liability for individual cases of cancer.

In developed countries, the intensity of formal regulation of health-endangering exposures has increased during the last 30 years. Quantitation of cancer risks assists the control of cancer hazards by providing policy-makers with information about the magnitude and gradient of risk across a range of exposure levels. Furthermore, this information, coupled with population exposure profiles, enables an assessment to be made of the relative importance of each carcinogen in relation to other carcinogens and other hazards "competing" for regulatory attention and resources. No community can afford to eliminate exposure to all known carcinogens, and policy-makers must deal with some carcinogenic exposures that cannot be eliminated (e.g. ultraviolet radiation, exposure to domestic radon).

Increasingly, governments at the local, national and international levels are making policy and regulatory choices in the fields of energy production, industrial practices, food safety and waste management. The health risks and environmental consequences of a particular activity are usually weighed against its economic and social benefits (Lave, 1985; McMichael, 1991). The combination of increased public concern over environmental hazards to health and a more open regulatory process means that, more than ever before, policy-makers are under pressure to make decisions about tolerable levels of exposure to environmental agents.

The data available for quantifying cancer risks to humans are often sparse. Scientists may therefore feel uncomfortable inferring dose–response relationships from meagre data sets such as the epidemiological data currently available for cancer associated with exposure to chlorinated drinking-water. Particular difficulties arise when the level (or range) of exposure of greatest public health relevance to some population is below that for which adequate quantitative empirical data are available, as is the case for most domestic radon exposure and lung cancer risk (Samet & Nero, 1989; Lubin, 1994; see also Chapter 8). In these situations, the primary scientific question may be whether or not there is a detectable increase in cancer risk at those levels of exposure, and this question must be answered before attempting to quantify the dose–response relationship. Difficulties of another kind arise when no information is available on cancer risks in humans, and inferences must be drawn from studies of animals. Extrapolation from animals to humans is a major issue in quantitative estimation and prediction of cancer risk, and is discussed later in this book.

The burden of cancer does not fall equally on all members of a population. Rather, there is a distribution of cancer risks over members of the population, some of whom are much more likely to develop cancer than others because not all individuals in the population are exposed at the same level of exposure. Additionally, the susceptibility of individuals to developing cancer depends upon both environmental and genetic factors, so that susceptibility to specific cancers varies among individuals. These ideas are illustrated schematically in Figure 1.1. When sufficient information is available, these factors, which determine the total burden of cancer in a population, can be investigated. In particular, information about dose–response relationships in various segments of the population may be used to formulate exposure guidelines or standards.

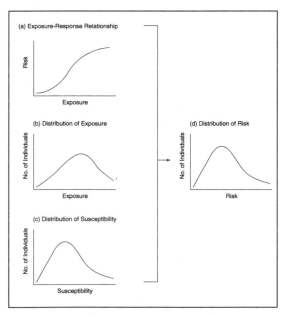

Figure 1.1. Factors influencing the distribution of risk in the population: (a) exposure–response relationship; (b) distribution of exposure; (c) distribution of susceptibility; (d) distribution of risk, which depends upon (a), (b) and (c)

Quantitative estimates of risk may be subject to many sources of uncertainty. For example, experimental and sampling error as well as random and systematic measurement error in both exposure and response variates all contribute to uncertainty in risk estimation. Risk can also vary appreciably among individuals in the population of interest, as illustrated in Figure 1.1. Even though estimates of cancer risk are subject to both uncertainty and variability, quantitative analyses can often provide a clearer basis for risk-management decisions than qualitative evaluations of (known, possible or probable) carcinogens.

1.2 Historical background

Since the 1940s, industrialization and the proliferation of synthetic organic chemicals have resulted in a myriad of actual and potential health-endangering exposures. In many industrialized countries, cancer, vascular disease and other chronic conditions have now replaced infectious diseases as the major causes of mortality. This has led to a new emphasis in public health on the risks, particularly cancer risks, posed by exposure to chemical agents (Paustenbach, 1989).

Initially, scientists and regulators used a qualitative assessment, based on toxicity testing, and invoking a binary "Yes–No" classification of agents as human health hazards. However, the setting of permissible exposure limits for the workplace, systematized by industrial hygienists in the USA during the 1940s, introduced the less absolute concept of "acceptable" levels of exposure to toxic agents (Paustenbach & Langner, 1986). The rudimentary quantitative risk-assessment methods that evolved during the 1940s and 1950s included the use, for health outcomes other than cancer, of dose–response graphs to identify a "no-observed-adverse-effect level" (NOAEL), i.e. a dose below which no adverse effect was apparent (Krewski et al., 1984; Paustenbach, 1989). This "no-effect dose" approach to risk assessment sought to identify a so-called safe level. However, for cancer risks, the notion of a "virtually safe dose" (Mantel & Bryan, 1961) soon came to be preferred, since any exposure to carcinogens was assumed to cause some increment in cancer risk. More recently, the term "risk-specific dose" has come into use in order to avoid implying the acceptability of specific levels of risk. Radiation standards, which historically have been designed primarily to protect against cancer, illustrate the changing view of "safe" exposures. The standards were first described in terms of a "tolerance dose", then a "maximum permissible dose", and now a "dose limit" accompanied by explicit advice to keep exposures as low as reasonably possible (Walker, 1989).

Mathematical models were used to estimate the dose-related excess lifetime cancer risks (including the estimated upper-bound excess risk) for humans, based on the dose–response curve obtained in animal bioassays and taking into account differences in species sensitivity to carcinogen exposure (Crump *et al*, 1976). Subsequent improvements in cancer modelling have come about through awareness of the processes involved in carcinogenesis and improved modelling of tissue dosimetry. Increasingly, knowledge about the mechanisms of carcinogenesis is facilitating the quantitative estimation of cancer risks, as illustrated in Chapter 7. This subject is discussed in detail in a previous IARC Scientific Publication (Vainio *et al.*, 1992).

A number of criticisms have been made of the use of quantitative estimation of cancer risk in setting policy (Lave, 1985; Rushefsky, 1986; Perera, 1987). It has been argued that the quality of the primary epidemiological and toxicological data is often not good enough to sustain the complex and seemingly robust estimates of risk cited by policy-makers. Estimations of cancer risks have been criticized for not acknowledging fully the underlying uncertainties. The sources of uncertainty in risk estimation include not only statistical error, but also judgements that must frequently be made in science where evidence is incomplete. For example, the magnitude of estimated cancer risks may be affected substantially by the selection of data sets, the method of extrapolation of risk between species or choice of outcomes (such as the inclusion or exclusion of benign tumours in risk assessment), yet none of these critical choices can be settled solely by measurement and observation. Furthermore, the extent of interindividual variation in susceptibility to some particular carcinogen, even if known, will render the estimation of risk more complex.

Ideally, the "upstream" scientifically based quantitation of cancer risk would be distinguishable from the "downstream" value judgements, trade-offs and political choices that must be made when formulating regulations. However, the boundary between the two is not always easy to define. Scientific data do not exist in a social vacuum but must be interpreted, and it is often difficult to distinguish between interpretation of a technical kind (which, anyway, is affected by the prevailing biological theories and choice of statistical models) and interpretation that is affected by values and other considerations from outside the realm of science (Landy *et al.*, 1990).

1.3 Definitions of terms and concepts

The primary purpose of this volume is to assess formal methods for the quantitative estimation and prediction of human cancer risks. Whereas the term "hazard" refers to a potential cause of illness or injury, "risk" expresses the probability that some specified adverse outcome will occur in a person or a group exposed to a particular concentration of a hazardous agent over specific time intervals (Paustenbach, 1989). Quantifying that risk entails a mix of formal procedures and judgements, depending on the range of data available.

For risk management, it may be important to distinguish between two exposures that may entail the same "lifetime risk" but that induce death at different ages. For this purpose, predictions of "years of life lost", defined as the difference in life expectancy between an unexposed person and one exposed at a certain age, may be derived.

In practice, the terms "exposure" and "dose" are often used interchangeably in quantitative estimation and prediction (QEP), in particular in the context of QEPs based on epidemiological studies. Throughout this book, these terms will be used in a more rigorous manner (see Chapter 4 for a more detailed discussion), with:

• "exposure" referring to the quantity of the agent in the individual's environment: for example the amount of tobacco smoke in the immediate environment of a non-smoker or the ^{131}I activity present in the environment, water and food products following the Chernobyl accident; and

• "dose" referring to the quantity that has been taken up by the individual: for example, the amount of smoke in the bronchi of the non-smoker exposed to passive smoke or the amount of energy deposited by ß and γ radiation in the target cells of the thyroid,which will depend on age, iodine-deficiency status, consumption of food and time spent out of doors.

The data available for risk quantification are derived from epidemiological studies of human populations and from toxicological studies conducted in the laboratory. Epidemiological studies have the advantage of providing direct information on cancer risks in humans, but are subject to various types of bias that can occur in observational studies of human populations (see Chapters 3 and 4). They are also subject to limitations in statistical sensitivity to the point where individual studies are often insensitive to small risks. These limitations can be overcome in a controlled laboratory environment using high doses to enhance statistical sensitivity, but at the expense of introducing the need for uncertain extrapolations from laboratory animals to humans and from high to low doses. It is within this research framework that a distinction is deliberately made between the words "estimation" and "prediction" as used throughout this volume.

An estimate is a value for an unknown quantity (e.g. the true risk of cancer), calculated according to sound statistical principles, and inferred from data that directly pertain to the specified exposure circumstance. The word "estimate" is used because the observations of any single study represent only a sample of all the observations that could, potentially, be made. Estimates are of varying degrees of precision and accuracy, depending on the nature of the data and on the inference methods upon which they are based. Precision will be influenced by sample size, and can be expressed in terms of standard errors or confidence intervals. Accuracy, or the degree to which the estimate is unbiased, is more difficult to evaluate, and requires consideration of potential sources of systematic as well as random error (see Chapter 4).

The term "prediction" is used here to refer to estimates of risk under conditions different from those under which the original data were obtained. It includes, in particular, extrapolation

outside the range of the original data, both to different species and to different exposure circumstances with the same species. One might expect that the greater the extrapolation, the greater the degree of uncertainty associated with predictions of risk. An understanding of the biological processes leading to carcinogenic effects in the original study population can strengthen confidence in extrapolated predictions. If such knowledge is available, the likelihood of similar mechanisms operating in other circumstances can be evaluated. As an example of another type of extrapolation, epidemiological data on lung cancer risks experienced by active smokers have been used to predict potential risks associated with a different but related exposure, namely passive smoking. Epidemiological studies of passive smoking have addressed this issue directly, and have been useful for evaluating the predictions of risk derived by extrapolation from studies of active smokers (Wald *et al.*, 1986; US Environmental Protection Agency, 1992).

Although reliable estimates of risk based on relevant data are most desirable, predictions of risk can also be useful. Direct estimates of risk are possible in epidemiological studies of human populations subjected to unusually high levels of exposure, and in animal experiments where high doses are used to enhance the probability of detecting a response. In order to predict the risks for humans exposed at lower levels, it is essential to do one or more of the following:

(i) Extrapolate the high-exposure human data to lower dose levels.
(ii) Estimate the risks for animals at high exposures, extrapolate that to low doses, and then extrapolate that prediction to humans.
(iii) Extrapolate from low-exposure observations in animals to humans.

As will be seen later in this volume, quantitative estimates of risk can be expressed in different ways. In regulatory applications of cancer risk assessment, risk is often expressed in terms of the lifetime probability of developing a cancer in a particular population under specified conditions of exposure. To make this concept precise, it is necessary to specify the expected life span over which risk accumulates. Such estimates can be adjusted for intercurrent mortality, or standardized with respect to patterns of mortality from causes other than cancer. Epidemiologists often summarize their quantitative estimates of risk in terms of age-specific cancer incidence rates, which reflect the number of new cancer cases occurring in a particular exposed population of a specified age over a specified period. Risks may also be described in terms of number of years of life lost, which may be adjusted for quality of life. Various quantitative measures of risk are discussed in more detail in Chapters 3 and 6, including measures to evaluate the effect of an exposure on an entire population.

This volume focuses on scientific principles for the quantitative estimation and prediction of cancer risks in humans. In some cases, estimates of risk under conditions prevailing in the original data will be of primary interest; in others, predictions of risk under other conditions will be required. Estimates of risk may be based on empirical models that provide a reasonable description of the available data, or on models developed on the basis of plausible assumptions about the mechanisms of carcinogenesis. Throughout this volume, established scientific principles of carcinogenesis will be used to support methods proposed for the quantitative estimation and prediction of risk.

The term "quantitative estimation and prediction of cancer risks" was chosen here for several reasons. Firstly, the authors of the volume wanted to focus on scientific approaches to the estimation and prediction of risk. Secondly, the term "risk assessment" was avoided since in certain countries it includes public policy considerations involved in risk management. Finally, the term "quantitative risk assessment" was also avoided since it is sometimes considered as being synonymous with low-dose extrapolation of animal bioassay data.

1.4 Regulation and control of cancer risks

Ideally, the unequivocal identification of a carcinogenic hazard would precede QEP. The strength of the evidence for carcinogenicity can be assessed by using carcinogen classification schemes such as that employed by the International Agency for Research on Cancer. Candidate chemicals for QEP would include known carcinogens (Group 1) and could also include probable (Group 2A) and possible (Group 2B) carcinogens. A further condition for QEP is the existence of sufficient data to permit characterization of the exposure–response relationship under relevant conditions of exposure, or under other conditions that permit predictions of risk to be made.

The perceived magnitude of a health risk depends not only on its numerical probability but also on the severity of the outcome for the affected person. The evaluation of such a risk—and therefore the type of social response to it—is influenced by such characteristics as whether the risk is experienced voluntarily, whether it occurs catastrophically or gradually, whether any benefits accompany the risk, and whether the source of the risk is familiar (Slovic et al., 1981).

The assessment of the aggregate risk that applies to a population with a known profile of exposure to some particular agent entails addressing four questions:

(i) Is exposure to the agent a hazard to health?
(ii) How does the health risk vary with level of exposure?
(iii) What is the profile of exposure to the agent within the population?
(iv) What, then, is the aggregate public health risk within that population?

The second of these steps seeks to determine the dose–response relationship, and is the critical one for quantitation of the cancer risk for individuals (or groups of individuals) at specified levels of exposure. The subsequent two steps are important within a public health context, when the aggregate risk (and the intrapopulation distribution of that risk) is being predicted for a particular population.

Quantitative information about cancer risks in humans (as summarized in the dose–response relationship) could be used in setting exposure standards or guidelines, or estimating the magnitude of public health risk (i.e. the excess cancer burden). Two idealized processes are shown in Figure 1.2:

(i) A limit to how far exposure levels can be lowered, within the available technical and financial resources, may determine the level of risk that will have to be tolerated.

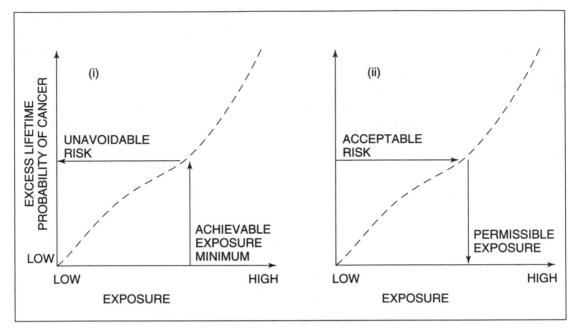

Figure 1.2. Two ways in which exposure–response information can be used to guide the formulation of social policy. For explanation, see text

(ii) Society or regulatory authorities may pre-specify a level of "acceptable risk" for a given situation, which would then determine the maximal permissible level of exposure.

Countries differ in the way that terms pertaining to the scientific assessment and social management of risk are used. The elements in this overall process are: hazard identification, risk estimation, consideration of risk management (i.e. control) options, choice of an option, implementation, and monitoring and review. Collectively, these six elements make up the processes of "risk assessment" and "risk management", although there is no agreement on the subgrouping and labelling of these steps. A widely cited definition of risk assessment is that of the US National Academy of Sciences (1983), as follows:

"risk assessment [is] the characterization of the potential adverse health effects of human exposures to environmental hazards. Risk assessments include several elements:

- description of the potential adverse health effects based on an evaluation of results of epi-

demiologic, clinical, toxicologic, and environmental research;

- extrapolation from those results to predict the type and estimate the extent of health effects in humans under given conditions of exposure;

- judgements as to the number and characteristics of persons exposed at various intensities and durations; and

- summary judgements on the existence and overall magnitude of the public health problem.

Risk assessment also includes characterization of the uncertainties in the process of inferring risk."

This definition which elaborates the four-step sequence previously mentioned, embraces the quantitative estimation and prediction of cancer risk, both for individuals exposed at specified levels and for a population with a given exposure profile. Once such an analysis has been conducted, society can evaluate a risk in relation to the social and economic costs of its reduction and in relation to community perceptions of the nature of that risk. This will lead to a risk management strategy, often entailing guidelines or exposure standards. Ideally, the setting of an exposure standard would indicate that society is satisfied either that there are no adverse health risks below that level of exposure, or that the estimated risk is less than some previously specified "acceptable" level of risk. In the latter case, a certain level of adverse health effects may be tolerated in return for the use of various hazardous agents deemed useful to society. The degree of tolerance may be influenced by the relative political clout of those who experience the adverse health effects and of those who benefit from the agent's use. Exposure standards typically entail single (or just several) numbers to facilitate regulatory activity, and are inevitably a somewhat arbitrary and reductionist version of a complex reality.

For at least the following reasons, the quantitative estimation of risk is often difficult and may yield a simplified or misleading result:

1. Even where population exposures are well recorded, individual exposures may be inadequately documented. Interindividual differences in the uptake or metabolism of carcinogens further complicate the construction of dose–response relationships.

2. The epidemiological estimation of the actual risk of exposed humans may be inaccurate, particularly at low levels of exposure, where there is likely to be insufficient statistical power in typical epidemiological studies, or where there is the possibility of unmeasured or inadequately measured confounding variables.

3. The quantification of risk usually works best when there is a constant level of exposure to a single agent over time. It is much more difficult for changing complex exposures and exposures to multiple agents and mixtures.

4. The setting of exposure limits for specific exogenous agents usually ignores the fact that individuals may encounter the same agent via several routes and from several sources. This problem applies particularly to exposures encountered within the wider ambient environment.

5. Typically, the risk of occurrence of some particular type of cancer is increased by exposure to several different agents, some of which may occur together in the same environment. What is actually important for the exposed individual is the cumulative effect of the composite exposure, especially where the risks due to multiple exposures combine in a synergistic fashion.

6. The risk that results from one particular exposure may depend on factors such as the sex or age of the subjects or on various other inherited or acquired host characteristics. These interactive effects may be particularly important when including a safety margin in exposure standards since a level of exposure which carries little risk for one person may carry an unacceptable risk for another similarly exposed but more susceptible person. For example, exposures in childhood to ionizing radiation may lead to a greater risk of cancer than exposures occurring later in life (United Nations Scientific Committee on the Effects of Atomic Radiation, 1994).

7. While risk may be expressed in relation to total "dose", or perhaps "average dose rate", variations in the temporal pattern of exposure may significantly influence the net risk. (For example, the periodicity of exposure or the peak exposure rates may be important.)

1.5 Risk prediction

As will be discussed in detail later in this volume, many uncertainties surround the estimation of dose–response relationships (Karstadt, 1988; Houk, 1989). These include, in particular, uncertainty about how to extrapolate from high-dose to low-dose exposure and how to extrapolate from non-human species to humans. Additional difficulties, foreshadowed in the previous section, concern the handling of variability in individual response and those posed by interactive effects between two or more coexisting exposures.

Often, a no-threshold model, linearized at low dose, has been assumed. This model enables one to calculate the "lifetime unit risk", i.e. the incremental risk of some specified health outcome associated with a lifetime of exposure to one unit of concentration (e.g. 1 µg/m^3 benzo[a]pyrene in air). Such an approach has been used in setting air quality criteria for Europe in relation to the risk of disease associated with a range of air pollutants (World Health Organization, 1987).

To predict the risk of cancer at low doses, the linearized multistage procedure (see Chapter 6) is commonly used. This procedure is based on the multistage model first proposed by Armitage & Doll (1954) to explain the observation that the age-specific incidence curves of many human carcinomas are roughly proportional to a power of age. This model posits that cancer results from the accumulation, within a single susceptible cell, of a sequence of heritable and irreversible alterations. Current laboratory research leaves little doubt that cancer is the result of an accumulation of critical mutations by such a cell. Additionally, a disruption of cell division kinetics is also believed to play an important role in the carcinogenic process. A discussion of the Armitage–Doll model and others that have been developed more recently to take explicit account of cell division kinetics (Moolgavkar & Venzon, 1979; Moolgavkar & Knudson, 1981) will be found in Chapter 7.

The linearized model, which assumes linearity of carcinogenic responses at low doses, has often been used in QEP of carcinogenic risk. A number of theoretical and practical arguments have been put forward in support of this assumption. Crump et al. (1976) and Hoel (1980) argue that, for agents that act by accelerating an already ongoing process in a dose-wise additive fashion, the dose–response relationship will be linear in the low-dose region, regardless of the precise mechanism of the acceleration. Other arguments in support of the hypothesis of linearity at low doses include the observed linearity of DNA adduction at very low doses of DNA-reactive carcinogens (Beland et al., 1988; Lutz, 1990). Consequently, low-dose linearity has been used as a default assumption by the US Environmental Protection Agency (Perera, 1987) in the absence of evidence to the contrary. QEP methods requiring no assumptions other than low-dose linearity are discussed by Krewski et al. (1991).

The basic linearized model does not include dose rate (although changes can be made to include this variable), and makes no allowance for interaction with other exposure variables. The occurrence of such interactive effects may cause this model to underestimate the risk at low dose, and variations in individual susceptibility can produce large errors in the predictions of average effect (Perera, 1987). Scientists and regulators need to tread carefully in this area, as we learn more and develop better techniques. Houk (1989) cautions that: "So-called conservative assumptions will not suffice. We must also strive to learn how far and in what direction these assumptions differ from the truth."

Methodological difficulties aside, there are various environmental exposures such as environmental tobacco smoke and additional ultraviolet radiation due to ozone layer depletion where the policy decision is likely to be one of elimination of the cause of the problem, rather than limitation of the exposure. In such circumstances, precise prediction of personal cancer risk at some nominated low-level exposure is not the primary concern of the decision-maker. It is more likely that calculation of the increment in population-attributable risk caused by the exposure, and therefore entirely avoidable by its elimination, will be the more relevant piece of information.

1.6 Conclusions

This book is concerned with the quantitative estimation and prediction of cancer risk; it does not deal with other elements of public health decision-making, which include evaluation and perception of risk, risk communication and risk management. The regulation and control of causes of cancer entail reviewing the interventions that may be made to prevent disease and selecting among the options available. The quantification of risk provides essential scientific information for use in risk management, but risk estimates are ultimately interpreted in terms of social, economic, political and value judgements.

QEP is an inexact science, particularly when it is necessary to predict risks well outside the range of the available data. Despite its limitations, however, it can be an important tool for public health decision-making. In the presence of a sufficiently rich database, useful estimates of risk can often be obtained using currently available QEP techniques. More reliable risk estimates will be possible as our knowledge about the mechanisms of carcinogenesis increases, and as more accurate measures of exposure and dose to the individual become available. In the mean time, it is important to understand and describe the uncertainties associated with quantitative summaries of carcinogenesis data, and to define the limitations of science in characterizing cancer risks. This is one of the primary objectives of this volume.

The quantitative estimation of cancer risks evolved first in the USA, the Netherlands and Canada, and has emerged more recently in other countries. However, the reasons for using this approach apply wherever decisions must be made on the best means of allocating resources to control disease. Cancer is a substantial public health problem for many developing countries, and is likely to become more important in the future as populations age and industrialization proceeds (Tomatis, 1991). In countries with fewer resources than those that the developed countries currently possess, cost-effective programmes to control cancer are especially important. Countries that cannot afford the specialized expertise, person–time and physical facilities needed to conduct their own quantitative estimation of cancer risk will depend increasingly on international agencies, such as the World Health Organization. A desire to understand how best to meet the needs of the world community for quantitative estimation and prediction of cancer risk and to promote development and understanding in a scientifically sound way are the motivations for this book.

References

Armitage, P. & Doll, R. (1954) The age distribution of cancer and a multistage theory of carcinogenesis. *Br. J. Cancer*, **8**, 1–12

Beland, F.A., Fullerton, N.F., Kinouchi, T. & Poirier, M.C. (1988) DNA adduct forming during continuous feeding of 2-acetylaminofluorene at multiple concentrations. In: Bartsch, H., Hemminki, K. & O'Neill, I.K., eds, *Methods for Detection of DNA Damaging Agents in Humans: Applications in Cancer Epidemiology and Prevention* (IARC Scientific Publications No. 89), Lyon, International Agency for Research on Cancer, pp. 175-180

Crump, K.S., Hoel, D.G., Langley, C.H. & Peto, R. (1976) Fundamental carcinogenic processes and their implications for low dose assessment. *Cancer Res.*, **36**, 2973-2979

Hoel, D.G. (1980) Incorporation of background in dose–response models. *Fed. Proc.*, **39**, 73-75

Houk, V.N. (1989) The risk of risk assessment. *Reg. Toxicol. Pharmacol.*, **9**, 257-262

Karstadt, M. (1988) Quantitative risk assessment: qualms and questions. *Teratog. Carcinog. Mutag.*, **8**, 137-152

Krewski, D., Brown, C. & Murdoch, D. (1984) Determining 'safe' levels of exposure: safety factors or mathematical models. *Fundam. Appl. Toxicol.*, **4**, S383-S394

Krewski, D., Gaylor, D.W. & Szyszkowicz, M. (1991) A model-free approach to low dose extrapolation. *Environ. Health Perspect.*, **90**, 279-285

Landy, M., Roberts, M. & Thomas, S. (1990) *The Environmental Protection Agency: Asking the Wrong Questions*, New York, Oxford University Press

Lave, L.B. (1985) The role of quantitative risk assessment in environmental regulations. In: Hoel, D.G., Merrill, P.A. & Perera, F.P., eds, *Risk Quantitation and Regulatory Policy* (Banbury Report 19), Cold Spring Harbor, NY, CSH Press, pp. 3-13

Lubin, J.H. (1994) Invited commentary: Lung cancer and exposure to residential radon. *Am. J. Epidemiol.*, **140**, 323-332

Lutz, W.K. (1990) Dose–response relationship and low dose extrapolation in chemical carcinogenesis. *Carcinogenesis*, **11**, 1243-1247

Mantel, N. & Bryan, W.R. (1961) 'Safety' testing of carcinogenic agents. *J. Natl Cancer Inst.*, **27**, 455-460

McMichael, A.J. (1991) Setting environmental exposure standards: current concepts and controversies. *Int. J. Environ. Health Res.*, **1**, 2-13

Moolgavkar, S.H. & Knudson, A.G. (1981) Mutation and cancer: A model for human carcinogenesis. *J. Natl Cancer Inst.*, **84**, 1037-1052

Moolgavkar, S.H. & Venzon, D.J. (1979) Two-event models for carcinogenesis: Incidence curves for childhood and adult tumors. *Math. Biosci.*, **47**, 55-77

Paustenbach, D.J. (1989) A survey of environmental risk assessment. In: Paustenbach, D.J., ed., *The Risk Assessment of Environmental Hazards*, New York, NY, Wiley, pp. 27-124

Paustenbach, D.J. & Langner, R. (1986) Corporate occupational exposure limits: the state of the art. *Am. Ind. Hyg. Assoc. J.*, **47**, 809-818

Perera, F. (1987) Quantitative risk assessment and cost-benefit analysis for carcinogens at EPA: a critique. *J. Public Health Policy*, **8**, 202-221

Rushefsky, M.E. (1986) *Making Cancer Policy*, Albany, NY, State University of New York Press

Samet, J.M. & Nero A.V. (1989) Indoor radon and lung cancer. *New Engl. J. Med.*, **320**, 591-594

Slovic, P., Fischhoff, B. & Lichtenstein, S. (1981) Perceived risk: psychological factors and social implications. *Proc. R. Soc. Lond.*, **376**, 17-34

Tomatis, L. (1991) Poverty and cancer. *Cancer Epidemiol. Biomarkers Prev.*, **1**, 167-175

United Nations Scientific Committee on the Effects of Atomic Radiation (1994) *Sources and Effects of Ionizing Radiation*, New York, United Nations

US Environmental Protection Agency (1992) *Respiratory Health Effects of Passive Smoking: Lung Cancer and Other Disorders*, Washington, DC

US National Academy of Sciences (1983) *Risk Assessment in the Federal Government: Managing the Process*, Washington, DC, National Academy Press

Vainio, H., Magee, P., McGregor, D. & McMichael, A.J., eds (1992) *Mechanisms of Carcinogenesis in Risk Identification* (IARC Scientific Publications No. 116), Lyon, International Agency for Research on Cancer

Wald, N.J., Nanchahal, K., Thompson, S.G. & Cuckle, H.S. (1986) Does breathing other people's tobacco smoke cause lung cancer? *Br. Med. J.*, **293**, 1217-1222

Walker, J.S. (1989) The controversy over radiation safety. A historical overview. *J. Am. Med. Assoc.*, **262**, 664-668

World Health Organization (1987) *Air Quality Guidelines for Europe*, Copenhagen, WHO Regional Office for Europe

Quantitative Estimation and Prediction of Human Cancer Risks
S. Moolgavkar, D. Krewski, L. Zeise, E. Cardis and H. Møller
IARC Scientific Publications No. 131
International Agency for Research on Cancer, Lyon, 1999

2: Quantitative Estimation and Prediction of Cancer Risk: Review of Existing Activities

Lauren Zeise, Elisabeth Cardis, Kari Hemminki and Michael Schwarz

2.1 Introduction

Nearly all quantitative estimation and prediction (QEP) of cancer risk is undertaken for the ultimate purpose of decision-making, typically by regulatory agencies, for mitigating carcinogenic risks. The aim is to generate reproducible, objective bench marks to guide decisions. The derivation of a measure of carcinogenic activity (e.g. the cancer potency or "unit risk") is common to most QEP. This is often taken as the slope of the cancer dose–response curve at low doses. Risk predictions are frequently derived by multiplying dose averaged over lifetime by the slope. Population exposure profiles make it possible to predict the total burden of exposure-induced cancers (see Figure 1.1 of Chapter 1). In theory, the decision-maker assesses the impacts of different control strategies on the exposure profiles, and consequently the cancer burden, and selects those that are technically, economically and politically achievable in attempting to reduce risks to acceptable levels. This is the conceptual framework for evaluating environmental and occupational exposures which, in practice, is followed by few regulatory programmes worldwide.

This chapter reviews existing QEP activities, as practised by international and national institutions. Developments in response to recent efforts to improve on existing techniques are also described. The lack of uniformity in the approaches taken by different bodies typically reflects the different policy choices which are made in the absence of adequate data. Efforts are under way to harmonize QEP guidelines and practices across institutions, while at the same time introducing techniques to improve cancer risk prediction. The chapter concludes by describing initiatives to develop improved QEP for specific agents using non-standard techniques.

A distinction is made here between the terms "prediction" and "estimation" (see section 1.3) in order to differentiate extrapolation outside the range of data (prediction) from direct estimations from data pertaining to the specified human exposure of concern. Typically, these distinctions are not made by many people involved in QEP, who generally use the term "estimation" interchangeably with "extrapolation". In practice, the vast majority of QEP applications involve risk prediction.

Various types of quantitative information on cancer risk can help decision-makers. For example, a "no-observed-effect level" (NOEL) for increased incidence of a specific tumour in a cancer bioassay may be divided by adjustment and uncertainty factors; a ratio of a human exposure to an estimated "tumorigenic 50% dose" (TD_{50}) may be given; values of TD_{50} estimated from data sets on different chemicals can be compared; cancer risks may be predicted by fitting a dose–response model to animal bioassay data and assuming that the same relationship holds for humans; cancer risks may be estimated or predicted based on the analysis of data from occupational studies. This publication emphasizes quantitative estimations and predictions of human risk and, by definition, considers only the last two items as examples of QEP. However, because institutions may specifically select the NOEL/uncertainty factor (UF) or other quantitative approaches rather than QEP to provide information for decision-making on carcinogens, these alternative approaches are also discussed in this chapter for completeness.

The application of a NOEL/uncertainty factor approach in some instances depends on a decision by the relevant institution to characterize an agent as "non-genotoxic" as opposed to "genotoxic". There is no universally accepted definition of these terms (Vainio *et al.*, 1992), and they are used here only when given in the specific guidelines and documents discussed.

2.2 QEP by international bodies using standardized approaches

QEP is practised by international bodies to establish guidelines or standards to protect against specific chemical and radioactive risks from occupational, consumer, and general environmental exposures. Formal guidelines of varying detail have been adopted by several organizations for the conduct of QEP. QEP practices and guidelines adopted by the World Health Organization, international bodies concerned with protection against ionizing radiation, and other international bodies are described below.

2.2.1 World Health Organization

The World Health Organization (WHO), in collaboration with other specialized agencies of the United Nations, develops quantitative descriptions of carcinogenesis data for use in establishing guidance values for carcinogen exposures. WHO has published guidelines on methods to be used in assessing the risks of exposure to carcinogens in ambient air (World Health Organization, 1987a), drinking-water (World Health Organization, 1993a, 1996a), food additives (World Health Organization, 1987b) and pesticide residues (World Health Organization, 1990), and in general (World Health Organization, 1994a) (see Table 2.1).

Quantitative assessments of carcinogens are made by the International Programme on Chemical Safety (IPCS)[1]. The International Agency for Research on Cancer provides qualitative evaluations, but few quantitative assessments to date (e.g. benzene and benzidine (International Agency for Research on Cancer, 1982)). IPCS has a small staff and convenes panels of outside experts to evaluate specific chemicals and to develop and review the methods used. Through these panels IPCS has formulated "guiding principles for exposure limits, such as acceptable daily intakes [ADIs] for food additives and

pesticide residues, and tolerances for toxic substances in food, water, air, soil and the working environment" (World Health Organization, 1987b, 1990). The methodological guidance developed and the practice of QEP at WHO are described below.

2.2.1.1 Drinking-water

WHO has updated its 1984–1985 *Guidelines for Drinking-water Quality* (World Health Oganization, 1993a). The guidelines are intended to be used as the basis for establishing national regulatory standards. A guideline value "represents the concentration of a constituent that does not result in any significant risk to the health of the consumer over a lifespan of consumption" (World Health Organization, 1993a). The revised WHO procedure requires classifying carcinogens as "genotoxic" or "non-genotoxic". A standardized QEP procedure is used in predicting the risks of "genotoxic" carcinogens, which includes application of the linearized multistage model to animal bioassay data. Animals and humans are assumed to be equally sensitive to the same daily dose in mg/kg; in comparison, the regulatory bodies in the USA use surface area or 3/4 power scaling (see section 2.3.2 below). For "non-genotoxic" agents, tolerable daily intakes (TDIs) are derived by dividing NOELs by uncertainty factors and multiplying by adjustment factors (e.g. to change to appropriate units).

The World Health Organization (1993a, 1996a) recommended guidance values corresponding to a 10^{-5} risk for roughly a dozen chemicals identified as genotoxic and carcinogenic (e.g. acrylamide, benzene, vinyl chloride, 1,2-dibromo-3-chloropropane). For benzo[*a*]pyrene, the recommended level corresponded to a risk of 10^{-5} derived from a two-stage "birth–death–mutation" model. Levels identified as "provisional" corresponding to risks greater than 10^{-5} were adopted for some chemicals because practical treatment methods could not be used to achieve lower levels, or disinfection was likely to result in the value being exceeded (e.g. arsenic and bromate). For some chemicals identified as genotoxic and carcinogenic, data were found to be insufficient for QEP and no guidance values were recommended

---

[1] WHO is the executing agency of IPCS, which is operated jointly with the International Labour Organisation (ILO) and the United Nations Environment Programme (UNEP).

Table 2.1. WHO Guidelines for quantitative carcinogenicity assessment		
Guideline and reference	**Responsible body or assessment programme**[a]	**Method of assessment**
Guidelines for Drinking-water Quality (World Health Organization, 1993a, 1996a)	WHO Regional Office for Europe; International Programme on Chemical Safety; WHO Prevention of Environmental Pollution	Perform QEP on carcinogens characterized as "genotoxic" Use a NOEL/UF[b] approach on "non-genotoxic" substances Use an extra uncertainty factor of 10 for some agents with limited evidence in animals
Air Quality Guidelines for Europe (World Health Organization, 1987a)	WHO Regional Office for Europe	IARC Groups 1, 2A: perform QEP using epidemiological data IARC Groups 2B, 3: base numerical guidance values on non-cancer end-point; cite cancer risk estimates
Principles for the Safety Assessment of Food Additives and Contaminants in Food (World Health Organization, 1987b)	Joint FAO/WHO Expert Committee on Food Additives (JECFA)	QEP not recommended[c]
Principles for the Toxicological Assessment of Pesticide Residues in Food (World Health Organization, 1990)	Joint FAO/WHO Meeting on Pesticide Residues	QEP not recommended NOEL/UF approach adopted[d]
Assessing Human Health Risks of Chemicals: Derivation of Guidance Values for Health-based Exposure Limits (World Health Organization, 1994a)	International Programme on Chemical Safety	"Non-threshold" effects: "Characterize the dose–response relationship to the extent possible" "Threshold" effects: use a NOEL/UF approach

[a] At the time of writing.
[b] NOEL/UF; the "no observed effect level" divided by the uncertainty and adjustment factors.
[c] In general, JECFA has not condoned the use of carcinogenic food additives. The safety factor approach is used for determining safe levels, but has been applied to carcinogens only in exceptional instances (World Health Organization, 1987b). See text for further explanation.
[d] The result is a level of pesticide that "can be ingested by man without appreciable risk" (World Health Organization, 1990).

(e.g. ethylene dibromide). Epichlorohydrin was noted to be an IARC 2A agent, and "genotoxic" but a NOEL/UF approach was employed "because tumours are only seen at the site of administration, where EHC is highly irritating." An extra safety factor of 10 was applied in derivations for some IARC 2B agents characterized as "non-geno-toxic" (e.g. perchloroethylene, lindane), but this was not always the case (e.g. di(2-ethylhexyl) phthalate, 1,4-dichlorobenzene). Similarly, for agents with suggestive evidence of carcinogenicity not found to be "sufficient in animals", an extra safety factor of 10 was included (e.g. simizine, hexachlorobutadiene), with some exceptions (e.g. di(2-ethylhexyl) adipate, mono-chlorobenzene).

2.2.1.2 Ambient air

Air Quality Guidelines for Europe (World Health Organization, 1987a) was published to provide criteria values (e.g. recommended maximal average air concentrations) to aid national and local regulatory bodies in establishing standards and controls for air pollutants. Criteria are not provided for agents identified by IARC as having "limited" or "sufficient" epidemiological evidence for carcinogenicity. Instead, unit risk values are given and it is noted that "The decision on the acceptability of a certain risk should be taken by the national authorities in the context of a broader risk management process. Risk estimate figures should not be applied in isolation when regulatory decisions are being made ..." (World Health Organization, 1987a, p. 30). A standardized QEP procedure to predict risks from epidemiological data is given for the derivation of unit risk values for chemicals with "sufficient" or "limited" human evidence. (Cancer potency or "unit risk" based on epidemiological data is obtained by subtracting 1.0 from the estimated relative risk, multiplying it by the background lifetime cancer incidence, and dividing the product by the lifetime average exposure.) Animal carcinogens (with sufficient evidence for effects in animals but with inadequate or insufficient evidence in humans) are treated in the same way as non-carcinogens: air quality guidelines are derived by applying a NOEL/UF approach to dose–response data for a non-cancer end-point. Thus, the guideline value of 3 mg/m^3 (24-h exposure) for the animal carcinogen methylene chloride is based on experimental results on increases in carboxyhaemoglobin (COHb) levels in humans exposed for 24 h. (At the guideline level, COHb was observed to be increased by 0.1%, a percentage characterized as insignificant by WHO.)

Risk predictions, generally derived using linear extrapolation procedures, are given for animal carcinogens in the health risk evaluation as scientific background information, "However, these estimates, based on animal data only, would not be incorporated into the guideline recommendations because of various uncertainties in this connection" (World Health Organization, 1987a, p. 13). No comments were made on the uncertainties associated with applying a NOEL/UF approach for a non-cancer end-point in deriving guidelines on acceptable exposures for carcinogens.

2.2.1.3 Food residues and additives

Pesticide residues are assessed by WHO Expert Groups, which are the responsibility of IPCS, in collaboration with expert panels of the Food and Agriculture Organization of the United Nations (FAO) at the Joint FAO/WHO Meeting on Pesticide Residues (JMPR). The Joint FAO/WHO Expert Committee on Food Additives (JECFA), which assesses food additives, contaminants, and residues of veterinary drugs, is similarly constituted. An inventory of pesticide evaluations has recently been published (World Health Organization, 1997a). WHO Expert Groups conduct toxicological evaluations for use in setting maximum residue levels, which are then used by the Codex Alimentarius Commission to establish international standards. JEFCA reports are published in the WHO Technical Report Series and JMPR reports in the FAO Plant Production and Protection Paper Series. "Acceptable daily intakes" (ADIs) or "tolerance intakes" (TIs) for food additives and pesticide residues and other environmental contaminants are published by WHO in the Environmental Health Criteria series. An inventory of evaluations performed on pesticides by WHO expert committees has been released (World Health Organization, 1997); Summaries of evaluations by JMPR (e.g. World Health Organization, 1994b) and JEFCA (e.g. World Health Organization, 1996b) are issued or published from time to time.

Under guidelines developed for evaluating pesticides and food additives (World Health Organization, 1987b, 1990), QEPs are not recommended for carcinogens. Quantitative analyses leading to recommended ADIs for carcinogenic food additives have been uncommon and, when used, a NOEL/UF approach has been taken: "... it would be appropriate to consider the use of a carcinogenic substance as an intentional food additive only under very restricted circumstances. For example, if cancer is shown to be a secondary effect, such as bladder tumours occurring secondary to the induction of bladder stones, and there is evidence of a threshold below which the additive is safe, then it would be appropriate to use a safety factor for determining the safe level of use of the additive" (World Health Organization, 1987b, 1990). As in earlier evaluations by JMPR of ethylene oxide, WHO (1985) declined to provide an ADI and recommended that "its levels in the environment should be kept as low as feasible", since it found it to be an agent with "overwhelmingly positive *in vivo* responses in mutagenic and clastogenic assays, [the] reproductive positive carcinogenic findings in animals, and the epidemiological findings suggesting an increase in the incidence of human cancer ..." The WHO Expert Group on Pesticide Residues (Food and Agriculture Organization, 1986) withdrew a temporary ADI set earlier on the basis of positive carcinogenicity findings: "In view of the established carcinogenic potential of this compound, the meeting recommended that captafol should not be used where its residues in food can arise (p.11)." In contrast, for lindane, WHO (1991) notes that "the results of studies on initiation–promotion, on mode of action, and on mutagenicity indicate that the tumorigenic effect of gamma-HCH [lindane] in mice results from non-genetic mechanisms", and it derived a maximal ADI of lindane in humans (0.008 mg/kg body weight per day) from a NOEL in rodents (0.75 mg/kg body weight per day in rats) at the 1989 JEFCA meeting (World Health Organization, 1991, p. 150). WHO (1970, 1979) also used a margin of safety approach to establish a "conditional ADI" for DDT (at 0.005 mg/kg body weight per day), after evaluating data from intake, exposure, and levels in populations and comparing them with toxicological and epidemiological data. Subsequently, however, the WHO Expert Group on Pesticide Residues (Food and Agriculture Organization, 1985) noted that "repeated exposure of workers for 25 years at an average doseage of 0.25 mg/kg/day is without any adverse effect, and this may be taken as a no-effect level for man." WHO then established an ADI at roughly a factor of 10 below that value, at 0.02 mg/kg per day. More recently this value was confirmed and characterized as the "provisional tolerable daily intake" (Food and Agriculture Organization, 1995).

2.2.1.4 General environmental evaluations

IPCS, in the Environmental Health Criteria series, provides "evaluated information, including guidance for exposure limits, for the protection of human health and the maintenance of environmental integrity against the possible deleterious effects of chemical and/or physical agents" (World Health Organization, 1994a). The most recent guidance for conducting quantitative evaluations on carcinogens (World Health Organization, 1994a) is contained in procedures used to address "threshold effects" and "non-threshold effects." For agents producing "threshold effects," a NOEL/UF approach has been adopted, and for those producing "non-threshold effects," the procedure calls for characterizing the dose–response relationship "to the extent possible" through mathematical modelling, relative ranking of potencies or division of effect levels by a (large) uncertainty factor, especially when dose–response data are limited.

Examples of the newer procedures are found in the Environmental Health Criteria published subsequent to the 1994 guidelines. IPCS, after finding tris(2,3-dibromopropyl)phosphate (World Health Organization, 1995a), ethylene dibromide (World Health Organization, 1996c), and ethylene dichloride (World Health Organization, 1995b) to be clearly genotoxic and, on the basis of animal studies, carcinogenic, declined to derive tolerable daily intake levels but instead called for human exposures to be eliminated or minimized. Slopes of linear dose–response relationships for carcinogenicity and corresponding risks to workers are being considered for chrysotile asbestos, an agent tentatively found to be non-threshold in an ongoing IPCS process and for which human data exist. In contrast, for short-chain chlorinated paraffins, IPCS noted that they "did not mediate carcinogenic effects via direct action with DNA" and divided the dose estimated to cause 5% tumour incidence by 1000 to establish a TDI for neoplastic effects (World Health Organization, 1996d). "Since the induction of tumours by acetaldehyde has not been well studied," guidance values for neoplasia were reported for two approaches: (1) fitting a linearized multistage model to bioassay data to obtain a concentration associated with 10^{-5} cancer risk; and (2) dividing an effect level (for irritancy) by an uncertainty factor of 1000 (World Health Organization, 1995c). The tolerable intake for chlorthalonil, an agent for which there is limited evidence of carcinogenicity in animals, was developed by applying an uncertainty factor of 100 to an effect level for an end-point unrelated to carcinogenicity (World Health Organization, 1996e).

Prior to the 1994 guidance, IPCS had adopted the stratagem of assigning ADIs to carcinogens believed to act by secondary mechanisms, while not assigning ADIs to those judged genotoxic, but this was not strictly followed. For example, WHO did not establish ADIs for polychlorinated biphenyls (PCBs) or terphenyls (PCTs), noting that "no levels of PCBs or PCTs exposure that can provide an absolute assurance of safety can be identified on the basis of the available data" (World Health Organization, 1993b, p.22), and that "in an ideal situation, it would be preferable not to have these compounds in food at any level" (p.21). Yet it found that "PCBs are not genotoxic ... PCBs do act as tumour promoters. It can be concluded that the toxicity of PCB mixtures can be evaluated on a threshold basis" (p.41).

The specialized agencies of the United Nations rely on the work of IPCS. Thus ILO relies on IPCS health evaluations in providing information on occupational safety (US Office of Technology Assessment, 1993), and the International Labour Conference establishes international standards for occupational exposure, primarily for use by developing countries which lack the resources to develop such standards themselves or to monitor occupational exposures. The Pan American Health Organization/WHO Regional Office for the Americas generally refers to values developed by IPCS and the Codex Alimentarius Commission when evaluating health risks quantitatively (US Office of Technology Assessment, 1993).

2.2.1.5 Developments in the practice of QEP at WHO

While not entirely consistent in approach within and across programmes, the above overview suggests that the use of, and reliance on QEP is increasing in WHO. A little over a decade ago none of the guidance-setting procedures used by WHO incorporated QEP analyses. Currently, WHO guidelines for establishing guidance values provide for the application of QEP in considering ambient air hazards (World Health Organization, 1987a), recommending drinking-water quality guidelines (World Health Organization, 1993a), and establishing tolerable daily intake levels for environmental contaminants (World Health Organization, 1994a). QEP is more extensively integrated into the procedures of the two most recent guidelines (World Health Organization, 1993a, 1994a) and the practices in the associated

programmes are more similar. Whereas, for the air contaminants, a major factor in using QEP to support guidance values was the presence of human evidence of carcinogenicity, for IPCS it was the existence of a "non-threshold effect," and for drinking-water, the characterization of an agent as "genotoxic."

In moving towards the use of QEP, WHO has been careful to point out the inaccuracy in the overall approach or the lack of reliability of low-dose risk predictions. Thus in *Air Quality Guidelines for Europe*, it is pointed out that: "The risk estimates in this book should not be regarded as being equivalent to the true cancer risk" (World Health Organization, 1987a, p.17). Similarly, in the *Guidelines for Drinking-water Quality*, in which guidance values are established for a dozen carcinogens primarily on the basis of low-dose risk predictions, it is stated that: "It should be emphasized, however, that if guideline values for carcinogenic compounds have been computed using mathematical models, these values must be considered at best as rough estimates of cancer risk." IPCS has been cautious in its application of QEP for developing numerical guidelines in the Environmental Health Criteria series, reporting cancer risk predictions for only a couple of agents so far. In its guidelines document (World Health Organization, 1994a) IPCS states that: "...crude expression of risk in terms of excess incidence or numbers of cancers per unit of the population at doses or concentrations much less than those on which the estimates are based may be inappropriate, owing to the uncertainties of quantitative extrapolation over several orders of magnitude." Such precautionary notes are not provided when NOEL/UF approaches are applied, despite the large uncertainty about the cancer risks posed by exposures indicated as being safe under such procedures.

2.2.2 International bodies that assess radiation risks

Over the last 40 or so years, the United Nations Scientific Committee on the Effects of Atomic Radiation (UNSCEAR) has provided estimates of radiation doses and risks in general populations worldwide (United Nations Scientific Committee on the Effects of Atomic Radiation, 1994). It has published radiation potency figures for various cancer sites (e.g. United Nations Scientific Committee on the Effects of Atomic Radiation, 1977) and reviews of dose–response relationships for radiation-induced cancers to provide the basis for its risk estimates (e.g. United Nations Scientific Committee on the Effects of Atomic Radiation, 1977, 1986). In 1988, UNSCEAR summarized the "main ideas underlying the Committee's assessments and how these assessments have changed with time and as a result of increasing scientific knowledge" (United Nations Scientific Committee on the Effects of Atomic Radiation, 1988), tabulated UNSCEAR's cancer risk coefficients for fatal cancers at various sites presented in previous reports, and published an updated list of cancer risk coefficients. (Cancer risk coefficients, when multiplied by radiation dose, give cancer risk estimates or predictions). In doing so, it noted that "...the problems in deriving risk coefficients at low doses and for low dose rates remain", and considered the division of the potencies presented by a reduction factor in the range 2–10 when they are used to predict risks at low doses and low dose rates. Regarding the use of the values presented to estimate cancer deaths, it noted that "Unfortunately any estimate of a finite number of cancer deaths is soon taken out of context and the qualifications forgotten. For these reasons, the Committee prefers to follow its previous practice of comparing collective dose commitments from the main radiation sources rather than estimated detriments [e.g. cancer risks]."

The International Commission on Radiological Protection (ICRP) was established in 1928 by the Second International Congress of Radiology (International Commission on Radiological Protection, 1991). ICRP provides guidance within the field of protection against exposures to ionizing radiation by making recommendations on dose limits, comments on the risks associated with them, and recommendations on procedures to use in controlling exposure to radiation. ICRP recommendations are published in the *Annals of the ICRP*. In its 1977 recommendations, it noted that "A practical radiation protection system needs to be based on certain simplifying assumptions if it is to be applied effectively" (International Commission on Radiation Protection, 1977, p.8). It recommended the assumption of proportionality between dose and

effect, which "over the range of doses of concern in radiation protection imply certain principles that can be applied to important practical problems such as those relating to significant volumes and areas and the rate at which doses may be accumulated" (e.g. use of mean tissue dose "over all cells of uniform sensitivity in a particular tissue or organ" except the skin). A "system of dose limitation" was recommended "to ensure that no source of exposure is unjustified in relation to its benefits or those of any available alternative, and that dose equivalents received do not exceed certain specified limits" (p. 14). To test their recommended limit for occupational exposure, ICRP calculated the average risk in industries adhering to its limit (50 mSv). The mean exposures in these industries were roughly a factor of 10 below the limit value. ICRP concluded that the average risk to the workers concerned was comparable with the "average risk in other safe industries" (International Commission on Radiation Protection, 1977, pp. 20–21). The "1990 recommendations of the ICRP" (International Commission on Radiation Protection, 1991) bring the 1977 report up to date and provide revised dose limits for public and occupational exposures. To account for non-linearities in the dose response, probability coefficients for low linear energy transfer (LET) radiation when derived from high-dose data are divided by a "dose and dose rate effectiveness factor" of 2.

2.2.3 Other international bodies

As the European Union (EU) moves towards the creation of a market where goods and services can cross national boundaries with few or no restrictions, it has tried to harmonize national policies on worker and environmental exposures. The administrative body of the EU, the European Commission, has issued a number of directives in this regard (see, e.g. Skov *et al.*, 1992), including Commission Directive 93/67/EEC (European Commission, 1993) "laying down the principles for assessment of risks to man and the environment ..." The Directive notes that the responsibility for risk assessment lies with the Member States, but that it is "appropriate that general principles be adopted at Community level to avoid disparities between Member States which not only affect the functioning of the internal market but also do not guarantee the same level of protection of man and the environment throughout the Community." In addition, "... the results of a risk assessment should be the principal basis of decisions under appropriate legislation to reduce risks arising from placing substances on the market ..."

The Commission adopted the same risk-assessment procedure as that chosen by a US National Research Council committee (US National Research Council, 1983): "The risk assessment shall entail hazard identification and, as appropriate, dose (concentration)–response (effect) assessment, exposure assessment and risk characterization" (Commission Directive 93/67/EEC, Article 3, paragraph 1). Dose–response assessment is required only for "non-genotoxic" carcinogens; "For mutagenicity and carcinogenicity, it shall be sufficient to determine whether the substance has an inherent capacity to cause such effects. However, if it can be demonstrated that a substance identified as a carcinogen is non-genotoxic, it will be appropriate to identify a NOAEL/LOAEL ..." (Commission Directive 93/67/EEC, Annex IB). As part of the risk characterization of "non-genotoxic" carcinogens, "an exposure level/N(L)OAEL ratio shall be derived."

The assessment is also required to include a finding regarding the degree of concern and the need to request further information pertaining to the assessment (Commission Directive 93/67/EEC, Article 3, paragraph 4), i.e. it must find that the substance is: (i) "of no concern and need not be considered again until further information is made available...", or is "of concern" and (ii) "the competent authority shall decide what further information is required", but shall defer the request until the quantity on the market "reaches the next tonnage threshold", when (iii) "further information shall be requested immediately"; or (iv) "the competent authority shall immediately make recommendation for risk reduction." In deciding which conclusion to reach, the "competent authority" is to take into account uncertainty, including that arising from intraspecies variation and variability in experimental data (Commission Directive 93/67/EEC, Annex 1, Part B, 4.3).

In 1971 the Governing Council of the Organization for Economic Co-operation and Development (OECD) (composed of representatives of 23 member countries and the EU) established the Chemicals Programme, intended primarily to identify hazards and strategies to manage them. Typically, the Chemicals Programme does not perform risk assessments. OECD is working with WHO and IPCS to develop harmonized risk assessment guidelines and explore risk assessment methodologies (US Office of Technology Assessment, 1993). OECD is, however, in the process of considering a harmonized scheme for classifying carcinogens, and as part of the proposed scheme notes the importance of considering cancer potency and the need for a harmonized method of potency estimation (Organization for Economic Co-operation and Development, 1996).

2.3 QEP by national institutions using standardized approaches

Some national bodies have been increasingly using QEP and related procedures to guide the treatment of carcinogens in their regulatory programmes. While not exhaustive, the review below illustrates the procedures used by various national institutions to account for the activity of agents characterized as having carcinogenic potential. In some countries (e.g., Netherlands, Canada and the USA), risk prediction has become an integral part of the regulatory process for establishing environmental controls, and the discussion has been extended to describe how risk predictions have been used in a few cases. Risk assessment practices and uses are reviewed for these countries first.

2.3.1 Netherlands

In 1978, a commission of the Health Council of the Netherlands (HCN) established an approach to QEP for certain types of carcinogens. It decided "that it was vital to distinguish two types of carcinogenic substances according to the mechanism of their action. For practical reasons, a subdivision of four categories was made" (Health Council of the Netherlands, 1980, p. 4) as follows: I "Substances that cause an irreversible self-replicating effect ... the complete carcinogens and the initiators"; II "Substances that are different from those given for category I" (e.g. those found to be non-DNA-reactive); III "Substances upon which suspicion has fallen on the basis of the results of adequate chronic animal assays or other relevant test arrangements, so that further studies are usually necessary" and IV "Unclassifiable substances which extensive investigations have failed to show to be complete carcinogens or initiators" (Health Council of the Netherlands, 1980, p. 101). For carcinogens falling into categories I and III, "the Commission's preference is for the first-order kinetics of extrapolation (the 1-hit method)" (p. 102). For categories II and IV, a NOEL/safety factor approach is recommended, with a greater safety factor applied to category IV carcinogens.

Specific guidance is given on the approach to deriving risk estimates. Risk is extrapolated linearly from lower doses in the animal bioassay "... by applying the 1-hit method to the lowest dose for which an effect can be detected in a chronic animal trial." An additional factor to account for interspecies differences is not recommended; animals and humans are assumed to be equally sensitive if they receive the same exposure in mg/kg per day throughout life (Health Council of the Netherlands, 1980, pp. 77, 143). Adjustments are made for human exposures of short duration (Health Council of the Netherlands, 1980, p. 130), and experiments lasting less than a lifetime (Health Council of the Netherlands, 1980, p. 131).

In 1988, a committee of the HCN published an update to the 1978 guidelines. This did not substantially alter the approach adopted in 1978, although it did allow for the use of non-linear models "providing there is sufficient understanding of the biological process to provide a proper basis for scientifically sound extrapolation." Thus the HCN explicitly provided for the use of approaches other than the one-hit when scientifically justified. More recently, the HCN re-evaluated and affirmed the 1978 approach to estimating risk (Health Council of the Netherlands, 1994). In its re-evaluation, the HCN reviewed recent developments in carcinogenesis biology and modelling. Regarding mathematically more sophisticated models, the committee noted that "assessment is not improved, however, by incorporating mathematically more complicated models that suggest a scientific accuracy that is not available." The HCN committee advised the use of "the lowest tumorigenic dose for extrapolation

to low exposure levels provided that this dose is not toxic to the experimental animals."

The Netherlands (Health Council of the Netherlands, 1994) is unique in providing explicitly for the quantitative assessment of untested agents. "About 100,000 chemicals are produced commercially ... Quantitative assessment of the risk of exposure to each of these compounds would be an almost impossible task. Consequently, relative risk assessment might provide a solution for setting priorities and predicting the risk of exposure to such a multitude of compounds ..." using structurally related genotoxic compounds as reference substances.

Several agencies in the Netherlands use the results of quantitative risk assessments developed by expert advisory committees in establishing regulations (US Office of Technology Assessment, 1993). The risk assessments for vinyl chloride (Health Council of the Netherlands, 1987) and benzene (Health Council of the Netherlands, 1989) are examples of the application of the HCN approach.

2.3.2 USA

Results of QEP are used extensively by the US Environmental Protection Agency (US EPA) and State and other US Federal regulatory agencies for establishing regulatory priorities, and are a major consideration in the development of numerical standards for controlling exposure to carcinogens. The term frequently used in the USA for quantitative predictions and analyses is "risk assessment", with risk most often meaning the lifetime risk of developing cancer. The Agency (1986b) has published guidelines on the methods to be used in QEP analyses. These guidelines, which are undergoing revision (US Environmental Protection Agency, 1988a, 1992a, 1996a), are followed by the US EPA programmes which develop QEPs to implement a variety of statutes (e.g. the Clean Water Act). The US National Institute for Occupational Safety and Health (NIOSH) currently makes risk estimates for some carcinogens when recommending occupational standards to the US Occupational Safety and Health Administration (1980) but has not formally adopted guidelines for doing so. The US Food and Drug Administration (US FDA) began using quantitative risk assessments for environmental contaminants in food in the 1970s, and in the 1980s began applying the same techniques to food and colour additives. US FDA has made several guideline proposals for QEP methods but none has been adopted in final form (US Office of Technology Assessment, 1993). Advisory committees such as the US National Research Council (1977, 1980, 1986a, 1987, 1989, 1990) and the US National Council on Radiation Protection and Measurements (1980) rely on QEP for developing guidance values and have published descriptions of the methods they use. Some states (e.g., State of California, 1985) have adopted formal risk-assessment guidelines for carcinogens which are followed in regulatory approaches for controlling exposures to carcinogens in drinking-water, ambient air, consumer products and hazardous waste.

2.3.2.1 Default risk prediction

As in the Netherlands, the guidelines adopted for QEP in the USA address a number of science policy decisions regarding procedures to follow when scientific knowledge is lacking. Typically, these include procedures for modelling the dose response, accounting for parameter instability in modelling, and interspecies extrapolation. In addition, some guidelines also address the use of pharmacokinetic data, correcting for exposures of short duration, and counting animals with tumours. The specific assumptions made to bridge gaps in scientific knowledge in deriving cancer potency values are often referred to as the "default assumptions"; the term "inference guidelines" has also been used (US National Research Council, 1983). In general, exceptions to default assumptions have been allowed when there is sufficient evidence to convince an agency that another approach is justified.

Most hotly debated is the assumption of low-dose linearity in extrapolating from high to low dose. In estimating the carcinogenic risk of low-level ionizing radiation, the US NCRP and other institutions in the USA have typically assumed non-threshold dose–response relationships (US National Council on Radiation Protection and Measurement, 1980; Sinclair, 1981; Rall *et al.*, 1985). The application of this procedure, once adjustments have been made to account for dose-dependent pharmacokinetics, has been the default in chemical risk assessment in the USA

since the mid-1980s. To predict cancer potency or unit risk values in one species from those in another, it has been assumed in several programmes that different species were equally susceptible when dose was expressed in mg per unit surface area. A modification to this default assumption, namely, $^3/_4$ power scaling, has been proposed by a working group of Federal regulatory agencies (US Environmental Protection Agency, 1992b), and has been adopted by the US EPA (1996a) and by a least one other Federal institution (US Agency for Toxic Substances and Disease Registry, 1993).

A committee of the US National Research Council (US National Research Council, 1994) was statutorily charged (Under Section 112(o) of the Clean Air Act Amendments of 1990) to review US EPA methods for risk assessment, including cancer potency estimation, and indicate revisions needed in its guidelines. The committee supported continued use of "the agency's non-threshold extrapolation practice (i.e., the linear multistage procedure)" and other default assumptions in the absence of adequate information to do otherwise, and encouraged the development of formal criteria for departure from defaults. It called for greater rigour in establishing the predictive accuracy and uncertainty of the methods used. Noting that interindividual variability is typically not addressed in US EPA assessments, it recommended the adoption of a default adjustment factor to account for differences in susceptibility among humans. The committee called for formal uncertainty assessments, but cautioned US EPA to "appropriately reflect the difference between uncertainty and variability."

The US EPA in its 1996 *Proposed Guidelines for Carcinogen Risk Assessment* decided not to follow the above-mentioned committee's recommendation that an adjustment factor to account for differences in human susceptibility should be used in its linear extrapolations, but noted that, where data on interindividual variability are available, they may be used. Furthermore, the Agency decided to change its procedure for low-dose extrapolation: The first step entails a quantitative analysis of carcinogenicity data and the establishment of a "point of departure for extrapolation", i.e. "either a data point or an estimated point that can be considered to be in the range of observation." The LED_{10}, a lower 95% confidence limit on a dose associated with 10% extra risk, is the standard "point of departure"; others will be considered case by case. Use of a specific mathematical model for estimating the LED_{10} is not required. In some cases, the point of departure will not be derived from tumorigenicity data, but instead, for example, from data providing evidence on the mode of action. The dose associated with the point of departure is adjusted to a human equivalent dose when animal data are used. The second step involves a decision regarding the mode of action. "When the evidence supports a mode of action of gene mutation due to DNA reactivity" or another anticipated to follow a linear dose–response relationship, risk is predicted by linear extrapolation ("a straight line is drawn from the point of departure to the origin.") When there is sufficient evidence to support non-linear extrapolation outside the range of observation (e.g. "the carcinogenicity may be a secondary effect of toxicity"), risks are not predicted, and a margin of exposure approach is used: the LED_{10} (or other "point of departure") is compared with the environmental exposure of interest. Decisions regarding the appropriateness of a specific margin of exposure are left to the individuals making the risk management decisions. When the evidence indicates a threshold, the analysis follows that for non-cancer end-points (with the establishment of reference doses (RfDs) or concentrations (RfCs).

2.3.2.2 Use of QEPs

QEPs in the USA have been used in various ways to guide environmental decision-making. For example, QEP is a critical component in the development of numerous recommendations by the US NCRP on controlling radiation exposures in occupational settings and of the general public. These recommendations are made in accordance with its mandate, set out in the Congressional charter in 1964, to establish an organization for the development and dissemination of information on radiation protection and measurement in the public interest.

In part on the basis of risk predictions, national and state groups in the USA have compared and ranked environmental problems (such as air pollution from automobiles, drinking-water cont-

amination from hazardous waste sites) with respect to one another to evaluate priorities for regulation (US Environmental Protection Agency 1987a; US Environmental Protection Agency Science Advisory Board, 1990; California Comparative Risk Project, 1994; Vermont Agency of Natural Resources, 1991; Washington State 2010 Action Strategies Analysis Committee, 1990). Priority setting on the basis of risk alone has been criticized because, as practised, it typically does not take into account the disproportionate risk burden on some segments of the population, particularly the poor; economic efficiency; and public views and perceptions (Resources for the Future, 1993).

A major use of QEPs for carcinogens has been to provide information for regulatory decisions. The extent to which such QEPs have resulted in stringent and costly regulations and pervade decision-making on environmental pollutants has been the subject of debate (Ames & Gold, 1990; US Office of Management and Budget, 1990; Harvard Center for Risk Analysis, 1991; Pease, 1992a). Concerns regarding carcinogenicity have been a factor in the design and implementation of a number of environmental statutes. Regulatory actions under these statutes range in stringency from information disclosure requirements, to standards controlling exposure levels, and to bans on chemical use (Pease, 1992a). In general, the more stringent the rule, the more difficult it is to support and implement, and hence the scope of application is smaller. Occupational regulations demonstrate the trade-off between stringency and scope: warnings are required for all identified carcinogens, but limits on exposure to protect against cancer risk have been established for only 10% of them, and the estimated or predicted risk levels for some workers under these standards can be quite high (e.g. 1% or 10% of exposed workers develop cancer) (Pease, 1992a), although the trigger for action to control workplace exposures to carcinogens is typically quoted as 10^{-3} (US Occupational Safety and Health Administration, 1987). Failures to establish adequate safeguards for exposures to carcinogens in some areas have in part been attributed to unrealistic demands for evidence and rigour in risk assessments and associated opportunities for delay (Latin, 1988; Pease, 1992b; Cranor, 1993) in order to demonstrate that regulatory proposals are not "arbitrary or capricious". Latin (1988) notes that corresponding risk assessments can be extremely resource-intensive, the associated process of review, debate, revision and re-review quite protracted, and regulatory controls delayed. Ruttenberg & Bingham (1981) found a need for generic regulation for setting workplace standards in order to "eliminate one of the major factors that inhibited the issuance of regulations to control workplace carcinogens in the past: the need to cover the same ground in every rule making proceeding."

In the 1970s, a stringent approach to standard setting based on health considerations alone was established under laws governing pollutant releases to air and water (the Clean Air Act of 1970 and the Federal Water Pollution Control Act of 1972; for review, see Robinson & Pease, 1991; Pease, 1992a). These acts called for chemical-by-chemical control of hazardous air emissions and water effluents from manufacturing facilities that provided an "ample margin of safety". For carcinogens considered to pose a risk at any dose, this could be interpreted as a ban. Through a series of legal challenges and court rulings, an intermediate position was reached whereby US EPA would consider an air emission "safe" if the excess/lifetime risk of cancer to the "maximally exposed individual" remained below 1/10 000 and that to the general population, below 1/1 000 000. US EPA was given the discretion to select chemicals for control by placing them on a hazardous air pollutant list, but in 20 years only six chemicals were identified as hazardous, due to difficulties in establishing risk assessments, concerns regarding overregulation, and other factors. To effect greater risk reduction, the most recent Clean Air Amendments of 1990 replaced stringent "health-based" (risk-based) standards by the technology-based requirement of "maximum achievable control technology" (MACT). Because significant residual risks may remain, a second requirement (scheduled to begin in 2001) calls for further reductions beyond MACT for sources posing cancer risks above 1/10 000 for the most highly exposed individuals and above 1/1 000 000 for the general exposed population. Thus, the results of QEP are scheduled to be addressed in the second stage of implementation of the amended Act.

Other Federal programmes employ QEP and have adopted risk levels ranging from 10^{-6} to 10^{-3}, which elevate the level of concern and may trigger regulatory action when exceeded. The legislation which regulates pesticide residues that are present in raw agricultural commodities and that are not concentrated in the course of food processing provides for a balancing of risks and benefits (US National Research Council, 1993a): "The economic, social and environmental costs as well as the potential benefits" of pesticide use must be considered (7 US Code Section 136(a)). In practice, if predicted cancer risk to the consumer exceeds 10^{-4}, prohibition of pesticide use is seriously considered and is a possibility, and if risk falls below 10^{-6}, a tolerance is rarely questioned (Pease, 1992a). Restrictions on land disposal are designed to minimize predicted risks so that they fall between 10^{-6} and 10^{-4}, and on hazardous site clean-ups to between 10^{-7} and 10^{-4}. Technical and economic considerations rather than health concerns determine the level of control for risks falling within these ranges (Pease, 1992a). The goal established for drinking-water by legislation is zero risk, but in practice calculated risks less than 10^{-6} are treated as not of concern. Technical and economic feasibility are major factors in the establishment of standards, with roughly one-half of existing standards corresponding to calculated risks above 10^{-5}, and one-fourth above 10^{-4} (Pease, 1992a). At the State level, a warning is required in California when "in the course of doing business" risks of 10^{-5} are exceeded for any agent listed as "known to the State to cause cancer" (California Health and Safety Code Section 25249.5 et seq.) Thus, risk predictions are used extensively in establishing regulatory goals in the USA but only in a few instances are regulatory controls required when a particular threshold for predicted risk is exceeded.

2.3.3 Canada

Risk analysis plays a critical role in the regulation of chemicals under the Canadian Environmental Protection Act, which provides the legal framework for assessing and controlling substances present in the Canadian environment (Hickman & Toft, 1989; Health Canada, 1994). The guidance document *Carcinogen Assessment*, produced by Health and Welfare Canada (1991), gives general directions on the conduct of a carcinogen risk analysis. In addition, risk-management guidelines (Health and Welfare Canada, 1990) outline the structure for environmental regulatory decision-making in Canada in which "risk analysis" is defined as the processes of hazard identification and risk estimation taken together. "Risk assessment" includes risk analysis and the process of evaluating various options available for controlling risk (Health and Welfare Canada, 1990; Krewski et al., 1993).

In Carcinogen Assessment, a "carcinogen" is defined as "an agent that increases the rate of formation of malignant tumours, or under appropriate circumstances both benign and malignant tumours, in a population", and is evaluated using a weight-of-evidence approach. Agents considered to be carcinogenic or probably carcinogenic to humans are those for which there is sufficient or limited evidence of carcinogenicity in humans, or "with sufficient animal evidence of carcinogenicity in two species, combined with positive in vitro or in vivo genotoxicity data" (Health and Welfare Canada, 1991, p.66). Regarding "non-genotoxic" animal carcinogens, "there is some room for further experimentation to demonstrate whether or not the agent is likely to be carcinogenic to humans." Under the Act, the distinction between "genotoxic" and "non-genotoxic" carcinogens is recognized in the scheme for classification of the weight of evidence of carcinogenicity (Health Canada, 1994; Meek et al., 1994)

Quantitative risk evaluation for an agent considered to be a "non-genotoxic" carcinogen "possibly carcinogenic to humans" under the Act follows the practice used for "threshold toxicants", in which a TDI is developed by a NOEL/UF approach (Health and Welfare Canada, 1992). If the estimated daily intake of an agent by certain subpopulations exceeds the TDI, the agent is considered to be "toxic" under the Act, and the process of evaluating mitigating strategies is initiated. Agents that are "carcinogenic to humans" or "probably carcinogenic to humans" are considered to be "non-threshold toxicants". However, because of the "tenuous nature of low-dose extrapolation procedures", "risks are not specified in terms of predicted incidence or numbers of excess deaths..." Instead, carcinogenic activity is

characterized by a TD_{05}, or that dose which induces a 5% increase in the incidence of tumours associated with exposure (Health Canada, 1994). The dose–response relationship may be "modelled using appropriate mathematical models such as the multistage model". TD_{05} is referred to as the "cancer potency" (Health and Welfare Canada, 1992). Considerations of options for control are a high priority when the ratio of the TD_{05} to estimated exposures exceeds 5000. For comparison with US EPA evaluations if body-weight or surface area scaling (see section 6.7.2) is used to adjust for interspecies differences in deriving the TD_{05}, the ratio 5000 would roughly correspond to a risk of 10^{-5} calculated via the procedures used in the USA and, without interspecies adjustment, a risk of 10^{-4}. The priority for evaluating control options is moderate for agents with exposure to TD_{05} ratios between 2×10^{-6} and 2×10^{-4} (corresponding to risk estimates in the USA of between 10^{-4} and 10^{-6}, if no surface area scaling is applied in TD_{05} derivation). Agents with TD_{05} ratios lower than 2×10^{-6} are considered to be of low priority.

The use of pharmacokinetic and metabolic information in dose–response evaluations is encouraged by the Canadian authorities in both the generic and specific guidance documents (Health and Welfare Canada, 1991, 1992; Krewski et al., 1995). With respect to default approaches to interspecies extrapolation, Carcinogen Assessment provides some scientific rationale for surface area scaling, or alternatively 3/4 power scaling (in contrast to body weight scaling), without stating a preference. In practice, a scaling factor is used when evidence indicates that the agent is "direct acting" (M.E. Meek, 1996, personal communication). Regarding the use of the classical two-stage or other biological models, Carcinogen Assessment notes that, before they can be used routinely, statistical properties need to be understood, especially with regard to low-dose extrapolation. This issue is not discussed in the guidelines under the Act, presumably because the use of TD_{05} obviates the need for a more complicated modelling approach. Krewski et al. (1993), in discussing the Canadian approach, note the value of "biologically based models" in understanding the carcinogenic mechanism.

2.3.4 Norway

QEP is beginning to be used in Norway to provide information for governmental decisions on exposures to carcinogens. For example, the leukaemia burden of consumers from filling their petrol tanks has been estimated, and the potential risk of different occupational exposures has been discussed for use in making decisions on occupational health (E. Dybing & T. Sanner, personal communication, 1991). Unit risk figures developed by the US EPA and US OSHA were used in making the calculations (T. Sanner, personal communication, 1996). Risk assessments to address acrylamide in cosmetics (Dybing & Sanner, 1997) and indoor residential exposure to radon have also been performed (Sanner et al., 1988). Based on measurements by the Norwegian National Institute of Radiation Hygiene and dose–response evaluations in the literature, Sanner et al. (1988) estimated that approximately 240 deaths from lung cancer annually in Norway were due to radon, although it was noted that indoor levels of radon and its decay products have probably increased in recent years. This estimate was later corrected to 75–225 annual deaths, corresponding to 5–15% of all lung cancer deaths in Norway (Sanner & Dybing, 1990). The Norwegian Advisory Board on Food Toxicology, Directorate of Health (1987) similarly estimated cancer risks in evaluating the health consequences of radioactivity in food as a result of fallout from the Chernobyl accident. The Board estimated that, over the next 50 years, the deaths due to ionizing radiation from the accident would be 36 using dose–response figures from the ICRP, and 81 if figures from US EPA were used. On the basis of their analyses, the Board made a number of recommendations regarding action levels for radioactive caesium in reindeer and other wild game.

The Norwegian Scientific Group for Identification of Carcinogens, (1993, 1994) has developed a scheme similar to that considered in the Netherlands (Willems et al., 1990) to rank agents based on their carcinogenic activity. A similar approach is used in Sweden (Sanner et al., 1996). The chemical rankings are used to designate labelling requirements for consumer products (Sanner et al., 1996; Institute for Cancer Research, Norway, 1995). All chemicals with sufficient evidence of carcinogenicity are ranked as having "high", "medium" or "low" potency. The Norwegian scheme was based on measures of carcinogenic activity, as well other factors, namely the availability of epidemiological data, mechanistic information and toxicokinetics. The scheme is based on a proposal of a working group supervised by the Nordic Council of Ministers. The measure of carcinogenic activity selected was the lowest daily dose inducing an increased tumour incidence, referred to as the "TDx, where x denotes the percentage of animals with tumors." Because of the small numbers of animals typically used in cancer bioassays, for statistically significant increases in tumours "x" in most cases exceeds 15%. In addition, the usual differences between TD_{15} and TD_{100} for a given agent are small compared to the enormous variation in carcinogenic potency among chemicals. Follow-up research by some of the authors found that TD_{25} was a practical measure of carcinogenic activity (Dybing et al., 1997). In distinguishing high- from low-potency agents, as much as a 600-fold variation in TD_{50} values for the same agent can result from differences in factors in experimental design and protocol, such as strain of animal tested, route of exposure employed, and tumour site. TD_{50} values estimated from the different available experiments varied by a factor of 100–150. On the basis of these considerations, high-potency carcinogens were those substances with TD_x values less than 15 mg/kg per day; carcinogens of intermediate/medium potency had TD_x values between 15 and 600 mg/kg per day; and those of low potency, TD_x values greater than 600 mg/kg per day. Caveats regarding the use of this scheme were related to borderline cases, (e.g. TD_x in the range 150 – 600 mg/kg per day). Ranking is never determined solely by TD_x values; other factors must always be taken into account.

2.3.5 United Kingdom

In the United Kingdom, the Committee on Carcinogenicity of Chemicals in Food, Consumer Products and the Environment of the Department of Health has developed guidelines for the evaluation of potential human carcinogens for regulatory purposes (Department of Health, 1991) (e.g. to establish maximal residue levels for pesticides in food). To assess exposures to carcinogens, the Committee recommends first characterizing an agent as "genotoxic" or "non-genotoxic". Those characterized as "non-genotoxic" are presumed to have a threshold exposure below which there is no carcinogenic hazard. A safety factor approach is used in deriving estimates of safe levels for these agents. The guidelines state that, as a matter of prudence, genotoxic agents are presumed not to have a threshold. However, because QEP "models may give an impression of precision which cannot be justified from the approximations and assumptions upon which they are based", QEP is not endorsed. Instead, the "broadly based approach adopted by the Committee ... uses all the available data and ... draws on expertise and information from a wide range of medical and scientific opinion" (Department of Health, 1991, p.69).

2.3.6 Germany

In Germany, QEP is rarely employed in the establishment of regulatory controls for carcinogens, although both its use for this purpose and its methodology are being intensely debated (US Office of Technology Assessment, 1993). German environmental law aims to eliminate dangers to public health, which is not consonant with the concept of determining levels associated with small, acceptable risks (US Office of Technology Assessment, 1993). Nevertheless, the Federal Committee for Protection against Pollution (1992) has published a list of maximal tolerable levels for air pollutants that includes those for seven agents derived using a unit risk approach similar to that of the US EPA. These levels were associated with a 1/2500 risk of cancer. In contrast, the 1992 lists of Maximale Arbeitsplatzkonzentrationen (maximal workplace concentrations) and Biologische Arbeitsstofftoleranzwerte (biological tolerance values for occupational substances) developed by the Deutsche Forschungsgemeinschaft as a recommendation to the Ministry of Labour ensure that permissible exposure levels cannot be given for demonstrated human carcinogens.

2.3.7 Denmark

In Denmark, at the request of the National Agency for Environmental Protection, the National Food Agency of Denmark, Institute of Toxicology (1990) explored the possibility of carrying out QEP and discussed the strengths and weaknesses of existing methods. Assessments were made for acrylonitrile, perchloroethylene and aflatoxin B_1. The National Food Agency found that "the final mathematical extrapolation to the low-dose range can now best be performed by using different simplified versions of Knudson and Moolgavkar's multi-stage model. For genotoxins, this model can often be approximated by the two-hit or one-hit model. For the substances that act by means of promoter mechanism, the expression must be simplified to a model requiring special data for the substance's organ toxicity. If such data are not available, it may be possible to use the Mantel–Bryan model instead."

Perchloroethylene was characterized as a promoter, "but the possibility of the substance also having a fairly weak genotoxic effect cannot be excluded". Subsequently, the analysis was based on the model of Mantel & Bryan (1961), a probit model (Finney, 1952) which implicitly assumes that there is a threshold dose that differs among individuals in a population, below which carcinogens will not cause cancer. For acrylonitrile, it was noted that "there is thus every probability that ACN is primarily a procarcinogen with genotoxic metabolites", and one- and two-hit models were applied to the animal data to derive risk estimates. The same models were applied to animal and human data sets to estimate risks from aflatoxin.

2.4. Standard approaches to QEP for carcinogens

Results of quantitative risk assessments for carcinogens play a major role in the development of standards and guidelines by organizations concerned with radiation hazards, by WHO committees on drinking-water, ambient air, and general environmental risks, and by regulatory agencies in some countries (e.g. the Netherlands and the USA) (Table 2.2), all of which have adopted standardized approaches for deriving risk estimates and predictions. In Canada, a quantitative procedure based on standard QEP methods is used to establish regulatory priorities for agents classified as "known" carcinogens or "probably carcinogenic to humans" and "genotoxic". Agencies in Germany, Denmark and Norway have begun to consider quantitative risk predictions, and in some cases have employed

Table 2.2. Standard approaches used by various countries or bodies to characterize dose–response relationships for carcinogens	
Procedure	**Country or body**
"Genotoxic": no quantitative assessment "Non-genotoxic": NOEL/UF	European Union United Kingdom WHO/FAO (JECFA and JMPR)[a]
Non-threshold dose–response model	UNSCEAR (radiation) NCRP (radiation) ICRP (radiation) USA[b]
"Genotoxic": "non-threshold" modelling "Non-genotoxic": NOEL/UF	WHO (drinking-water) Netherlands[c]
"Genotoxic": "one-hit" or "two-hit" model "Promoters": Mantel–Bryan procedure or "Knudson–Moolgavkar multistage" (data permitting)	Denmark

Carcinogens with mode of action:
Low-dose linear: linear extrapolation below the "point of
   departure" (e.g. ED_{10})
Low-dose non-linear: margin of exposure comparison
   between "point of departure" and environmental level
	US EPA 1996 (*Proposed Guidelines*)

"Non-threshold" effect: "characterize the dose–response
   relationship" (by mathematical modelling, ranking the
   relative potencies or division of effect levels by (large)
   uncertainty factor)
"Threshold" effect: NOEL/UF approach
	IPCS

Known human or probable human and "genotoxic": calcu-
   late exposure:TD_{05} ratio
Possible human or "non-genotoxic" probable human
   carcinogen: NOEL/UF approach
	Canada

IARC Groups 1, 2A: QEP using epidemiological data	WHO Regional Office for Europe (air)
Rank carcinogens on the basis of their TD_x and other factors[d]	Norway

[a] In a few instances, WHO (JECFA/JMPR) has used NOEL/UF for agents found to act via genotoxic mechanisms.
[b] When data are sufficient to support different dose–response models, exceptions occur.
[c] For agents with an unknown mode of action, "non-threshold" modelling is applied.
[d] TD_x is the lowest daily dose inducing increased tumour incidence.

QEPs in making decisions. The United Kingdom has specifically decided against using QEP for "genotoxic" carcinogens, uses a quantitative assessment method (NOEL/UF approach) for "non-genotoxic" carcinogens, and makes the case for this decision in its guidelines for evaluating chemical carcinogenicity. Similarly, an EU Directive embracing the use of risk assessment in environmental decision-making precludes quantitative assessment for carcinogens not characterized as "non-genotoxic". Agents considered to be "non-genotoxic" are assessed using a NOEL/UF approach. In general, exposures characterized as "tolerable" are considerably lower if derived from risk predictions using the standard QEP techniques based on the assumption that no threshold exists than if obtained by the NOEL/UF approach. Typically, institutions in the USA have adopted the default assumption that carcinogens are without thresholds for all but those few agents for which scientific data strongly support an alternative hypothesis. US EPA in its 1996 *Proposed Guidelines* has decided to establish a dose, or "point of departure" within the observable range, such as that associated with a 10% lifetime cancer risk, and then to extrapolate linearly below that dose for carcinogens with modes of action consistent with the low-dose linearity assumption. For agents with sufficient evidence of non-linearity at low doses, a margin of exposure approach is used ("point of departure" and environmental doses are compared), and risk predictions are not made.

Inconsistencies in guidance result from differences in the treatment of carcinogens found to be "non-genotoxic", as shown by the different guidance values given for 2,3,7,8-tetrachlorodibenzo-*p*-dioxin (TCDD). In contrast, the Netherlands, Norway, several state and federal institutions in the USA, as well as the International Agency for Research on Cancer (1982), have produced similar risk estimates and predictions for benzene. Such predictions have been considered in numerous environmental decisions in Europe and North America.

Regular application of the standard approaches by national and international bodies has resulted in tabulations and databases of carcinogenicity values for individual agents which can then be applied in a variety of risk-assessment situations. Examples include the unit risk and cancer potency tabulations of US EPA (1996b, 1997) and of the California Environmental Protection Agency (1995), some tabulations in the WHO air quality guidelines (World Health Organization 1987a), the WHO drinking-water standards associated with 10^{-5} risk (World Health Organization 1996a), and the no significant risk levels of California's Proposition 65 (*California Code of Regulations*, Title 22, Section 12705). An expedited procedure based on a routine data-set selection approach applied to a large compendium of carcinogenicity bioassay results (the Cancer Potency Database of Lois Gold, Bruce Ames and colleagues at Lawrence Livermore National Laboratories), and subsequent curve fitting with a multistage model has also been used to rapidly generate standardized cancer potency values (Hoover *et al.*, 1995).

When used, QEP is typically an initial step in establishing regulatory controls, economic and technical feasibility and political considerations coming into play once risks of concern are found. The same holds true when a NOEL/UF approach is used. The uncertainties associated with the assumptions made in risk extrapolations are often emphasized when justifying the rejection of QEP. Analogous concerns have also been noted for the NOEL/UF approach, for the characterization of an agent as "non-genotoxic" is subject to error, and there is no assurance that all "non-genotoxic" agents have thresholds. Some proposals for changes in QEP have included a provision for non-threshold responses for certain classes of agents characterized as "non-genotoxic" (e.g. Cohen & Ellwein, 1990). Crump *et al.* (1976) noted that, if spontaneous tumours are associated with an effective background dose to which exposure from environmental carcinogens is added, then under almost any model the response will be linear at low doses (see also US Environmental Protection Agency, 1986b). The usual concerns associated with the use of the NOEL/UF approach for non-cancer end-points also remain. For example, the NOEL divided by the uncertainty factor has been characterized as an estimate of the population no effect level, which does not provide absolute assurance of safety (Crump, 1984; US National Research Council, 1993b). "Larger and better studies can demonstrate effects at lower doses, but the size of the uncertainty factor is not directly related to sample size. Therefore, smaller and poorer experiments tend to lead to larger ADIs" (US National Research Council, 1993b, p. 326). In addition, the uncertainty factors typically employed "are not based on validated biological models" (US National Research Council, 1993b). In part because safety is not guaranteed, the terms "ADI" and "acceptable intake" have been replaced by "reference dose", "tolerable intake" and "tolerable daily intake" by various institutions. To address the concern regarding study size, a "benchmark dose" approach has been proposed as a replacement for the NOEL/UF approach (Crump, 1984; Crump *et al.*, 1991;

California Environmental Protection Agency, 1993; US Environmental Protection Agency, 1993). US EPA (1996a) has adopted a similar approach for carcinogens with sufficient evidence of a mode of action associated with a non-linear dose response at low doses, because of the large uncertainty in low-dose risk predictions for such agents.

Concerns over the accuracy of the risk predicted by standard QEP procedures and the appropriateness of applying the NOEL/UF approach to carcinogens have provided the incentive to develop more reliable approaches. Several examples of attempts to provide improved assessments are described below.

2.5 Attempts to Improve QEP

A variety of activities aimed at improving routine cancer risk assessment procedures have been undertaken in an effort to derive more reliable estimates of risk for specific agents, and are indicative of the evolving discipline and practice of QEP. The goal is to generate, through experimentation and analysis, principles of extrapolation to replace the default assumptions necessarily made as a matter of policy due to limited scientific information. Examples of such activities are given here, and include approaches reported to be more "biologically based" than the standard methodology, or more scientifically sound because they incorporate more data in the analysis. Because of the reliance on QEP by regulatory agencies in the USA, and the related economic impact, many of the initiatives discussed here originated in the USA.

In "biologically based" approaches, the dose–response relationship is divided into three components: (i) a model of pharmacokinetics and physiology (typically a compartmental "physiologically based pharmacokinetic (PBPK)" model) describing the relationship between the exposure to the agent and the resultant critical exposure in the target organ; (ii) a pharmacodynamic model describing the interaction of the agent with target cellular components; and (iii) a model of cell kinetics which describes the transformation to tumorigenic cells, and palpable tumour (see Chapter 7 for details). Examples of attempts to model one or more of the components of "biologically based" approaches given

below indicate the limitations and insights afforded by this modelling activity as applied to TCDD, saccharin, formaldehyde, methylene chloride and perchloroethylene; for benzene, see Section 2.5.3. These approaches require numerous assumptions to be made about model structure and parameters. Thus examples of uncertainty and sensitivity analyses are given for two of the substances considered (perchloroethylene and methylene chloride). A common criticism of assessments using epidemiological or animal bioassay data is that they rely on a single study to the exclusion of all others. Examples of risk estimates based on meta-analyses of a number of epidemiological studies on environmental tobacco smoke and ionizing radiation are given in Section 2.5.2. For numerous substances, lack of direct observations of dose–response for carcinogenicity in epidemiological studies and animal bioassay preclude assessments of cancer potency. Examples of cases where ancillary data are used to predict cancer potency are given in Section 2.5.4 (complex mixtures of polynuclear aromatic hydrocarbons (PAHs) and dioxins; ethylene).

2.5.1 "Biologically based" approaches

2.5.1.1 Integrated modelling of physiology, pharmacokinetics, pharmacodynamics and cell dynamics: 2,3,7,8-tetrachlorodibenzo-p-dioxin (TCDD)

The mechanisms of TCDD carcinogenicity have been better studied and are better understood than those of most other environmental contaminants. As discussed in detail in Chapters 7 and 8, analyses of varying complexity (Sielken, 1987; Thorslund, 1987; Leung et al., 1988; Andersen et al., 1993; Kohn et al., 1993) have been performed to improve upon the standard analyses used by regulatory agencies in establishing the cancer potency of TCDD (Portier et al., 1984; US Environmental Protection Agency, 1985a; California Department of Health Services, 1986; US Environmental Protection Agency, 1989; California Department of Health Services, 1990). These include: the fitting of a two-stage model on the assumption that TCDD induces the proliferation of initiated cells and is without genotoxic activity (Thorslund, 1987); re-evaluation of the histopathological slides serving as the basis of the US EPA (1985a) unit risk derivation

(Pathology Working Group, 1990); use of the re-evaluated histopathology for unit risk derivations using time-dependent multistage (Zeise *et al.*, 1990) and two-stage (Paustenbach *et al.*, 1991) models; use of data on liver concentration in the rat to obtain maximum likelihood estimates with the linearized multistage model (Sielken, 1987); the development of physiological pharmacokinetic models to estimate tissue dose of TCDD in the liver (Kissel & Robarge, 1988; Leung *et al.*, 1988, 1989, 1990a,b; Mills *et al.*, 1992) and in breast-feeding infants (Smith, 1987; Hoover *et al.*, 1991). More recently a coupled pharmacodynamic/pharmacokinetic model ("receptor-mediated physiologically based pharmacokinetic model") has also been developed (Andersen *et al.* 1993).

Using TCDD as the model compound, the US National Institute of Environmental Health Sciences and US EPA have undertaken the most extensive and costly risk assessment effort to date (Greenlee *et al.*, 1991; Lucier *et al.*, 1993; US National Research Council, 1996). These agencies chose as the basis for human risk prediction the female rat liver, one of several sites of TCDD carcinogenesis, and developed the following detailed models: rat physiology and pharmacokinetics, emphasizing the liver; human physiology and pharmacokinetics; pharmacodynamics; cell kinetics. In addition, extensive laboratory work was performed to support the modelling. In contrast to what was anticipated, their modelling and research results were consistent with the linearity extrapolation assumption. The data are mathematically consistent with the assumption that TCDD is a significant creator of mutated cells, and is not a pure, "non-genotoxic" promoter (Portier *et al.*, 1996; Moolgavkar *et al.*, 1996). Despite the magnitude of the effort, the pharmacokinetic and pharmacodynamic mechanisms of liver carcinogenesis are consistent with either a low-dose linear or a non-linear dose–response relationship.

The case of TCDD is of particular interest from the risk-assessment point of view in that it represents one of the most comprehensive attempts at biologically based cancer risk assessment conducted to date (US National Research Council, 1996). Information is available on the pharmacokinetics of TCDD, receptor-mediated induction of the liver enzymes CYP1A1 and CYP1A2, and cancer occurrence in both animals and humans. Despite the richness of this database, some critical gaps in the data remain. For example, quantitative information on the number and size of preneoplastic lesions in rodent liver as a function of both time and dose would be useful in developing realistic models of TCDD carcinogenesis. In addition, uncertainty remains about the full range of biological events involved in TCDD carcinogenesis. In particular, the sequence of events involved in the induction and proliferation of liver foci in rodents is not known. Another issue relates to the emphasis on liver cancer, to the exclusion of other cancers, such as cancer of the lung, a site associated with TCDD exposure in the most informative epidemiological studies (International Agency for Research on Cancer, 1997). Nevertheless, this case has served to promote the use of biologically based approaches to cancer risk assessment, making use of the full spectrum of available data.

2.5.1.2 Mechanistic modelling assuming cancer induced by chronic irritation: saccharin

Exposure of male rats *in utero* or at time of birth to sodium saccharin and then continued exposure throughout their lives results in the induction of bladder tumours (Arnold *et al.* 1980) with a non-linear dose–response (Taylor *et al.*, 1980; Schoenig *et al.*, 1985). The tumorigenic response is thought to be specific to the rat (Chappel, 1992), although saccharin has generally not been studied in other species exposed before weaning. To explain these results and to provide the basis for assessing the safety of saccharin as a food additive, a number of laboratory investigations have been performed, as reviewed elsewhere (Arnold *et al.*, 1983; Renwick, 1985, 1993). A variety of hypotheses have been put forward to explain the findings in the cancer bioassays and follow-up investigations (Sweatman & Renwick, 1980; Renwick & Sims, 1983; Anderson, 1985; Lawrie *et al.*, 1985; World Health Organization, 1987b; Anderson *et al.*, 1988).

Cohen, Ellwein and colleagues have proposed a unifying hypothesis for saccharin bladder carcinogenesis and ancillary data (Cohen, 1985; Cohen & Ellwein, 1990), which they model mathematically using a two-stage cancer model

(Greenfield *et al.*, 1984; Ellwein & Cohen, 1988, 1989; Cohen & Ellwein, 1989; Ellwein & Cohen, 1992). They hypothesize that exposure to high dietary concentrations of sodium saccharin leads to the formation of silicate microcrystals in the urine (Cohen *et al.*, 1989), and that tumour incidence is greater in male rats because of the high concentrations of urinary proteins, particularly α_{2u}-globulin (Cohen *et al.*, 1991). They suggest that saccharin bound to urinary protein is a nidus for the formation of silicate crystals. The crystals act as microabrasives causing mild focal regenerative hyperplasia, and the increased cell turnover results in an increase in the rate of mutation.

In the Cohen and Ellwein two-stage model for saccharin, cancer occurs through initiation and transformation to malignancy, with normal, initiated and transformed cell populations increasing or decreasing in number according to mitotic, birth, death and transition rates which vary with time. (For a full description of the two-stage models, see Chapter 7). Values for each model parameter are specified, and tumour response is then simulated in computer runs. The simulations do not consider cell division and cell death explicitly. Rather, the net rate of cell proliferation, i.e. the difference between the rate of division and the rate of death, is modelled. Moolgavkar (1991) has pointed out that this approach can lead to the wrong incidence function. Instead of using formal statistical techniques to select model parameters or test goodness of fit, parameter values are varied until the simulation and data match. Another criticism of the approach is therefore the lack of clear criteria for selecting trial values for the parameters or for determining goodness of fit because the most appropriate parameters may not be found, results may not be reproducible, and uncertainty in parameter estimates is poorly understood (US National Research Council, 1993b). The approach has, however, provided important biological insights into the mechanisms of carcinogenesis by saccharin.

2.5.1.3 Use of information on DNA cross-links as a measure of dose: formaldehyde

Inhaled formaldehyde produces squamous-cell carcinomas of the nasal cavity in rats (e.g. Albert *et al.*, 1982) with a markedly non-linear dose–response relationship (Kerns *et al.*, 1983; Monticello, 1990). Application of standard methodology results in high risk estimates for occupational exposure and for exposure of the general public through offgassing of consumer products (Tancrede *et al.*, 1987; US Environmental Protection Agency, 1987c). A major effort was made by the Chemical Industry Institute of Toxicology to develop alternative approaches for estimating risk (Casanova & Heck, 1991). Non-default approaches for extrapolations from high to low dose and across species have addressed two aspects of formaldehyde inhalation toxicology: (i) the significant non-linear formation of DNA–protein cross-links; and (ii) sustained tissue damage and cell proliferation associated with exposure to high concentrations. DNA–protein cross-links are used as a surrogate measure of concentration in the target cells (US Environmental Protection Agency, 1991; California Environmental Protection Agency, 1992), and the potential contribution of cell proliferation to the tumorigenic response is explored through modelling (California Environmental Protection Agency, 1992). To address interspecies differences, the US EPA (1991) considered the formation of cross-links in monkeys as the best surrogate for human exposure. The US EPA's resulting unit risk estimate $(3.3 \times 10^{-7}/\text{ppb})$ is a factor of 50 lower than its 1987 estimate $(1.5 \times 10^{-5}/\text{ppb})$, which was based on standard methodology. The California Environmental Protection Agency estimate $(7 \times 10^{-6}/\text{ppb})$ is a factor of two lower because it employed the rat DNA cross-link data to address the non-linearity in the dose–response relationship for the rat, but did not use the monkey data as the basis for extrapolating to humans.

2.5.1.4 Uncertainty and variability analysis in PBPK models: methylene chloride and perchloroethylene

Methylene chloride and perchloroethylene are treated as carcinogens by regulatory agencies in the USA, and risk estimates based on animal bioassay data guide the degree of environmental control required. PBPK models have been developed for assessing the risks of methylene chloride (e.g. Angelo & Prichard, 1984; Angelo *et al.*, 1984; Dankovic & Bailar, 1984; Gargas *et al.*,

1986; Angelo et al., 1986a,b; Andersen et al., 1987; US Environmental Protection Agency, 1987b; Reitz et al., 1988; California Department of Health Services, 1989; Andersen et al., 1991; Casanova et al., 1996) and perchloroethylene (e.g. Reitz & Nolan, 1986; US Environmental Protection Agency, 1986a; Hattis et al., 1986; Chen & Blancato, 1987; Bogen & McKone, 1988; Ward et al., 1988; Bois et al., 1990; Gearhart et al., 1993; Dallas et al., 1994a,b; Bois et al., 1996a). The models are used to describe and predict species-, dose- or route-dependent differences in pharmacokinetics. Incorporation of the PBPK approach into the assessment by some researchers has resulted in risk estimates for these compounds significantly lower by one to two orders of magnitude than those derived by standardized methods. However, once uncertainties in model parameters were considered, the extent of the difference from the standard approach diminished substantially.

PBPK models are described in detail in Chapter 7, and briefly here for the purposes of discussion. In these PBPK examples, the body is divided into compartments (typically a fat group, a richly perfused tissue group, a poorly perfused tissue group, and a liver metabolizing group), characterized by volumes and blood:tissue partition coefficients (Gargas et al., 1989). For modelling perchloroethylene, the lung is included as a volumeless gas-exchange unit, described by the alveolar ventilation rate and blood:air partition coefficient; metabolism occurs via the mixed-function oxidase (MFO) pathway in the liver only. For methylene chloride, both the lung and liver are assumed to have metabolic capacity (glutathione-S-transferase (GST) and saturable MFO pathways), with the lung described by a lung compartment with metabolic capacity coupled in series with a gas-exchange unit. The lung and the other compartments are linked in parallel. The model consists of a series of differential equations describing the change in tissue concentration over time due to transport to tissue compartments via blood flow, uptake by, and elimination from tissue in accordance with the relevant partition coefficients, and metabolism within the tissue. The average daily concentrations of the metabolite hypothesized to be the active proximate carcinogen serve

as the surrogate measure of carcinogenic dose. The source of the carcinogenic intermediate is assumed to be the GST pathway for methylene chloride and the MFO pathway for perchloroethylene.

The models require identification of the activation pathway, and the biochemical and physiological data needed to estimate the following parameters for the animal tested in the cancer bioassay serving as the basis of the risk estimate: (i) tissue:air partition coefficients; (ii) blood flows to compartments and tissue volumes of compartments; and (iii) biochemical constants for critical metabolic pathways. In addition, if used for across-species extrapolation, a human model together with estimates of physiological and pharmacokinetic parameters for humans are required.

Limitations of the models for perchloroethylene and methylene chloride and areas in which they could be improved have been extensively discussed (see e.g. US Environmental Protection Agency, 1987b; California Department of Health Services, 1989; Portier & Kaplan, 1989; Bois et al., 1990; Hattis et al., 1990; Bois et al., 1996a). Concerns have been raised about a variety of aspects of the modelling exercise, and include the following. Data are lacking or limited to such an extent that a number of model parameters are not well defined. For example, partition coefficients are determined in vitro using tissue homogenates, and are often assumed to be the same in different species; however, they may not reflect in vivo partitioning into the organ, and there can be significant species differences for some tissues (see e.g. Dallas et al., 1994b; Pelekis et al., 1995). Proper statistical optimization procedures are frequently not used to derive pharmacokinetic parameters from in vivo studies, and measurements of such parameters from in vitro studies can be quite inaccurate, particularly for human tissue. The models have not been adequately validated experimentally, and basic model structure may be misspecified (Andersen et al., 1994; Clewell et al., 1994). The data used to develop an animal pharmacokinetic model for methylene chloride have been used in some exercises designed to validate it. For perchloroethylene, it is assumed that metabolism occurs in the liver and that the active metabolite is too unstable to be transported far, yet leukaemia is observed in the rat. Typically, perchloroethylene has been assumed to be activated only to an epoxide via the cytochrome P-450 pathway, whereas the glutathione pathway has been observed to produce DNA-binding metabolites (see Hattis *et al.*, 1990 for discussion). Finally, the variability in metabolic parameters among humans may be substantial for some pathways, and single values are typically assigned to them and assumed to be representative of the human population.

To account for some of the limitations listed above, uncertainty analyses using a statistical approach have been performed for both methylene chloride (Portier & Kaplan, 1989) and perchloroethylene (e.g. Bois *et al.*, 1990). The cancer and pharmacokinetic models were linked and the model parameters were described by probability distributions, rather than assigned fixed values. Monte Carlo sampling over these distributions was used to generate a distribution of the risk estimate. For perchloroethylene, parameters were assumed to correlate with body size, not to be independent. In addition, due to the experimental design, the metabolic parameters V_{max}, the maximal metabolic rate, and K_m, the Michaelis–Menton coefficient, could not be estimated independently, and were assumed to follow the joint distribution derived by fitting the PBPK model to *in vivo* data. In sensitivity analyses, model prediction was most sensitive to the metabolic parameters. A more descriptive approach to evaluating uncertainties in the pharmacokinetic modelling for perchloroethylene has also been undertaken (Hattis *et al.*, 1990).

The extent of human metabolism of perchloroethylene at low doses has been a critical area of uncertainty. Published estimates of the fraction of inhaled perchloroethylene metabolized for air concentrations of 1 ppm have ranged from 2 to 86% (Hattis *et al.*, 1990). Physiological and pharmacokinetic data on six healthy adult male volunteers exposed to high doses (72 and 144 ppm) in chamber studies for four hours and followed for four days (Monster *et al.* 1979) provide information on high-dose kinetics near the time of exposure, and over the subsequent days of follow-up on low-dose kinet-

ics. Bois *et al.* (1996a) fitted these data to a hierarchical model of population toxicokinetics, developed to account for individual variability and parameter uncertainty, in order to describe the dose-dependent pharmacokinetics for these six individuals. The two most different of the six individuals differed by roughly a factor of 2. The mean fraction metabolized at 50 ppm was 1.7% (95%CI 0.52–4.1), as compared with 36% (95%CI 15–58) at 1 ppb. This provided an explanation for the wide range of values for fraction metabolized reported in the literature, since the low values correspond to those derived from high-dose experiments and the assumption of linear kinetics.

For the methylene chloride uncertainty analysis (Portier & Kaplan, 1989), all model parameters were assumed to be independent in the simulations. Both this analysis and that for perchloroethylene showed that upper bounds of cancer risk can be underestimated if uncertainty in parameters of the pharmacokinetic model are not taken into account. In this case, the underestimation was found to be substantial. In a sensitivity analysis undertaken on the methylene chloride PBPK model (Clewell *et al.*, 1994), the importance of model parameters was found to depend markedly on the conditions simulated (e.g. concentration and species) and the dose surrogate considered. Model structure also had a significant impact. As far as the assessment of variability among exposed individuals is concerned, the impact of exercise and variation in enzyme activities (Dankovic & Bailar, 1994) as well as of age and prior exposure to methylene chloride (in mice; Thomas *et al.*, 1996) has been described.

Another issue that arose in these examples was the degree to which PBPK analysis accounts for interspecies differences in cancer potency. Currently, some regulatory agencies in the USA consider humans and animals to have the same sensitivity to a carcinogenic dose given over a lifetime, when the dose is expressed as amount per surface area (the so-called "surface area scaling" assumption) or amount per body weight to the 3/4 power. The assumption is incorporated by applying an adjustment factor to the cancer potency (typically expressed in mg/kg per day). It has been argued (Andersen *et al.*, 1987; Reitz *et al.*, 1988) that pharmacokinetic analysis accounts for interspecies differences in potency, and that, if one has been performed, an interspecies correction should not be applied. A counter-argument (US Consumer Product Safety Commission, 1978; US Environmental Protection Agency, 1986a; California Department of Health Services, 1989; Rhomberg, 1995) is that, even if the pharmacokinetics in different species were accounted for precisely, interspecies differences in cell kinetics, pharmacodynamics, and other factors have not been addressed; thus, much of the potentially considerable difference in species susceptibility to cancer may remain, and not be taken into account in the overall analysis.

2.5.2 Meta-analyses of epidemiological data: Ionizing radiation and environmental tobacco smoke

2.5.2.1 Ionizing radiation

Current estimates of cancer risk associated with external exposure to low LET ionizing radiation are derived primarily from studies of the mortality of atomic bomb survivors in Hiroshima and Nagasaki and of patients irradiated for therapeutic purposes (US National Research Council, 1990; International Commission on Radiological Protection, 1990; United Nations Scientific Committee on the Effects of Atomic Radiation, 1994). Both these groups were exposed primarily at high dose rates. Radiation protection recommendations for environmental and occupational exposures have generally been based on the use of these estimates in conjunction with models to extrapolate the effects of such acute (or short-term) high-level exposures to the relatively low-dose, low-dose-rate exposures of environmental and occupational concern, and across populations with different baseline cancer risks (International Commission on Radiological Protection, 1990). These models, which are generally based on linear or linear–quadratic extrapolations and sometimes on the use of dose and dose-rate effectiveness factors (DDREF), are inevitably, subject to uncertainties.

A direct assessment of the carcinogenic effects of long-term, low-level radiation exposure in humans can be made from studies of cancer risk among workers in the nuclear industry. Published studies have covered cohorts of nuclear industry workers in Canada, the United Kingdom and the United States of America (see, for example, Cardis *et al.* 1995a, the full study report, for a review). Most of these studies have provided little evidence of any dose-related increase in all cancer mortality. The statistical power of individual studies was, however, low and in most cohorts the confidence intervals of the risk estimates were compatible with a range of possibilities, from negative effects to risks an order of magnitude greater than those on which current radiation protection recommendations are based.

In order to increase the power to estimate small risks and the precision of the resulting estimates, formal national and international combined analyses of original data from these studies have been carried out (Gilbert *et al.*, 1993; Carpenter *et al.*, 1994; IARC Working Group, 1994; Cardis *et al.*, 1995b). The comparability of dosimetric information was also assessed. The combined analyses covered a total of 2 124 526 person–years at risk (PY) and 15 825 deaths, 3976 of which were due to cancer.

The resulting excess relative risk estimates (ERR) for all cancers excluding leukaemia, and leukaemia excluding chronic lymphocytic leukaemia (CLL), the two main groupings of causes of deaths for which risk estimates have been derived from studies of atomic bomb survivors, were -0.07 per Sv (90 % CI: -0.4–0.3) and 2.18 per Sv (90 % CI: 0.1–5.7), respectively. These values correspond to a relative risk of 0.99 for all cancers excluding leukaemia for a cumulative protracted dose of 100 mSv compared with zero mSv. For leukaemia excluding CLL, the corresponding value was 1.22 and the number of leukaemia deaths attributed to radiation exposure in this cohort was 9.7 (8%). These estimates, which did not differ significantly across cohorts nor between men and women, are the most comprehensive and precise direct estimates obtained to date. Although they are lower than the linear estimates obtained from studies of atomic bomb survivors, they are compatible with a range of possibilities, from a reduction of risk at low doses to risks twice those on which current radiation protection recommendations are based. Overall, the results of this study do not suggest that current radiation risk estimates for cancer at low levels of exposure are appreciably in error.

2.5.2.2 Environmental tobacco smoke

Lung cancer risks posed by environmental tobacco smoke (ETS) have been derived from epidemiological studies on non-smokers exposed to their spouse's smoking. After adjusting for systematic biases, the estimates of relative risk are applied to the general population to predict lung cancer mortality in non-smokers associated with exposure to ETS (Blot & Fraumeni, 1986; Wald et al., 1986; Wells, 1988; US National Research Council, 1986b; Robins et al., 1989; Saracci & Riboli, 1989; US Environmental Protection Agency, 1992c). Adjustments are made to account for smoker misclassification and for exposures to ETS in addition to that for which the smoking spouse is responsible. In the meta-analysis, the relative risk is derived from a large subset of available studies, rather than from a particular study, as is typical in risk assessments. A critical assumption in using the relative risk estimate to calculate lung cancer mortality is the extent to which background exposure from sources other than spouse's smoke occurs (US National Research Council, 1986b; US Environmental Protection Agency, 1992c). An expression incorporating the ratio of total ETS exposure to ETS exposure from non-spousal sources is used to adjust relative risk for background exposures. To address the issue of exposure to ETS outside the home, a variant of this approach was developed. The lung cancer risks of Seventh Day Adventists are compared with those of non-Seventh Day Adventists who never smoked (Repace & Lowrey, 1985). It is argued that, because of differences in lifestyle, Seventh Day Adventists are far less likely to be exposed outside the home. From estimates of the age-specific differences in lung cancer mortality rates of the two populations, the number of lung cancer deaths in the general population was derived. This approach was applied using American (Repace & Lowrey, 1985) and Canadian (Wigle et al., 1987) life tables to estimate the impact of passive smoking in the two countries.

The main criticism of the meta-analyses of ETS and lung cancer relates to the quality of the studies providing the basis for the analysis (see, e.g. Fleiss & Gross, 1991). The main deficiencies of these studies have been misclassification and publication bias, and confounding (Lee, 1992; for discussion, see Woodward & McMichael (1991) and California Environmental Protection Agency (1997)). Of particular concern is the misclassification as non-smokers of current and former smokers. Two recent studies found that, while misclassification of smokers as non-smokers does occur, it is unlikely to explain the observed associations between lung cancer and ETS exposure. A large multicentre international study to validate self-reported exposure to ETS by analysis of urinary cotinine found a small proportion of participants to be deceivers (1.5%) (Riboli et al., 1995). An investigation of misclassification rates in two large Swedish cohorts, for which smoking habits were assessed after an interval of 6–10 years, found, as in other studies, that most of the ever-smokers misclassified as non-smokers had quit smoking and had smoked less than average smokers (Nyberg et al., 1997). Overall, the study suggested that misclassification bias was at a level which could not explain the lung cancer risk associated with ETS exposure. Well conducted studies of ETS exposure and lung cancer released subsequent to the publication of the meta-analyses by the US National Research Council (1986b) and US Environmental Protection Agency (1992c) have been designed to minimize misclassification bias (Stockwell et al., 1992; Fontham et al., 1994). Clear dose–response relationships between ETS exposure and lung cancer are observed in these studies, and in the large multicentre study (Fontham et al., 1994), which was designed to address many of the limitations of earlier studies, the overall estimates of relative risk for exposure to spouse's smoke are consistent with those found in the meta-analyses, providing some validation of, and further support for the earlier findings.

The dose–response relationship derived for active smokers has also been used to predict risks for the ETS-exposed on the basis of cigarette equivalents (Vutuc, 1984; Repace & Lowrey, 1985; Russell et al., 1986; Arundel et al., 1987; Robins et al., 1989). Cigarette equivalents are calculated from surrogate measures of exposure common to both active and passive smoking. Those used in the extrapolations have included urinary nicotine concentrations (Russell *et al.*, 1986), mg tar per day (Repace & Lowrey, 1985), and mg of particulates (Arundel *et al.*, 1987). Because mainstream and sidestream smoke differ in physical and chemical composition and in characteristics of intake, the validity of the overall approach has been questioned (US Department of Health and Human Services, 1986; Woodward & McMichael, 1991; US Environmental Protection Agency, 1992c).

2.5.3 Experimental and epidemiological efforts to improve estimates of benzene cancer potency

Benzene is known to cause leukaemia in humans (International Agency for Research on Cancer, 1982), particularly acute myelogenous leukaemia (AML), and appears to cause other haematological neoplasms (see e.g. Hayes *et al.*, 1997). The possibility that other sites in humans may also be at risk is indicated by an elevated risk of lung cancer mortality observed in a large cohort study (Hayes *et al.*, 1997) and by findings from animal bioassays: cancers at multiple sites are observed after oral exposures (Huff *et al.* 1989; Maltoni *et al.*, 1983, 1989), including squamous-cell carcinomas of lip, palate, tongue, Zymbal gland, skin, preputial gland, ovary, mammary gland, Harderian gland, lung, and haematopoietic system. Similarly, inhalation exposures (Maltoni *et al.*, 1989; Cronkite *et al.* 1989) give rise to squamous-cell carcinomas of the Zymbal gland, oral and nasal cavity, Harderian gland, lung, mammary gland and haematopoietic system. Benzene cancer potencies currently used to establish regulatory controls in the USA have been derived from epidemiological or animal bioassay data by means of standard methods (California Department of Health Services, 1984; Crump & Allen, 1984; US Environmental Protection Agency 1985b; A. Kelter, personal communication, 1988). The International Agency for Research on Cancer (1982, p.395) has also published a dose–response characterization of benzene. In potency derivations from animal data (California Department of Health Services, 1984; for a review, see Crump, 1992), the polynomial form of the multistage model (see Section 6.3.1) was fitted to data from bioassays performed via inhalation (Maltoni *et al.*, 1983) or gavage (Maltoni *et al.*, 1983; US National Toxicology Program, 1986). The potency value currently used by the US EPA (1993, 1985) is the geometric mean of four maximum likelihood point estimates derived from the pooled dose incidence data for leukaemia from two occupational data sets (Ott *et al.* (1978); Rinsky *et al.* (1981)) and adjusted for the results of a third, a study by Wong and colleagues that was unpublished at the time. The four estimates correspond to different assumptions regarding benzene interaction with background factors (i.e. additive versus relative risk models) and of timing of exposure.

A number of attempts have been made to improve the basis for the estimation of benzene cancer potency, one of which is the development of biological models. Progress has been made in modelling the dose-, dose-rate- and species-dependent metabolism of benzene (see e.g. Sabourin *et al.*, 1987; Henderson *et al.* 1989; Medinsky *et al.* 1996). Models of leukaemogenesis which account for the biological effects of benzene have been the subject of extensive research, but a clear understanding of the mechanisms is still elusive (Goldstein, 1989; Smith, 1996), so that the development of "biologically based" multistage models which can be reliably used for the prediction of benzene risks is seen as premature (Smith & Fanning, 1997). Empirical approaches to improving potency estimates have included retrospective analyses of exposures for the cohort of Rinsky *et al.* (1981, 1987) and reassessing the corresponding dose–response relationship, as well as collecting detailed exposure and outcome information for a large cohort of workers in China (74 828 exposed to benzene and 35 805 unexposed) (Dosemeci *et al.*, 1994; Hayes *et al.*, 1996, 1997). A third area of development entails efforts to characterize interindividual variation in benzene risk include epidemiological study of risks in terms of variation in activation and detoxification enzymes (e.g. CYP2E1, NQ01; Rothman *et al.*, 1997) and developing models of population toxicokinetics of benzene based on human metabolic data (e.g. Bois *et al.*, 1996b).

2.5.3.1 Modelling of benzene pharmacokinetics

Pharmacokinetic models of varying complexity have been developed for the prediction of benzene and metabolite levels in experimental animals (Bailar & Hoel, 1989; Medinsky et al., 1989; Travis et al., 1990; Spear et al., 1991; Cox & Ricci, 1992). In a classical (non-PBPK) approach (Bailar & Hoel, 1989), the Michaelis–Menten equation (see Chapter 7) was fitted to data from pharmacokinetic experiments to obtain estimates of metabolic parameters. These were used to estimate, as a measure of "internal dose", the amount of benzene metabolized in the gavage bioassay of benzene of the US National Toxicology Program (1986) at the doses administered. Estimates of "internal" dose were used in place of administered doses to derive cancer potency from the US National Toxicology Program bioassay. Predicted lower bounds on internal dose associated with minimal risk were then expressed in terms of administered dose to estimate "safe [administered] doses". Depending on the species and target site serving as the basis of the prediction, the doses associated with a one per million lifetime risk of cancer were between one and five times lower than those predicted by standard methods. A similar analysis was also performed on the basis of individual benzene metabolites, since these may be a better indicator of risk than fraction of benzene metabolized. However, because species differ considerably in the levels of particular metabolites produced, risk predictions based on internal dose of metabolite are strongly dependent on the species assumed to be the human surrogate and the metabolite assumed to be active. A simplified approach to assessing dose-dependent pharmacokinetics is supported by in vivo studies of benzene adducts with rat nucleic acids (Mazzullo et al., 1989), which suggest a linear relationship between benzene exposure and reactive species for a wide range of doses below the high doses where metabolic saturation is observed.

A four-compartment PBPK model (poorly perfused tissues, richly perfused tissues, fat and liver (metabolizing)) was used to examine major pathways of benzene metabolism in mice and rats subsequent to the formation of benzene oxide (Medinsky et al., 1989). Model simulations showed that, for mice and rats, the activation pathways leading to more toxic metabolites represented a larger fraction of total benzene metabolized at lower than at higher concentrations. At higher concentrations, both mice and rats produced relatively more conjugates of phenol, a less toxic metabolite. Mice were found to metabolize more benzene than rats at a given air concentration, and a greater proportion of the metabolites formed were associated with activation in mice. A five-compartment PBPK model (fat, bone marrow (metabolizing), muscle, organ and liver (metabolizing)) was also developed and used to estimate total benzene metabolites produced by rats, mice and humans, and to investigate the relative metabolic capacities of bone marrow and liver (Travis et al., 1990). The model has been used to derive a dose–response relationship between internal dose and probability of cancer (Cox & Ricci, 1992); this was found to produce lower estimates of risk than would be obtained by the use of standard methods. The end-point used was all squamous-cell carcinomas in male mice. This risk derivation has been criticized (Crump et al., 1993) because internal target tissue dose "may be different for the various possible tumor types in such a general category as 'all squamous cell carcinomas'". Also, an end-point "more closely related to the observed human cancer endpoint, which is leukemia" was not selected. Crump et al. (1993) applied the method to two additional end-points, namely malignant lymphoma and alveolar/bronchiolar carcinoma in male mice. Significantly higher human risks were estimated because, whereas the dose–response for squamous-cell carcinoma increases with dose roughly to the power of three, it increases linearly with dose for alveolar/bronchiolar carcinoma and for lymphoma.

Metabolic parameters used in the two PBPK models previously mentioned were adjusted, and adopted when visual inspection indicated a good fit between experimental results and model output. In addition, a statistical approach has been taken to study the sensitivity of these and other benzene PBPK model predictions to parameter selection and data set (Spear et al., 1991). It was found that "the regions of the parameter space associated with various inhalation and gavage experiments are distinct, and the model[s] as presently structured cannot adequately represent the outcomes of all experiments." Also, in simulation studies, the predictions derived by using the parameters from the PBPK models were found to be significantly different from the best statistical result in the sensitivity study (Woodruff et al., 1992).

Beyond providing a means of adjusting for high dose saturation of pharmacokinetic processes, the PBPK models described above, which were designed to predict internal dose for the animal bioassays, have been found to have limited application for QEP. Many metabolites are probably involved in benzene carcinogenesis (Smith, 1996; Smith & Fanning, 1997), and the role of particular metabolites in the process is uncertain. There is also the issue of across-species extrapolation, while disagreements over the use of animal models of haematopoietic malignancies for human leukaemia (especially acute myelogenous) are a further complication. Human risk predictions by direct extrapolation from occupational studies have therefore been judged to be more reliable than those derived from animal bioassays and related pharmacokinetic analyses. Better understanding of the relationship between administered dose and internal levels of metabolites may significantly improve the accuracy of potency estimates. Such models of human pharmacokinetics are under development (Bois et al., 1996b).

2.5.3.2 Cohort exposure reconstruction and related dose–response evaluations

Another attempt to improve benzene risk predictions involves the re-evaluation of data on the cohort of Rinsky et al. (1981, 1987). Because of the importance of this cohort, regulated industries in the USA have conducted or sponsored retrospective exposure evaluations (Kipen et al., 1989; Paustenbach et al., 1992) and reanalyses of the dose–response relationship (Thorslund et al., 1988; Crump, 1992, 1993; Crump et al., 1993; Crump, 1994; Paxton et al., 1994; Crump, 1996; Paxton, 1996; Schnatter et al., 1996). The reanalysis of exposures in the cohort by Paustenbach et al. (1992) resulted in some cases in considerably higher exposures than those estimated by Rinsky and colleagues. Paustenbach et al. assumed short-term, high-level exposure to benzene vapours and

substantial dermal exposure, and made a variety of assumptions regarding industrial hygiene controls, long working weeks in the 1940s, and effectiveness of gloves and respirators. An extensive critical evaluation of this analysis has been published by Utterback & Rinsky (1995), who conclude that the analysis used "selected information, sometimes improperly cited, to adjust previously reported benzene exposure estimates" and that the method used "multiple adjustments ... by a number of factors that are apparently based on worse case assumptions ... determined through extrapolation of data collected under substantially different conditions." Thus the extent of exposure in the cohort of Rinsky et al. continues to be a subject for debate.

Several of the recent re-evaluations of the cancer dose–response relationship for benzene (e.g. Crump, 1996; Paxton, 1996; Schnatter et al., 1996) are based on the Paustenbach exposure assessment; results are compared with those based on the exposure assessments of Crump & Allen (1984), the basis of the US EPA evaluation of benzene carcinogenic activity, and of Rinsky et al. For linear models, risk predictions based on the Paustenbach exposure analysis are generally a factor of two lower than those based on the exposure assessments of Crump & Allen (1984), which in turn are roughly a factor of two lower than those based on those of Rinsky et al. As noted by Synder et al. (1993), the uncertainty in the exposures received by the Rinsky cohort is small in comparison with other factors contributing to uncertainty in the dose–response relationship. Schnatter et al. (1996) listed long-term average concentrations associated with the maximally exposed jobs in the cohort of Rinsky et al., and reported a critical concentration between 20 and 60 ppm below which effects are not observed; however, more formal analyses by Crump (1996) of the relationship between exposure intensity and risk in the cohort found a quadratic term only marginally significant ($p = 0.085$ for AML) and only for the Paustenbach and not the Crump & Allen exposure estimates. Also, for the large Chinese cohort, Hayes et al. (1997) reported relative risks of 3.2 (95% CI 1.0–10.3) for AML/myelodysplastic syndromes combined for "constant low level exposures" (<10 ppm).

Recent epidemiological and biomarker data on the Chinese cohort hold the promise of further resolution of the dose–response curve in the range 1–10 ppm in the workplace, and perhaps below that range, as well as better characterizations of the extent of interindividual variation (see e.g. Rothman *et al.*, 1997).

2.5.4 Predictions of cancer potency without cancer bioassay or epidemiological data

2.5.4.1 Ethylene cancer potency inferred from metabolite ethylene oxide

Ethylene, an important industrial gas, is also produced endogenously in plants, mammals and humans (International Agency for Research on Cancer, 1985). Since ethylene has been demonstrated to be metabolized to ethylene oxide in mice (Ehrenberg *et al.*, 1977), rats (Filser & Bolt, 1983a,b) and humans (Törnquist, 1989; Filser *et al.*, 1992) and since ethylene oxide is mutagenic (Ehrenberg & Hussein, 1981) and carcinogenic in rodents (Dunkelberg, 1982; Lynch *et al.*, 1984; Snellings *et al.*, 1984; Garman *et al.*, 1985; US National Toxicology Program, 1987) and probably in humans (International Agency for Research on Cancer, 1985; Hogstedt *et al.*, 1986), there is concern about the potential risk of exposure of humans to ethylene. In a two-year inhalation study with ethylene in rats, no dose-related tumour response was observed for concentrations up to 3000 ppm in air (Hamm *et al.*, 1984). It has been pointed out, however, that this negative result may be misleading for pharmacokinetic reasons (Bolt & Filser, 1987): while the rate of metabolism of ethylene to ethylene oxide may be described by first order kinetics at concentrations below 80 ppm, saturation kinetics are observed at higher concentrations, reaching a plateau at about 1000 ppm. This corresponds to 5.6 ppm of ethylene oxide (Bolt & Filser, 1987). The tumour incidence in rats at this dose of internally formed ethylene oxide would not be expected to be more than 2% greater than that in controls, and carcinogenic effects would therefore not be easily detectable in small groups of rats (Bolt & Filser, 1987).

Ethylene oxide alkylates cellular macromolecules including protein and DNA (Ehrenberg & Osterman-Golkar, 1980; Ehrenberg & Hussein, 1981; Segerbäck, 1983). In experiments involving short-term exposure to ethylene oxide, the rate of alkylation of haemoglobin was shown to be directly related to alkylation of DNA as measured in several different organs (Osterman-Golkar *et al.*, 1983; Segerbäck, 1983; Potter *et al.*, 1989). Determinations of hydroxyethyl-adducts to amino acids in haemoglobin have therefore been used to estimate the tissue DNA dose levels of ethylene in humans. This approach has been questioned, however, since, due to differences in formation, persistence, repair and chemical depurination, the relationships between hydroxyethyl adducts to haemoglobin and to DNA have been demonstrated to vary with length of exposure, interval since exposure, species and tissue (Walker *et al.*, 1992, 1993). The body burden of ethylene oxide from ethylene has also been calculated for rats and humans using pharmacokinetic models (Filser & Bolt, 1984; Bolt & Filser, 1987) and was found to correlate well with data on haemoglobin binding (Filser *et al.*, 1992).

Several risk estimations for ethylene oxide have been performed by allometric extrapolation of carcinogenicity data obtained in experimental animals (Beliles & Parker, 1987; Hattis, 1987; Hertz-Picciotto *et al.*, 1987) or using the rad-equivalence approach (Törnquist, 1989). This latter approach was developed by Ehrenberg (1980) to express the capacity of a defined target dose of a genotoxic chemical (in this case ethylene oxide) to induce genetic damage in terms of "rad equivalents", which are then the basis of estimates of total cancer morbidity or mortality risks. A cancer risk estimation for ethylene based on target dose (haemoglobin/ethylene oxide adducts) and the "rad equivalence" approach was published by Törnquist & Osterman-Golkar (1991). For an average exposure of 15 ppm of ethylene in the environment (an estimated value for Sweden), the cancer morbidity risk was calculated to be 2×10^{-5} per year. A similar study was performed by Denk (1990) (see also Denk & Filser, 1990). Using the "rad equivalence" approach and pharmacokinetic models, these authors estimated the lifetime cancer morbidity risks for an endogenous average concentration of 0.44 mmol/kg body weight of ethylene (equivalent to 0.17 mmol/kg body weight of resulting ethylene oxide) to be 10.4×10^{-4}, and for an occupational ethylene exposure to 20–70 ppm (40 h/per week; 45 years) to be 850×10^{-4}. Somewhat lower estimates (1.25×10^{-4} and 104×10^{-4}, respectively) were obtained by replacing the "rad equivalence" approach by the allometric extrapolation of ethylene oxide carcinogenicity data from rats to humans.

The concept of "rad equivalence" of a chemical was introduced (Ehrenberg, 1980) by analogy to the concept of the "relative biological effectiveness" (RBE) of one radiation type compared with the reference radiation. The RBE indicates the quantity of a given radiomimetic agent needed to induce the same amount of biological damage (number of forward mutations for rad equivalence) as the reference radiation. This concept has been criticized for a number of reasons including the unknown relevance of forward mutations to human cancer risks, and the fact that the "rad equivalence", like the relative biological effectiveness of radiations, is not a single quantity, but most probably a function of dose, dose-rate and biological end-points.

2.5.4.2 Use of toxicity equivalency factors: complex mixtures

Mixtures of many different compounds, or "complex mixtures", represent a special challenge for QEP. Exposure to the ubiquitous heterocyclic compounds derived from incomplete combustion exemplifies the problem. As shown in Table 2.3, the composition of a mixture of polycyclic aromatic hydrocarbons (PAHs) varies widely depending on its source (International Agency for Research on Cancer, 1983; Carmichael et al., 1990). For example, the concentration of benzo[a]pyrene, a commonly used indicator of PAHs, varies from 0.7 to 38% in PAH mixtures. In addition to PAHs, combustion products always contain a number of biologically active heterocyclic compounds, making extrapolations even more complicated.

Coal-tar is a historical example of a complex mixture. After the publication of the first animal carcinogenicity studies by Yamagiwa & Ichikawa in 1915, in which tumours were induced on rabbit ears by coal-tar, a systematic search for the active principle was started (Phillips, 1983). By 1930, purified benz[a]anthracene was tested on mouse skin and tumours were observed. During the same period, dozens of new PAHs were isolated and many of them were found to be carcinogenic in mouse skin (Phillips, 1983). Complex mixtures are often fractionated on the basis of their genotoxic activity.

The mutagenicity of complex mixtures has often been used as a measure of their genotoxic potential (Vainio et al., 1990). The approach has been described as "bioassay-directed fractionation and chemical characterization" (Lewtas & Gallagher, 1990), and has led to the characterization of classes of potent mutagenic compounds. Cooking-related heterocyclic amines, combustion-induced nitro-PAHs and chlorination-induced mutagens, such as 3-chloro-4-(dichloromethyl)- 5-hydroxy- 2(5H)- furanone (MX), were identified using this approach (Vainio et al., 1990). Another approach has been to test complex mixtures in various model systems and to derive risk estimates from such experiments. At US EPA, several complex mixtures have been tested in a number of systems, including mutagenicity in bacteria, DNA binding to mouse tissues and carcinogenicity in mouse skin (Lewtas & Gallagher, 1990). Experimental results for certain complex mixtures have been compared with carcinogenic potency using a "comparative potency method" (Lewtas, 1991). For three complex mixtures, namely coke oven emissions, roofing tar emissions and cigarette smoke, the bioassay data appear to predict the carcinogenic potency quite well. However, more complex mixtures must be assayed by means of the comparative potency method before its general validity can be assessed.

The "toxicity equivalency factor" (TEF) approach to assessing the risk posed by mixtures of polychlorinated dibenzo-p-dioxins (PCDDs), dibenzofurans (PCDFs) and biphenyls (PCBs) is a second well studied example. Most environmental sources of PCDDs, PCDFs and PCBs consist of mixtures of different isomers and congeners of these halogenated aromatic compounds. The most toxic of the family of compounds is 2,3,7,8-TCDD. A number of studies have indicated a common receptor-mediated mechanism of action for several classes of these halogenated aromatics (Poland & Knutson,

Table 2.3. Percentages of PAHs present in complex mixtures						
	Percentage of PAH in source					
Compound	Cigarette smoke	Used motor oil	Grilled meat	Processed food	Car exhaust	Polluted urban air
Phenanthrene	46	-	13	-	32	-
Pyrene	24	18	21	26	39	18
Benzo[g,h,i]perylene	2	26	5	3	2	-
Fluoranthene	12	11	24	44	23	8
Dibenzo[a,h]anthracene	4	4	0.2	0.7	-	6
Benzo[b]fluoranthene	0.5	8	-	3	0.4	4
Benzo[a]pyrene	4	5	7	1	0.7	38
Chrysene	5	11	17	20	1	6
Benzo[a]anthracene	4	16	5	3	0.7	11

1982; Safe, 1986). Structure/receptor-binding relationships have been established for different classes of halogenated aromatics, which correlate very well with their structure-activity (biological and toxic) relationships (Poland & Knutson, 1982; Safe, 1986). This observation forms the mechanistic basis for the development of TEFs for individual PCDDs, PCDFs and PCBs, thus providing a basis for risk assessment and regulation (US Environmental Protection Agency, 1988b; Safe, 1990). A variety of TEF schemes have been proposed for estimating the toxicological significance of complex mixtures of halogenated aromatics in terms of equivalent amounts of the most potent member of the family, namely 2,3,7,8-TCDD (US Environmental Protection Agency, 1988b; Safe, 1990). Table 2.4 lists the international TEFs for some selected PCDDs and PCDFs taken from the report of the NATO/CMMS Pilot Study on International Information Exchange on Dioxins and Related Compounds, prepared by the US Environmental Protection Agency (1988b). The utility of the TEF approach for the hazard and risk assessment of complex mixtures of halogenated aromatic compounds has been confirmed in several studies (see the review by Safe (1990)).

2.6 Conclusions

Quantitative assessments of carcinogenic activity are being increasingly used to guide decisions by national and international organizations. Standardized approaches have been employed by a number of governments and scientific advisory institutions. In most instances the schemes employed distinguish between carcinogens in terms of the assumed mode of action, and the procedures for agents characterized variously as "(low dose) linear", "genotoxic," or "non-threshold", differ from those for carcinogens identified as "(low dose) non-linear", "threshold", or "non-genotoxic". However, the levels of evidence required to make these distinctions can vary considerably from one organization to another and within an organization. For the "genotoxic" or "(low dose) linear" carcinogens, some groups decline to make quantitative assessments, while others use standardized QEP techniques. The approach used for the second class of carcinogens ("(low dose) non-linear") for most organizations involves the application of uncertainty and adjustment factors to a "no observed effect level" in judging the potential harm of certain exposures. Questions regarding the accuracy of the risk predicted by standard QEP procedures

Table 2.4. International toxicity equivalency factors (I-TEFs) for some toxic halogenated aromatics[a]			
PCDD	**I-TEF**	**PCDF**	**I-TEF**
2,3,7,8-TCDD	1	2,3,7,8-TCDF	1
1,2,3,7,8-PeCDD	0.5	2,3,4,7,8-PeCDF	0.5
1,2,3,4,7,8-HxCDD	0.1	1,2,3,7,8-PeCDF	0.05
1,2,3,7,8,9-HxCDD	0.1	1,2,3,4,7,8-HxCDF	0.1
1,2,3,6,7,8-HxCDD	0.1	1,2,3,7,8,9-HxCDF	0.1
1,2,3,4,6,7,8-HpCDD	0.01	1,2,3,6,7,8-HxCDF	0.1
OCDD	0.001	2,3,4,6,7,8-HxCDF	0.1
		1,2,3,4,6,7,8 HpCDF	0.01
		1,2,3,4,7,8,9-HpCDF	0.01
		OCDF	0.001

[a] Source: US Environmental Protection Agency (1988b).

and the appropriateness of applying the NOEL/UF approach to certain carcinogens have provided the incentive for more detailed approaches to QEP.

Several different approaches designed to improve risk predictions have been presented in this Chapter. For some agents, tumorigenicity data are poor or unavailable, but structure activity and other mechanistic information indicate probable carcinogenic activity. In a handful of cases, rather than expend resources on testing such agents in bioassays, or wait for tumorigenicity data to appear, alternative approaches have been used to derive dose–response relationships. Toxic equivalency factors have been used to predict the cancer potencies of dibenzo-*p*-dioxins and furans, and such values have been used in estimating risks in a variety of settings (e.g. air emissions, hazardous waste sites). A similar approach has been suggested for evaluating the risks of carcinogenic polycyclic aromatic amines. Cancer potency predictions for untested substances have also been made by considering the rate of formation of carcinogenic metabolites (which have been tested). The prediction of cancer potency for ethylene, based on that of ethylene

oxide, was presented as an example. This approach may prove useful in evaluations of other agents, such as untested benzidine dyes and related materials and styrene.

Examples of trends in the use of epidemiological data in QEP were also provided. A problem frequently encountered is that available studies were not designed to detect small or moderate risks of public health concern (e.g. associated with relative risks less than two). Meta-analyses, which formally combine data from several epidemiological studies, have been used to improve the ability to identify carcinogenic hazards, but are less commonly attempted for risk predictions. The dose–response analyses for environmental tobacco smoke and low LET radiation were described as examples of meta-analyses employed for QEP. Large multicentre studies providing large numbers of subjects with good exposure and case ascertainment represent another approach to achieving better resolution for somewhat small relative risks. The multicentre study of environmental tobacco smoke conducted in the USA provided some validation for QEP estimates produced through earlier meta-analyses. Data useful for QEP are just being released from the very large multicentre study of benzene workers in China (e.g. Rothman *et al.*, 1997; Hayes *et al.*, 1997), and may make possible the resolution of the dose–response curve at lower levels than in previous occupational studies. The exposure reconstructions for the American benzene Pliofilm cohort are examples of other attempts to improve predictions based on epidemiological data, which have had only limited success.

Pharmacokinetic analyses are now being used extensively in QEP, and three examples have been provided. In the case of benzene, PBPK models have been used to reconcile results observed in different species, and also, to a limited extent, to describe variable human susceptibility. However because of incomplete understanding of benzene leukaemogenesis, the resulting conclusions for QEP have been viewed as premature. For perchloroethylene and methylene chloride, PBPK models have provided a rationale for reducing predictions of human risks based on animal data, which became less clear once uncertainties in model parameters and structure were assessed. Work is continuing on statistical approaches and more experimental data are being obtained, and are leading to considerable improvements to the PBPK models first introduced in the 1980s. The general problem of the validation of PBPK models and making predictions for humans is being addressed in part through the introduction of biomarker components in occupational epidemiological studies, e.g. in the large occupational study of benzene in China, and controlled exposures and measurements in humans. In a hierarchical population model of perchloroethylene pharmacokinetics, which formally accounted for uncertainty and interindividual variability, metabolite formation at different dose levels and rates and in different individuals was inferred from excretion data on humans exposed briefly and followed over a period of days (corresponding to several half-lives).

The costly attempt to improve risk predictions for TCDD was also described. Although initially considered to be an example in which further limited experimentation and modelling could provide resolution at low doses, and despite considerable research, fundamental questions remain regarding the risk to humans of relatively low doses, and the extent of that risk, if it does exist. Nevertheless, this case has served to promote the use of biologically based approaches to cancer risk assessment, making use of the full spectrum of data available. The long-term research on sodium saccharin has been more successful, although the problem was less difficult. The mechanistic data indicate that the standard approach may overestimate the low-dose risk for this agent, and the modelling to date has provided important biological insights into the mode of action of saccharin.

References

Albert, R.E., Sellakumar, A.R., Laskin, S., Kuschner, M., Nelson, N. & Snyder, D.A. (1982) Gaseous formaldehyde and hydrogen chloride induction of nasal cancer in the rat. *J. Natl Cancer Inst.*, **68**, 597-603

Ames, B.N. & Gold, L.S. (1990) Carcinogens and human health: Part 1—response. *Science*, **250**, 1645-1646

Andersen, M.E., Clewell, H.J., Gargas, M.L., Smith, F.A. & Reitz, R.H. (1987) Physiologically based pharmacokinetics and the risk assessment process for methylene chloride. *Toxicol. Appl. Pharmacol.*, **87**, 185-205

Andersen, M.E., Clewell, H.J., Gargas, M.L., MacNaughton, M.G., Reitz, R.H., Nolan, R.J. & McKenna, M.J. (1991) Physiologically based pharmacokinetic modeling with dichloro-methane, its metabolite, carbon monoxide, and blood carboxyhemoglobin in rats and humans. *Toxicol. Appl. Pharmacol.*, **108**, 14-27

Andersen, M.E., Mills, J.J., Gargas, M.L., Kedderis, L., Birnbaum, L.S., Neubert, D. & Greenlee, W.F. (1993) Modeling receptor mediated processes with dioxin: Implications for pharmacokinetic and risk assessment. *Risk Anal.*, **13**, 25-36

Andersen, M.E., Clewell, H.J., Mahle, D.A. & Gearhart, J.M. (1994) Gas uptake studies of deuterium isotope effects on dichloromethane metabolism in female B6C3F1 mice *in vivo*. *Toxicol. Appl. Pharmacol.*, **128**, 158-165

Anderson, R.L. (1985) Some changes in gastrointestinal metabolism and in the urine and bladders of rats in response to saccharin ingestion. *Food Chem. Toxicol.*, **23**, 457-464

Anderson, R.L., Lefever, F.R. & Maurer, J.K. (1988) The effect of various saccharin forms on the gastrointestinal tract, urine and bladder of male rats. *Food Chem. Toxicol.*, **26**, 665-669

Angelo, M.J. & Pritchard, A.B. (1984) Simulations of methylene chloride pharmacokinetics using a physiologically based model. *Reg. Toxicol. Pharmacol.*, 4:329-339

Angelo, M.J., Bischoff, K.B., Pritchard A.B., & Presser M.A. (1984) A physiological model for the pharmacokinetics of methylene chloride in B6C3F1 mice following iv administration *J. Pharmacokinet. Biopharm.*, **12**, 413-436

Angelo, M.J., Pritchard, A.B., Hawkins, D.R., Waller, A.R. & Roberts A. (1986a) The pharmacokinetics of dichloromethane I. Disposition in B6C3F1 mice following intravenous and oral administration. *Food Chem. Toxicol.*, **24**, 965-974

Angelo, M.J., Pritchard, A.B., Hawkins, D.R., Waller, A.R. & Roberts A. (1986b) The pharmacokinetics of dichloromethane II. Disposition in Fischer 344 rats following intravenous and oral administration. *Food Chem. Toxicol.*, **24**, 975-980

Armstrong V.C. & Newhook R. (1992) Assessing the health risks of priority substances under the Canadian Environmental Protection Act. *J. Reg. Toxicol. Phamacol.*, **15**, 111-121

Arnold, D.L., Moodie, C.A., Grice, H.C., Charbonneau, S.M., Stavric, B., Collins, B.T., McGuire, P.F., Zawidzka, Z. & Munroe, I.C. (1980) Long term toxicity of ortho-toluenesulfonamide and sodium saccharin in the rat. *Toxicol. Appl. Pharmacol.*, **52**, 113-152

Arnold, D.L., Krewski, D. & Munroe, I.C. (1983) Saccharin: a toxicological and historical perspective. *Toxicology*, **27**, 179-256

Arundel, A., Sterling, T. & Weinkam, J. (1987) Never smoker lung cancer risks from exposure to particulate tobacco smoke. *Environ. Int.*, **13**, 409-426

Bailar, A.J. & Hoel, D.G. (1989) Metabolite based internal dose used in a risk assessment of benzene. *Environ. Health Perspect.*, **82**, 177-184

Beliles, R.P. & Parker, J.C. (1987) Risk assessment and oncodynamics of ethylene oxide as related to occupational exposure. *Toxicol. Ind. Health*, **3**, 317-382

Blot, W.J. & Fraumeni, J.F., Jr (1986) Passive smoking and lung cancer. *J. Natl Cancer Inst.*, **77**, 993-999

Bogen, K.T. & McKone, T.E. (1988) Linking indoor air and pharmacokinetic models to assess tetrachloroethylene risk. *Risk Anal.*, **8**, 509-520

Bois, F.Y., Zeise, L. & Tozer, T.N. (1990) Precision and sensitivity of pharmacokinetic models for cancer risk assessment: tetrachloroethylene in mice, rats, and humans. *Toxicol. Appl. Pharmacol.*, **102**, 300-315

Bois, F.Y., Gelman, A., Jiang, J., Maszle, D.R., Zeise, L. & Alexeef, G.(1996a) Population toxicokinetics of tetrachloroethylene. *Arch. Toxicol.*, **70**, 347-355

Bois, F.Y., Jackson, E.T., Pekari, K., & Smith, M.T. (1996b) Population toxicokinetics of benzene. *Environ. Health Perspect.*, **104**, Suppl.6, 1405-1411

Bolt, H.M. & Filser, J.G. (1987) Kinetics and disposition in toxicology. *Arch. Toxicol.*, **60**, 73-76

California Comparative Risk Project (1994) *Toward the 21st Century: Planning for the Protection of California's Environment*, Sacramento, CA, Office of Environmental Health Hazard Assessment

California Department of Health Services (1984) *Health Effects of Benzene*, Berkeley, CA

California Department of Health Services (1986) *Health Effects of Chlorinated Dioxins and Dibenzofurans*, Berkeley, CA

California Department of Health Services (1989) *Health Effects of Methylene Chloride*, Berkeley, CA

California Department of Health Services (1990) *2,3,7,8-Tetrachlorodibenzo(p)dioxin*, Berkeley, CA

California Environmental Protection Agency (1992) *Final Report on the Identification of Formaldehyde as a Toxic Air Contaminant*, Part B, *Health Assessment*, Berkeley, CA, Office of Environmental Health Hazard Assessment, Air Toxicology and Epidemiology Section

California Environmental Protection Agency (1993) *Safety Assessment for Non-cancer Endpoints: The Benchmark Dose and Other Possible Approaches*, Sacramento, CA, Office of Environmental Health Hazard Assessment, Reproductive and Cancer Hazard Assessment Section

California Environmental Protection Agency (1995) *Criteria for Carcinogens*, Sacramento, CA, Cal/EPA Standards and Criteria Workgroup, Office of Environmental Health Hazard Assessment

California Environmental Protection Agency (1997) *Health Effects of Exposure to Environmental Tobacco Smoke*, Berkeley, CA, Cal/EPA Office of Environmental Health Hazard Assessment

Cardis, E., Gilbert, E.S., Carpenter, L., Howe, G., Kato, I., Fix, J., Salmon, L., Cowper, G., Armstrong, B.K., Beral, V., Douglas, A., Fry, S.A., Kaldor, J., Lave, C., Smith, P.G., Voelz, G., & Wiggs, L. (1995a) *Combined Analysis of Cancer Mortality in Nuclear Workers in Canada, the United Kingdom and the United States of America* (International Agency for Research on Cancer Technical Report No. 25), Lyon, International Agency for Research on Cancer

Cardis, E., Gilbert, E.S., Carpenter, L., Howe, G., Kato, I., Armstrong, B.K., Beral, V., Cowper, G., Douglas, A., Fix, J., Fry, S.A., Kaldor, J., Lave, C., Salmon, L., Smith, P.G., Voelz, G.L. & Wiggs, L.D. (1995b) Effects of low doses and low dose rates of external ionizing radiation: cancer mortality among nuclear industry workers in three countries. *Radiat. Res.*, **142**, 117-132.

Carmichael, P.L., Jacob, J., Grimmer, X. & Phillips, D.P. (1990) Analysis of the polycyclic aromatic hydrocarbon content of petrol and diesel engine lubricating oils and determination of DNA adducts in topically treated mice by ^{32}P-postlabelling. *Carcinogenesis*, **11**, 2025-2032

Carpenter, L., Higgins, C., Douglas, A., Fraser, P., Beral, V. & Smith, P. (1994) Combined analysis of mortality in three United Kingdom nuclear industry workforces, 1946–1988. *Radiat. Res.*, **138**, 224-238

Casanova, M. & Heck, H. (1991) The impact of DNA–protein cross-linking studies on quantitative risk assessment of formaldehyde. *CIIT Act.*, **11**, 1-7

Casanova, M., Conolly, R.B. & Heck, H. (1996) DNA–protein cross-links (DPX) and cell proliferation in B6C3F1 mice but not Syrian golden hamsters exposed to dichloromethane: pharmacokinetics and risk assessment with DPX as dosimeter. *Fundam. Appl. Toxicol.*, **31**, 103-116

Chappel, C.I. (1992) A review and biological risk assessment of sodium saccharin. *Reg. Toxicol. Pharmacol.*, **15**, 253-270

Chen, C.W. & Blancato, J.N. (1987) Role of pharmacokinetic modeling in risk assessment: perchloroethylene as an example. In: National Research Council, *Pharmacokinetics in Risk Assessment, Drinking Water and Health*, Vol. 8, Washington, DC, National Academy Press, pp.369–390

Clewell, H.J., Lee, T.S. & Carpenter, R.L. (1994) Sensitivity of physiologically based pharmacokinetic models to variation in model parameters: Methylene chloride. *Risk Anal.*, **14**, 521-531

Cohen, S.M. (1985) Multistage carcinogenesis in the urinary bladder. *Food Chem. Toxicol.*, **23**, 521-528

Cohen, S.M. & Ellwein, L.B. (1989) Cell growth dynamics in bladder carcinogenesis: implications for risk analysis. *J. Am. Coll. Toxicol.*, **8**, 1103-1114

Cohen, S.M. & Ellwein, L.B. (1990) Cell proliferation in carcinogenesis. *Science*, **249**, 1007-1011

Cohen, S.M., Cano, M., Garland, E.M. & Earl, R.A. (1989) Silicate crystals in the urine and bladder epithelium of male rats fed sodium saccharin. *Proc. Am. Assoc. Cancer Res.*, **30**, 205

Cohen, S.M., Cano, M., Earl, R.A., Carson, S.C. & Garland, E.M. (1991) A proposed role for silicates and protein in the proliferative effects of saccharin on the male rat urothelium. *Carcinogenesis*, **12**, 1551-1555

Cox, L.A. & Ricci, P.F. (1992) Reassessing benzene cancer risk using internal doses. *Risk Anal.*, **12**, 401-410

Cranor, C. (1993) *Regulating Toxic Substances. A Philosophy of Science and the Law*, Oxford, Oxford University Press

Cronkite E.P., Drew, R.T., Inoue, T., Hirabayashi, Y. & Bulls, J.E. (1989) Hematotoxicity and carcinogenicity of inhaled benzene. *Environ. Health Perspect.*, **82**, 97-108

Crump, K.S. (1984) A new method for determining allowable daily intakes. *Fundam. Appl. Toxicol.*, **4**, 854-871

Crump, K.S. (1992) Risk assessment for benzene-induced leukemia—a review. In: Zervos, C., ed., *Oncogene and Transgenic Correlates of Cancer Risk Assessments*, New York, Plenum, pp.241–262

Crump, K.S. (1994) Risk of benzene-induced leukemia: A sensitivity analysis of the pliofilm cohort with additional follow-up and new exposure estimates *J. Toxicol. Environ. Health,* **43**, 219-242

Crump, K.S. (1996) Risk of benzene induced leukemia predicted from the pliofilm cohort, *Environ. Health Perspect.*, **104**, Suppl.6, 1437-1441

Crump, K. & Allen, B. (1984) *Quantitative Estimates of the Risk of Leukemia from Occupational Exposure to Benzene. Final Report to the Occupational Safety and Health Administration*, Ruston, LA, Science Research Systems

Crump, K.S., Hoel, D.G., Longley, C.H. & Peto, R. (1976) Fundamental carcinogenic processes and their implications for low dose risk assessment. *Cancer Res.*, **36**, 2973-2979

Crump, K.S., Allen, B.C. & Faustman, E. (1991) *The Use of the Benchmark Dose (BMD) Approach in Health Risk Assessment* (Draft Final Report prepared for the US Environmental Protection Agency Risk Assessment Forum), Ruston, LA, K.S. Crump Associates, Clement International Corp.

Crump, K., Allen, B. & Clewell, H. (1993) Limitations to benzene cancer risk assessment by Cox and Ricci. *Risk Anal.*, **13**, 145-146

Dallas, C.E., Chen, X.M., O'Barr, K., Muralidhara, S., Varkonyi, P. & Bruckner, J.V. (1994a) Development of a physiologically based pharmacokinetic model for perchloroethylene using tissue concentration–time data. *Toxicol. Appl. Pharmacol.*, **128**, 50-59

Dallas, C.E., Chen, X.M., Muralidhara, S., Varkonyi, P., Tackett, R.L. & Bruckner, J.V. (1994b) Use of tissue disposition data from rats and dogs to determine species differences in input parameters for a physiological model for perchloroethylene. *Environ. Res.*, **67**, 54-67

Dankovic. D.A. & Bailar, A.J. (1994) The impact of exercise and intersubject variability on dose estimates for dichloromethane from a physiologically based pharmacokinetic model. *Fundam. Appl. Toxicol.*, **22**, 20-25

Denk, B. (1990) *Abschätzung des kanzerogenen Risikos von Ethylen und Ethylenoxid für den Menschen durch Speziesextrapolation von der Ratte unter Berücksichtigung der Pharmakokinetik*, Doctoral Thesis, Munich, University of Munich

Denk, B. & Filser J. (1990) Abschätzung des durch Ethylen und Ethylenoxid bedingten kanzerogenen Risikos für den Menschen—Vergleich mit dem Risiko durch endogenes Ethylen. In: Schuckmann, F. & Schopper-Jochum, S., eds, *Berufskrankheiten, Krebserzeugende Arbeitsstoffe, Biological-Monitoring*, Stuttgart, Gentner-Verlag, pp. 397-401

Department of Health (1991) *Guidelines for the Evaluation of Chemicals for Carcinogenicity* (Report on Health and Social Subjects No. 42), London, Her Majesty's Stationery Office

Dosemeci M., Li, G-L, Hayes, R.B., Yin, S-N, Linet, M., Chow, W-H, Wang, Y-Z, Jiang, Z-L, Dai, T-R, Zhang, W-U, Chao, X-J, Ye, P-Z, Kou, Q-R, Fan, Y-H, Zhang, X-C, Lin, X-F, Meng, J-F, Zho, J-S, Wacholder, S., Kneller, R. & Blot, W.J. (1994) A cohort study among workers exposed to benzene in China. 2: Exposure Assessment. *Am. J. Ind. Med.*, **26**, 401-411

Dunkelberg, H. (1982) Carcinogenicity of ethylene oxide and 1,2-propylene oxide upon intragastric administration to rats. *Br. J. Cancer*, **46**, 924-933

Dybing, E. & Sanner, T. (1997) *Risk Assessment for Acrylamide*, Oslo, National Institute for Public Health

Dybing, E., Sanner, T., Roelfzema, H., Kroese, D. & Tennant, R.W. (1997) T25: A simplified carcinogenic potency index: Description of the system and study of correlations between carcinogenic potency and species/site specificity and mutagenicity. *Pharmacol. Toxicol.* **80**, 272-279

Ehrenberg, L. (1980) Purposes and methods of comparing effects of radiation and chemicals. In: *Radiobiological Equivalents of Chemical Pollutants, Proceedings of the Advisory Group Meeting on Radiobiological Equivalents of Chemical Pollutants Organized by the International Atomic Energy Agency and held in Vienna 12–16 December 1977*, Vienna, International Atomic Energy Agency, pp. 23-36

Ehrenberg, L., & Hussain, S. (1981) Genetic toxicity of some important epoxides. *Mutat. Res.*, **86**, 1-113

Ehrenberg, L. & Osterman-Golkar, S. (1980) Alkylation of macromolecules for detecting mutagenic agents. *Teratog. Carcinog. Mutag.*, **1**, 105-127

Ehrenberg, L., Osterman-Golkar, S., Segerbäck, D., Svensson, K. & Calleman, C.J. (1977) Evaluation of genetic risks of alkylating agents. III. Alkylation of hemoglobin after metabolic conversion of ethene to ethylene oxide *in vitro. Mutat. Res.*, **45**, 175-184

Ellwein, L.B. & Cohen, S.M. (1988) A cellular dynamics model of experimental bladder cancer: Analysis of sodium saccharin in the rat. *Risk Anal.*, **8**, 215-221

Ellwein, L.B. & Cohen, S.M. (1989) Comparative analyses of the timing and magnitude of genotoxic and nongenotoxic cellular effects in urinary bladder carcinogenesis. In: Travis, C.C., ed., *Biologically Based Methods for Cancer Risk Assessment*, New York, Plenum, pp. 181-192

Ellwein, L.B. & Cohen, S.M. (1992) Simulation modeling of carcinogenesis. *Toxicol. Appl. Pharmacol.*, **113**, 98-108

European Commission (1993) Commission Directive 93/67/EEC of 20 July 1993. Laying down the principles for assessment of risks to man and the environment of substances notified in accordance with Council Directive 67/548/EEC. *Off. J. Eur. Communities*, **L227**, 9-18

Federal Committee for Protection against Pollution (Länderausschuss für Immissionsschutz) (1992) *Krebsrisiko durch Luftverunreinigungen*, Düsseldorf, Ministerium für Umwelt, Raumordnung und Landwirtschaft des Landes Nordrhein-Westfalen

Filser, J.G. & Bolt, H.M. (1983a) Exhalation of ethylene oxide by rats on exposure to ethylene. *Mutat. Res.*, **120**, 57-60

Filser, J.G. & Bolt, H.M. (1983b) Inhalation pharmacokinetics based on gas uptake studies IV. The endogenous production of volatile compounds. *Arch. Toxicol.*, **52**, 123-133

Filser, J.G. & Bolt, H.M. (1984) Inhalation pharmacokinetics based on gas uptake studies. *Arch. Toxicol.*, **55**, 219-223

Filser, J.G., Denk, B., Törnqvist, M., Kessler, W. & Ehrenmann, L. (1992) Pharmacokinetics of ethylene in man; body burden with ethylene oxide and hydroxyethylation of hemoglobin due to endogenous and environmental ethylene. *Arch. Toxicol.*, **66**, 157-163

Finney, D.J. (1952) *Probit Analysis*, 2nd ed., London, Cambridge University Press

Fleiss, J.L. & Gross, A.J. (1991) Meta-analysis in epidemiology, with special reference to studies of the association between exposure to environmental tobacco smoke and lung cancer: A critique. *J. Clin. Epidemiol.*, **44**, 127-139

Fontham, E.T.H., Correa, P., Reynolds, P., Wu-Williams, A., Buffler, P.A., Greenberg, R.S., Chen, V.W., Alterman, T., Boyd, P., Austin, D.F. & Liff, J. (1994) Environmental tobacco smoke and lung cancer in nonsmoking women. *J. Am. Med. Assoc.*, **271**, 1752-1759

Food and Agriculture Organization of the United Nations (1985) *Pesticide Residues in Food—1984. Data and Recommendations of the Joint Meeting of the FAO Panel of Experts on Pesticide Residues in Food and the Environment and the WHO Expert Group on Pesticide Residues. Rome, 24 September–3 October 1984* (FAO Plant Production and Protection Paper 67), Rome

Food and Agriculture Organization of the United Nations (1986) *Pesticide Residues in Food—1985. Data and Recommendations of the Joint Meeting of the FAO Panel of Experts on Pesticide Residues in Food and the Environment and the WHO Expert Group on Pesticide Residues. Geneva, 23 September–2 October 1985* (FAO Plant Production and Protection Paper 68), Rome

Food and Agriculture Organization of the United Nations (1995) *Pesticide Residues in Food—1994. Report of the Joint Meeting of the FAO Panel of Experts on Pesticide Residues in Food and the Environment and a WHO Expert Group on Pesticide Residues* (FAO Plant Production and Protection Paper 127), Rome

Gargas, M.L., Clewell, H.J. & Andersen, M.E. (1986) Metabolism of inhaled dihalomethanes *in vivo*: differentiation of kinetic constants for two independent pathways. *Toxicol. Appl. Pharmacol.*, **82**, 211-223

Gargas, M.L., Burgess, R.J., Voisard, D.E., Cason, G.H. & Andersen, M.E. (1989) Partition coefficients of low-molecular-weight volatile chemicals in various liquids and tissues. *Toxicol. Appl. Pharmacol.*, **98**, 87-99

Garman, R.H., Snellings, W.M. & Maronpot, R.R. (1985) Brain tumors in F344 rats associated with chronic inhalation exposure to ethylene oxide. *Neurotoxicology*, **6**, 117-138

Gearhart, J.M., Mahle, D.A., Greene, R.J., Seckel, C.S., Flemming, C.D., Fisher, J.W. & Clewell, H.J. (1993) Variability of physiologically based pharmacokinetic (PBPK) model parameters and their effects on PBPK model predictions in a risk assessment for perchloroethylene (PCE). *Toxicol. Lett.*, **68**, 131-144

Gilbert, E.S., Cragle, D.L. & Wiggs, L.D. (1993) Updated analyses of combined mortality data for workers at the Hanford Site, Oak Ridge National Laboratory, and Rocky Flats Weapons Plant. *Radiat. Res.*, **136**, 408-421

Goldstein, B.D. (1989) Introduction: Occam's razor is dull. *Environ. Health Perspect.*, **82**, 3-6

Greenfield, R.E., Ellwein, L.B. & Cohen, S.M. (1984) A general problabistic model of carcinogenesis: analysis of urinary bladder cancer. *Carcinogenesis*, **5**, 437-445

Greenlee, W.F., Andersen, M.E. & Lucier, G.W. (1991) A perspective on biologically-based approaches to dioxin risk assessment. *Risk Anal.*, **11**, 437-445

Hamm, T.E., Guest, D. & Dent, J.G. (1984) Chronic toxicity and oncogenicity bioassay of inhaled ethylene in Fischer 344 rats. *Fundam. Appl. Toxicol.*, **4**, 473-478

Harvard Center for Risk Analysis (1991) *OMB vs. the Agencies. The Future of Cancer Risk Assessment. Summary and Highlights of Discussion for March 6–7, 1991 Workshop to Peer Review the OMB Report on Risk Assessment and Risk Management.* Boston, MA, Harvard University School of Public Health

Hattis, D. (1987) *A Pharmacokinetic/mechanism-based Analysis of the Carcinogenic Risk of Ethylene Oxide*, Cambridge, MA, Center for Technology, Policy and Industrial Development, Massachusetts Institute of Technology

Hattis, D., White, P., Marmorstein, L. & Koch, P. (1990) Uncertainties in pharmacokinetic modeling for perchloroethylene. I. Comparison of model structure, parameters, and predictions for low-dose metabolism rates for models derived by different authors. *Risk Anal.*, 10, 449-458

Hattis, D., Tuler, S., Finkelstein, L. & Luo, Z.Q. (1986) *A Pharmacokinetic/Mechanism-based Analysis of the Carcinogenic Risk of Perchloroethylene* (CTPID 86-7), Cambridge, MA, MIT Center for Technology, Policy, and Industrial Development

Hayes, R.B., Yin, S-N, Dosemeci, M., Li, G-L, Wacholder, S., Chow, W-H, Rothman, N., Wang, Y-Z, Dai, T-R, Chao, X-J, Jiang, Z-L, Ye, P-Z, Zhao, H-B, Kou, Q-R, Zhang, W-Y, Meng, J-R, Zho, J-S, Lin, X-F, Ding, C-Y, Li, C-Y, Zhang, Z-N, Li, D-G, Travis, L.B., Blot, W.J. & Linet, M.S. (1996) Mortality among benzene-exposed workers in China. *Environ. Health Perspect.*, 104, Suppl.6, 1349-1352

Hayes, R.B., Yin, S-N, Dosemeci, M., Li, G-L, Wacholder, S., Travis, L.B., Li, C-Y, Rothman, N., Hoover, R.N. & Linet, M.S. (1997) Benzene and dose related incidence of hematologic neoplasms in China. *J. Natl Cancer Inst.*, 89, 1065-1071

Health Canada (1994) *Human Health Risk Assessment for Priority Substances*, Ottawa, Environmental Health Directorate

Health and Welfare Canada (1990) *Risk Management in the Health Protection Branch*, Ottawa, Health Protection Branch

Health and Welfare Canada (1991) *Carcinogen Assessment: A Research Report to the Department of National Health and Welfare* (Cat H49-69/1991), Ottawa, Minister of Supply and Services

Health and Welfare Canada (1992) *Determination of 'Toxic' under Paragraph (11c) of the Canadian Environmental Protection Act*, 1st ed., Ottawa, Bureau of Chemical Hazards, Environmental Health Directorate, Health Protection Branch

Health Council of The Netherlands (1980) *Report on the Evaluation of the Carcinogenicity of Chemical Substances* (Report No. 1978/19) Rijswijk

Health Council of The Netherlands (1987) A scientific basis for the risk assessment of vinyl chloride. *Reg. Toxicol. Pharmacol.*, 7, 120-127

Health Council of The Netherlands (1988) *Carcinogenicity of Chemical Substances* (Report No. 1988/04), The Hague

Health Council of The Netherlands (1989) Carcinogenic risk assessment of benzene in outdoor air. *Reg. Toxicol. Pharmacol.*, 9, 175-185

Health Council of The Netherlands (1994) Risk Assessment of Carcinogenic Chemicals in The Netherlands. *Reg. Toxicol. Pharmacol.*, 19,14-30

Henderson, R.F., Sabourin, P.J., Bechtold, W.E., Griffith, W.C., Medinsky, M.A., Birnbaum, L.S. & Lucier, G.W. (1989) The effect of dose, dose rate, route of administration, and species on tissue and blood levels of benzene metabolites. *Environ. Health Perspect.*, 82, 9-18

Hertz-Picciotto, I., Neutra, R.R. & Collins, J.F. (1987) Ethylene oxide and leukemia. *J. Am. Med. Assoc.*, 257, 2290

Hickman, J.R. & Toft, P. (1989) *The Development of Chemical Safety Programs in Canada*. Paper presented at the Department of Health and Social Security/IPCS, Risk Assessment Seminar, London, 13–24 February 1989

Hogstedt, V.C., Aringer, L. & Gustavsson, A. (1986) Epidemologic support for ethylene oxide as a cancer-causing agent. *J. Am. Med. Assoc.*, 255, 1575-1578

Hoover, S.M., Zeise, L. & Krowech, G. (1991) Exposure to environmental contaminants through breast milk. In: Travis, C.C., ed., *Advances in Risk Analysis*, New York, NY, Plenum, pp.257–266

Hoover, S.M., Zeise, L., Pease, W.S., Lee, L.E., Hennig, M.P., Weiss, L.B. & Cranor C. (1995) Improving the regulation of carcinogens by expediting cancer potency estimation. *Risk Anal.*, **15**, 267-280

Huff, J.E., Haseman, J.K. DeMarini, D.M., Eustis, S., Maronpot, R.R., Peters, A.C., Persing, R.L., Chrisp, C.E. & Jacobs AC (1989) Multiple site carcinogenicity of benzene in Fischer 344 rats and B6C3F1 mice. *Environ. Health Perspect.*, **82**, 125-163

IARC Working Group (1994) Direct estimates of cancer mortality due to low doses of ionising radiation: an international study. *Lancet*, **344**, 1039–1043

Institute for Cancer Research, Norway (1995) *Classification of Carcinogens by Different Countries and Organizations*, Oslo, Laboratory for Environmental and Occupational Cancer, Radiumhospitalet

International Agency for Research on Cancer (1982) *IARC Monographs on the Evaluation of the Carcinogenic Risk of Chemicals to Humans*, Vol.29, *Some Industrial Chemicals and Dyestuffs*, Lyon

International Agency for Research on Cancer (1983) *Monographs on the Evaluation of the Carcinogenic Risk of Chemicals to Humans*, Vol. 32, *Polynuclear Aromatic Compounds, Part 1, Chemical, Environmental and Experimental Data*, Lyon

International Agency for Research on Cancer (1985) *IARC Monographs on the Evaluation of the Carcinogenic Risk of Chemicals to Humans*, Vol. 36, *Allyl Compounds, Aldehydes, Epoxides and Peroxides*, Lyon

International Agency for Research on Cancer (1997) *Monographs on the Evaluation of the Carcinogenic Risk of Chemicals to Humans*, Vol. 69, *Polychlorinated Dibenzo-para-dioxins and polychlorinated dibenzofurans*, Lyon

International Commission on Radiological Protection (1977) *Recommendations of the International Commission on Radiological Protection*, Oxford, Pergamon Press (ICRP Publication 26; *Annals of the ICRP*, Vol. 1, No. 2)

International Commission on Radiological Protection (1990) *Age-dependent Doses to Members of the Public from Intake of Radionuclides: Part 1. A Report of a Task Group of Committee 2 of the International Commission on Radiological Protection.*, Oxford, Pergamon Press

International Commission on Radiological Protection (1991) *1990 Recommendations of the International Commission on Radiological Protection*, Oxford, Pergamon Press (ICRP Publication 60; *Annals of the ICRP*, Vol. 21, No. 1–3).

Kerns, W.D., Pavkov, K.L., Donofrio, D., Gralla, E.J. & Swenberg, J.A. (1983) Carcinogenicity of formaldehyde in rats and mice after long-term inhalation exposure. *Cancer Res.*, **43**, 4382-4392

Kipen, H.M., Cody R.P. & Goldstein, B.D. (1989) Use of longitudinal analysis of peripheral blood counts to validate historical reconstructions of benzene exposure. *Environ. Health Perspect.*, **82**, 199-206

Kissel, J.C. & Robarge, G.M. (1988) Assessing the elimination of 2,3,7,8-TCDD from humans with a physiologically based pharmacokinetic model. *Chemosphere*, **17**, 2017-2027

Kohn, M.C., Lucier, G.W., Clark, G.C., Sewell, C., Tritscher, A.M. & Portier C.J. (1993) A mechanistic model of effects of dioxin on gene expression in the rat liver. *Toxicol. Appl. Pharmacol.*, **120**, 138-154

Krewski D., Zielinski, J.M., Goddard, M. & Blakey, D. (1995). Environmental health risk assessment: a Canadian perspective. In: Greenwald, P., Kramer, B.S. & Weed, D.L., eds, *Cancer Prevention and Control*, New York, NY, Marcel Dekker, pp.161–179

Latin, H. (1988) Good science, bad regulation and toxic risk assessment. *Yale J. Reg.*, **4**, 89-148

Lawrie, C.A., Renwick, A.G. & Sims, J. (1985) The urinary excretion of bacterial amino acid metabolites by rats fed saccharin in the diet. *Food Chem. Toxicol.*, **23**, 445-450

Lee, P.N. (1992) *Environmental Tobacco Smoke and Mortality*, Basel, Karger

Leung, H.W., Ku, R.H., Paustenbach, D.J. & Andersen, M.E. (1988) A physiologically based pharmacokinetic model for 2,3,7,8-tetra-chlorodibenzo-*p*-dioxin in C57BL/6J and DBA/2J mice. *Toxicol. Lett.*, **42**, 15-38

Leung, H.-W., Paustenbach, D.J. & Anderson, M.E. (1989) A physiologically based pharmaco-kinetic model for 2,3,7,8-tetrachloro-di-benzo-*p*-dioxin. *Chemosphere*, **18**, 659-664

Leung, H.-W., Poland, A., Murray, F.J., Paustenbach, D.J. & Anderson, M.E. (1990a) Pharmacokinetics of [^{125}I]-2-iodo-3,7,8-trichloro-dibenzo-*p*-dioxin in mice: analysis with a physio-logical modeling approach. *Toxicol. Appl. Pharmacol.*, **103**, 411-419

Leung, H.-W., Paustenbach, D.J., Murray, F.J. & Anderson, M.E. (1990b) A physiological pharmacokinetic description of the tissue distribution and enzyme inducing proper-ties of 2,3,7,8-tetrachlorodibenzo-*p*-dioxin in the rat. *Toxicol. Appl. Pharmacol.*, **103**, 399-410

Lewtas, J. (1991) *Carcinogenic Risks of Polycyclic Organic Matter (POM) from Selected Emission Sources. Development of a Comparative Potency Method* (Deliverable Report No. 3128), Research Triangle Park, NC, US Environmental Protection Agency

Lewtas, J. & Gallagher, J. (1990) Complex mix-tures of urban air pollutants: Identification and comparative assessment of mutagenic and tumorigenic chemicals and emission sources. In: Vainio, H., Sorsa, M. & McMichael, A.J., eds, *Complex Mixtures and Cancer Risk* (IARC Scientific Publications No. 104), Lyon, International Agency for Research on Cancer, pp. 252-260

Lucier, G. Portier, C. & Gallo, M.A. (1993) Receptor mechanisms and dose–response models for the effects of dioxins. *Environ. Health Perspect.*, **101**, 36-44

Lynch, D.W., Lewis, T.R., Moorman, W.J., Burg, J.R., Groth, D.H., Khan, A., Ackerman, L.J. & Cockrell, B.Y. (1984) Carcinogenic and toxicolog-ic effects of inhaled ethylene oxide and propylene oxide in F344 rats. *Toxicol. Appl. Pharmacol.*, **76**, 85-95

Maltoni, C., Conti, B. & Cotti, G. (1983) Benzene: a multipotential carcinogen. Results of long-term bioassays performed at the Bologna Institute of Oncology. *Am. J. Ind. Med.*, **4**, 589-630

Maltoni C., Ciliberti, A., Cotti, G., Conti, B., & Belpoggi, F. (1989) Benzene, an experimental mul-tipotential carcinogen: Results from long-term bioassays performed at the Bologna Institute of Oncology. *Environ. Health Perspect.*, **82**,109-124

Mantel, N. & Bryan, W. (1961) "Safety" testing of carcinogenic agents. *J. Natl Cancer Inst.*, **27**, 445–470

Mazzullo, M., Bartoli, S., Bonora, B., Colacci, A., Grilli, S., Lattanzi, G., Niero, A., Turina, M.P. & Parodi, S. (1989) Benzene adducts with rat nucle-ic acids and proteins: Dose–response relationship after treatment *in vivo*. *Environ. Health Perspect.*, **82**, 259-266

Medinsky, M.A., Sabourin, P.J., Lucier, G., Birnbaum, L.S. & Henderson R.F. (1989) A physi-ological model for simulation of benzene metab-olism by rats and mice. *Toxicol. Appl. Pharmacol.*, **99**, 193-206

Medinsky, M.A., Kenyon, E.M., Seaton, M.J. & Schlosser, P.M. (1996) Mechanistic considerations in benzene physiological model development. *Environ. Health Perspect.*, **104**, Suppl.6, 1399-1404

Meek, M.E., Newhook, R., Liteplo, R.G. & Armstrong, V.C. (1994) Approach to assessment of risk to human health for priority substances under CEPA. *J. Environ. Sci. Health*, Part C, **12**(2), 105-134

Mills, J.J., Gargas, M.L. & Andersen, M.E. (1992) Biological and physiological factors involved in disposition of dioxin and related compounds. *Chemosphere*, 25, 3-6

Monster, A.C., Boersma, G. & Steenweg H. (1979) Kinetics of tetrachloroethylene in volunteers; influence of exposure concentrations and work load. *Int. Arch. Occup. Environ. Health*, 42, 303-309

Monticello, T.M. (1990) *Formaldehyde Induced Pathology and Cell Proliferation*, PhD Dissertation, Durham, NC, Duke University

Moolgavkar, S.H. (1991) Carcinogenesis models. *Science*, 251, 143

Moolgavkar, S.H., Luebeck, E.G., Buchmann, A. & Bock K. (1996) Quantitative analysis of enzyme-altered foci in rats initiated with diethylnitrosamine and promoted with 2,3,7,8-tetrachlorodibenzo-*p*-dioxin or 1,2,3,6,7,8-heptachlorodibenzo-*p*-dioxin. *Toxicol. Appl. Phamacol.*, 138, 31-41

National Food Agency of Denmark, Institute of Toxicology (1990) *Quantitative Risk Analysis of Carcinogens* (Publication No. 190), Copenhagen, Ministry of Health

Norwegian Advisory Board on Food Toxicology, Directorate of Health (1987) *Helserisiko i forbindelse med radionuklider i naeringsmidler. Forholdene etter reaktorulykken i Tsjernobyl* (Rapport 1/87), Oslo

Norwegian Scientific Group for Identification of Carcinogens (1993) *Guidelines for the Scientific Evaluation of Carcinogens* (TS/ED 13.10.93; utr. 303), Oslo, State Pollution Control Authority and Directorate of Labour Inspection

Norwegian Scientific Group for Identification of Carcinogens (1994) *Guidelines for the Scientific Evaluation of Carcinogens* (TS/ED 20.09.95; Vtr.303), Oslo, State Pollution Control Authority and Directorate of Labour Inspection

Nyberg, F., Isaksson, I., Harris, J.R. & Pershagen, G. (1997) Misclassification of smoking status and lung cancer risk from environmental tobacco smoke in never-smokers. *Epidemiology*, 8, 304-309

Organization for Economic Co-operation and Development (1996) *A Proposal for a Harmonized Scheme for the Classification of Chemicals which Cause Cancer in Humans* (OECD 604), Paris

Osterman-Golkar, S., Farmer, P.B., Segerbäck, D., Bailey, E., Calleman, C.J., Svensson, K. & Ehrenberg, L. (1983) Dosimetry of ethylene oxide in the rat by quantitation of alkylated histidine in hemoglobin. *Teratog. Carcinog. Mutag.*, 3, 395-405

Ott, G.M., Townsend, J.C., Fishbeck, W.A. & Langner, R.A. (1978) Mortality among individuals occupationally exposed to benzene. *Arch. Environ. Health*, 33, 3-10

Pathology Working Group (1990) *2, 3, 7, 8-Tetrachlorodibenzo-p-dioxin in Sprague Dawley rats*. Submitted to the Maine Scientific Advisory Panel by Pathco, Inc., 10075 Tyler Place, # 16, Ivansville, MD 21754, March 13

Paustenbach, D.J., Layard, M.W., Wenning, R.J. & Keenan, R.E. (1991) Risk assessment of 2,3,7,8-TCDD using a biologically based cancer model: A reevaluation of the Kociba *et al.* bioassay using 1978 and 1990 histopathology criteria. *J. Toxicol. Environ. Health* 34, 11-26

Paustenbach, D.J., Price, P.S., Ollison, W., Blank, C., Jernigan, J.D., Bass, R.D. & Peterson H.D. (1992) Reevaluation of benzene exposure for the Pliofilm (rubberworker) cohort (1936–1976). *J. Toxicol. Environ. Health*, 36, 177-231

Paxton, M.B. (1996) Leukemia risk associated with benzene exposure in the pliofilm cohort. *Environ. Health Perspect.* 104, Suppl.6, 1431-1436

Paxton, M.B., Chinchilli, VM.., Brett, S.M. & Rodericks, J.V. (1994) Leukemia risk associated with benzene exposure in the pliofilm cohort. II. Risk Estimates. *Risk Anal.*, 14, 155-157

Pease, W.S. (1992a) The role of cancer analysis in the regulation of industrial pollution. *Risk Anal.*, 12, 253-265

Pease, W.S. (1992b) *Strategies for Reforming Toxic Chemical Regulation: An Assessment of California's Proposition 65*, PhD Thesis, Berkeley, CA, University of California

Pelekis, M., Poulin, P. & Krishnan, K. (1995) An approach for incorporating tissue composition data into physiologically based pharmacokinetic models. *Toxicol. Ind. Health*, **11**, 511-522

Phillips, D.H. (1983) Fifty years of benzo(a)pyrene. *Nature*, **303**, 468-472

Poland, A. & Knutson, J. (1982) 2,3,7,8-Tetrachlorodibenzo-*p*-dioxin and related halogenated aromatic hydrocarbons: examination of the mechanism of toxicity. *Ann. Rev. Pharmacol. Toxicol.*, **22**, 517-554

Portier, C.J. & Kaplan, N.L. (1989) Variability of safe dose estimates when using complicated models of the carcinogenic process. A case study: methylene chloride. *Fundam. Appl. Toxicol.*, **13**, 533-544

Portier, C.J., Hoel, D.G. & Van Ryzin, J. (1984) Statistical analysis of the carcinogenesis bioassay data relating to the risks from exposure to 2,3,7,8-tetrachlorodibenzo-*p*-dioxin. In: Lowrence, W.W., ed., *Public Health Risks of the Dioxins. Symposium Proceedings at Rockefeller University, New York, NY, October 19–20, 1983*, Los Altos, CA, William Kauffmann, pp. 99-119

Portier, C., Sherman, C. Kohn, M., Edler, L., Kopp-Schneider, A., Maronpot, R. & Lucier, G. (1996) Modeling the number and size of hepatic focal lesions following exposure to 2,3,7,8-TCDD. *Toxicol. Appl. Pharmacol.*, **138**, 20-30

Potter, D., Blair, D., Davies, R., Watson, W.P. & Wright, A.S. (1989) The relationship between alkylation of hemoglobin and DNA in Fischer 344 rats exposed to [14-C] ethylene oxide. *Arch. Toxicol.*, Suppl.13, 254-257

Rall, D., Beebe, G.W., Hoel, D.G., Jablon, S., Land, C.E., Nygaard, O.F., Upton, A.C., Yalow, R.S. & Zeve, V.H. (1985) *Report of the National Institute of Health Working Group to Develop Radioepidemiological Tables* (NIH Publication No. 85-2748), Washington, DC, US Government Printing Office

Reitz, R.H. & Nolan, R.J. (1986) *Physiological Pharmacokinetic Modeling for Perchloroethylene Dose Adjustment: Draft Comments on US Environmental Protection Agency's Addendum to the Health Assessment Document for Tetrachloroethylene*, Midland, MI, Dow Chemical Company

Reitz, R.H., Mendrala, A.L., Park, C.N., Andersen, M.E. & Guengerich, F.P. (1988) Incorporation of *in vitro* enzyme data into the physiologically based pharmacokinetic (PB-PK) model for methylene chloride: implications for risk assessment. *Toxicol. Lett.*, **43**, 97-116

Renwick, A.G. (1985) The disposition of saccharin in animals and man—a review. *Food Chem. Toxicol.*, **23**, 429-435

Renwick, A.G. (1993) A data-derived safety (uncertainty) factor for the intense sweetener, saccharin. *Food Addit. and Contaminants*, **10**(3), 337-350

Renwick, A.G. & Sims, J. (1983) Distension of the urinary bladder in rats fed saccharin containing diet. *Cancer Lett.*, **18**, 63-68

Repace J.L. & Lowrey, A.H. (1985) A quantitative estimate of nonsmokers' lung cancer risk from passive smoking. *Environ. Int.*, **11**, 3-22

Resources for the Future (1993) *Setting National and Environmental Priorities: The EPA Risk-based Paradigm and its Alternatives*, Washington, DC, Center for Risk Management

Rhomberg, L. (1995) Use of quantitative modelling in methylene chloride risk assessment. *Toxicology*, **102**, 95-114

Riboli, E., Haley, N.J., Tredaniel, J., Saracci, R., Preston-Martin, S. & Trichopoulos, D. (1995) Misclassification of smoking status among women in relation to exposure to environmental tobacco smoke. *Eur. Respir. J.*, **8**, 285-290

Rinsky, R.A., Young, R.J. & Smith, A.B. (1981) Leukemia in benzene workers. *Am. J. Ind. Med.*, **2**, 217-245

Rinsky, R.A., Smith, A.B., Hornung, R., Filloon, R.G., Young, R.J., Okun, A.H., & Landrigan, P.J. (1987) Benzene and leukemia. An epidemiological risk assessment. *New. Engl. J. Med.*, **316**, 1044-1050

Robins, J.M., Blevins, D. & Schneiderman, M. (1989) The effective number of cigarettes inhaled daily by passive smokers: are epidemiologic and dosimetric estimates consistent? *J. Hazard. Mater.*, **21**, 215-238

Robinson, J.C. & Pease, W.S. (1991) From health based to technology based standards for hazardous air pollutants. *Am. J. Public Health*, **81**, 1518-1523

Rothman, N., Smith, M.T., Hayes, R.M., Traver, R.D., Hoener, B., Campleman, S., Li, G-L, Dosemeci, M., Linet, M., Zhang, L., Xi, L., Wacholder, S., Lu, W., Meyer, K.B., Titenko-Holland, N., Stewart, J.T., Yin, S. & Ross, D. (1997) Benzene poisoning, a risk factor for hematological malignancy, is associated with the NQ01 $^{609}C \rightarrow T$ mutation and rapid fractional excretion of chlorzoxazone. *Cancer Res.*, **57**, 2839-2842

Russell, M.A.H., Jarvis, M.J. & West, R.J. (1986) Use of urinary nicotine concentrations to estimate exposure and mortality from passive smoking in non-smokers. *Br. J. Addict.*, **81**, 275-281

Ruttenberg, R. & Bingham, E. (1981) A comprehensive occupational carcinogen control policy as a framework for regulatory activity. *Ann. N.Y. Acad. Sci.*, **363**, 13-27

Sabourin , P.J., Chen, B.T., Lucier, G., Birnbaum, L.S., Fisher, E. & Henderson, R.F. (1987) Effects of dose on the absorption and excretion of [14C] benzene administered orally or by inhalation in rats and mice. *Toxicol. Appl. Pharmacol.*, **87**, 325-336

Safe, S.H. (1986) Comparative toxicology and mechanism of action of polychlorinated dibenzo-*p*-dioxins and dibenzofurans. *Ann. Rev. Pharmacol. Toxicol.*, **26**, 371-399

Safe, S.H. (1990) Polychlorinated biphenyls (PCBs), dibenzo-*p*-dioxins (PCDDs), dibenzofurans (PCDFs), and related compounds: environmental and mechanistic considerations which support the development of toxic equivalence factors (TEFs). *CRC Crit. Rev. Toxicol.*, **21**, 51-88

Sanner, T., Dybing, E. & Stranden, E. (1988) Indoor radon exposure and lung cancer. *Tidsskr. Nor. Laegeforen.*, **25**, 2023-2025

Sanner, T., Dybing, E., Kroese, D., Roelfzema, H. & Hardeng, S. (1996) Carcinogen classification systems: Similarities and differences. *Reg. Toxicol. Pharmacol.*, **23**, 2128-138

Saracci, R. & Riboli, E. (1989) Passive smoking and lung cancer: current evidence and ongoing studies at the International Agency for Research on Cancer. *Mutat. Res.*, **222**, 117-127

Schnatter, A.R., Nicolich, M.J. & Bird, M.G. (1996) Determination of leukemogenic benzene exposure concentrations: Refined analyses of the pliofilm cohort. *Risk Anal.*, **16**, 833-840

Schoenig, G.P., Goldenthal, E.I., Geil, R.G., Frith, C.H., Richter, W.R. & Carlborg, F.W. (1985) Evaluation of the dose response and *in utero* exposure to saccharin in the rat. *Food Chem. Toxicol.*, **23**, 475-490

Segerbäck, D. (1983) Alkylation of DNA and hemoglobin in the mouse following exposure to ethene and ethene oxide. *Chem.-Biol. Interactions*, **45**, 139-151

Sielken, R.L. (1987) Quantitative cancer risk assessments for 2,3,7,8-tetrachlorodibenzo-*p*-dioxin. *Food Chem. Toxicol.*, **25**, 257-267

Sinclair, W.K. (1981) The scientific basis for risk quantification. In: *Quantitative Risk in Standard Setting, Proceedings of the Sixteenth Annual Meeting of the National Council on Radiation Protection and Measurements*, (Proceedings No. 2), Bethesda, MD, National Council on Radiation Protection and Measurements, pp.3-33

Skov, T., Hermind, B. & Lynge, E. (1992) *EC Legislation on Carcinogens*, Copenhagen, Danish Cancer Society

Smith, A. (1987) Infant exposure assessment for breast milk dioxins and furans derived from waste incineration emissions. *Risk Anal.*, 7, 347-353

Smith, M.T. (1996) The mechanism of benzene-induced leukemia: A hypothesis and speculations on the causes of leukemia. *Environ. Health Perspect.*, 104, Suppl.6, 1219-1225

Smith, M.T. & Fanning E.W. (1997) Report on the workshop entitled: "Modeling chemically-induced leukemia—Implications for benzene risk assessment" *Leukemia Res.*, 21, 361-374

Snellings, W.M., Weil, C.S. & Maronpot, R.R. (1984) A two-year inhalation study of the carcinogenic potential of ethylene oxide in Fischer 344 rats. *Toxicol. Appl. Pharmacol.*, 75, 105-117

Spear, R.C., Bois, F.Y., Woodruff, T., Auslander, D., Parker, J. & Selvin, S. (1991) Modeling benzene pharmacokinetics across three sets of animal data: parameter sensitivity and risk implications. *Risk Anal.*, 11, 641-654

State of California (1985) *Guidelines for Chemical Carcinogen Risk Assessments and Their Scientific Rationale*, Sacramento, CA, Department of Health Services

Stockwell H.G., Goldman A.L., Lyman G.H., Noss C.I., Armstrong A.W., Pinkham P.A., Candelora E.C. & Brusa M.R. (1992) Environmental tobacco smoke and lung cancer risk in nonsmoking women. *J. Natl Cancer Inst.*, 84, 1417-1422

Sweatman, T.W. & Renwick, A.G. (1980) The tissue distribution and pharmacokinetics of saccharin in the rat. *Toxicol. Appl. Pharmacol.*, 55, 18-31

Synder, R., Witz, G. & Goldstein, B.D. (1993) The toxicology of benzene. *Environ. Health Perspect.*, 100, 293-306

Tancrede, M., Wilson, R., Zeise, L. & Crouch, E.A.C. (1987) The carcinogenic risk of some organic vapors indoors. A theoretical survey. *Atmos. Environ.*, 21, 2187-2205

Taylor, J.M., Weinberger, M.A. & Friedman, L. (1980) Chronic toxicity and carcinogenicity to the urinary bladder of sodium saccharin in the *in utero* exposed rat. *Toxicol. Appl. Pharmacol.*, 54, 57-75

Thomas, R.S., Yang, R.S., Morgan, D.G., Moorman, M.P., Kermani, H.R., Sloane, R.A., O'Conner, R.W., Adkins, B., Gargas, M.L. & Andersen, M.E. (1996) PBPK modeling/Monte Carlo simulation of methylene chloride kinetic changes in mice in relation to age and acute, subchronic, and chronic inhalation exposure. *Environ. Health Perspect.*, 104, 858-865

Thorslund, T. (1987) *Quantitative Dose Response Model for Tumor-Promoting Activity of TCDD. Appendix A: A Cancer Risk Specific Dose Estimate for 2, 3, 7, 8-TCDD* (Report for the Carcinogen Assessment Group), Washington, DC, ICF Clement Associates

Thorslund, T.W., Anver, M. & Wegner, R.E. (1988) *Quantitative Re-evaluation of the Human Leukemia Risk Associated with Inhalation Exposure to Benzene*, Fairfax, VA, ICF Clement Associates

Törnquist, M. (1989) *Monitoring and Cancer Risk Assessment of Carcinogens, Particularly Alkenes in Urban Air*, Doctoral Thesis, Stockholm, University of Stockholm

Törnquist, M. & Osterman-Golkar, S. (1991) Monitoring of *in vivo* dose by macromolecular adducts: usefulness in risk estimation. In: Groopman, J.D. & Skipper, P.L., eds, *Molecular Dosimetry and Human Cancer: Analytical, Epidemiological and Social Considerations*, Boca Raton, FL, CRC Press, pp. 89-102

Travis, C.C., Quillen, J.L. & Arms, A.D. (1990) Pharmacokinetics of benzene. *Toxicol. Appl. Pharmacol.*, 102, 400-420

United Nations Scientific Committee on the Effects of Atomic Radiation (1977) *Sources and Effects of Ionizing Radiation. 1977 Report to the*

General Assembly, with Annexes, New York, United Nations

United Nations Scientific Committee on the Effects of Atomic Radiation (1986) *Genetic and Somatic Effects of Ionizing Radiation. 1986 Report to the General Assembly, with Annexes*, New York, United Nations

United Nations Scientific Committee on the Effects of Atomic Radiation (1988) *Sources, Effects and Risks of Ionizing Radiation*, New York, United Nations

United Nations Scientific Committee on the Effects of Atomic Radiation (1994) *Sources and Effects of Ionizing Radiation: UNSCEAR 1994 Report to the General Assembly*, New York, United Nations

US Agency for Toxic Substances and Disease Registry (1993) *Cancer Policy Framework*, Atlanta, GA, Centers for Disease Control, Public Health Service, US Department of Health and Human Services

US Consumer Product Safety Commission (1978) Interim statement of policy and procedures for classifying, evaluating, and regulating carcinogens in consumer products. *Fed. Reg.*, **43**, 25658-25665

US Department of Health and Human Services (1986) *The Health Consequences of Involuntary Smoking. A Report of the Surgeon General* (US DHHS Publication No. (PHS) 87-8398), Washington, DC, Public Health Service, Office of Smoking and Health

US Environmental Protection Agency (1985a) *Health Assessment Document for Polychlorinated Dibenzo-p-dioxins* (EPA 600/8-84-014F), Washington, DC, Office of Health and Environmental Assessment

US Environmental Protection Agency (1985b) *Interim Quantitative Cancer Unit Risk Estimates Due to Inhalation of Benzene* (EPA 600/X-85-022), Washington, DC, Carcinogen Assessment Group, Office of Health and Environmental Assessment

US Environmental Protection Agency (1986a) *Addendum to the Health Assessment Document for Tetrachloroethylene (Perchloroethylene). Updated Carcinogenicity Assessment for Tetrachloroethylene (Perchloroethylene, PERC, PCE)* (EPA/600/8-2/005FA) (draft), Washington, DC, Office of Research and Development

US Environmental Protection Agency (1986b) Guidelines for carcinogen risk assessment. *Fed. Regist.*, **51**, 33992-34054

US Environmental Protection Agency (1987a) *Unfinished Business: A Comparative Assessment of Environmental Problems*, Appendix I, *Report of the Cancer Risk Group* (EPA/230/2-87/025b), Washington, DC, Office of Policy Analysis

US Environmental Protection Agency (1987b) *Update to the Health Assessment Document and Addendum for Dichloromethane (Methylene Chloride): Pharmacokinetics, Mechanism of Action, and Epidemiology. Review Draft* (EPA 600/8-87-030A), Washington, DC, Office of Health and Environmental Assessment

US Environmental Protection Agency (1987c) *Assessment of Garment Workers and Certain Home Residents from Exposure to Formaldehyde*, Washington, DC, Office of Pesticides and Toxic Substances

US Environmental Protection Agency (1988a) Intent to review guidelines for carcinogen risk assessment. *Fed. Regist.*, **53**, 32656-32658

US Environmental Protection Agency (1988b) *Pilot Study on International Information Exchange on Dioxins and Related Compounds* (North Atlantic Treaty Organization/Committee on the Challenges of Modern Society Report No. 176), Washington, DC

US Environmental Protection Agency (1989) *Review of Draft Documents "A Cancer Risk-specific Dose Estimate for 2,3,7,8-TCDD" and "Estimating Exposure to 2,3,7,8-TCDD"*, Washington, DC, Ad Hoc Dioxin Panel, Science Advisory Board

US Environmental Protection Agency (1991) *Formaldehyde Risk Assessment Update*, Washington, DC, Office of Toxic Substances

US Environmental Protection Agency (1992a) *Working Paper for Considering Draft Revisions to the US EPA Guidelines for Cancer Risk Assessment* (EPA/600/AP-92/003), Washington, DC, Office of Health and Environmental Assessment, Office of Research and Development

US Environmental Protection Agency (1992b) Draft report: A cross species scaling factor for carcinogen risk assessment based on equivalence of mg/kg3/4/day. *Fed. Regist.*, **57**, 24152-24174

US Environmental Protection Agency (1992c) *Respiratory Health Effects of Passive Smoking: Lung Cancer and Other Disorders* (EPA/600/6-90/006), Washington, DC, Office of Research and Development, Office of Air and Radiation

US Environmental Protection Agency (1993) *Integrated Risk Information System: 'Benzene'*, Cincinnati, OH, Environmental Criteria Office

US Environmental Protection Agency (1996a) *Proposed Guidelines for Carcinogen Risk Assessment* (EPA/600/P-92/003C), Washington, DC, Office of Research and Development

US Environmental Protection Agency (1996b) *Integrated Risk Information System*, Washington, DC, Office of Research and Development

US Environmental Protection Agency (1997) *Health Effects Assessment Summary Tables* (PB97-921199), Washington, DC, Office of Solid Waste and Emergency Response

US Environmental Protection Agency Science Advisory Board (1990) *The Report of the Human Health Subcommittee. Relative Risk Reduction Project, Reducing Risk*, Appendix B (USEPA SAB-EC-90-021B), Washington, DC

US National Council on Radiation Protection and Measurement (1980) *Influence of Dose and Its Distribution in Time on Dose Response Relationships for Low-LET Radiations* (NCRP Report No. 64), Bethesda, MD

US National Research Council (1977) *Drinking Water and Health*, Vol. 1, Washington, DC, Safe Drinking Water Committee

US National Research Council (1980) *Drinking Water and Health*, Vol. 3, Washington, DC, Safe Drinking Water Committee

US National Research Council (1983) *Risk Assessment in the Federal Government: Managing the Process*, Washington, DC, National Academy Press

US National Research Council (1986a) *Drinking Water and Health*, Vol. 6, Washington, DC, Safe Drinking Water Committee

US National Research Council (1986b) *Environmental Tobacco Smoke: Measuring Exposures and Assessing Health Effects*, Washington, DC, National Academy of Sciences, National Academy Press,

US National Research Council (1987) *Regulating Pesticides in Food. The Delaney Paradox. US NRC Committee on Scientific and Regulatory Issues Underlying Pesticide Use Patterns and Agricultural Innovation*, Washington, DC, Board on Agriculture, National Academy Press

US National Research Council (1989) *Drinking Water and Health*, Vol. 9, Washington, DC, Safe Drinking Water Committee

US National Research Council (1990) *Health Effects of Exposure to Low Levels of Ionizing Radiation*, Washington, DC, Committee on the Biological Effects of Ionizing Radiation, NRC Board on Radiation Effects Research, Commission on Life Sciences, National Academy Press

US National Research Council (1993a) *Pesticides in the Diets of Infants and Children*, Washington, DC, US NRC Committee on Pesticides in the Diets of Infants and Children, Board on Agriculture and Board on Environmental Studies and Toxicology, National Academy Press

US National Research Council (1993b) *Issues in Risk Assessment*, Washington, DC, Committee on Risk Assessment Methodology, Commission on Life Sciences, National Academy Press

US National Research Council (1994) *Science and Judgment in Risk Assessment*, Washington, DC, Committee on Risk Assessment of Hazardous Air Pollutants, Commission on Life Sciences, National Academy Press

US National Research Council (1996) *Understanding Risk: Informing Decisions in a Democratic Society*, Washington, DC, Committee on Risk Characterization, Commission on Behavioral and Social Sciences and Education, National Academy Press

US National Toxicology Program (1986) *Toxicology and Carcinogenesis Studies of Benzene in F344/N Rats and B6C3F1 Mice* (NTP Technical Report Series, No. 289), Washington, DC

US National Toxicology Program (1987) *Toxicology and Carcinogenesis Studies of Ethylene Oxide in B6C3F1 Mice (Inhalation Studies)* (NTP Technical Report 326; NIH-88-2582), Research Triangle Park, NC

US Occupational Safety and Health Administration (1980) Identification, classification and regulation of potential occupational carcinogens. *Fed. Regist.*, 45, 5002-5202

US Occupational Safety and Health Administration (1987) Occupational exposure to benzene. *Fed. Regist.*, 52, 34460-34579

US Office of Management and Budget (1990) *Regulatory Program of the United States Government April 1, 1990–March 31, 1991*, Washington, DC, Office of the President

US Office of Technology Assessment (1987) *Identifying and Regulating Carcinogens*, Washington, DC, Congress of the United States p. 68

US Office of Technology Assessment (1993) *Researching Health Risks* (OTA-BS-570), Washington, DC, US Government Printing Office

Utterback, D.F. & Rinsky, R.A. (1995) Benzene exposure assessment in rubber hydrochloride workers: A critical evaluation of previous estimates. *Am. J. Ind. Med.*, 27, 661-676

Vainio, H., Sorsa, M. & McMichael, A.J. (1990) *Complex Mixtures and Cancer Risk* (IARC Science Publications No. 104), Lyon, International Agency for Research on Cancer

Vainio, H., Magee, P.N., McGregor, D.B. & McMichael, A.J., eds (1992) *Mechanisms of Carcinogenesis in Risk Identification* (IARC Scientific Publication No. 116), Lyon, International Agency for Research on Cancer

Vermont Agency of Natural Resources (1991) *Environment 199a: Risk to Vermont and Vermonters*, Montpelier, VT

Vutuc, C. (1984) Quantitative aspects of passive smoking and lung cancer. *Prev. Med.*, 13, 698-704

Wald, N.J., Nanchahal, K., Thompson, S.G. & Cuckle, H.S. (1986) Does breathing other people's tobacco smoke cause lung cancer? *Br. Med. J.*, 293, 1217-1222

Walker, V.E., Fennell, T.R., Upton, P.B., Skopek, T.R., Prevost, V., Shuker, D.E.G. & Swenberg, J.A. (1992) Molecular dosimetry of ethylene oxide: formation and persistence of 7-(2-hydroxyethyl)guanine) in DNA following repeated exposures of rats and mice. *Cancer Res.*, 52, 4328-4334

Walker, V.E., Fennell, T.R., Upton, P.B., MacNeela, J.P. & Swenberg, J.A. (1993) Molecular dosimetry of DNA and hemoglobin adducts in mice and rats exposed to ethylene oxide. *Environ. Health Perspect.*, 99, 11-17

Ward, R.C., Travis, C.C, Hetrick, D.M., Andersen, M.E. & Gargas, M.L. (1988) Pharmacokinetics of tetrachloroethylene. *Toxicol. Appl. Pharmacol.*, 93, 108-117

Washington State Environment 2010 Action Strategies Analysis Committee (1990) *Environment 2010 Action Agenda: Compilation of Background Analysis for Action Strategies*, Olympia, WA

Wells, A.J. (1988) An estimate of adult mortality in the United States from passive smoking. *Environ. Int.*, 14, 249-265

Wigle, D.T., Collishaw, N.E., Kirkbride, J. & Mao, Y. (1987) Deaths in Canada from lung cancer due to involuntary smoking. *J. Can. Med. Assoc.*, **136**, 945-951

Willems, M.I., Blijleven, W.G.H., Splinter, A., Roelfzema, H. & Feron, V.J. (1990) *Classification of Occupational Genotoxic Carcinogens on the Basis of their Carcinogenic Potency*, The Hague, Ministry of Social Affairs and Employment, Directorate General of Labour

Woodruff, T.J., Bois, F.Y., Auslander, D. & Spear, R.C. (1992) Structure and parametrization of pharmacokinetic models: their impact on model predictions. *Risk Anal.*, **12**, 189-201

Woodward A. & McMichael, A.J. (1991) Passive smoking and cancer risk: The nature and uses of epidemiological evidence. *Eur. J. Cancer*, **27**, 1472-1479

World Health Organization (1970) *Pesticide residues in food*. Report of the 1969 Joint Meeting of the FAO/WHO Meeting of Experts on Pesticide Residues (WHO Technical Report Series, No.458), Geneva

World Health Organization (1979) *DDT and Its Derivatives* (Environmental Health Criteria 7), Geneva

World Health Organization (1985a) *Ethylene Oxide* (Environmental Health Criteria 55), Geneva

World Health Organization (1987a) *Air Quality Guidelines for Europe*, Copenhagen, WHO Regional Office for Europe

World Health Organization (1987b) *Principles for the Safety Assessment of Food Additives and Contaminants in Food* (Environmental Health Criteria 70), Geneva

World Health Organization (1990) *Principles for the Toxicological Assessment of Pesticide Residues in Food* (Environmental Health Criteria 104), Geneva, pp 52-53

World Health Organization (1991) *Lindane* (Environmental Health Criteria 124), Geneva

World Health Organization (1993a) *WHO Guidelines for Drinking-water Quality*, Vol. 1, *Recommendations*, Geneva

World Health Organization (1993b) *Polychlorinated Biphenyls and Terphenyls*, 2nd ed. (Environmental Health Criteria 140), Geneva

World Health Organization (1994a) *Assessing Human Health Risks of Chemicals: Derivation of Guidance Values for Health-Based Exposure Limits*. (Environmental Health Criteria 170), Geneva

World Health Organization (1994b) *Summary of the Toxicological Evaluations Performed by the Joint FAO/WHO Meeting on Pesticide Residues (JMPR)* (WHO/PCS/94.1), Geneva

World Health Organization (1995a) *Tris(2,3-dibromo propyl) Phosphate and Bis(2,3-dibromopropyl) Phosphate* (Environmental Health Criteria 173), Geneva

World Health Organization (1995b) *1,2-Dichloroethane*, 2nd ed. (Environmental Health Criteria 176), Geneva

World Health Organization (1995c) *Acetaldehyde* (Environmental Health Criteria 167), Geneva

World Health Organization (1996a) *WHO Guidelines for Drinking-water Quality*, Vol. 2, *Health Criteria and Other Supporting Information*, Geneva

World Health Organization (1996b) *Summary of Evaluations Performed by the Joint FAO/WHO Expert Committee on Food Additives (JECFA). 1956–1995 (First Through Forty-first Meetings and Update Through Forty-fourth Meeting)*. Geneva

World Health Organization (1996c) *1,2-Dibromoethane* (Environmental Health Criteria 177), Geneva

World Health Organization (1996d) *Chlorinated Paraffins* (Environmental Health Criteria 181), Geneva

World Health Organization (1996e) *Chlorthalonil* (Environmental Health Criteria 183), Geneva

World Health Organization (1997) *Inventory of IPCS and other WHO Pesticide Evaluations and Summary of Toxicological Evaluations Performed by the Joint Meeting on Pesticide Residues (JMPR) through 1996* (WHO/PCS/97.3), Geneva

Zeise, L., Huff, J.E., Salmon, A.G. & Hooper, N.K. (1990) Human risks from 2,3,7,8-tetra-chlorodibenzo- *p*-dioxin and hexachloro-dibenzo-*p*-dioxins. *Adv. Mod. Environ. Toxicol.*, **17**, 293-342

Zeise, L., Crouch, E.A.C. & Wilson, R. (1987) Dose response relationships for carcinogens: a review. *Environ. Health Perspect.*, **73**, 259-308

Quantitative Estimation and Prediction of Human Cancer Risks
S. Moolgavkar, D. Krewski, L. Zeise, E. Cardis and H. Møller
IARC Scientific Publications No. 131
International Agency for Research on Cancer, Lyon, 1999

3: Principles of the Epidemiological Approach to QEP[1]

Suresh H. Moolgavkar, Henrik Moller and Alistair Woodward

3.1 Introduction

In its broadest sense, epidemiology is the study of diseases in populations. Although veterinary epidemiology is a rapidly growing field, we are concerned here with human epidemiology and its role in the quantitative estimation and prediction (QEP) of cancer risk. Intervention trials, in which individuals are randomly assigned to one or another "treatment" group, are becoming more common in epidemiology. Such trials are conducted to determine the efficacy of some intervention, such as lowering fat intake or ingesting β-carotene, on subsequent cancer risk, and have limited usefulness in QEP. For ethical reasons, the randomized experiments with putative carcinogens that are routinely conducted in the laboratory cannot be conducted on human populations. The traditional epidemiological approach to study design, analysis and interpretation, is influenced heavily by the fact that epidemiology is largely an observational discipline.

For QEP, epidemiological studies offer two obvious major advantages over experimental studies. Firstly, the studies are done in the species of ultimate interest, i.e. the human. The difficult problem of interspecies extrapolation is thus avoided, but that of the representativeness of the study population must still be addressed. This problem, however, is much more tractable than the interspecies extrapolation problem. Even if the representativeness problem is not explicitly addressed, the resulting uncertainty in QEP is likely to be small compared with that introduced by interspecies extrapolation. Secondly, estimates of risk can be directly obtained for levels of exposure that are close to those typical of "free-living" human populations. Epidemiological studies are often conducted in industrial cohorts, which are typically exposed to higher levels of the agent of interest than the general population. Nevertheless, the levels of exposure even in such cohorts are much closer to those in the general population than those used in experimental studies. Some of what epidemiological studies gain in the way of relevance over experimental studies is lost in precision, however. It is generally true that both exposures and disease outcomes are measured with less precision in epidemiological studies than in laboratory studies, leading, possibly, to bias in the estimate of risk. Exposure measurement is discussed in Chapter 4. Another, potentially serious, problem arises from the fact that human populations, particularly populations of industrial workers, are rarely exposed to single agents. When exposure to multiple agents is involved, the effect of the single agent of interest is often difficult to investigate.

Conventionally, epidemiology is often thought of as encompassing "descriptive" and "analytical" activities. While there is no well defined line distinguishing these two types of activities, descriptive studies generally report the distribution of disease or exposure, whereas analytical studies are designed to quantify associations. Broadly speaking, analytical studies can be divided into three categories. Of these, the cohort study is, at least conceptually, close to the traditional experimental study in that groups of exposed and non-exposed individuals are followed in time, and the occurrence of disease in the different groups compared. In the case–control study, relative risks are estimated from cases of the disease under investigation and suitably chosen controls. In these two types of study, information on exposures and disease is available on an individual basis. In a third type of study, namely the ecological study, information is available only on a group basis. Ecological studies have

---

[1] We are grateful to Sander Greenland for careful reading and constructive criticism of this chapter.

generally been looked upon with disfavour by epidemiologists. They can provide useful information, however (see the aflatoxin example in Chapter 8). We briefly discuss these three types of studies in this chapter. Because epidemiological studies are observational, careful attention must be paid to controlling for factors that may bias estimates of risk. Thus, controlling for what epidemiologists call "confounding" is of paramount importance both in the design and analyses of epidemiological studies. We shall briefly discuss the concept of confounding.

Within the last two decades, sophisticated statistical tools have been developed for the analysis of epidemiological data, and are briefly discussed in this chapter; a more comprehensive discussion can be found in Chapter 6. Finally, epidemiological studies are often not large enough to detect the small risks associated with typical human exposures. For example, studies of residential radon and lung cancer have yielded equivocal results. When many such inconclusive studies are available, it may be possible to increase statistical power by combining the information from all of them. Recently, there has been much discussion in the literature on such meta-analyses in epidemiology. We shall briefly discuss some of the important issues in combining information from different studies.

For detailed discussions of epidemiological study design and data analyses the reader is directed to the work of Breslow & Day (1980, 1987), Kleinbaum et al. (1982), Rothman (1986), Checkoway et al. (1989), Kelsey et al. (1996), and Rothman & Greenland (1997).

3.2 Measures of disease frequency and measures of effect

One of the tasks of descriptive epidemiology is to estimate the frequency of disease in populations. Perhaps the most fundamental measure of disease frequency is the incidence rate (also called the hazard rate by biostatisticians) which measures the rate (per person per unit time) at which new cases of a disease appear in the population under study. For example, because the incidence rates of many chronic diseases vary strongly with age, a commonly used measure of frequency is the age-specific incidence rate. Usually, five-year

age groups are used: the age-specific incidence rate per year of a cancer in the five-year age group 35–39, for instance is the ratio of the number of new cases of cancer occurring in that age group in a single year and the number of individuals in that age group who are cancer free at the beginning of the year. Strictly speaking, the denominator should be, not the total number of individuals who are cancer-free at the beginning of the year, but the person–years at risk during the year. This is because some individuals contribute less than a full year of experience to the denominator, either because they enter the relevant population after the year has begun (e.g. an individual may reach the age of 35 some time during the year) or because they may leave the population before the year is over (e.g. an individual may reach the age of 40 or die during the year). For a more detailed consideration of the concept of person–years, see Rothman (1986). We note here that the concept of incidence rate is an instantaneous concept, and is most precisely defined in terms of the differential calculus. For a definition of hazard rate, see any standard text on survival analysis (e.g. Kalbfleisch & Prentice, 1980; Cox & Oakes, 1984).

Another commonly used measure of disease frequency is the probability that an individual will develop the disease in a specified period of time. In QEP, one is often interested in the lifetime probability (often called lifetime risk) of developing cancer, and the impact of environmental agents on this probability. If the incidence rate is known as a function of age, the probability of developing the disease during any age interval can easily be derived. Conversely, if the probability of developing the disease is known as a function of age, the incidence rate as a function of age can easily be computed. In this sense, the incidence rate and the probability of disease are completely equivalent. The relationship between incidence rate and probability of disease is expressed by the following equation:

$$P(t)=1-\exp(-\int_0^t I(s)\mathrm{d}s),$$

where $P(t)$ is the probability of developing the disease by age t, and $I(s)$ is the incidence rate at age s. We note that what we have called the probability of disease is called cumulative incidence in the book by Rothman (1986), whereas the integral

$\int_0^t I(s)ds$ is called cumulative incidence in the statistical literature. When the incidence rate is small, as is true for most chronic diseases including cancer, then the above expression for $P(t)$ simplifies to

$$P(t) = \int_0^t I(s)ds.$$

The impact of an environmental agent on the risk of disease can be measured on either the absolute or the relative scale. The last two decades have seen an explosion of statistical literature on relative measures of risk, which can be estimated in both case–control and cohort studies. Let I_e be the incidence rate in the exposed population and I_u be the incidence rate in the unexposed population. Then the relative incidence, i.e the relative risk (RR) is defined by RR = I_e/I_u. A closely related measure is excess relative risk (ERR), which is defined as ERR = $(I_e - I_u)/I_u$ = RR - 1. Yet another measure of risk is the attributable or aetiological fraction (AF), which is defined as AF = $(I_e - I_u)/I_e$ = (RR - 1)/RR. AF is the fraction of incident cases in the exposed population that would not have occurred in the absence of exposure, and "can be interpreted as the proportion of exposed cases for whom the disease is attributable to the exposure" (Rothman, 1986). In most regression analyses of epidemiological data, RR is modelled either as a "multiplicative" or an "additive" function of the covariates of interest. More details are given below and in Chapter 6. Since RR is readily estimated from both case–control and cohort studies, the various measures of effect discussed above, which are functions of RR alone, can be estimated.

On the absolute scale, the impact of an agent can be measured simply by the difference between the incidence rates (or probabilities) in exposed and non-exposed subjects. Absolute measures of risk cannot be estimated from case–control studies without ancillary information (see, e.g. Rothman & Greenland, 1997).

The impact of an environmental agent on the risk of disease in a population will depend not only on the strength of its effect in the exposed subpopulation but also on how large this subpopulation is. Even if the agent is a very potent carcinogen, its impact on the cancer burden of the entire population will be small if only a small fraction of the population is exposed. On the other hand, if exposure to a weak carcinogen is widespread, the population impact could be substantial. A measure of risk that attempts to quantify the population burden of disease due to a specific exposure is the population-attributable fraction (PAF), which is defined as the fraction of all cases in the population that can be attributed to the exposure, and is given by the expression PAF = $(I_T - I_u)/I_T$, where I_T is the incidence in the total population. In addition to the RR, estimation of PAF requires information on the fraction of the population exposed to the agent of interest (see Rothman, 1986). PAF can be estimated directly from case–control data only if the controls are a random sample of the population (Rothman & Greenland, 1997). When the RR associated with exposure to an agent is high and the exposure is widespread, a major fraction of disease in the population can be attributed to the agent. For example, it has been estimated that, in England and Wales during the period 1971–1975, approximately 80% of all bladder cancer deaths among males and 25% among females could be attributed to cigarette smoking (Moolgavkar & Stevens, 1981).

The calculation of PAF can be extended to situations where there are multiple levels of exposure (by considering each level in turn and adding up the PAFs) or where the exposure is a continuous variable rather than a categorical one (by creating discrete categories, such as quartiles or quintiles, of exposure, or by using regression models). Joint effects of several exposures may be considered similarly. In the case of two or more exposures, the separate PAFs may be calculated for each exposure while ignoring the other exposures, or a combined PAF may be calculated by considering all possible combinations of exposures, calculating the PAF for each and adding them up. When two or more exposures are involved, the sum of the separate PAFs will frequently exceed the combined PAF calculated in this way and may actually exceed 100%. The reason for this is clear; cases that occur in the joint exposure categories are counted several times when PAFs for single exposures are computed, namely once for each exposure in the joint exposure category. Attribution of causation in the case of joint exposures is best done by considering all possible combinations of exposures. For example, with two exposures, attribution of causation may be done by subdividing the cases into those that can be considered as being caused by the combination of the two agents, each agent exclusively, and neither agent. For a more advanced treatment of PAFs see, for example, Bruzzi *et al.* (1985), Wahrendorf (1987), Benichou (1991), and Greenland & Drescher (1993).

3.3 Confounding

The concept of confounding is of central importance in the design and analysis of epidemiological studies. Suppose one is interested in alcohol as a possible cause of oral cancer, and that an epidemiological study shows an association between alcohol consumption and oral cancer, i.e. that the incidence of oral cancer in the subpopulation of individuals that imbibes alcohol is higher than that in the subpopulation of teetotallers. The crucial question then is the following. Could the association between alcohol consumption and oral cancer be "spurious" in the sense that it is due to another agent that is itself a cause of oral cancer, and more likely to be found in the subpopulation of alcohol imbibers than in that of teetotallers? One example of such an agent is tobacco smoke. Individuals who imbibe alcohol are more likely than teetotallers to be smokers. Moreover, smoking is a strong risk factor for oral cancer. Thus the observed association between alcohol consumption and oral cancer may actually be due to the association between smoking and alcohol consumption. In a study of oral cancer and alcohol, tobacco smoke is a confounder.

As we have seen by way of a specific example, confounding is the distortion of the effect of the agent of interest by an extraneous factor. To be a confounder, a factor must satisfy two conditions. First, the putative confounder must be a risk factor for the disease in the absence of the agent of interest. Second, the putative confounder must be associated with the exposure of interest in the population in which the study is conducted. Sometimes a third condition (Rothman & Greenland, 1997) is added: the putative confounder must not be an intermediate step in the pathway between exposure and disease. While these three criteria define a confounder for most epidemiologists, other definitions, which are

close, but not identical, to the definition given here have been given by biostatisticians. These are usually couched in terms of collapsibility of contingency tables. For a more detailed discussion, see Greenland & Robins (1986), and Rothman & Greenland (1997).

Confounding in epidemiological studies can be addressed in one of two ways: it can be prevented by appropriate study design or controlled for by appropriate analyses. The specific method used depends upon the type of epidemiological study, which we now briefly discuss.

3.4 Types of epidemiological study

Although randomized trials, which are similar to experimental studies, are becoming more common in epidemiology, particularly in the area of disease prevention, the mainstays of epidemiological investigations are cohort (or follow-up) studies and case–control studies. A third type of study, the ecological study, is also being increasingly used, especially in the area of air pollution epidemiology.

3.4.1 Cohort studies

The observational study that is closest in form to an experiment is the cohort study. In this type of study, cohorts or groups of individuals, defined in terms of their level of exposure to the agent of interest, are followed over time, and the occurrence of cancer (or other diseases) is noted. The objectives of the study are to investigate the frequency and timing of cancer occurrence as functions of the levels of exposure to the agent of interest. For example, for a cohort study of chemical exposures in the workplace and the risk of cancer, levels of occupational exposures to various chemicals could be determined by personal interviews and by consideration of the specific jobs performed by the individual. Exposures in various job categories could be verified by actual measurements in the workplace. Information on factors, such as smoking and dietary habits, that could confound the association between the agent of interest and cancer could also be collected. Increasingly, questionnaires are being supplemented by the acquisition of biological samples, such as blood fractions, nail clippings and samples of subcutaneous fat, because measurements on such samples may provide improved assessments of occupational, dietary and other exposures.

Cohort studies allow the estimation of incidence rates in the various subcohorts. Additionally, information can be obtained on a variety of disease end-points. Thus substantial advantages are offered by the cohort study over the case–control study. Unfortunately when rare diseases, such as cancer, are the primary focus of interest, the cohort study must enroll a large number of subjects and follow them up for a long period of time in order to ensure that a sufficient number of cases occur to satisfy the requirements of statistical power and precision. This makes the cohort study an expensive and time-consuming exercise. One of the best known examples of a cohort study is the follow-up study of the atomic bomb survivors in Hiroshima and Nagasaki. That study has been going on for almost 50 years.

A type of cohort study that is widely used in occupational epidemiology is the historical (or retrospective) cohort study. In this type of study, the members of the study cohort are not followed up from the time of the initiation of the study. Rather, the cohort is defined by historical records and is followed up to the present. This means that all, or a substantial part of the follow-up period has occurred in the past. Information on exposures and on occurrence of disease among cohort members is obtained from multiple sources, such as employment records, disease registries, and interviews with survivors. Only limited exposure information may be available, and duration of employment may have to be used as a surrogate for cumulative exposure. In the occupational setting, information on the jobs performed by each subject and the probable exposures within specific job categories is often available, as is information on cause of death. Exposure to multiple agents is the rule rather than the exception, so that the effect of single agents may be difficult to assess. Often, information on potential confounding factors, such as tobacco smoking, dietary habits and previous occupational exposures, is not available. In the absence of an identifiable unexposed comparison group, the incidence among cohort members is often compared to that in a reference population, which may be other workers or the regional or national population.

Occupational cohort studies are susceptible to a type of bias commonly called the healthy worker effect. If individuals with a particularly low risk of disease tend to be selected for employment, or if individuals with poor health terminate employment or are reassigned to jobs with low exposures, the estimated risks associated with employment may be biased downwards. This effect has received much attention in the literature (e.g. McMichael, 1976; Robins, 1986; Steenland & Stayner, 1991; Pearce, 1992). Various practical methods have been proposed to adjust for the effect (Pearce, 1992). A complete theoretical treatment of the problem has been given in a series of papers by Robins and colleagues (1986, 1989, 1992, 1994).

Three variants of the cohort study are worthy of mention, all three of which are based on special sampling from the cohort. With all three designs, information needs to be collected only on a small subset of individuals in the cohort, so that each method can lead to a substantial reduction in the cost of the cohort study. One is the case–control study nested within a cohort, sometimes called a nested case–control study. In this type of study, when a subject being followed up develops the disease, a random sample of controls is chosen from among individuals in the cohort who are "at risk" at that time, i.e. from among individuals who are free of disease at that time. Typically, from one to several controls are selected for each case. This approach is known as "riskset" or density sampling. Inferences regarding the association of the exposure with the disease are based on a comparison of exposures among cases and controls after adjustment for confounders. Multivariate methods based on the so-called relative risk regression models are generally used for analyses of the data. A second variant of the cohort study is the so-called case–cohort design (Prentice et al., 1986). In this design, a subcohort of individuals is chosen at the beginning of the study to serve as controls. Of course, individuals in this subcohort may themselves become cases. Inferences are based on a comparison of the exposure history of cases with those of the individuals within the subcohort who are disease-free at the time that the case occurs. An advantage of the case–cohort design over the nested case–control design is that the same group of controls can be used for multiple disease end-points. A third variant is the two-stage study. In this design, it is assumed that some, but not all, the desired exposure or confounder information is available on all cohort members. This full-cohort information is used to sample efficiently the remainder of the cohort to obtain further information (Breslow & Cain, 1988; Flanders & Greenland, 1991; Zhao & Lipsitz, 1992). All three of the designs usually focus on estimation of relative risk, but can be used to estimate incidence rates via special analytical methods.

Confounding can be addressed in cohort studies either by appropriate design strategies to prevent its occurrence or by the use of appropriate statistical techniques to control for it during analyses. If the study size is large enough, one of the best ways to prevent confounding by known and unknown confounders is to randomize individuals to either the intervention (exposed) or the control group. While this approach can and should be used with intervention and clinical trials, it cannot be used in a strictly observational study. An effective way to prevent confounding in cohort studies is by restriction. As Rothman (1986) points out "Confounding cannot occur if the potentially confounding variate is prohibited from varying." Therefore, if the admissibility criteria for the study allow only subjects at a single level of the potentially confounding variable, confounding by that variable will be avoided. For example, age is a confounder in a study of tobacco smoke and lung cancer. Confounding by age can be avoided, however, if the entire study is restricted to individuals in a single age group, where the age group is defined by a range of ages within which the incidence of lung cancer is reasonably homogeneous. Another method for the prevention of confounding is matching on potentially confounding variables.

Confounding can be controlled for during analyses of cohort studies either by stratification or by the use of multivariate statistical methods. In practice, both methods are often employed simultaneously. Stratification during analysis corresponds to the ideas of restriction and matching during design of the study. The data are stratified by level of a potential confounder, and analyses are conducted on each of the strata separately. While this is an effective way to control for confounding, the number of subjects in some of the strata may be too small for meaningful analyses. One way to get around this "sparse-data" problem is to use multivariate methods of analyses, which are briefly discussed below and in greater detail in Chapter 6. It should be kept in mind, however, that multivariate methods avoid the problems of sparse data by making explicit assumptions regarding the variation of disease risk by levels of the covariates entered into the analysis. The interpretation of the results of such analyses requires good judgement. For example, the method of Poisson regression is often used for analyses of cohort data. This method is based on the assumption that the logarithm of relative risk (associated with a particular covariate) is a linear function of the level of exposure. This assumption may not be correct and could lead to a distorted view of the true relationship between exposure and response.

3.4.2 Case–Control Studies

Better understanding of the methodology of the case–control study is certainly one of the most important developments in the observational study of diseases in populations. In the case–control study, data from cases of the disease under investigation and persons at risk of the disease (controls) are obtained and then analysed to yield effect estimates, usually relative risks. Thus, information is available on exposure conditional on disease status. The crucial observation that allows relative risks to be estimated from case–control studies is that the controls can serve as substitutes for the population denominators if they are sampled using the risk-set (density) method described earlier for nested case-control studies (Rothman & Greenland, 1997).

Consider a population of individuals that is being followed forward in time. Whenever the disease of interest occurs, information on the exposures under investigation and on potential confounding variables is obtained from the case and from randomly selected controls from the subcohort of individuals who are disease-free at that time. Of course, in practice, there is no follow-up of the cohort. Rather, all cases occurring during a given time period in a suitably defined population are identified. Matched controls, consisting of individuals who are disease-free at that time, are randomly chosen from the same population. Generally, between one and a few controls are chosen per case. Age is usually the most important matching variable, so that the ages of the controls fall in fairly narrow bands around the ages of the cases. Matching may also be used on other, potentially confounding, covariates. The larger the number of matching variables, the more difficult it is to find suitable controls, however. It is usually best to match on a few variables (age, sex and race, for example) and to control for potential confounding by other covariates by multivariate techniques during analysis. Information on exposures of interest is usually obtained by means of questionnaires administered by trained interviewers; see Chapter 4 and Breslow & Day (1980), Kelsey *et al.* (1996), and Rothman & Greenland (1997) for more details.

The main advantage of the case–control study over the cohort study is that the former can be completed with a much smaller expenditure of time and money. The disadvantages are that only a single disease can be investigated in a given study and, without ancillary information, the incidence of the disease in exposed and unexposed individuals cannot be estimated from the results of the study. Additionally, unbiased selection of controls to provide a representative profile of exposures in the general population can be difficult to achieve. The principal weakness of the case–control study is the quality of the exposure data. People's memory of past exposures may be inaccurate, and actual measurements of exposure may no longer be possible. Biases, such as recall bias (a case may remember events in the past differently from a control) and subconscious interviewer bias that results in the phrasing of questions or recording of answers differently for cases and controls must also be guarded against. Example of such biases in recent case–control studies are discussed by Johnson (1992). Methods of improving the accuracy of exposure data in case–control studies include blinding of interviewers to study hypotheses, use of supplementary data sources (e.g. historical records, interviews with relatives or colleagues) and simulations of exposure circumstances; see Chapter 4 and Armstrong *et al.* (1994) for more details.

Case–control studies provide an efficient means of identifying cancer hazards in human populations. Their role in the quantitative estimation and prediction of cancer risk is limited by the quality of the exposure data available. Sometimes, case–control studies record no more than the presence or absence of exposure. Where quantitative information on exposure is available, it is often relatively sparse, or subject to uncertainties associated with recall.

3.4.3 Ecological Studies

In both cohort and case–control studies, the unit of observation is the individual: exposure and covariate information is available on individuals in the study, and the outcome, whether it is the occurrence of disease or death, is also observed on individuals. During analyses, individuals with similar exposures and who developed disease at about the same age may be combined into strata, but persons in different exposure–disease categories (e.g. exposed and diseased, unexposed and diseased, etc.) remain separate.

In ecological studies, by contrast, the unit of observation is a group of people. Information on individuals is not available. Exposure is generally measured in terms of some overall index, such as the total number of cigarettes smoked or the amount of alcohol consumed, estimated from tax or other data. Outcomes are also measured on a group basis, generally in terms of the number of cases of a disease occurring in the group in a specified period of time. The numbers in each exposure–disease category remain unknown. Thus, the major problem in interpreting the results of an ecological study is that, because both exposure and outcome are measured at the group level, there is no assurance that the individuals who are exposed are actually those who develop the disease. Failure to account for this feature of the ecological study is often referred to as the ecological fallacy. Ecological studies also present special problems with respect to the control of confounding. In ecological studies, this is particularly difficult in the presence of non-linear effects, as has been illustrated by the analysis of ecological data relating to lung cancer risk, exposure to radon progeny, and cigarette smoking (Greenland & Robins, 1994). See Greenland & Morgenstern (1989) and Greenland & Robins (1994) for further details.

Despite their limitations, ecological studies have an important role to play in epidemiology.

They are inexpensive because they can usually be carried out with data available from public sources. For some exposures, individual data are simply too difficult to obtain with currently available monitoring technology. In some circumstances, individual exposures vary little, so that group-level data are suitable for epidemiological analysis. A good example on both counts is exposure to the various components of air pollution. Important insights into the adverse health effects of air pollution have been obtained from ecological studies (Dockery & Pope, 1994; Moolgavkar & Luebeck, 1996). In these studies, daily mortality counts or number of hospital admissions in a particular geographical area are regressed against levels of air pollution as measured at central monitoring stations in that area. Inferences regarding the association of air pollution with mortality, for example, depend upon relating fluctuations in daily mortality counts to levels of air pollution on the same or earlier days.

Ecological studies have been used to generate hypotheses which can subsequently be tested by cohort or case–control studies. For example, an intriguing finding is the strong correlation between cancer rates at several sites and total fat consumption. Thus Armstrong (1976) showed that rates of breast cancer, colon cancer and endometrial cancers in various populations were highly correlated with total fat consumption. These and similar observations led to case–control and cohort studies of the relation.

Ecological data can also be used to investigate time-trends in disease incidence, and to relate these time-trends to trends in exposure to risk factors thought to be associated with the disease. If the evolution of rates of a specific disease appears to follow changes in a known risk factor, then the search for other causes is not urgent. For example, Armstrong & Doll (1974) used graphical methods to conclude that the increase in bladder cancer mortality in English males born after 1870 can be attributed to cigarette smoking. On the other hand, if disease rates are increasing, and if the increase cannot be explained by changes in known risk factors, the search for new causes acquires greater urgency. For example, analyses using population fertility data have not convincingly demonstrated that trends in the incidence and mortality of female breast cancer are linked to changes in fertility (MacMahon, 1958; Armstrong, 1976; Hahn & Moolgavkar, 1989).

A specific type of time-trends analysis, sometimes called cohort analysis (or age–cohort–period analysis) has often been used in epidemiology. In this type of analysis, age-specific incidence rates of cancer (or other diseases) are modelled as functions of age, birth epoch and period of occurence of the disease (Roush et al., 1987). The goal of such analyses is to estimate separately the effects of age, birth cohort (epoch of birth) and calendar time (period of occurrence) on disease incidence rates. A serious problem with cohort analysis when all three factors—age, birth cohort and period—are included in the model is that the parameter estimates are not uniquely determined. When population-based information on specific risk factors is available, and these factors are known to have been introduced in a cohort-wise fashion or during specific time periods, then it may be possible to replace the non-specific cohort or period effects by modelled effects of the risk factors. This approach may alleviate the non-uniqueness problem just described. For example, the cigarette habit was taken up in England and Wales in a cohort-wise fashion. In an analysis of some smoking-related cancers in the English population, it was possible to replace non-specific cohort effects with smoking-specific effects, and to estimate relative risks associated with smoking for carcinomas of the lung, bladder and pancreas (Moolgavkar & Stevens, 1981; Stevens & Moolgavkar, 1984). The relative risks estimated in this fashion from ecological data were in good agreement with those obtained from case–control and cohort sudies. Unfortunately, the kind of information required for this approach is not often available.

3.5 Data analysis

The last quarter of a century, since the publication of Mantel & Haenszel's pioneering paper in 1959, has seen an explosion of statistical methodology in chronic disease epidemiology. The classical methods introduced in that paper, which are based on crude (unstratified) and stratified analyses of 2 by 2 contingency tables, have been supplemented by the introduction of multivariate methods, many of them based on an important paper by Cox (1972). Additionally, biologically based carcinogenesis models have been used for the analysis of cohort studies, but have seen only limited use in the analysis of case–control studies. For a discussion of the classical methods, see Breslow & Day (1980, 1987), Checkoway et al. (1989), Kelsey et al. (1996), and Rothman & Greenland (1997). Information on multivariate statistical models, including Poisson regression and relative risk regression, can be found in Chapter 6, and on biologically based models in Chapter 7.

3.6 Combined and meta-analysis

QEPs are conducted for the purpose of predicting the risk resulting from low levels of exposure to putative carcinogens in the environment. Much of the information on the magnitude of the risks associated with exposure, however, comes from studies of relatively high levels of exposure in settings that may not necessarily be relevant to environmental exposures, e.g. radiation exposures resulting from the atomic bombs in Hiroshima and Nagasaki or from radiotherapy. Risk following low-dose exposures can theoretically be assessed in two ways: (1) by prediction from studies of the effect of higher exposure levels, i.e. by low-dose extrapolation; or (2) by direct estimation from studies of populations receiving the low doses of concern. In the latter case, individual studies usually produce risk estimates too imprecise to be used for risk-management purposes.

Because studies of populations receiving low-level exposure provide the most direct assessment of the risk associated with such exposure, methods have been developed for combining the results of individual studies in order to enhance statistical power. Two approaches can be used: (1) meta-analyses, in which a single measure of effect is derived by combining measures of effect over studies; and (2) combined analyses, in which the original data of the studies are combined formally to obtain more precise estimates of effect. This latter approach allows a more thorough investigation of the comparability of the data being combined. Formal combined analyses are, however, considerably more costly and more time-consuming than meta-analyses, and are often impossible because raw data may not be available. Be that as it may, for

low-dose chronic exposures to carcinogenic agents, a careful large-scale combined analysis is probably the most useful tool for the direct estimation of risk and for testing the adequacy of extrapolations.

An excellent example of a formal combined analysis is provided by the recently completed international study of workers in the nuclear industry (Cardis et al., 1995). This study of mortality among nuclear industry workers in Canada, the United Kingdom, and the USA covered over 95 000 workers with over 2 000 000 person–years of observation, and was undertaken in order to obtain direct assessment of the carcinogenic effects of protracted low-level exposure to external, predominantly γ, radiation. Although the estimated risks of cancer following protracted exposure to low levels of γ radiation were lower in this study than those predicted by linear extrapolation from studies of atomic bomb survivors, they are compatible with a range of possibilities, from a reduction of risk at low doses, to risks twice those on which current radiation protection recommendations are based.

Much has recently been written on meta-analysis in epidemiology (Greenland, 1987; Fleiss & Gross, 1991; Dickersin & Berlin, 1992; MacClure, 1993; Greenland, 1994). The problems faced by the meta-analyst can be summed up in one word: heterogeneity. Whether it is heterogeneity in the probability of publication (publication bias), in the quality of studies, in the measures of exposures and response used, in the presence of factors modifying the effect of exposure on disease outcome, or in the control of confounders, the analyst has been warned in recent publications to guard against it. In the face of such heterogeneity and in the absence, often, of sufficient data to detect it, Greenland (1994) has suggested that an analytical approach that treats meta-analysis as a "study of studies" is vastly preferable to a synthetic approach, which attempts to arrive at a single estimate of risk derived from the studies considered. The two approaches are not mutually exclusive, however. Sometimes, after a careful review of the various studies, it may be possible to select a subset that satisfies some predetermined criteria of excellence, and arrive at a consensus estimate of risk from these studies, if there is no evidence of heterogeneity among the estimates of risk made in them. At the very least, meta-analysis should improve the quality of judgements in QEP of cancer risk, since it requires that comparisons and combinations of study findings be made in a structured and explicit fashion.

Meta-analyses for QEP present special problems. Because QEP is performed largely for purposes of risk management and the protection of public health, it may be appropriate to adopt a "risk-sensitive" approach, and allow some latitude in combining risk estimates from studies that appear to be discrepant. Often risk-management decisions must be taken even before it is firmly established that the agent under investigation is a human carcinogen. There are at least three distinct situations in which evidence from various studies may have to be combined, as follows:

1. The aim may be to determine whether an agent is a human carcinogen. For example, both the International Agency for Research on Cancer and the US Environmental Protection Agency place considerable weight on the epidemiological evidence in evaluating the carcinogenicity of an agent in human populations. In this case, the most stringent criteria should be applied in carrying out any kind of meta-analysis. Careful consideration should be given to the quality of individual studies and to the consistency of results from study to study. In short, the basic principles of meta-analysis summarized above should be adhered to. An example of such a meta-analysis is provided by a recent review of dioxin by the US Environmental Protection Agency. Epidemiological evidence of the carcinogenicity of dioxin was evaluated from occupational cohort studies, case–control studies of soft-tissue sarcomas and lymphomas, and from studies of populations exposed to dioxin as a result of industrial accidents or poisoning of food.

2. Sometimes adequate, or even compelling, human evidence is available that an agent is carcinogenic at high doses, but the effects at low doses are not well understood. Low-level

exposures to such agents are often ubiquitous, and control measures may therefore impose a large economic burden on society. Exposure to radon is an example of such an exposure. Although studies among miners, who are exposed to high levels of radon, leave little doubt that, at high doses, it is a human carcinogen, ecological and case–control studies of household radon and lung cancer have yielded inconsistent results. The challenge here is to use all the information in appropriately selected cohort and case–control studies to obtain an exposure–response curve for radon and lung cancer.

3. With most agents for which QEPs are required, little direct human evidence of carcinogenicity is available. Sometimes QEPs are required on closely related agents, and some information may be available for only one, or a few, of a group of agents. For example, the polycyclic aromatic hydrocarbons (PAHs) are a group of organic compounds that have been shown to be carcinogenic in experimental systems and are constituents of known human carcinogens, such as cigarette smoke. The carcinogenic potencies of the different PAHs are different, however. Similarly, a number of polychlorinated biphenyls (PCBs) are strong tumour promoters and are known to have dioxin-like effects on biological systems. Typically, human exposures occur, not to single compounds, but to mixtures of compounds. QEPs are then sometimes based on the concept ot toxicity equivalents, i.e. an easily measured biological end-point is used as a surrogate measure of carcinogenic potency. For example, with the dioxin-like PCBs, a toxicity equivalence factor (TEF) is estimated based on the efficiency, relative to dioxin, with which the agents induce the cytochrome P-450s. The carcinogenic potency of the mixture is then assumed to be directly proportional to the total TEF of the mixture. When some human data are available, one can use a Bayesian approach originally proposed by DuMouchel & Harris (1983), and used by the US National Academy of Sciences/National Research Council Committee on the Biological Effects of Ionizing Radiation (1988)

to estimate the risk of bone cancer in humans following exposure to two isotopes of plutonium.

3.7 Conclusions

The main strength of the epidemiological approach to QEP is the relevance of the investigated exposures and the unit of study to the ultimate purpose of QEP, which is the control of cancer-causing exposures in human populations. In epidemiological studies, the exposure circumstances and dose levels, although often not characterized in great detail, are commonly typical of the exposure situations relevant to human health and of concern to policy-makers.

The major problems of the epidemiological method are uncontrolled confounding and inaccuracy in the measurements of exposure. Various design and analytical strategies have been developed to address the first problem (confounding), as briefly discussed above. Measurement error is discussed in Chapter 4.

Free-living human populations are not homogeneous in their susceptibility to disease. Yet, every epidemiological study begins (wrongly) with the implicit assumption that, at least for the purposes of the study, populations can be divided into homogeneous subgroups. Later information may reveal that, in fact, the assumptions of homogeneity were unjustified. For instance, it is now becoming increasingly clear that interindividual variations in metabolic phenotype, as exemplified by debrisoquine metabolism and the rate of metabolism of aromatic amines (acetylator phenotype), greatly influence the risk associated with exposure to carcinogenic agents. Studies have shown approximately five-fold increases in lung cancer risk among extensive metabolizers of debrisoquine (Ayesh et al., 1984; Caporaso et al., 1990). Slow acetylators are at increased risk of bladder cancer (Mommsen et al., 1985). As information on interindividual variation in cancer risk becomes available, it can be used to quantify more accurately the risks in subpopulations. Immediate consequences of the heterogeneity of human populations are that estimates of risk derived from assumptions of homogeneity may not reflect true underlying risks in subpopulations and, moreover, estimates of risk derived in one population may not apply to another.

References

Armstrong, B. (1976) Recent trends in breast cancer incidence and mortality in relation to changes in possible risk factors. *Int. J. Cancer,* **17,** 204-211

Armstrong, B.K. (1977) The role of diet in human carcinogenesis with special reference to endometrial cancer. In: Hiatt, H.H., Watson, J.D. & Winsten, J.A., eds, *Origins of Human Cancer,* New York, NY, Cold Spring Harbor Laboratory, pp. 55-565

Armstrong, B. & Doll, R. (1974) Bladder cancer mortality in England and Wales in relation to cigarette smoking and saccharin consumption. *Br. J. Prev. Soc. Med.,* **28,** 233-240

Armstrong, B., White, E. & Saracci, R. (1994) *Principles of Exposure Measurement in Epidemiology.* (Monographs on Epidemiology and Biostatistics, Vol. 21), New York, Oxford University Press

Ayesh, R., Idle, J.R., Ritchie, J.C. & Crothers, M.J. (1984) Metabolic oxidation phenotypes as markers for susceptibility to lung cancer. *Nature,* **312,** 169-170

Benichou, J. (1991) Methods of adjustment for estimating the attributable risk in case–control studies: a review. *Stat. Med,* **10,** 1753-1773

Breslow, N.E. & Cain, K.C. (1988) Logistic regression for two-stage case–control data. *Biometrika,* **75,** 11-20

Breslow, N.E. & Day, N.E. (1980) *Statistical Methods in Cancer Research,* Vol. 1, *The Analysis of Case–control Studies* (IARC Scientific Publications No. 32), Lyon, International Agency for Research on Cancer

Breslow, N.E. & Day, N.E. (1987) *Statistical Methods in Cancer Research,* Vol. II, *The Design and Analysis of Cohort Studies* (IARC Scientific Publications No. 82), Lyon, International Agency for Research on Cancer

Bruzzi, P., Green, S.B., Byar, D.P., Brinton, L.A. & Schairer, C. (1985) Estimating the population attributable risk for multiple risk factors using case–control data. *Am. J. Epidemiol.,* **122,** 904-914

Caporaso, N.E., Tucker, M.A., Hoover, R.N., Hayes, R.B., Pickle, L.W., Issaq, H.J., Muschik, G.M., Green-Gallo, L., Buivys, D., Aisner, S. *et al.* (1990) Lung cancer and the debrisoquine metabolic phenotype. *J. Natl Cancer Inst.*, **82**, 1264-1272

Cardis, E., Gilbert, E.S., Carpenter, L., Howe, G., Kato, I., Armstrong, B.K., Beral, V., Cowper, G., Douglas, A., Fix, J. *et al.* (1995) Effects of low doses and low dose rates of external ionizing radiation: cancer mortality among nuclear industry workers in three countries. *Radiat. Res.*, **142**, 117-132

Checkoway, H., Pearce, N. & Crawford-Brown, D.J. (1989) *Research Methods in Occupational Epidemiology*, New York, NY, Oxford University Press

Cox, D.R. (1972) Regression models and life tables. *J. R. Stat. Soc. (B)*, **34**, 187-220

Cox, D.R. & Oakes, D. (1984) *Analysis of Survival Data* (Monographs on Statistics and Applied Probability 21), New York, NY, Chapman and Hall

Dickersin, K. & Berlin, J.A. (1992) Meta-analysis: state-of-the-science. *Epidemiol. Rev.*, **14**, 154-176

Dockery, D.W. & Pope, C.A., III. (1994) Acute respiratory effects of particulate air pollution. *Ann. Rev. Public Health*, **15**, 107-132

DuMouchel, W.H. & Harris, J.E. (1983) Bayes methods for combining the results of cancer studies in humans and other species. *J. Am. Stat. Assoc.*, **78**, 293-315

Flanders, W.D. & Greenlands, S. (1991) Analytic methods for two-stage case–control studies and other stratified designs. *Stat. Med.*, **10**, 729-747

Fleiss, J.L. & Gross, A.J. (1991) Meta-analysis in epidemiology, with special reference to studies of the association between exposure to environmental tobacco smoke and lung cancer: a critique. *J. Clin. Epidemiol.*, **44**, 127-139

Greenland, S. (1987) Quantitative methods in the review of epidemiologic literature. *Epidemiol. Rev.*, **9**, 1-30

Greenland, S. (1994) Invited commentary: A critical look at some popular meta-analytic methods. *Am. J. Epidemiol.*, **140**, 290-296

Greenland, S. & Drescher, K. (1993) Maximum likelihood estimation of the attributable fraction from logistic models. *Biometrics*, **49**, 865-872

Greenland, S. & Morganstern, H. (1989) Ecological bias, confounding, and effect modification. *Int. J. Epidemiol.*, **18**, 269-274

Greenland, S. & Robins, J. (1986) Identifiability, exchangeability, and epidemiological confounding. *Int. J. Epidemiol.*, **15**, 413-419

Greenland, S. & Robins, J. (1994) Invited commentary: Ecologic studies—biases, misconceptions and counterexamples. *Am. J. Epidemiol.* **139**, 747-759

Hahn, R.A. & Moolgavkar, S.H. (1989) Nulliparity, decade of first birth, and breast cancer in Connecticut cohorts, 1855 to 1945: An ecological study. *Am. J. Public Health*, **79**, 1503-1507

Johnson, E.S. (1992) Human exposure to 2,3,7,8-TCDD and risk of cancer. *Crit. Rev. Toxicol.*, **21**, 451-463

Kalbfleisch, J.D. & Prentice, R.L. (1980) *The Statistical Analysis of Failure Time Data* (Wiley Series in Probability and Mathematical Statistics), New York, NY, Wiley

Kelsey, J.L., Whittemore, A.S., Evans, A.S. & Thompson, W.D. (1996) *Methods in Observational Epidemiology*, 2nd ed. (Monographs in Epidemiology and Biostatistics, Vol. 26), New York, NY, Oxford University Press

Kleinbaum, D.G., Kupper, L.L. & Morgenstern, H. (1982) *Epidemiologic Research. Principles and Quantitative Methods*, New York, NY, Van Nostrand-Reinhold

Maclure, M. (1993) Demonstration of deductive meta-analysis: ethanol intake and risk of myocardial infarction. *Epidemiol. Rev.*, **15**, 328-351

MacMahon, B. (1958) Cohort fertility and increasing breast cancer incidence. *Cancer*, **11**, 250-254

Mantel, N. & Haenszel, W. (1959) Statistical aspects of the analysis of data from retrospective studies of disease. *J. Natl Cancer Inst.*, **22**, 719-748

McMichael, A.J. (1976) Standardized mortality ratios and the 'healthy worker effect': scratching beneath the surface. *J. Occup. Med.*, **18**, 165-168

Mommsen, S., Barfod, N.M. & Aagaard, J. (1985) *N*-acetyltransferase phenotypes in the urinary bladder carcinogenesis of a low-risk population. *Carcinogenesis*, **6**, 199-201

Moolgavkar, S.H. & Luebeck, E.G. (1996) A critical review of the evidence on particulate air pollution and mortality. *Epidemiology*, **7**, 420-428

Moolgavkar, S.H. & Stevens, R.G. (1981) Smoking and cancers of bladder and pancreas: risks and temporal trends. *J. Natl Cancer Inst.*, **67**, 15-23

Moolgavkar, S.H., Dewanji, A. & Luebeck, G. (1989) Cigarette smoking and lung cancer: rcanalysis of the British doctors' data. *J. Natl Cancer Inst.*, **81**, 415-420

Pearce, N. (1992) Methodological problems of time-related variables in occupational cohort studies. *Rev. Epidemiol. Santé Publique*, **40**, S43-S54

Prentice, R.L., Self, S.G. & Mason, M.W. (1986) Design options for sampling within a cohort. In: Moolgavkar, S.H. & Prentice, R.L., eds, *Modern Statistical Methods in Chronic Disease Epidemiology*, New York, NY, Wiley, pp. 50-62

Robins, J.M. (1986) A new approach to causal inference in mortality studies with a sustained exposure period—applications to control of the health workers survivor effect. *Math. Model.*, **7**, 1393-1512

Robins, J.M. (1989) The analysis of randomized and non-randomized AIDS treatment trials using a new approach to causal inference in longitudinal studies. In: Sechrest, L., Freeman, H. &

Mulley, A., eds, *Health Service Research Methodology: A Focus on AIDS*, Washington, DC, US Public Health Service, pp. 113-159

Robins, J.M. & Greenland, S. (1994) Adjusting for differential rates of prophylaxis therapy for PCP in high- versus low-dose AZT treatment arms in an AIDS randomized trial. *J. Am. Stat. Assoc.*, **89**, 737-749

Robins, J.M., Blevins, D., Ritter, G. & Wulfsohn, M. (1992) *G*-estimation of the effect of prophylaxis therapy for *Pneumocystis carinii* pneumonia on the survival of AIDS patients. *Epidemiology*, **3**, 319-336

Rothman, K.J. (1986) *Modern Epidemiology*, Boston, MA, Little, Brown

Rothman, K.J. & Greenland, S. (1997) *Modern Epidemiology*, 2nd ed., New York, NY, Lippincott-Raven

Roush, G.C., Holford, T.R., Schymura, M.J. & White, C. (1987) *Cancer Risk and Incidence Trends: The Connecticut Perspective*, New York, NY, Hemisphere

Steenland, K. & Stayner, L. (1991) The importance of employment status in occupational cohort mortality studies. *Epidemiology*, **2**, 418-423

Stevens, R.G. & Moolgavkar, S.H. (1984) A cohort analysis of lung cancer and smoking in British males. *Am. J. Epidemiol.*, **119**, 624-641

US National Academy of Sciences/National Research Council Committee on the Biological Effects of Ionizing Radiations (1988) *Health Risks of Radon and Other Internally Deposited Alpha Emitters*, BEIR IV, Washington, DC, National Academy Press

Wahrendorf, J. (1987) An estimate of the proportion of colo-rectal and stomach cancers which might be prevented by certain changes in dietary habits. *Int. J. Cancer*, **40**, 625–628

Zhao, L.P. & Lipsitz, S. (1992) Design and analysis of two-stage studies. *Stat. Med.*, **11**, 769–782

Quantitative Estimation and Prediction of Human Cancer Risks
S. Moolgavkar, D. Krewski, L. Zeise, E. Cardis and H. Møller
IARC Scientific Publications No. 131
International Agency for Research on Cancer, Lyon, 1999

4: Measurement of Exposure and Outcome in Epidemiological Studies used for Quantitative Estimation and Prediction of Risk

Bruce Armstrong and Paolo Boffetta

4.1 Introduction

Making the right measurements of the exposure (including agents confounded with it and modifiers of its effect) and of the outcome of interest (usually cancer, a preneoplastic lesion or another intermediate step between exposure and cancer), and making them accurately, are crucial to the valid quantitative estimation and prediction (QEP) of cancer risk. These requirements are the two sides of the same coin: if the right measurements are not made, the consequences for QEP will be the same as if inaccurate measurements are made: the dose–response relationship will be biased and predictions made from it may be far from the truth. They are both errors in measurement.

Theoretically, error in measurement of exposure and outcome will have similar effects on the dose–response relationship. In the simplest kind of study, investigating the association between a binary exposure variable and a binary outcome variable in the absence of confounding or other intervening variables, error in measurement of either the exposure or the outcome variable has the same effect on the estimate of association between exposure and outcome. In practice, however, the measurement of exposure is usually more complex than that of outcome, mainly because of the problem of measuring past exposures, the need to measure exposure to several agents (the agent of interest, confounders and effect modifiers), and the multiplicity of methods available to measure exposure. As a result, greater attention is usually paid to the correct measurement of exposure than to that of outcome. In addition, the study of the effect of exposure measurement error has presented more interesting theoretical problems than that of outcome measurement error, and has received more attention in the relevant literature.

In principle, error in the measurement of exposure is a concern only for observational research. Error in measurement of outcome, on the other hand, is probably of equal concern in both observational and experimental research. In well designed and conducted experiments, the exact exposure of each subject to the agent should be known and controlled by the investigator, and randomization should prevent confounding. In practice, it is usually desirable to measure key confounding variables and control for them in the analysis because of the possibility that, by chance, important confounding may be present. In addition, measurement error again becomes an issue when, in an experimental study, it is desirable to estimate exposure within the body at the level of the target tissue or target molecules. In these experimental situations, the problems and issues related to error in measurement of exposure are the same as they are in observational research.

In this chapter, we shall consider in detail aspects of the measurement of exposure from the perspective of observational epidemiological research; we shall outline the exposure measurements that should be made, the effects of error in exposure measurement on QEP, the prevention of error in exposure measurement and the control of its effects when it has not been prevented. These issues will also be considered in a more limited way for outcome measurement in epidemiological studies. The book *Principles of Exposure Measurement in Epidemiology* (Armstrong et al., 1992) is acknowledged as a major source of material for this chapter.

4.2 Making the right exposure measurements

4.2.1 Nature of exposure measurements

Exposure variables should be *specific* in the sense that they measure indivisible agents of exposure. Thus, for example, it is better to measure the different forms of tobacco smoking (cigarettes, pipes, cigars, etc.) separately than generically as "smoking". The dose–response relationship of smoking-related lung cancer differs by method of smoking (see, for example, Higgins *et al.*, 1988) and use of a non-specific variable will lead to a dose–response relationship that cannot readily be interpreted in terms of any individual exposure and therefore used to undertake specific QEP. Similarly, the exposure variables measured should permit the distinction of the exposure of interest from possibly confounding exposures. In this regard, it is relevant to note that, in evaluations of the evidence for the carcinogenicity of chemicals in humans made by the International Agency for Research on Cancer, the commonest reason for applying a "limited" or "inadequate" evidence classification was that exposure to the agent of interest had not been distinguished from exposure to other potentially carcinogenic agents in the environment in which it had occurred (Armstrong, 1985). If such data cannot support qualitative assessment of risk, they will be even less useful for QEP.

The exposure variables should also be *sensitive* in the sense that they include all ways by which subjects may be exposed to the agent of interest. For example, in examining the relationship between environmental tobacco smoke (passive smoking) and lung cancer a number of studies in non-smoking women have used the spouses smoking habits as the sole exposure variable. This variable excludes home exposures prior to marriage, home exposures other than to the spouse's smoke, and workplace, social and other exposures outside the home at any time. The importance of multiple sources of exposure to environmental tobacco smoke has been shown in recall of lifetime exposure (Cummings *et al.*, 1989) and in comprehensive analyses of the determinants of current exposure (Coghlin *et al.*, 1989; Riboli *et al.*, 1990). A complete history of exposure is necessary, therefore, to obtain accurate measurements of exposure to environmental tobacco smoke. Variation in the error caused by incomplete (or insensitive) measurement of passive smoking may explain some of the variation in the strength of the relationship that has been observed between it and lung cancer in non-smoking women (see, for example, Garfinkel, 1981; Hirayama, 1981). More recent studies have attempted more comprehensive coverage of passive exposure to tobacco smoke (see, for example, Fontham *et al.*, 1991; Stockwell *et al.*, 1992).

4.2.2 Measurement of dose

For QEP, the dose should be measured in quantitative terms, preferably as a dose rate (rather than the dose accumulated over, e.g. the whole of the period of exposure), in the most fundamental units in which the agent is usually measured. For example, to obtain an accurate quantitative measure of dose of the combined oral contraceptive pill, a complete history covering the nature and period of use of each kind of pill used should be obtained. Provided the exact formulations are identified (and this is not impossible; UK National Case–Control Study Group, 1989), not only can use of combined oral contraceptives be measured in terms of, say, years of use but also in actual weights of the oestrogenic and progestagenic components consumed. Information on dose rate would allow measurement of intake in specific periods of time within the whole exposure period (see below).

A number of levels at which dose may be measured are important to QEP (Figure 4.1). The *exposure*, sometimes called the available dose, is measured in the environment external to the subject, e.g. the concentration of asbestos fibres per ml of ambient air over a small time interval. The exposure is often the measurement used for regulatory purposes, and may therefore be the quantity most relevant to QEP. It does not usually coincide with the *administered dose* or intake, i.e. the actual amount of the agent coming into contact with the human body. How much of the exposure becomes administered dose depends on the subject's physiology and behaviour, e.g. the respiratory volume at rest and during activity and the quantities of food, drinks, and medications actually ingested. From a biological viewpoint, even the administered dose can usually only be regarded as a proxy measurement of the *absorbed dose* or uptake, i.e. the dose that actually enters the body.

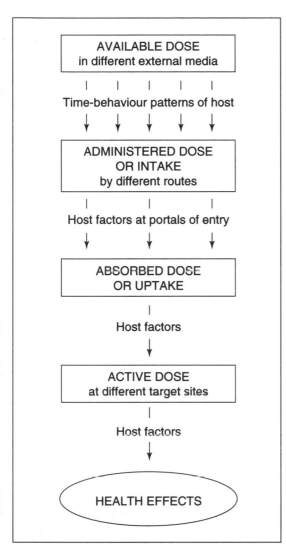

Figure 4.1. Levels at which dose may be measured

The absorbed dose, in turn, is a proxy for the dose that really matters in terms of causing the disease, the *active or biologically effective dose* at the sites in the body (organs, tissues, cells, molecules) which are the specific targets of action of the agent.

It could be argued that, for accurate quantitative estimation of risk, the most appropriate dose to measure would be the biologically effective dose at the level of interaction with the cellular targets (e.g. specific DNA adducts or exposure-specific mutations) because it is measured after all preceding sources of variation (environmental conditions influencing available dose, behaviours affecting the administered dose, physiological factors affecting the absorbed dose and metabolic factors affecting the active dose) have been taken into account. On the other hand, available dose is the measurement most commonly (although not invariably) subject to public health regulation and therefore the one for which QEP is required. There is, then, a conflict between what might be best for estimation and what is needed for prediction.

If, as may be hoped, measurements of biologically effective dose are able to fulfill their promise as accurate, quantitative predictors of risk of human cancer, at least in some circumstances, it may be that measurement of the biologically effective dose of some agents in exposed humans may become the most appropriate variable for public health regulation. In the meantime, it will still be important to strive for accurate measurement of available dose as well as to develop and evaluate the predictive capacities of absorbed and biologically effective doses and to understand better the relationships between these various levels of dose.

4.2.3 Measurement of variation in exposure with time

As far as possible, each exposure should be characterized by when it first began, when it finally ended (if at all), and how the dose rate varied during the period of exposure. The time relationships of exposure are important for several reasons. Thus, duration of exposure is a critical determinant of the total amount of exposure that has occurred. Then, for a cancer occurring at a particular time, there exists a "critical" (or effective) time window (the aetiologically relevant exposure period) during which exposure can be relevant to its causation (Rothman, 1981). Inclusion of exposure outside that time window will lead to error in the exposure measurement (a case of non-specificity in the terms outlined above), and therefore to error in the estimation of dose–response. We do not generally know when the effective time window for exposure occurred for any particular exposure–cancer combination. The matter is further complicated by the possibility of multiple effective time windows for an agent when, for example, it has both early- and late-stage effects. For epithelial cancers, it has been commonly assumed that the effective time window was at least 10 years ago, and exposure in the last 10 or so years is therefore excluded from the analysis. This approach ignores late-stage effects. An alternative approach, such as that exemplified by the "serially additive expected dose model" (Smith *et al.*, 1980), may be used to seek the location of the effective time window empirically. This allows for the possibility that more than one such time window will be found. Full data on the time relationships of exposure may allow the construction of more complete and potentially more informative mechanistic exposure–response models for QEP than are currently available (see Chapter 6).

Finally, pattern of exposure during the exposure period may also be important. For example, to explain the apparently anomalous occurrence of a higher incidence of malignant melanoma of the skin in indoor workers than in outdoor workers, it was postulated that a particular total dose of sunlight may be more effective in causing melanoma if it is received intermittently or irregularly rather than frequently or continuously (Holman *et al.*, 1983). There is empirical evidence supporting this hypothesis (Armstrong, 1988). Unless such pattern effects are taken into consideration, QEP may produce misleading results.

Measurement of duration, dose rate, and pattern of exposure will permit the maximum flexibility in defining exposure in a biologically relevant way when analysing the relationship between exposure and disease. Alternatively, if there is no prior hypothesis regarding which representation of dose and time would be the most appropriate, the representation that best predicts disease incidence may then be sought empirically. In practice, however, it may be difficult to distinguish between different, possibly appropriate representations of dose, especially when many different characteristics of dose are included in statistical dose–response models.

Lee-Feldstein (1989) has given an example of an empirical search for the most appropriate representation of dose in relation to time. She examined the quantitative relationships between exposure to arsenic in a copper smelter and risk of lung cancer in two cohorts of men, one first employed before 1925 and the other employed between 1925 and 1947. Exposure was defined in terms of job with maximum exposure to arsenic (a "peak" exposure definition), cumulative exposure based on arithmetic or geometric mean levels of arsenic in specific job areas, and time-weighted average exposures based on arithmetic or geometric means. Analyses were carried out with and without exclusion of exposure in the last 10 years before death. Table 4.1 shows the results obtained for both cohorts with three different definitions of expo-

---

Table 4.1 Relationship of risk of lung cancer with arsenic exposure under different definitions of exposure in two cohorts of copper smelters[a]

Definition of exposure	First cohort			Second cohort		
	$\hat{\beta}$[b]	SE of $\hat{\beta}$[b]	Likelihood ratio statistic for $\beta = 0$	$\hat{\beta}$[b]	SE of $\hat{\beta}$[b]	Likelihood ratio statistic for $\beta = 0$
Maximum exposure category	0.55	0.13	18.5	0.30	0.14	4.5
Cumulative exposure	0.68×10^{-4}	0.20×10^{-4}	10.4	0.65×10^{-4}	0.34×10^{-4}	3.2
Time-weighted average exposure	0.026	0.0075	10.8	0.021	0.0075	7.0

[a] Based on data from Lee-Feldstein (1989).
[b] $\hat{\beta}$ = estimated logistic regression coefficients for models in which each variable was fitted as a continuous variable. SE = standard error.

sure. The cumulative and time-weighted average exposures shown are those based on the arithmetic means since they gave slightly higher likelihood ratio statistics than those based on geometric means. In the first cohort, using the likelihood ratio statistic in each case as a criterion, maximum exposure statistically showed the strongest association with lung cancer, whereas time-weighted average and cumulative exposure were similar in their association. In the second cohort, however, the time-weighted average appeared to be more strongly associated with lung cancer than cumulative exposure, and the maximum exposure category was intermediate between the two. It appears, in this case, that some measure of intensity of exposure over time was important in determining risk. The values in Table 4.1 were little affected by removing the last 10 years of exposure from the exposure estimates.

With respect to time, it is relevant to note that some measurement instruments relate only to comparatively short periods of exposure and are therefore of limited use for QEP of cancer, unless multiple measurements can or have been taken over the aetiologically relevant exposure period or exposure can be considered to be reasonably constant over time. For example, measurement of the concentration of asbestos fibres in air relates, strictly speaking, only to the period of time over which the air sample was taken, measurement of urinary cotinine reflects exposure to tobacco smoke only within the past 3–4 days (Riboli *et al.*, 1990), and measurement of adducts of aflatoxin B_1 with serum albumin reflects intake of aflatoxin B_1 over the preceding several weeks to a few months (Wild *et al.*, 1990). Unless records exist, such measurements may be of little value in documenting exposure in a case–control study of cancer in which the aetiologically relevant exposure period may have been 20 or 30 years ago. Similarly, they are of limited value in prospective cohort studies unless they are repeated at intervals during the follow-up period. If repeated, they could provide the best possible data on dose rate and pattern of exposure obtainable. Such data, however, may bring additional problems, such as the non-independence of the multiple measures in any individual and the possibility that the errors in measurement may vary with time, e.g. because of changes in the technology used.

Methods that purport to be able to measure exposure over long periods of time also have limitations. First, even if accurate (as, for example, measurements of UV-specific mutations of the *p53* gene in normal skin might be for UV exposure; Nakazawa *et al.*, 1994), they may provide information on cumulative exposure only and tell us nothing about dose rate and pattern of exposure. Second, when based on human recall, as commonly they must be, they are usually of uncertain, if not doubtful, accuracy.

4.3 Effects of exposure measurement error on QEP

Measurement error can be simply conceived as follows:

$$X_i = T_i + b + E_i$$

where the observed measure, X_i, differs from the true value T_i by the systematic error or bias, b, which occurs, on average, in the measurements of all measured subjects, and the non-systematic error, E_i, that varies unpredictably from subject to subject (Armstrong *et al.*, 1992). X, T, and E are variables with distributions; their expectations are denoted by μ_X, μ_T and μ_E and their variances by σ^2_X, σ^2_T and σ^2_E respectively. Because the average measurement error in X is expressed as a constant, b, it follows that μ_E, the population mean of the non-systematic measurement error, is assumed to be zero.

When two or more groups of subjects are being compared, measurement error can be either differential or non-differential. It is differential if the value of b (the bias) differs between the groups or if the precision of X (the observed measurements) differs between the groups (due to differences between the groups in the value of σ^2_E), or if both are true. If neither is true, the error is non-differential.

4.3.1 Effect of exposure measurement error on the dose–response relationship

The effect of error in the measurement of the primary exposure on the empirical dose–response relationship depends on (i) the type of study, namely whether it is analytical (cohort or case–control) or ecological; (ii) the type of measurement, namely whether it is continuous or categorical; and (iii) whether the error is differential or non-differential.

4.3.1.1 Analytical epidemiological studies

In general terms, it can be said that, when a continuously distributed measure of exposure is related to disease outcome in a logistic model and there is differential error in measurement of the exposure, the observable odds ratio (OR_O) for the disease, per unit of exposure, bears no predictable relationship to the true odds ratio (OR_T). In other words, it may be closer to the null value, further from the null value, or on the other side of the null value (e.g. below 1.0 instead of above 1.0) from the true value.

If error in measurement of a continuous variable is non-differential its effects may be more predictable. If it is assumed that the degree of measurement error is uncorrelated with the true value of the measurement and the true values are normally distributed and have the same variance in subjects with and without disease, it can be shown that non-differential error in exposure measurement causes flattening of the curve of the relationship of the odds ratio with exposure towards the null value (odds ratio constant at 1.0 with increasing exposure; see Figure 4.2). The relationship between the observable logistic regression coefficient, β_O (which is related to the observable odds ratio for u units of exposure as follows, $OR_O = \exp(\beta_O u)$, is:

$$\beta_O = \rho^2_{TX}\beta_T$$

In this expression, T and X are the true and observed values of the measurement, respectively, and ρ is the coefficient of correlation of T with X, the validity coefficient, and β_T is the true logistic regression coefficient. Thus β_O, and therefore OR_O, falls as the value of ρ falls. For example, when ρ has a value of 0.5, an OR_T of 2.0 for one unit of exposure is attenuated substantially to an OR_O of 1.19.

When the assumptions of the preceding paragraph are not true, the odds ratio curve shown in Figure 4.2 can take a variety of shapes including convex upwards, convex downwards with the lowest odd ratios falling below the null value, or even sigmoid.

When the exposure variable is categorical, the effects of measurement error on the exposure–disease and dose–response relationships

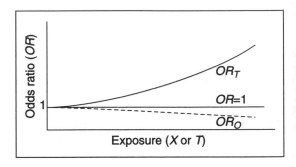

Figure 4.2. Relationship between observable logistic regression coefficient and true logistic regression coefficient for different values of true and observed measurement (see text for details)

are analogous to those when the variable is continuous. If there is differential error in measurement, the observable odds ratio (or odds ratios if there are more than two exposure categories) may bear almost any relationship to its true value.

If there is non-differential measurement error, the effect depends on whether there are two or more than two exposure categories. When there are two exposure categories, OR_O will be biased towards the null value relative to OR_T but will not cross over the null value provided that the measurement classifies a truly exposed person as exposed with the same or a greater probability than it classifies a truly unexposed person as exposed.

The position is more complex and less predictable when there are more than two exposure categories (Birkett, 1992). Briefly, when risk of disease truly increases monotonically with increasing exposure, the OR_O for the most extreme exposure category will always be biased towards the null while that for intermediate categories may be biased away from it. Values of OR_O for lower levels of exposure can cross over the null value, and all values of OR_O can be so biased that the apparent direction of the relationship can be reversed. If it is assumed that misclassification occurs only between adjacent exposure categories, the overall direction of the relationship cannot be reversed. However, OR_O for the lowest category can cross over the null, and a monotonic dose–response relationship may thus appear as a U- or J-shaped curve.

4.3.1.2 Ecological studies

The effect of measurement error on dose–response estimation in ecological studies has only recently been considered (Brenner *et al.*, 1992). For an ecological study in which exposure was measured by the proportion of individuals in each population who were exposed, it was shown that bias in estimated relative risks was always away from, rather than towards the null value and that the bias could be quite large. It appears, however, that when the exposure of each population is estimated by a single common measure (e.g. area air pollution), as would be the most useful for the quantitative estimation of risk, the bias would usually be towards the null value (Brenner *et al.*, 1992). This case, however, has not been rigorously worked out.

4.3.2 Measurement error in confounding

Error in the measurement of a confounding variable influences the results of statistical control of the effects of this variable on the dose–response relationship of the primary exposure variable with disease.

4.3.2.1 Analytical epidemiological studies

When the confounder is measured with non-differential error and the exposure is measured perfectly, the effects of the confounder will be incompletely controlled and the effects of the exposure, independent of the confounder, will appear greater or smaller than they really are, depending on the direction of confounding. When the exposure is measured with non-differential error and the confounder is measured perfectly, the adjusted disease–exposure association may be biased towards the null value to an even greater degree than the crude association. When both are measured with error, the adjusted disease–exposure association may, with reference to the true disease–exposure association, be biased towards or away from the null.

4.3.2.2 Ecological studies

Confounding in ecological studies is more complex than in analytical studies, its effects are potentially much greater, and its control more difficult (Greenland & Morgenstern, 1989; Greenland, 1992). The effects of error in the measurement of confounders on the results of ecological studies has not been described.

4.3.3 Example of effects of exposure measurement error on QEP

Much work has been carried out to evaluate and take into account sources of systematic and random error in the radiation dosimetry of the atomic bomb survivors. Around 1986, a new dosimetry system, "DS86", was introduced to replace the dose estimates, referred to as "T65D", which had previously been used for risk estimation in studies of atomic bomb survivors. Correlations of doses with chromosome aberration data indicate that DS86 doses are more accurate than T65D doses, particularly for some groups of survivors with complicated shielding patterns. DS86 doses were estimated for a number of specific target organs and are also more accurate than T65D doses, which were based only on the application of a set of organ transfer factors. Overall, DS86 neutron doses were less than the corresponding T65D ones. DS86 doses from γ-rays, however, were generally larger than the corresponding T65D ones, the difference increasing with distance from the epicentre and varying with the characteristics of shielding, irrespective of whether the survivor was a child or an adult at the time of the bombing and the target organ.

The introduction of DS86 in risk estimates coincided with a change in the risk models used to estimate and predict risk from data on atomic bomb survivors and with the analysis of extended follow-up data. The results of the life-span study follow-ups (Preston *et al.*, 1987; Shimizu *et al.*, 1990) are therefore not strictly comparable. However, Preston & Pierce (1988) carried out analyses to evaluate the impact of the change in dosimetry on risk estimates. Their results indicate that the improvement in the accuracy of the dose estimate resulted in a 75–85% increase in estimates of radiation-induced mortality from leukaemia and from all other cancers.

Following this, methods were developed (Pierce *et al.*, 1990, 1992) to adjust risk estimates for the biases resulting from random errors in individual dose estimates. The magnitude of the random errors varied with dose, being greatest for survivors with doses above 4 Gy. It was concluded that random errors of 30–40% can lead to underestimation of the risk of solid cancers by 7–11% and of leukaemia by 4–7%.

The adequacy of neutron dosimetry, particularly in Hiroshima, has recently been questioned (Straume *et al.*, 1992). It appears that DS86 does not fully account for the neutrons probably present at Hiroshima, particularly at the greater distances, and additional work will need to be carried out to improve the dosimetry.

4.3.4 Conclusions

Error in measurement of exposure can have substantial and largely unpredictable effects on the direction and shape of dose–response relationships. The consequences of exposure measurement error for QEP are potentially serious, therefore, unless the effects of error can be controlled or error can be prevented from occurring in the first place.

4.4 Prevention of exposure measurement error

To the extent that an economically and logistically feasible way exists to achieve the prevention of errors in measurements of the primary exposure and potential confounders, this is the best way to control the effects of measurement error and therefore to minimize its effects on QEP. There are two general approaches to the prevention of measurement error: (i) quality in the design of measurement instruments; and (ii) quality control in making and using measurements.

4.4.1 Quality in the design of measurement instruments

Instruments for measuring exposure to carcinogens for the purposes of QEP should be designed to make the right measurements accurately. There are few general prescriptions for accuracy at the design stage as its determinants vary from one kind of measurement instrument to another. The removal of human subjectivity, however, is a desirable characteristic of all measurement processes. In the administration of a questionnaire by interview, for example, this will require the use of carefully trained interviewers, a highly structured questionnaire, and keeping the interviewers ignorant, in the specific situation, of whether they are interviewing a person with or without disease or with or without exposure. In laboratory measurements on environmental or biological samples, it will require the processing of all samples without those concerned knowing whether they come from subjects with or without disease.

Some specific procedures for ensuring high quality in the design of instruments for the field collection of epidemiological data, including the collection of biological samples, are summarized in Table 4.2.

Table 4.2 Quality in the design of measurement procedures for the collection of data on exposure in epidemiological studies[a]

Design of forms:

Include all items needed to compute dose, timing of exposure, etc.

Include adequate subject identifiers—at least an identity number and a check digit or alphabetic code on all forms

Use separate forms for each method of exposure measurement

Make instructions clear and data collection items unambiguous

Use different typefaces for instructions, data collection items and responses

Provide mutually exclusive and exhaustive response categories for closed-ended items

Make forms self-coding for simple items, e.g. data collector circles a number corresponding to the appropriate response category

Make response codes consistent within and across forms, e.g. 1 = yes, 2 = no

Provide for coding without loss of information, i.e. do not design forms so that continuous data are categorized at the coding stage

---

Table 4.2 (Contd) Quality in the design of measurement procedures for the collection of data on exposure in epidemiological studies[a]

Design of forms (contd):

Do not require computation by data collectors, rather make provision on the form for entry of raw data into the computer

Design forms for direct entry of data into the computer

Design of specimen collection:

Design procedures for specimen collection, identification, transport and storage in consultation with specialists in the laboratory procedures

Study procedures manual:

Always have a study procedures manual

Include at least the following in the study procedures manual:

* *Description of the study in general terms*
* *Sample selection, recruitment and tracking procedures*
* *Data forms*
* *General methods of data collection*
* *Item by item clarification of questions and responses on forms and questionnaire, including special cases*
* *Detailed procedures for the collection of biological samples*
* *Editing procedures*
* *Coding instructions for items not self-coded on form*
* *Codebooks*

Update manual and distribute updated pages whenever procedural changes are made

Pretesting instruments:

Have instruments reviewed by other researchers

Pretest instruments on samples of convenience

Train data collectors and pretest instruments on samples similar to study subjects

Identify problems through feedback from pretested subjects and data collectors and by monitoring data collection (e.g. observing interviews, reabstracting records) and make appropriate changes as early as possible

Review frequencies of responses to identify items with little variation in responses

Modify instrument

Pretesting instruments:

Discuss importance of complete and accurate data

Review study manual

Practise data collection

Monitor initial data collection by each data collector

Resolve problems

[a] Source: Armstrong *et al.,* (1992)

4.4.2 Quality control in making and using measurements

The most important steps in quality control in making and using measurements are ensuring that the measurement procedures are written down, that specific quality-control measures form part of these procedures, and that all staff involved in making measurements are adequately trained. Table 4.3 summarizes specific quality-control procedures in the field collection, processing and statistical analysis of epidemiological data. Some major aspects of quality control in the laboratory analysis of biological or environmental samples collected as part of an epidemiological study are also listed. More comprehensive coverage of quality control in analytical laboratories can be found in Westgard & Klee (1986) and Copeland (1989).

Table 4.3 Quality control in making and using exposure measurements in epidemiological studies[a]

QUALITY CONTROL DURING DATA COLLECTION

Supervision of data collectors:

Assign cases and controls in a case–control study (or exposed and unexposed subjects, where this is known in advance, in a cohort study) in the same proportion to each data collector

Maintain ignorance of data collectors to case–control (exposed-unexposed) status of subjects, as far as possible

Replicate some proportion of data collection (e.g. 10% of subjects) to identify fictitious data, items with poor reliability, data collectors with errors on certain items, etc.

Compare the distribution of study variables among data collectors

Compare distributions of study variables over time

Address problems identified through monitoring immediately with the relevant data collector(s)

Conduct staff meetings for retraining, discussion of problems and motivation

Editing and coding:

Have data collectors edit data forms immediately to clarify responses and check for missing items

Have supervisor perform a second edit soon after data collection to check for missing items, inadmissible codes, inconsistencies among responses, illegible responses, etc.

Have editor code open-ended questions and query those inadequately answered

Correct errors by call back to subjects (or check-backs to records)

Have one staff member maintain an editors' log to ensure consistency of recording and coding of unanticipated responses, and to record comments and responses coded as "other"

Handling and analysis of biological samples:

Ensure as far as possible that samples are collected at around the same time from matched subjects with and without disease, or numerically balanced samples of subjects with and without disease, so that their storage and analysis times can be similar

Record time and conditions of collection, initial storage, transport, entry into secondary storage, and removal for laboratory processing. review periodically and investigate reasons for departure from agreed standards

Reasons should be given by the laboratory for rejection of samples as unacceptable and investigated in case they point to errors in collection, storage and transport procedures that can be corrected

Table 4.3 (Contd) Quality control in making and using exposure measurements in epidemiological studies[a]

Handling and analysis of biological samples (contd):

Ensure, as far as possible, that matched subjects with and without disease, or numerically balanced samples of subjects with and without disease, are included in each batch of laboratory analyses

Undertake all laboratory analyses without knowledge of which samples come from subjects with and without disease

Implement local, within-batch quality control and standardization procedures according to best laboratory practise. Optimally, participate also in a programme of external standardization of the analyses. If reference sample are not available, assay blind duplicates of some samples in the same batch and in different batches

QUALITY CONTROL DURING DATA PROCESSING

Key entry:

Create a codebook with format and code of "raw" data

Enter data contemporaneously with data collection

Double enter (verify) all data

Edit data by computer by performance of range and logic checks contemporaneously with data entry

Correct errors and feed back findings of relevance to data collection

Creation of new variables:

Check and recheck the programming code used to create new variable

Check the correctness of new variables by manual computation from a sample of original records, whenever reasonably possible

Review distributions of original and created variables

Create a codebook with detailed descriptions of new variables created including original variables and programming code used to create them

[a]　Source: Armstrong et al., (1992)

4.4.3 Other factors

Much good advice can be given about the prevention of error in measurement of exposure and it is self-evident that at least some of the procedures proposed above will lead to its reduction. How free from error measurements may become when all of these procedures are adopted will depend very much on the exposure being measured and the options available for its measurement.

Some exposures, such as the smoking of cigarettes, are comparatively easy to measure. This is so because, traditionally, cigarette smoking has been a habit commenced in youth and indulged in more or less continuously until the habituee relinquishes it, usually in middle life, or dies. Its adoption and relinquishment are important events and are therefore easily remembered. Moreover, the number of cigarettes smoked per day is reasonably constant and also easily remembered because the smoker must regularly purchase fresh supplies. However, while empirical data indicate that cigarette consumption is recalled well if constant, it may be recalled with bias if consumption has changed (Persson & Norell, 1989). Prospectively collected data on cigarette consumption have been used to produce plausible QEPs (see, e.g. Doll & Peto, 1978; Doll et al., 1994).

However, the measurement of cigarette smoking and, in particular, the consequential exposure to carcinogens, has become more complicated over the past 30 years because of changes resulting from concerns about the health effects of smoking. The use of filter cigarettes has become almost universal in industrialized countries, cigarettes that deliver smaller amounts of tar have been designed and their use has increased substantially. Thus, to estimate the intake of tar from tobacco smoke retrospectively now requires that smokers recall when they took up the use of filter cigarettes and the brands that they smoke—a rather more demanding task. Smokers may now also tend to underestimate their cigarette consumption because of social disapproval of their habit. While none of these problems is insurmountable, it is now more difficult to obtain an accurate measure of intake of tobacco smoke carcinogens (a complex mixture for which simple cigarette consumption was a proxy) than it used to be.

Some other exposures are extremely difficult to measure no matter how carefully they are approached. For example, dietary intake of sodium cannot be measured accurately by any form of dietary assessment except the observation, weighing and sampling, for analysis, of all food eaten in some defined period of time. Much simpler than this, although by no means easy, is the measurement of urinary sodium excretion which, if carried out over 14 periods of 24 h, provides a reasonably accurate reflection of present sodium intake (Liu et al., 1979). Neither of these approaches can provide a measure of anything other than present intake of sodium unless repeated. Thus accurate retrospective measurement of individual intake of sodium for, say, a case–control study of cancer of the stomach (with which it may be associated) must be considered to be impossible unless it can be assumed that dietary sodium intake is reasonably constant over time. This assumption is unlikely to be true.

Between these two extremes lie most other exposures of interest in quantitative estimation and prediction of risk of cancer. All are measured with some error. Thus steps must be taken to control the effects of the error or it will influence the results of QEP.

4.5 Control of the effects of exposure measurement error

Issues relating to the control of the effects of exposure measurement error have been discussed by Willett (1989). There are three possible approaches to control when measurement error has not been prevented (Greenland & Robins, 1985; Armstrong et al., 1992): (i) the use of multiple measures of exposure; (ii) the adjustment of study results for the effects of measurement error; and (iii) in some circumstances, adjustment in the analysis for a covariate which is related in some way to the occurrence of error in the exposure measurement. In principle, each of these approaches can produce a more accurate representation of the dose–response relationship and therefore allow more accurate QEP.

4.5.1 Multiple measures of exposure

The average or some other combination of the information in multiple measures of the same exposure for each individual in an analytical study (or population in an ecological study) is, in principle, a more accurate measure of exposure than a single measurement because of reduction in within-subject variability (Marshall, 1989; Brenner & Blettner, 1993). The multiple measures may be either repeated measures using the same (e.g. repeated collection of dietary diaries over a one-year period) or different instruments (e.g. a combination of measurements from a food frequency questionnaire and a period of collection of dietary diaries). There may be no advantage and may even be a disadvantage in the latter approach if one of the two instruments is substantially less accurate than the other. The average of the two measurements may then be less accurate than the measurement with the more accurate instrument.

The use of multiple measures of exposure is most unlikely to fully control the effects of measurement error. In the case of repeated applications of the same instrument, for example, no correction will be obtained for bias in measurements or in error which differs between subjects with and without disease. While some correction of both may be achieved if two different measurement instruments are used, full correction will only be possible if both instruments were perfect in the first place or had had exactly opposite biases, which is highly unlikely.

4.5.2 Adjustment of study results for the effects of measurement error

Table 4.4, taken from Armstrong *et al.* (1992), gives equations expressing the true logistic regression coefficients or odds ratios in terms of their observable values and exposure measurement error. In principle, these equations can be used to estimate the true values given the observed values and estimates of the error expressed in appropriate terms. Estimates of the error can be obtained by means of a validity study in a sample of the subjects in the epidemiological study.

Table 4.4. Equations for the true measure of association as a function of the observable measure of association and the exposure measurement error[a]

Equation[b]	Type of error
Continuous exposure, dichotomous outcome:	
$\beta_T = 1 - \left\lfloor \dfrac{b_D - b_N}{\mu_{X_D} - \mu_{X_n}} \right\rfloor \dfrac{\beta_O}{\rho^2_{TX}}$	Differential
$\beta_T = \beta_O / \rho^2_{TX}$	Non-differential
$OR_T = OR_O^{1/\rho^2_{TX}}$	Non-differential
Continuous exposure, continuous outcome:	
$\beta_T = \beta_O / \rho^2_{TX}$	Non-differential
Dichotomous exposure, dichotomous outcome:	
$OR_T = \dfrac{P_D(1 - P_N)}{P_N(1 - P_D)}$	Differential or non-differential
where $P_D = (p_D - 1 + \text{spec}_D)/(\text{sens}_D + \text{spec}_D - 1)$	
and $P_N = (p_N - 1 + \text{spec}_N)/(\text{sens}_N + \text{spec}_N - 1)$	

[a] Source: Armstrong *et al.* (1992).
[b] β_T and β_O are true and observable logistic regression coefficients, OR_T and OR_O are true and observable odds ratios, b_D and b_N are bias in the observable measurements in diseased (D) and non-diseased (N) subjects, μ_{X_D} and μ_{X_N} are expectations of the observable measurements in diseased and non-diseased subjects, ρ_{TX} is the correlation between the true and observable measurements (the validity coefficient), p_D and p_N are the observable proportions exposed in diseased and non-diseased subjects, spec_D and spec_N are the specificities of the observable measurements in diseased and non-diseased subjects, and sens_D and sens_N are the sensitivities of the observable measurements in diseased and non-diseased subjects.

In practice, the position is much more complex. First, there may be no satisfactory way of measuring the validity of the exposure measurements actually made because no perfect measure of exposure exists. A comparison of the method actually used with what is presumed to be a more accurate method may be made to provide an upper limit estimate of the validity coefficient, ρ_{TX}, in the case of a continuous measurement of exposure, and therefore a probably conservative correction for the effects of measurement error. Second, the equations in Table 4.4 assume, among other things, that the extent of measurement error is uncorrelated with the value of the true exposure. If this and other assumptions are not true, the adjustment will not be valid. Third, allowance needs to be made for sampling error in the observable disease–exposure association and the measurements of error. Finally, information on the multivariate measurement error structure of the primary exposure variable and the confounding variables is required if an adjustment for error in the measurement of all relevant variables is to be attempted.

While work has been done on a number of the problems listed above, and procedures are available that take account of some of them (Armstrong *et al.*, 1992; Thomas *et al.*, 1993), it will in most cases be difficult to overcome the difficulty that a source of true measurements against which a sample of the measurements actually obtained can be compared is lacking (Wacholder *et al.*, 1993). Therefore, while dose–response relationships adjusted for the effects of measurement error may be nearer the truth than the unadjusted relationships, they are unlikely to be close to perfect. Moreover, because the sensitivity and specificity or the validity coefficient will often have been derived from a small sample of subjects, the sampling error in any adjusted dose–response relationship or prediction of risk will be correspondingly large.

An example of the adjustment of a continuous dose–response relationship with reference to a validation study carried out in the same population of subjects is shown in Table 4.5, based on the US Nurses' Health Study (Rosner *et al.*, 1989). This examines the effect of using a comparison of calorie-adjusted, daily intake of saturated fat, measured both by food frequency questionnaire and by multiple daily records of weighed dietary intake in a sample of 173 nurses, to adjust the estimate of relative risk per 10 g increase in calorie-adjusted saturated fat intake based on the food frequency questionnaire. As would be expected, the adjusted relative risks are further from the null value (1.0) than the unadjusted estimates, and their 95% confidence intervals are wider because of the component of sampling error in the coefficient of regression of the the two estimates of adjusted saturated fat intake.

While the bias in the unadjusted estimate, in this example is apparently not large the adjusted estimate is open to question. First, while the recording of weighed dietary intake is probably the most accurate method of estimating nutrient intake, it is not perfect. For example, the close observation of diet that it entails is likely to change dietary intake in unpredictable ways. Second, while the 28 days of recording were spread throughout one year, they could only relate to diet in the recent past. The food frequency question-

---

Table 4.5 Use of results of a validation study to adjust for error in measurement of exposure:relationship of risk of breast cancer to calorie-adjusted saturated fat intake in a cohort of US nurses[a]

Validation study		Main cohort study	
Days of diet record	Estimate of regression coefficient (SE)[b]	Observed relative risk (95% CI)[c]	Adjusted relative risk (95% CI)[c]
28	0.468 (0.048)	0.92 (0.80–1.05)	0.83 (0.61–1.12)
2	0.540 (0.090)	0.92 (0.80–1.05)	0.85 (0.65–1.11)

[a] Based on data from Rosner *et al.* (1989).
[b] Coefficient of linear regression of estimated calorie-adjusted saturated fat intake from diet records on estimate from food frequency questionnaire. SE = standard error.
[c] Relative risk per 10g increase in saturated fat intake: CI = confidence interval.

naire, on the other hand, could, in principle, have related to diet over a much longer period. Neither, however, is likely to have been an accurate measure of the period of life in which dietary variables may be most important in breast cancer aetiology, namely, childhood (de Waard, 1986).

4.5.3 Control of a covariate related to measurement error

It is common in epidemiology to take steps either in the design or analysis of a study to ensure comparability in measurements on subjects with and without disease. For example, when multiple interviewers are used in a case–control study, each case and his or her matched controls may be interviewed by the same interviewer and at about the same time to equalize, between cases and controls, interviewer error and any error in response that may correlate with time. Similarly, when proxy respondents are necessary for some subjects (usually because they died before an interview could be obtained), a proxy may also be used for the matched controls, or the analysis may be stratified on whether the subject or a proxy was interviewed (Walker *et al.*, 1988). Such strategies will sometimes reduce bias in the effect measures. As a general rule, if misclassification is non-differential within levels of a covariate but varies across those levels, the validity of the effect measure will be improved by control of the covariate. In other circumstances, control of a covariate related to measurement error may increase bias in the effect measure (Greenland & Robins, 1985).

Walker *et al.* (1988) have given a hypothetical example of the effect of control of respondent status—self or proxy—in a case–control study of the relationship between smoking and a disease. They assumed that proxy responses were obtained for 50% of cases and 10% of controls, and used the matrix of proxy-reported versus self-reported smoking habits obtained by Rogot & Reid (1975). The results are summarized in Table 4.6. The effect of the differential measurement error introduced by the two different sources of exposure measurements is to slightly increase the relative risk of disease in smokers of more than one pack per day and to alter the shape of the dose–response relationship at the bottom of the distribution of cigarette use. Adjustment for respondent type corrects both of these biases, but increases slightly the width of the 95% confidence intervals about the relative risk estimates because of maldistribution of controls between the two groups of cases of equal size in the stratified analysis.

Table 4.6. Effect of adjustment for a source of exposure measement error, in this case use of proxy respondents, on bias due to the measurement error[a]

Risks	Current smoking habits								
	Non-smoker	Occasional smoker		< 1 pack per day		1 pack per day		> 1 pack per day	
		RR	95% CI	RR	95% CI	RR	95% CI	RR	95% CI
True relative risks	1.0	1.4	0.5–3.5	2.0	1.4–2.9	3.0	2.1–4.3	3.5	2.3–5.3
Crude observed relative risks	1.0	2.2	1.0–4.7	1.7	1.2–2.5	2.9	2.1–4.2	3.7	2.5–5.6
Observed relative risks adjusted for respondent	1.0	1.5	0.6–3.6	2.0	1.3–3.1	2.9	2.0–4.3	3.3	2.1–5.2

[a] Based on data from Walker et al. (1988). Hypothetical example of a case–control study of the relationship between a disease and current smoking habits in which 50% of exposure measurements in cases came from proxy respondents but only 10% in controls.

4.5.4 Resources for the control of exposure measurement error

Strategies to control the effects of exposure measurement error without actually preventing it can reduce the effects of both bias and random error on the dose–response relationship and therefore lead to more accurate QEP. None of these strategies is perfect, however, and it is unlikely that use of any or all of them will eliminate the effects of error entirely. In addition, two of them, namely the use of multiple measurements of exposure and adjustment of results with reference to a validity or reliability study, are expensive and may be difficult in practice or, in some cases (e.g. most historical cohort studies), impossible.

The allocation of resources to preventing or controlling the effects of exposure measurement error may well be cost-effective given the consequences of measurement error on the numbers of subjects needed to detect an effect or estimate it with some given precision. Freedman *et al.*, (1990) estimated the effects of error in the measurement of dietary fat intake on the numbers of subjects required in a cohort study to detect, with 90% power at $p<0.05$, relative risks of colorectal cancer of up to 2.3 over five levels of proportion of dietary calories derived from fat. If the correlation in the cohort between the measured and true proportion of dietary calories derived from fat was 0.65, they showed that a cohort of 141 000 subjects with an expected incidence of colorectal cancer of 200 per 100 000 person–years followed for five years would be required. The number required if the *true* exposure could be measured was nearly 10-fold less, namely 16 000.

To what should resources for the prevention or control of the effects of measurement error be allocated? In general, it appears that, when the proposed measure of exposure is reasonably accurate, a validation study on a sample of the study population, and use of its results to correct the risk estimates obtained in the whole population, is the most cost-effective approach. When the proposed measure is very inaccurate, it may be more efficient simply to use the criterion measurement proposed for the validation study as the measure to be applied in the whole population (Greenland, 1988; Spiegelman & Gray, 1991). Where there is no criterion measure, it may in some circumstances be more efficient to repeat the planned measure in all subjects and reduce the total sample size than to measure only once (Phillips & Davey Smith, 1993).

4.6 Error in the measurement of outcome

In cancer epidemiology, the outcome of interest is the occurrence of cancer in the subjects under study. However, although easy to conceptualize, occurrence of cancer is a difficult event to measure. As a result, the event actually measured may be more or less closely related to it.

The concept of occurrence of cancer is ambiguous. For example, how one considers a case of clinically silent cancer detected at necropsy will depend on the context of the study: it will be counted as a case in a study on the validation of death certificates by way of necropsy records but will be ignored in a study based solely on death certificates, and one could argue about its inclusion in a population-based case–control study. Even the most straightforward definition of a case of incident cancer, based on medical records reporting the results of diagnostic procedures and clinical reasoning, may be subject to ambiguity since medical procedures and diagnostic criteria differ among medical centres and among patients referred to the same centre (for a discussion on the comparability of data in cancer registries, see Parkin & Muir, 1992).

The most widely used outcome variables in cancer epidemiology, namely death from cancer, diagnosis of cancer, diagnosis of preneoplastic lesions, and molecular markers of early carcinogenic effect, can be seen as consecutive steps in a process corresponding to the putative natural history of the disease (for a review, see MacMahon & Pugh, 1970; Hulka *et al.*, 1990; and section 4.2.3).

4.6.1 Death from cancer

A fundamental source of error in outcome ascertainment is incorrect specification of vital status. In particular, deaths may be missed when death records are incomplete. For example, in studies involving record linkage with mortality records, vital status may be incorrectly specified when personal identifiers are insufficient to ensure that no linkage errors occur. Linkage errors lead to bias and additional uncertainty in commonly used statistics such as standardized mortality ratios (SMRs) and relative risk regression coefficients, with an excess (deficit) of deaths leading to upward (downward) bias in the estimated SMRs.

Information on death from cancer is based mainly on death certificates, which are issued for legal reasons in many countries. Additional sources of information on death from cancer may include medical records and interviews with next-of-kin (see, e.g. Chen et al., 1990). Most epidemiological studies of occupational cancer risk are based on mortality data from death certificates.

The main advantage of the use of death certificates is their availability in many populations and for relatively long periods, allowing long-term follow-up of large groups of exposed people and easy derivation of reference rates in population-based studies. Among the problems associated with their use are limitations in the data obtained from death certificates resulting, e.g. from differences in survival in different populations, failure to report cancer in patients dying from other causes, and limitations in the accuracy of the certificates themselves, including, in particular, errors in the reported cause of death and in the coding process. In a study of 1243 death certificates mentioning cancer, which were coded independently in nine countries, the proportion of certificates coded with cancer as the underlying cause of death varied from 88% to 96% (Percy & Muir, 1989).

4.6.2 Incidence of cancer

Data on cancer incidence are usually derived from established systems such as cancer registries reporting routinely all cases occurring in a particular population (see, e.g. Parkin et al., 1992), or from ad hoc surveys of medical or other records (e.g. in a hospital-based case–control study). The use of data from high-quality cancer registries has several theoretical advantages, such as ensuring control of the quality and completeness of registration and minimizing diagnostic misclassification (Parkin & Muir, 1992). However, quality of cancer registration is often unsatisfactory, and cancer registration covers less than 400 million individuals worldwide (Parkin et al., 1992). Studies using data on cancer incidence derived from ad hoc surveys are subject to additional problems because of their potential incompleteness, which may lead to bias with respect to the assumed population base, and because the information derived from sources other than medical records may not be correct (see, e.g. Steenland & Schnorr (1988) on diagnoses reported by next of kin).

One additional problem related to the use of data on cancer incidence is the fact that the degree of medical surveillance may vary among populations and groups, and thus lead to variable ascertainment of the true underlying incidence. Examples of such surveillance bias may be found in cancer patients followed up for incidence of secondary leukaemia (Kaldor et al., 1990) and occupational groups undergoing periodic medical examinations (Hiatt et al., 1993).

Whether the cases of cancer included in a study are obtained from mortality statistics, from a cancer registry or from an ad hoc survey (e.g. from the of pathology department of a hospital), measurement error can be introduced in the diagnosis of the neoplasm. In particular, there can be a diagnostic error when the true disease is not diagnosed, and a histopathological error when the measured histopathological class is not the true class. It should be noted that histopathological error is not necessarily less serious than diagnostic error: the inclusion of benign lesions in a series of malignant tumours, and similarly the exclusion of malignant lesions misdiagnosed as benign tumours, will have very important implications in a study on the quantification of the effect of a risk factor.

These errors can either be systematic or non-systematic, as discussed earlier for exposure measurement errors. Thus a systematic histopathological error exists, e.g. when a pathologist has a consistent tendency to call a benign melanocytic naevus a level I melanoma.

The major difficulty in assessing diagnostic or histopathological validity is the lack of a gold standard of the characteristics being measured. In other words, there is no way to determine the absolute truth with respect to the disease at the level of organ, tissue and cell type. For this reason, measurements of diagnostic and histopathological error have usually focused on reliability rather than validity, and have measured intraobserver and interobserver reliability.

Validity and reliability are related in the sense that valid measurements are also reliable.

Reliable measurements, however, are not necessarily valid, and the only certain conclusion is that an unreliable measurement is also invalid. Intraobserver reliability tends to be greater than the corresponding interobserver reliability because the single observer will repeat his or her own systematic error from observation to observation. Thus, the comparison of repeated measurements by one observer will be free from the effects of systematic error, whereas the often partly different systematic errors of different observers will be included in the assessment of interobserver agreement. Because systematic error is an important component of outcome measurement error, a measurement of interobserver reliability will be a better guide to validity (or at least to its upper limit) than a measurement of intraobserver reliability.

4.6.3 Preneoplastic lesions

Although there are many examples of preneoplastic lesions identified and measured in human populations, more important from the point of view of quantitative associations are those in which the preneoplastic lesions are used as surrogates for the cancer itself. In such cases, a quantitative estimation of risk can be made on the basis of the presence, or level, of the preneoplastic lesion. For example, melanocytic naevi are strong predictors of malignant melanoma of the skin (Armstrong & English, 1988), and genital warts and other manifestations of infection with human papilloma virus (HPV) are strongly associated with the risk of cervical cancer (Brinton, 1992).

Measurement of preneoplastic lesions, however, is also subject to random and systematic error. For example, in a study on the prevalence of melanocytic naevi in Western Australia in children assessed by two nurses, it was found that 4% of the variation in numbers of naevi of all sizes, and 8% of the variation in those of naevi of at least 2 mm in diameter was due to interobserver variation (English & Armstrong, 1994). Detection of HPV infection strongly depends on the method used, and recently developed methods based on the polymerase chain reaction have improved the sensitivity of the assay (Schiffman et al., 1991) and led to a reassessment of the quantitative aspects of the association between HPV infection and risk of cervical cancer (Muñoz et al., 1992).

4.6.4 Molecular markers of early carcinogenic effect

More recently, biological markers of early effects in the carcinogenic pathway have been used in studies in human populations (Perera & Weinstein, 1982). Such markers include non-specific lesions of the genome, such as sister chromatid exchanges (Wilcosky & Rynard, 1990), micronuclei (Vine, 1990) and chromosome aberrations (Schwartz, 1990), as well as more specific effects, such as activation of proto-oncogenes or inhibition of tumour-suppressor genes (Perera & Santella, 1993). In addition, biomarkers are now widely used to improve assessment of the biologically effective dose and to evaluate the role of individual susceptibility. It is clear, however, that when such methods are used, the traditional distinction between exposure and outcome becomes less clear, and the same event, such as the formation of a DNA adduct or the mutation of a relevant gene, can be considered either as a measure of exposure or as an effect.

Biomarkers of early carcinogenic effect may contribute greatly to knowledge of aetiological agents and the mechanism of tumour formation in humans (for review, see Hulka et al., 1990; Perera & Santella, 1993). In particular, from the point of view of quantitative estimation and prediction of risk, they may help to improve the classification of neoplastic lesions according to the genes that have been altered and the mutations in such genes, which may be risk-factor-specific. For example, it is possible to distinguish "spontaneous" mutations in the $p53$ tumour-suppressor gene from those caused by carcinogens such as benzo[a]pyrene or aflatoxin B_1 (Hollstein et al., 1991; Jones et al., 1991). There are also mutations of the $p53$ gene in skin cancer and normal skin which are almost completely specific to exposure to UV radiation (Ziegler et al., 1993; Nakazawa et al, 1994).

In addition, these biomarkers may help to identify critical steps in the carcinogenic process, and therefore to contribute to the definition of biologically relevant models of carcinogenicity to be used in quantitative human risk assessment (Perera et al., 1991; Hattis & Silver, 1993). The technical variability of biomarkers has been discussed by Vineis et al. (1993).

4.6.5 Sources, measurement and prevention of error in the measurement of outcome

The observer is not the only source of errors in the measurement of outcome in epidemiology, which can be classified as "preobserver", "observer", and "postobserver". Table 4.7 provides some examples of these sources of error in the histopathological classification of neoplastic lesions. The preobserver sources of error are important in relation to interobserver reliability and to validity in general, because they may contribute to measurement error by making the observer's task more difficult or increasing the likelihood of different biases between observers, and may also increase the level of variation seen between observers in a formal study of interobserver reliability (e.g. examination of different sections by different observers gives rise to the possibility of different errors in sampling from the tissue block and different quality of preparation of the mounted, stained section). A bibliography on observer variability has been published (Feinstein, 1985).

Table 4.7 Examples of sources of error in the histological classification of cancer

Preobserver sources:

State of preservation of tissue at the time of sampling

Location of biopsy (right site, right tissue)

Sampling of tissue for preservation and fixation

Trauma to tissue in the course of sampling or biopsy

Preservation and fixation of tissue

Sampling of tissue section to be mounted and stained

Preparation and processing of tissue section ready for examination

Quality and maintenance of microscope

"State of the art" of measurement of histopathological characteristics relevant to the tissue sample in question

Observer sources:

Familiarity with the "state of the art" of measurement of histopathological characteristics relevant to the tissue sample in question

Sampling of fields of the section for close examination

Thoroughness in making the observations necessary to classify the tissue (influenced by factors such as personality, state of mind, pressure of time)

Application of the classification rules implied in the "state of the art"

Postobserver sources:

Recording and transcription

Coding

Data processing

Communication

Integration of observations and classification rules into a diagnosis

Table 4.8 Requirements for the conduct of studies of interobserver reliabiltity in histopathology

1. A representative set of sections of the cancer(s) to be studied. Ideally this set will come from the real life practice of pathology in a whole population so that the results will reflect what may actually happen in practice rather than what can be achieved in ideal circumstances

2. Two or more willing pathologists. Again, ideally these pathologists will be involved in the general practice of histopathology of cancer rather than be particularly specialized in the cancer of interest

3. Circulation of the sections to be studied, in random order and with only numerical identification, to each pathologist who examines them without knowledge of the other pathologists' opinions of them. Ideally, because of the problem of sampling of the tissue block when taking a section and variation in the quality of the subsequent processing of the section, each pathologist should see the same section

4. Standardized recording on a specially prepared form of the histopathological observations of interest. An example of a form used in a study of interobserver variation in measurement of the histopathological characteristics of malignant melanoma is given in Figure 4.3

Interobserver reliability can be measured by means of ad hoc studies involving repeated independent measurements of the outcome based on the same, or at least very similar, material. It is obvious that in some instances a correct experimental design of the reliability study is not possible, since the measurement condition cannot be replicated (e.g. diagnosis based on macroscopic necropsy evidence). Some of the requirements for the conduct of a study of interobserver reliability in the histopathology of cancer are summarized in Table 4.8.

Several statistical methods have been proposed for use in measuring interobserver reliability. The simplest and most commonly used method is to determine the proportion of cases in which two (or more) observers agree. However, this method does not take into account the proportion of cases in agreement by chance only. It can be simply shown that this proportion varies with the prevalence of the outcome being measured, increasing as the prevalence increases to very high or decreases to very low values. A simple statistic corrected for chance agreement is the kappa statistic (Fleiss, 1971), which is the ratio of the difference between the observed proportion in agreement (p_o) and the proportion of agreement that can be expected by chance (p_e) to the proportion of agreement that cannot be attributed to chance ($1-p_e$), so that:

$$\text{kappa} = \frac{p_o - p_e}{1 - p_e}$$

An advantage of the kappa statistic is that is can be applied to nominal scale variables, which are common in pathology and histology. It can be interpreted like a correlation coefficient, i.e. its value varies from 0.0 (no agreement beyond that expected by chance) to 1.0 (perfect agreement) and to -1.0 (complete disagreement). While no strict rules exist, it has been stated that values of kappa in excess of 0.75 indicate very good agreement, and values below 0.40 indicate poor agreement (Landis & Koch, 1977). More information on the kappa statistic and on its limitations can be found in specialized papers (Maclure & Willett, 1987; Mazoyer & Mary, 1987; Dunn, 1989).

Alternatives to the kappa statistic include the intraclass correlation coefficient, which is less sensitive to changes in the number of categories, and the Pearson correlation coefficient (Snedecor & Cochran, 1980).

In principle, error in outcome measurement can be prevented or reduced by dealing with the sources discussed. While every effort should be made to minimize the error in any single set of measurements, error can be reduced further if multiple measurements are made. In practice, this means the use of multiple observers. The measurement to be taken as correct when multiple observers are used may be the majority position of the observers. There is value, however, in having the observers meet after they have made their measurements, discuss their findings, and reach a consensus position on the value of the measurement (Kraemer, 1992).

MELANOMA PROJECT PATHOLOGY ABSTRACT

1. **SERIAL NUMBER:** ☐☐☐☐ 4

2. **TUMOUR WIDTH & BREADTH IN MILLIMETERS:**
   (2 largest diameters)

   i. Total lesion ☐☐.☐ ☐☐.☐ 10

   ii. Nodular portion ☐☐.☐ ☐☐.☐ 16

3. **CROSS-SECTIONAL PROFILE:**
   1 Flat
   2 Dome
   3 Polypoid
   4 Plateau

   5 Verrucous ☐ 17

4. **HISTOLOGY:**
   (a) Premalignant intraepidermal lesion without invasion
   1 HMF type
   2 SSM type
   3 Mixed

   4 Other (specify below) ☐ 18

   (b) Premalignant intraepidermal involvement adjacent to invasive tumour
   1 HMF type
   2 SSM type
   3 Mixed
   4 Other (specify below)
   5 None ☐ 19

   (c) Cell type predominating
   1 Epithelioid
   2 Spindle
   3 Naevus cell-like

   4 Mixed ☐ 20

   (d) Degree of pigmentation
   1 Heavy
   2 Moderate to light

   3 None ☐ 21

   (e) Pre-existing or associated benign melanotic lesion

   Type.. ☐ 23

(f) Chronic inflammatory reaction

i. Intraepidermal component
   1 Severe
   2 Moderate
   3 Mild

   4 None ☐ 24

ii. Invasive component
   1 Severe
   2 Moderate
   3 Mild

   4 None ☐ 25

(g) Evidence of regression
   1 Yes

   2 No ☐ 26

(h) Mitotic activity in invasive component (HPF=high power field × 400)
   1 Less than 1 per 5 HPFs
   2 Between 1/HPF and 1/5 HPFs

   3 Greater than or equal to 1 per HPF ☐ 27

(i) Solar elastosis
   1 Severe or moderate
   2 Mild

   3 Absent ☐ 28

(j) Ulceration
   1 Yes

   2 No ☐ 29

5. **LEVEL OF INVASION:**
   1 Intraepidermal
   2 Papillary dermal
   3 Papillary-reticular interface
   4 Reticular dermal

   5 Subcutaneous fat ☐ 30

6. **TUMOUR DEPTH IN MILLIMETERS:**

   ☐☐.☐☐ 34

7. **PATHOLOGIST**
   .... ☐ 38

Figure 4.3. Form used for recording each pathologist's observations on each case in an interobserver reliability study of the measurement of features of the histopathology of malignant melanoma. Based on Heenan *et al.* (1984).

4.6.6 Effect of error in measurement of outcome on the dose–response relationship

The effect of outcome measurement error on the dose–response relationship is conceptually similar to the effect of exposure measurement error. When the outcome being measured is death from, or incidence of cancer, the outcome variable is invariably categorical, usually binary (i.e., presence or absence of cancer). If misclassification of a dichotomous outcome variable is independent of misclassification of exposure, the bias is always towards the null. In practice, however, misclassification of exposure and outcome might be correlated, resulting in a bias in an unpredictable direction, even with non-differential misclassification (Kristensen, 1992; Brenner *et al.*, 1993). When outcomes other than cancer are considered, there may be multiple categories, ordered, e.g. according to the severity of the disease (e.g. healthy, *in situ* carcinoma, invasive carcinoma) or reflecting multiplicity of a particular outcome in individual subjects (e.g. number of melanocytic naevi). The measurement of markers of early carcinogenic effect has added further complexity (Schulte *et al.*, 1993). While such markers are usually measured on two levels, it is now possible to identify several outcome categories based on combinations of them. For example, in a hypothetical study based on the measurement of cancer and a marker of early effect, such as activation of a proto-oncogene, four outcome categories can be considered: (1) healthy subjects without the activation; (2) healthy subjects with the activation; (3) cancer patients without the activation; and (4) cancer patients with the activation. In this example, categories 1, 2 and 4 can be seen as successive steps in the carcinogenic process, in which the presence of the early lesion is a required step. The implications of measurement error in studies based on more than two categories of outcome have not been investigated in any detail, and the effect of their misclassification on the risk estimate will be difficult to predict.

The major issue in outcome measurement error is whether the error is differential or non-differential across exposure categories. One example of differential measurement error is a cohort study in which the population under investigation (considered as exposed) is compared with a reference (e.g. national) population, considered as unexposed, where the members of the exposed cohort are more likely to be diagnosed with the cancer of interest than the reference population (see discussion on surveillance bias above).

In the case of non-differential error in measurement of outcome, by analogy with the effects of error in measurement of exposure (see section 4.3), the observed relative risk (RR) will be biased towards the null value relative to the true RR (and the dose–response curve will be flattened) provided that the probability that the measurement classifies a true case as a case is the same as, or greater than that with which it classifies a true non-case as a non-case. On the other hand, differential measurement error can cause a bias in any direction, and may even reverse the direction of the association (e.g. RR below 1 instead of above 1).

A good example of the effect of outcome measurement error deals with the risk of soft-tissue sarcomas (STS) among workers exposed to dioxin (see also Chapter 8). STS are rare malignant neoplasms originating in tissues of mesodermal origin, such as fat, muscle and connective tissue. However, although most STS originate from organs primarily containing mesodermal tissue, some originate from visceral organs, such as the stomach, that also contain mesodermal tissue, but such sarcomas represent only a small fraction of all neoplasms originating in these organs. Since the International Classification of Diseases (ICD), which is used in many countries to code causes of deaths from death certificates, is based on the topography of the neoplasms, STS arising from visceral organs are coded as neoplasms of those organs, and are therefore not identified in a mortality study, which will be based on the ICD category for malignant neoplasms of connective and other soft tissues. The net result is a 30–70% underestimation of the number of STS (Lynge *et al.*, 1987; Erikson & Gezelius, 1990).

Exposure to dioxin has been related to an increased risk of STS in a number of cohort studies in which the mortality of the exposed workers has been compared with the mortality of the national population (see section 9.2). In particular, a study of over 6000 workers in the USA has found a three-fold excess mortality from STS, based on four observed and 1.2 expected cases, although the result was not statistically significant (Fingerhut *et al.*, 1991). A careful examination of all death certificates of deceased cohort members and of the medical records of all those dying from cancers in sites where STS are likely to occur identified three additional cases of STS (Suruda *et al.*, 1993). Therefore, three[1] out of seven STS cases (43%) were missed in the analysis based on death certificates. The degree of misclassification in the reference population used in this study is not known, but one can reasonably assume that the misclassification in the original comparison was non-differential. The RR of 3.3 (4/1.2), although not biased, is then less precise than it would have been had it been possible to use all the cases of STS identified in the cohort in its estimation (95% confidence interval based on four cases, 0.9–8.7; based on seven cases, 1.4–6.9). A narrower confidence interval would allow a more precise quantitative estimation of risk based on these results. Had a comparison of the seven cases been made with the population expected value of 1.2, there would probably have been differential error in outcome measurement, with the RR biased away from the null.

4.7 Conclusions

Errors in measurement of exposure and outcome can have substantial and, to a large degree, unpredictable effects on the direction and shape of dose–response relationships. Measurement error can be prevented by careful selection and design of measurement instruments, and strict quality control in their use and in the processing and analysis of the measurement results. If not prevented, it can be controlled to some degree by the use of multiple measures of exposure and outcome, the adjustment of dose–response relationships for the effects of measurement error, and the control of covariates related to measurement error. While the application of these procedures may sometimes make the effects of measurement error negligible in QEP, this is probably rarely the case.

There are a number of areas of research that could lead to better measurements of exposure and outcome for QEP. First, development of accurate biological techniques to measure biologically effective dose may produce estimates of present exposure (e.g. DNA adducts) or of cumulative exposure (e.g. exposure-specific mutations) that are more accurate than any other measurements of exposure currently available. The use of the

first, however, is limited by the short exposure period that they cover, and the use of the second by the fact that they can give essentially no information about dose rate or pattern of exposure. To evaluate these problems and their significance, it would be desirable to incorporate in large cohort studies the periodic collection of biological samples for recurrent measurement of present exposure (to obtain information on dose rate, pattern of exposure and, ultimately, cumulative exposure over some period of time) and the collection, on a case–control basis within a cohort study, of biological measurements of cumulative exposure, ideally corresponding in some way to the measurements of present exposure.

Second, the development, as measures of outcome, of markers of early effects which are important in the process of cancer development may lead to studies that can be carried out sooner after exposure, more quickly, and with greater statistical power than those based on cancer incidence or mortality. The best way to investigate the significance and role of markers of early effect would be to make repeated collections of biological samples in prospective studies, and to carry out large surveys of these markers in high-risk populations with well characterized exposures.

Finally, there would be value in a thorough theoretical and empirical evaluation of the effects of measurement error on dose–response relationships and QEPs derived from them. The theory has been worked out only recently and, as yet, incompletely. Further substantial development and the exploration of its application to some of the more comprehensive data on dose–response in cancer epidemiology are possible.

References

Armstrong, B. (1985) The use of epidemiological data to assess human cancer risk. In: Vouk, V.B., Butler, G.C. & Peakall, D.B., eds, *Methods for Estimating Risk of Chemical Injury: Humans and Non-human Biota and Ecosystems*, Chichester, Wiley, pp. 289-301

Armstrong, B.K. (1988) Epidemiology of malignant melanoma: intermittent or total accumulated exposure to the sun. *J. Dermatol. Surg. Oncol.*, 14, 835-849

---

[1] Two were not STS.

Armstrong, B.K. & English, D.R. (1988) The epidemiology of acquired melanocytic naevi and their relationship to malignant melanoma. *Pigment Cell*, 9, 27-47

Armstrong, B.K., White, E. & Saracci, R. (1992) *Principles of Exposure Measurement in Epidemiology*, Oxford, Oxford University Press

Birkett, N.J. (1992) Effect of nondifferential misclassification on estimates of odds ratios with multiple levels of exposure. *Am. J. Epidemiol.*, 136, 356-362

Brenner, H. & Blettner, M. (1993) Misclassification bias arising from random error in exposure measurement: Implications for dual measurement strategies. *Am. J. Epidemiol.*, 138, 453-461

Brenner, H., Savitz, D.A., Jöckel, K.-H. & Greenland, S. (1992) Effects of nondifferential exposure misclassification in ecologic studies. *Am. J. Epidemiol.*, 135, 85-95

Brenner, H., Savitz, D.A. & Gefeller, O. (1993) The effects of joint misclassification of exposure and disease on epidemiologic measures of association. *J. Clin. Epidemiol.*, 46, 1195-1202

Brinton, L.A. (1992) Epidemiology of cervical cancer—overview. In: Muñoz, N., Bosch, F.X., Shah, K.V. & Meheus, A., eds, *The Epidemiology of Human Papillomavirus and Cervical Cancer* (IARC Scientific Publications No. 119), Lyon, International Agency for Research on Cancer, pp. 3-23

Chen, J., Campbell, T.C., Li, J. & Peto, R. (1990) *Diet, Lifestyle and Mortality in China: A Study of the Characteristics of 65 Chinese Counties*, Oxford, Oxford University Press

Coghlin, J., Hammond, S.K. & Gann, P.H. (1989) Development of epidemiologic tools for measuring environmental tobacco smoke exposure. *Am. J. Epidemiol.*, 130, 696-704

Copeland, B. (1989) Quality control. In: Kaplan, L.A. & Pesce, A.J., eds, *Clinical Chemistry: Theory, Analysis and Correlation*, 2nd ed., St Louis, MO, Mosby, pp. 279-289

Cummings, K.M., Markello, S.J., Mahoney, M.C & Marshall, J.R. (1989) Measurement of lifetime exposure to passive smoke. *Am. J. Epidemiol.*, 130, 122-132

de Waard, F. (1986) Body size, body mass and cancer of the breast. In: Ip, C., Birt, D.F. & Rogers, A.E., eds, *Dietary Fat and Cancer*, New York, NY, Alan R. Liss, pp. 33-41

Doll, R., Peto, R., Wheatley, K., Gray, R. & Sutherland, I. (1994) Mortality in relation to smoking: 40 years' observations on male British doctors. *Br. Med. J.*, 309, 901-911

Doll, R. & Peto, J. (1978) Cigarette smoking and bronchial carcinoma. Dose and time relationships among regular smokers and lifelong non-smokers. *J. Epidemiol. Commun. Health*, 32, 303-313

Dunn, G. (1989) *Design and analysis of reliability studies*. London, Edward Arnold, and New York, NY, Oxford University Press

English, D.R. & Armstrong, B.K. (1994) The epidemiology of benign melanocytic nevi in children. Observer variation in counting nevi. *Am. J. Epidemiol.*, 139, 402-407

Erikson, A. & Gezelius, C. (1990) Malignant diseases in cause-of-death autopsies in forensic medicine. *Nord. Med.*, 105(10), 264-265

Feinstein, A.R. (1985) A bibliography of publications on observer variability. *J. Chron. Dis.*, 38, 619-632.

Fingerhut, M.A., Halperin, W.E., Marlow, D.A., Piacitelli, L.A., Honchar, P.A., Sweeney, M.H., Greife, A.L., Dill, P.A., Steenland, K. & Suruda, A.J. (1991) Cancer mortality in workers exposed to 2,3,7,8-tetrachlorodibenzo-*p*-dioxin, *New. Engl. J. Med.*, 1991, 324(4): 212-218

Fleiss, J.L. (1971) Measuring nominal scale agreement among many raters. *Psychol. Bull.*, 76, 378-382

Fontham, E.T.H., Correa, P., Wu-Williams, A., Reynolds, P., Greenberg, R.S., Buffler, P.A., Chen,

V.W., Boyd, P., Alterman, T., Austin, D.F., Liff J & Greenberg, S.D. (1991) Lung cancer in nonsmoking women: a multicenter case–control study. *Cancer Epidemiol. Biomarkers Prev.*, **1**, 35-43

Freedman, L.S., Schatzkin, A. & Wax, Y. (1990) The impact of dietary measurement error on planning sample size requirements in a cohort study. *Am. J. Epidemiol.*, **132**, 1185-1195

Garfinkel, L. (1981) Time trends in lung cancer mortality among nonsmokers and a note on passive smoking. *J. Natl Cancer Inst.*, **66**, 1061-1066

Gilbert, E.S., Omohundro, E., Buchanan, J. & Holter, N.A. (1993) Mortality of workers at the Hanford site: 1945–1986. *Health Phys.*, **64**, 577-590

Greenland, S. (1988) Statistical uncertainty due to misclassification: importance for validation studies. *J. Clin. Epidemiol.*, **41**, 1167-1174

Greenland, S. (1992) Divergent biases in ecologic and individual-level studies. *Stat. Med.*, **11**, 1209-1223

Greenland, S. & Morgenstern, H. (1989) Ecological bias, confounding, and effect modification. *Int. J. Epidemiol.*, **18**, 269-274

Greenland, S. & Robins, J.M. (1985) Confounding and misclassification. *Am. J. Epidemiol.*, **122**, 495-506

Hattis, D. & Silver, K. (1993) Use of biomarkers in risk assessment. In: Schulte, P.A. & Perera, F.P., eds, *Molecular Epidemiology. Principles and Practices*, San Diego, CA, Academic Press, pp. 251-273

Heenan, P.J., Matz, L.R., Blackwell, J.B., Kelsall, G.R.H., Singh, A., ten Seldam, R.E.J. & Holman, C.D.J. (1984) Inter-observer variation between pathologists in the classification of cutaneous malignant melanoma in Western Australia. *Histopathology*, **6**, 581-589

Hiatt, R.A., Krieger, N., Sagebiel, R.W., Clark, W.H., Jr & Mihm, M.C. (1993) Surveillance bias and the excess risk of malignant melanoma

among employees of the Lawrence Livermore National Laboratory. *Epidemiology*, **4**, 43-47

Higgins, I.T.T, Mahan, C.M. & Wynder, E.L. (1988) Lung cancer among cigar and pipe smokers. *Prev. Med.*, **17**, 116-128

Hirayama, T. (1981) Non-smoking wives of heavy smokers have a higher risk of lung cancer: a study from Japan. *Br. Med. J.*, **282**, 183-185

Hollstein, M., Sidransky, D., Vogelstein, B. & Harris, C.C. (1991) *p53* mutations in human cancers. *Science*, **253**(5015): 49-53

Holman, C.D.J., Armstrong, B.K. & Heenan, P.J. (1983) A theory of the etiology and pathogenesis of human cutaneous malignant melanoma. *J. Natl Cancer Inst.*, **71**, 651-656

Hulka, B.S., Wilcosky, T.C. & Griffith, J.D. (1990) *Biological Markers in Epidemiology*, New York, NY, Oxford University Press

Jones, P.A., Buckley, J.D., Henderson, B.E., Ross, R.K. & Pike, M.C. (1991) From gene to carcinogen: a rapidly evolving field in molecular epidemiology. *Cancer Res.*, **51**(13), 3617-3620

Kaldor, J.M., Day, N.E., Clarke, E.A., van Leeuwen, F.E., Henry-Amar, M., Fiorentino, M.V., Bell, J., Pedersen, D., Band, P., Assouline, D. *et al.* (1990) Leukemia following Hodgkin's disease. *New Engl. J. Med.*, **322**, 7-13

Kraemer, H.C. (1992) How many raters? Toward the most reliable diagnostic consensus. *Stat. Med.*, **11**, 317-331

Kristensen, P. (1992) Bias from non-differential but dependent misclassification of exposure and outcome. *Epidemiology*, **3**, 210-215

Landis, J.R. & Koch, G.G. (1977) The measurement of observer agreement for categorical data. *Biometrics*, **33**, 159-174

Lee-Feldstein, A. (1989) A comparison of several measures of exposure to arsenic. *Am. J. Epidemiol.*, **129**, 112-124

Liu, K., Cooper, R., McKeever, J., McKeever, P., Byington, R., Soltero, I., Stamler, R., Gosch, F., Stevens, E. & Stamler, J. (1979) Assessment of the association between habitual salt intake and high blood pressure: methodological problems. *Am. J. Epidemiol.*, **110**, 219-226

Lynge, E., Storm, H.H. & Jensen, O.M. (1987) The evaluation of trends in soft tissue sarcoma according to diagnostic criteria and consumption of phenoxy herbicides. *Cancer*, **60**, 1896-1901

Maclure, M. & Willett, W.C. (1987) Misinterpretation and misuse of the kappa statistic. *Am. J. Epidemiol.*, **126**, 161-169

MacMahon, B. & Pugh, T.F. (1970) *Epidemiology. Principles and Methods*, Boston, MA, Little, Brown

Marshall, J.R. (1989) The use of dual or multiple reports in epidemiologic studies. *Stat. Med.*, **8**, 1041-1049

Mazoyer, B. & Mary, J.T. (1987) Kappa as an index of reproducibility: Distribution under the null-hypothesis. *Rév. Epidemiol. Santé Publ.*, **35**, 474-481

Muñoz, N., Bosch, F.X., de Sanjosé, S., Tafur, L., Izarzugaza, I., Gili, M., Viladiu, P., Navarro, C., Martos, C., Ascunce, N., Gonzalez, L.C., Kaldor, J.M., Guerrero, E., Lorincz, A., Santamaria, M., Alonso de Ruiz, P., Aristizabal, N. & Shah, K. (1992) The causal link between human papillomavirus and invasive cervical cancer: a population-based case–control study in Colombia and Spain. *Int. J. Cancer*, **52**, 743-749

Nakazawa, H., English, D., Randell, P.L., Nakazawa, K., Martel, N., Armstrong, B.K. & Yamasaki, H. (1994) UV and skin cancer: specific *p53* gene mutation in normal skin as a biologically relevant exposure measurement. *Proc. Natl Acad. Sci. USA*, **91**, 360-364

National Institutes of Health (1985) *Report of the National Institutes of Health Ad Hoc Working Group to Develop Radioepidemiological Tables* (NIH Publication No. 95-2748), Washington, DC, US Department of Health and Human Services

Parkin, D.M. & Muir, C. (1992) Comparability and quality of data. In: *Cancer Incidence in Five Continents*, Vol. VI (IARC Scientific Publications No. 120), Lyon, International Agency for Research on Cancer, pp 45-173

Parkin, D.M., Muir, C.S., Whelan, S.L., Gao, Y-T., Ferlay, J. & Powell, J., eds (1992) *Cancer Incidence in Five Continents*, Vol. VI (IARC Scientific Publications No. 120), Lyon, International Agency for Research on Cancer

Percy, C. & Muir, C. (1989) The international comparability of cancer mortality data. *Am. J. Epidemiol.*, **129**, 934-946

Perera, F.P. & Santella, R. (1993) Carcinogenesis. In: Schulte, P.A. & Perera, F.P., eds, *Molecular Epidemiology. Principles and Practices*, San Diego, CA, Academic Press, pp. 277-300

Perera, F.P. & Weinstein, I.B. (1982) Molecular epidemiology and carcinogen–DNA adduct detection—new approaches to studies of human cancer causation. *J. Chron. Dis.*, **35**, 581-600

Perera, F., Mayer, J., Santella, R.M., Brenner, D., Jeffrey, A., Latriano, L., Smith, S., Warburton, D., Young, T.L., Tsai, W.Y., Hemminki, K. & Brandt-Rauf, P. (1991) Biologic markers in risk assessment for environmental carcinogens. *Environ. Health. Perspect.*, **90**, 247-254

Persson, P.-G. & Norell, S.E. (1989) Retrospective versus original information on cigarette smoking. Implications for epidemiological studies. *Am. J. Epidemiol.*, **130**, 705-712

Phillips, A.M. & Davey Smith, G. (1993) The design of prospective epidemiological studies: more subjects or better measurement. *J. Clin. Epidemiol.*, **46**, 1203-1211

Pierce, D.A., Stram, D.O. & Vaeth, M. (1990) Allowing for random errors in radiation exposure estimates for the atomic bomb survivor data. *Radiat. Res.*, **123**: 275-284

Pierce, D.A., Stram, D.O., Vaeth, M. & Schafer, D.W. (1992) The errors in variables problem: considerations provided by radiation dose–response analyses of the A-bomb survivor data. *J. Am. Stat. Assoc.*, 87:351-359

Preston, D.L. & Pierce, D.A. (1988) The effect of changes in dosimetry on cancer mortality risk estimates in the atomic bomb survivors. *Radiat. Res.*, 114, 437-466

Preston, D.L., Kato, H., Kopecky, K. & Fujita, S. (1987) Studies of the mortality of A-bomb survivors. 8. Cancer mortality, 1950–1982. *Radiat. Res.*, 111, 151-178

Riboli, E., Preston-Martin, S., Saracci, R., Haley, N.J., Trichopoulos, D., Becher, H., Burch, J.D., Fontham, E.T.H., Gao, Y.-T., Jindal, S.K., Koo, L.C., Le Marchand, L., Segnan, N., Shimizu, H., Stanta, G., Wu-Williams, A.H. & Zatonski, W. (1990) Exposure of nonsmoking women to environmental tobacco smoke: a 10-country collaborative study. *Cancer Causes Control*, 1, 243-252.

Rogot, E. & Reid, D.D. (1975) The validity of data from next-of-kin in studies of mortality among migrants. *Int. J. Epidemiol.*, 4, 51-54

Rosner B., Willett, W.C. & Spiegelman, D. (1989) Correction of logistic regression relative risk estimates and confidence intervals for systematic within-person measurement error. *Stat. Med.*, 8, 1051-1069

Rothman, K.J. (1981) Induction and latent periods. *Am. J. Epidemiol.*, 114, 253-259

Schiffman, M.H. Bauer, H.M. Lörincz, A.T., Manos, M.M., Byrne, J.C., Glass, A.G., Cadell, D.M. & Howley, P.M. (1991) Comparison of Southern blot hybridization and polymerase chain reaction methods for the detection of human papillomavirus DNA. *J. Clin. Microbiol.*, 29, 573-577

Schulte, P.A., Rothman, N., & Schottenfeld, D. (1993) Design considerations in molecular epidemiology. In: Schulte, P.A. & Perera, F.P., eds, *Molecular Epidemiology. Principles and Practices*, San Diego, CA, Academic Press, pp. 159-198

Schwartz, G.C. (1990) Chromosome aberrations. In: Hulka, B.S., Wilcosky, T.C. & Griffith, J.D., eds, *Biological Markers in Epidemiology*, New York, NY, Oxford University Press, pp. 147-172

Shimizu, Y., Schull, W.J. & Kato, H. (1990) Cancer risk among atomic bomb survivors. The RERF Life Span Study. Radiation Effects Research Foundation comments. *J. Am. Med. Soc.*, 264, 601-604

Smith, A.H., Waxweiler, R.J. & Tyroler, H.A. (1980) Epidemiologic investigation of occupational carcinogenesis using a serially additive expected dose model. *Am. J. Epidemiol.*, 112, 787-797

Snedecor, G.W. & Cochran, W.G. (1980) *Statistical Methods*, Ames, IA, Iowa State University Press, pp. 243-244

Spiegelman, D. & Gray, R. (1991) Cost efficient designs for binary responses data with Gaussian covariate measurement error. *Biometrics*, 47, 851-869

Steenland, K. & Schnorr, T. (1988) Availability and accuracy of cancer and smoking data obtained from next of kin for decedents in a retrospective cohort study. *J. Occup. Med.*, 30, 348-353

Stockwell, H.G., Goldman, A.L., Lyman, G.H., Noss, C.I., Armstrong, A.W., Pinkham, P.A., Candelora, E.C. & Brusa, M.R. (1992) Environmental tobacco smoke and lung cancer risk in nonsmoking women. *J. Natl Cancer Inst.*, 84, 1417-1422

Straume, T., Egbert, S.D., Woolson, W.A., Finkel, R.C., Kubik, P.W., Gove, H.E., Sharma, P. & Hoshi, M. (1992) Neutron discrepancies in the DS86 Hiroshima dosimetry system. *Health Phys.*, 63:421-426

Suruda, A.J., Ward, E.M. & Fingerhut, M.A. (1993) Identification of soft tissue sarcoma deaths in cohorts exposed to dioxin and to chlorinated naphthalenes. *Epidemiology*, 4, 14-19

Thomas, D.C., Strom, D. & Dwyer, J. (1993) Exposure measurement error: Influence on exposure–disease relationships and methods of correction. *Ann. Rev. Public Health*, **14**, 69-93

UK National Case–Control Study Group (1989) Oral contraceptive use and breast cancer risk in young women. *Lancet*, **i**, 973-982

Vine, M.F. (1990) Micronuclei. In: Hulka, B.S., Wilcosky, T.C. & Griffith, J.D., eds, *Biological Markers in Epidemiology*, New York, NY, Oxford University Press, pp. 125-146

Vineis, P., Schulte, P.A. & Vogt, R.F. (1993) Technical variability in laboratory data. In: Schulte, P.A. & Perera, F.P., eds, *Molecular Epidemiology. Principles and Practices*, San Diego, CA, Academic Press, pp. 109-135

Wacholder, S., Armstrong, B. & Hartge, P. (1993) Validation studies using a gold standard. *Am. J. Epidemiol.*, **137**, 1251-1258

Walker, A.M., Velema, J.P. & Robins, J.M. (1988) Analysis of case–control data derived in part from proxy respondents. *Am. J. Epidemiol.*, **127**, 905-914

Westgard, J.O. & Klee, G.G. (1986) Quality assurance. In: Tietz, N.W., ed., *Textbook of Clinical Chemistry*, Philadelphia, PA, Saunders, pp. 424-458

Wilcosky, T.C. & Rynard, S.M. (1990) Sister chromatid exchange. In: Hulka, B.S., Wilcosky, T.C. & Griffith, J.D., eds, *Biological Markers in Epidemiology*, New York, NY, Oxford University Press, pp. 105-124

Wild, C.P., Jiang Y.-Z., Sabbioni, G., Chapot, B. & Montesano, R. (1990) Evaluation of methods for quantitation of aflatoxin–albumin adducts and their application to human exposure assessment. *Cancer Res.*, **50**, 245-251

Willett, W.C. (1989) An overview of issues related to the correction of non-differential exposure measurement error in epidemiologic studies. *Stat. Med.*, **8**, 1031-1040

Ziegler, A., Leffell, D.J., Kunala, S., Sharma, H.W., Gailani, M., Simon, J.A., Halpern, A.J., Baden, H.P. Shapiro, P.E., Bale, A.E. & Brash, D.E. (1993) Mutation hotspots due to sunlight in the *p53* gene of nonmelanoma skin cancers. *Proc. Natl Acad. Sci. USA*, **90**, 4216-4220

Quantitative Estimation and Prediction of Human Cancer Risks
S. Moolgavkar, D. Krewski, L. Zeise, E. Cardis and H. Møller
IARC Scientific Publications No. 131
International Agency for Research on Cancer, Lyon, 1999

5: Long- and Medium-term Carcinogenicity Studies in Animals and Short-term Genotoxicity Tests

Victor J. Feron, Michael Schwarz, Kari Hemminki and Daniel Krewski

5.1 General principles

The primary objective of carcinogenicity bioassays has been to identify agents that may induce cancer in humans. In the absence of human data, studies in laboratory animals (rodents) still remain the most reliable and most widely accepted means for the detection of carcinogenic hazards to public health (Faccini et al., 1992; Griesemer, 1992; Vainio et al., 1992). In addition to the screening of compounds for carcinogenic potential on a qualitative basis, a carcinogenicity study may be employed to determine dose–response relationships or to elucidate the mechanism of carcinogenic action (Gart et al., 1986; Krewski et al., 1992). Single-compound studies are performed mainly to identify the carcinogenic potential of the test substance or to determine dose–response relationships. Multiple-agent studies are focused on elucidating the mechanisms of action, viz. initiating, promoting, inhibiting or cocarcinogenic activity.

Studies that examine certain hypotheses concerning mechanisms of carcinogenesis need designs tailored to a particular hypothesis. A classical example of specific designs are initiation–promotion studies that most frequently use mouse skin or rat liver as experimental systems. Other examples are two-generation studies to distinguish between effects induced prenatally or postnatally, studies with exposure and non-exposure periods of varying duration to explore (ir)reversibility of hyper/preoplastic changes, and mixed-exposure studies to evaluate the possibility of synergistic or antagonistic potential (Gart et al., 1986; Griesemer & Tennant, 1992; Vainio et al., 1992). Important information such as dose– and time–response for cell proliferation in target and non-target tissues (Monticello et al., 1991), and presence or absence of DNA and protein adducts, proto-oncogene activation and tumour–suppressor gene inactivation can be obtained during or at the end of the study (Vainio et al., 1992). In particular, the use of biological markers may be of great importance in studies of carcinogenesis and quantitative estimation and prediction (QEP). When measuring DNA adducts, it is important to realise that the number of adducts will depend on repair reactions. On the other hand, when measuring protein adducts, the number will not be influenced by repair reactions and may thus give a measure of recent exposure. Measurement of different types of DNA adducts may give important information concerning the mechanism of action of the carcinogen under study. It is of particular importance to compare the dose–response curve for different biological markers at high and low doses with that for tumour incidences.

End-points of interest in a carcinogenicity study are primarily preneoplastic and neoplastic changes, but also include degree of malignancy, time to tumour appearance, multiplicity of (pre)neoplasia, and occurrence of metastases. Long-term bioassays are designed and conducted to detect all of these end-points. So-called medium-term bioassays are mainly based on the detection of putative preneoplastic lesions. The distinction between medium- and long-term studies is somewhat arbitrary, because, depending on the appearance of (pre)neoplasia, the duration of a medium-term bioassay in rodents may range from six to 18 or even 24 months, e.g. in mouse skin studies. Recent developments in carcinogenicity studies are the use of transgenic mice for screening and mechanistic purposes, and of biomarkers in both medium- and long-term animal studies.

Short-term genotoxicity tests have been the subject of intense research in the past few decades, and large numbers of compounds have been examined in existing test systems.

5.2 Design and analysis of cancer bioassays

While the different aspects of the design, conduct and analysis of carcinogenicity bioassays have been dealt with in extenso in several reviews (Gart et al., 1986; Montesano et al., 1986; Portier, 1991), elements of design and analysis of particular relevance to QEP of cancer risk will be discussed in this section.

5.2.1 Long-term studies

Considerable experience has now been accumulated with long-term bioassays for carcinogenicity. Since the 1970s, the US National Cancer Institute/National Toxicology Program (NTP) has evaluated the carcinogenic potential of over 400 chemicals in rats and mice. Of these, about 50% have shown some evidence of carcinogenic potential, with about 20% active in rodent liver. A recent meta-analysis of the NTP data conducted by Crump et al. (1998) provides statistical evidence that there are more liver carcinogens than have been identified by analysing the results of each study alone.

Gold et al. (1984) established a database on carcinogen bioassay, which now includes information on over 4000 individual experiments for over 1000 chemical carcinogens (cf. Gold et al., 1993). This information is of use both in identifying substances with carcinogenic properties, and in predicting cancer risks to humans.

5.2.1.1 Design and conduct

When planning a long-term bioassay, a large number of aspects must be considered, the most important being animal species and strain, route of administration, selection of doses, duration and interim sacrifices, ad libitum versus restricted feeding, and gross and microscopic pathology.

Dose. If the purpose of a long-term study is to find out whether or not the test substance is carcinogenic, a single high dose level may be sufficient. Such studies are useful for identifying carcinogenic hazards. If the bioassay is intended to provide dose–response data to be used in QEP, more dose levels are desirable. The greater the

number of dose levels, the greater the resolution of the dose–response curve. However, cost considerations normally dictate the conduct of relatively small studies involving one control and three or four different dose levels. As discussed in Chapter 7, information in addition to that from long- and medium-term bioassays is necessary in order to use biologically based models.

The high dose or estimated maximum tolerated dose (MTD) is one that is expected on the basis of prechronic studies to produce some toxicity when administered for the duration of the test period. The MTD should not, however, reduce the normal longevity of the treated animals from effects other than induced tumours, and body weight gain in treated animals should not be retarded too much. These criteria for selecting the high dose have been recommended even if the metabolic pathways at the high dose differ from those that operate at lower doses (International Agency for Research on Cancer, 1980; Stich, 1984; Feron & Kroes, 1986). An argument in favour of the MTD is that it compensates for a limited number of animals by increasing the doses that would express any carcinogenic potential and would therefore facilitate the detection of "weak carcinogens" (Faccini et al., 1992). It is also claimed that the MTD simulates extreme conditions that might be found, e.g. in occupational settings (Clayson et al., 1991). A recent evaluation of 216 chemicals found to cause tumours in rodents in studies conducted by the National Cancer Institute/National Toxicology Program showed that only 7% of these rodent carcinogens had led to increased tumour rates at the top dose alone (Haseman & Lockhart, 1994). The detection of chemicals inducing kidney tumours in male and female rats and in mice would have been particularly compromised if the top dose had not been included.

In recent years, the philosophy of choosing the MTD has been strongly criticized, to such an extent as even to cast doubt on the value of long-term rodent bioassays (Carr & Kolbye, 1991). These criticisms stem mainly from the argument that the MTD can cause tissue damage which may induce cell proliferation leading to mutations and eventually neoplasms. Thus, chemicals that induce tumours in rodents only at high doses may not present a carcinogenic risk to humans exposed to much lower, non-toxic doses (Ashby & Morrod, 1991). As a result, the concept of the maximum appropriate exposure (MAE) has been suggested as a substitute for the MTD (Faccini *et al.*, 1992). The MAE takes into account the pharmacokinetics and metabolism of a substance and, most importantly, avoids the use of doses that cause overt cyto- or histotoxicity likely to induce mitogenesis and physiological overloading.

The US National Research Council (1993) recently published a detailed review of the use of the MTD in animal cancer tests. While recognizing the difficulties in interpreting certain results observed at this dose, it nevertheless tended, with some reservations, to view the continued use of the MTD as desirable from the point of view of preserving the statistical power of the assay to detect carcinogenic agents.

In order to use tumour frequencies found at the MTD for QEP, it must be shown that the processes occurring at the MTD are also relevant at low doses, since tumour formation is often not seen at low doses due to the low sensitivity of animal studies. The problem of the relevance of the results of studies using the MTD to those obtained at low doses can also be investigated in toxicokinetic studies. Moreover, studies on the dose–relationship of surrogate markers, e.g. biological markers, may be useful in predicting effects at low doses from results obtained at high doses. Data from chronic toxicological studies may also be helpful in throwing light on this question.

Another complicating factor in animal studies is that the tumour frequency may be affected by the dose regime. Thus, even after oral administration, the tumour frequency has been found to depend on whether the substance has been added to the drinking-water or the food or given by gavage. How does the tumour frequency depend on the dosing regime? It is known from skin painting experiments with mice that the frequency of tumour formation depends on the dosing regime of the promoter. How should this be taken into account in QEP calculations? In studies of promotion in rodent liver, altered foci, which are often considered to be preneoplastic lesions, may regress when the dosing is stopped. Differences between animal experiments and humans have been found in the case of malignant melanoma and ultraviolet irradiation. In hairless mice, the

frequency of tumour formation is increased when the dose is given at a low rate, while, in humans, high doses at a young age, e.g. sunburn in children, appear to increase the risk of malignancy.

The problem of selecting the most suitable experimental design for prediction of low-dose risks has been the subject of several investigations (Portier & Hoel, 1983; Krewski *et al.*, 1984, 1986; Gaylor *et al.* 1985). The reader is referred to Portier (1991) for a review of these results. In general, the number of doses in an optimal experimental design depends on the number of parameters in the model used for low-dose extrapolation. With a three-parameter model, for example, the optimal designs for estimating the TD_{05} (defined as the dose inducing an excess lifetime risk of 5%) involve a control group, the MTD and an intermediate dose which depends on the degree of curvature in the dose–response relationship.

Experiments with vinyl chloride yield a dose–response curve which plateaus at high doses (Purchase *et al.*, 1985) owing to saturation of metabolic pathways, whereas that of formaldehyde exhibits sharp upward curvature (World Health Organization, 1989). Peto *et al.*, (1984, 1991) conducted a large-scale dose–response study of the carcinogenicity of several *N*-nitroso compounds, involving over 5000 rodents (rats, mice, and hamsters) and 16 different dose levels. In this study, the slope of the dose–response curve based on the lower dose levels was found to depend on the duration of exposure. Dewanji *et al.* (1993) showed that carcinogenic potency as measured by the TD_{50} also depended on duration of exposure in a large-scale bioassay of 2-acetylaminofluorene involving over 24 000 mice conducted by the US National Center for Toxicological Research (Littlefield *et al.*, 1980). In order to characterize the temporal aspects of cancer risk, both interim sacrifices and treatment groups involving exposures of different duration can be included in the experimental protocol.

A control group of untreated animals should always be included in a carcinogenicity study. When a compound is administered in a vehicle, the controls should also receive that vehicle. Historical control data, when used properly, may be of great value in evaluating the results of carcinogenicity studies. It is, however, questionable whether final conclusions can ever be based on the use of historical control tumour incidence data alone. Historical controls may not be compatible with concurrent controls because of genetic differences or differences in the laboratory environments in which the experiments were conducted (Haseman *et al.*, 1984). Based on a comparison with historical control data, the results of a study may be qualified as inconclusive, and a (costly and time-consuming) repeat study may then be necessary to reach an unequivocal conclusion (Maronpot, 1985; Feron & Kroes, 1986). Care should therefore be taken to ensure that historical controls are compatible with concurrent controls.

Duration and time to tumour appearance. Tumours appear in untreated rodents with increased frequency during the second half of their life span. As this is also the case in humans, this is an argument for quasi-lifetime studies, usually 24 months in rats and 18–24 months in mice. A strong argument for lifetime studies is that they also allow the maximum exposure to the test substance. A reason for extending studies beyond 24 months is that the carcinogenic effect might become visible only at some later time point. Obvious reasons for not extending the duration of a study include geriatric pathology that can complicate and obscure the assessment of carcinogenicity, loss of aging animals due to spontaneous death followed by autolysis and cannibalism, higher costs and animal welfare (Feron & Kroes, 1986; Faccini *et al.*, 1992). Very useful information can be obtained from histopathological examination of animals dying or being killed *in extremis* during the study, and also from interim sacrifices. For example, in a 24-month rat study, 10 animals per group may be killed at 12 or at 12 and 18 months. This will facilitate the collection of valuable information for the final interpretation of the results, e.g. such information could provide a better understanding of preneoplastic lesions and of hormonal or toxic effects (Faccini *et al.*, 1992). It is emphasized that a proper evaluation of the experimental results will take into account all animals included in the study regardless of whether or not they survived until the end of the study (Gart *et al.*, 1986).

Histopathology. It is imperative that pathological examinations meet the most stringent standards of quality, uniformity and objectivity, because conclusions concerning carcinogenicity are based on comparisons of patterns of tumour occurrence between exposed and unexposed animals (Ward & Reznik, 1983). An extensive discussion of the pathology as part of a carcinogenicity bioassay has recently been published by Faccini *et al.* (1992). The importance of accuracy of diagnosis and incidence of lesions cannot be overemphasized. The use of a standard nomenclature comprehensible to other pathologists and reviewers of a report is crucial. Standardized systems of nomenclature and diagnostic criteria guides for toxicological pathologists, and tumour pathology information systems for toxicologists are currently being published or are in preparation (Faccini *et al.*, 1992). From the statistical point of view, it is desirable that pathology is done "blind", i.e. histopathological evaluation should be performed without the pathologist knowing the treatment group. However, it is not recommended that pathologists ever undertake completely "blind" evaluation, i.e. without any knowledge of the animals from which the tissues originate or of the study, test compound, etc. What is advocated in toxicological pathology is a re-evaluation of the diagnosis by another pathologist who does not know whether a particular slide is from a treated or control animal.

While some form of "blind" reading of slides is recommended, the avoidance of "diagnostic drift" or time-related changes in the evaluation of histopathological changes is even more important (Arnold *et al.*, 1988). The best way of dealing with this problem is, at the end of the study, to re-examine all tissues in which there are important or statistically significant differences between groups. A practical way to minimize diagnostic drift is to evaluate a few animals from each group at a time, working across all groups rather than completing a whole group before starting the next (Faccini *et al.*, 1992).

The database for statistical analysis should include not only the pathologist's findings, but also the time at which the tumour was first noticed. This is feasible for visible or palpable (so-called observable) tumours; for internal (so-called occult) tumours, it will correspond to the time of necropsy. Whereas the analysis of observable tumours is relatively straightforward, that of occult tumours involves additional assumptions concerning the relationship between the observable outcome, age at death with a tumour, and age at onset of the tumour (McKnight & Crowley, 1984; Gart et al., 1986). It is also desirable to record whether each tumour was the underlying cause of death. The pathologist can be reasonably confident about this in some cases, but more often is unable to give a reliable answer. A practicable compromise is to categorize tumours as "definitely not", "probably not", "probably" or "definitely" responsible for the animal's death (Peto et al., 1980). Whenever possible, an effort should be made to determine the context of observation of each tumour. However, in many studies conducted to date, the contexts of observation are unknown for all or most tumours. As definitive information in this regard will probably remain incomplete in many future studies, a method for adjusting for differential survival rates which does not require the accurate categorization of individual tumours as incidental or fatal would be useful (Gart et al., 1986).

5.2.1.2 Statistical Analysis

The statistical analysis of long-term laboratory studies of carcinogenicity has been previously discussed in detail in an IARC publication (Gart et al., 1986). A fundamental objective of the analysis of such screening studies is to determine whether the administration of the test agent results in an increase in tumour occurrence rates as compared with those in unexposed controls (Bickis & Krewski, 1985). Tests for increased tumour occurrence rates among exposed animals may be based on pairwise comparisons between each treated group and the control group, or on increases in such rates with increasing dose.

Statistical tests of the null hypothesis of no effect of the test agent on the occurrence of a particular tumour may be based on the crude proportion of animals bearing that tumour, sometimes known as the "lifetime tumour incidence rate", defined as the ratio of the number of animals developing tumours during the course of the study in a given dose group to the number of animals initially assigned to that dose group. Pairwise comparisons of the proportion of tumour-bearing animals may be based on the usual chi-square test for 2 x 2 tables, or on Fisher's

exact test; the latter is recommended with rare tumours in order to maintain the desired type I (false-positive) error rate. Analogous procedures are available to test for an increase in the proportion of tumour-bearing animals with increasing dose: the Cochran–Armitage test is widely used to test for an increase in crude tumour rates with increasing dose, an exact permutation test being recommended when the observed number of tumours is small (Bickis & Krewski, 1989).

Statistical methods have been developed to take historical control information into account in tests for trend in lifetime tumour incidence rates. Historical controls from previous studies provide some information on the spontaneous rate of occurrence of the lesion of interest, and may therefore strengthen statistical tests for trend (Haseman et al., 1984). However, care should be taken to ensure that the historical controls are compatible with the concurrent controls in order to avoid distortion of the type I error rate (Krewski et al., 1988). Following the seminal paper by Tarone (1982) on tests for trend with historical controls, a number of different statistical tests designed to take historical control data into account have been proposed. Because historical experiments are unlikely to be identical in all respects to the study of current interest, allowances must be made for between-study variation in historical control tumour occurrence rates. These tests have recently been reviewed and evaluated by Fung et al. (1996). This study indicated that one of the tests proposed by Prentice et al. (1992) performed particularly well in terms of type I and type II (false-negative) error. The general tendency of tests on historical controls is to strengthen the evidence against the null hypothesis when the average historical control response rate is similar to that in the concurrent control group, and the historical controls do not demonstrate a high degree of variability. When they are highly variable, the use of historical control data has little effect on tests for trend in tumour occurrence rates.

Tests for increased tumour occurrence based on lifetime tumour incidence are most appropriate when survival rates do not differ appreciably in different dose groups (Gart et al., 1979; McKnight, 1988). For example, if the effect of treatment is to reduce survival, early mortality in the high-dose groups may preclude the development of tumours. In this case, reliance on crude lifetime tumour incidence rates may give the misleading impression that there is no increase in tumour occurrence, even in the presence of increased age-specific tumour incidence at all ages.

To avoid biases such as this due to differences in intercurrent mortality among treatment groups, Peto (1974) and Peto *et al.* (1980) proposed a test for differences in tumour occurrence rates due to treatment, taking into account the times at which tumours were observed. This procedure requires information on the cause of death of each animal, and is based on a time-stratified contingency table analysis of the prevalence of incidental tumours that did not kill their host and a similar analysis of fatal tumours that resulted in death prior to the termination of the study. These two analyses are then combined to arrive at an overall test for increasing trend in tumour occurrence rates allowing for differential survival rates among the treatment groups.

Theoretical justifications for this procedure were subsequently provided by Lagakos & Louis (1988) and Burnett *et al.* (1989). Such justifications involve certain assumptions, the most important of which is that the occurrence of a tumour does not alter the death rate from non-tumour causes (McKnight & Crowley, 1984).

Related statistical tests allowing for survival differences have been discussed by a number of authors. Dinse & Haseman (1986) and Finkelstein (1986) discuss parametric tests for non-lethal tumours. Dewanji & Kalbfleisch (1986) developed a non-parametric test designed for use with studies with serial sacrifices. Portier & Bailer (1989) proposed a simple method of adjusting lifetime tumour incidence data for intercurrent mortality; tests for trend in lifetime tumour incidence discussed previously can then be applied to the adjusted data. Tests requiring the availability of cause of death information have been developed by Dinse (1988a), Malani & Van Ryzin (1988), Archer & Ryan (1989) and McKnight & Wahrendorf (1992). Leroux *et al.* (1992) have developed a general class of non-parametric rank tests which involve minimal assumptions and do not require cause of death information. Other non-parametric tests are discussed by Kodell & Ahn (1997).

Since tests for increased cancer risk based on lifetime tumour incidence rates do not take into account the times at which tumours were observed, it is possible that such tests may be inefficient as compared with those based on time-to-tumour data even in the absence of differential intercurrent mortality. Ryan (1989) and Gart & Tarone (1987) show that this is in fact the case, but that the loss in efficiency is usually small.

Another important consideration in the statistical analysis of long-term animal experiments is multiple hypothesis testing. In a typical experiment, information may be available on the occurrence of 20–30 different types of tumours. Although tests for trend may be based on the number of tumour–bearing animals in each treatment group without regard to tumour type, separate tests for each type of tumour are generally conducted. Such tests are desirable because most carcinogens induce specific types of tumours; tests based on each tumour type are then generally more sensitive than those based on the aggregation of tumour types in terms of the number of tumour-bearing animals (Bickis & Krewski, 1989). Statistical tests based on multiple tumour types designed to control the overall false positive rate have been developed by Farrar & Crump (1988, 1990) and Westfall & Young (1989). For further discussion, see Chen (1996).

5.2.2 Medium-term studies

Medium-term bioassays have been developed primarily for the identification of carcinogens in a relatively short period of time, but are increasingly being used for obtaining information on carcinogenic action and for studying dose–response relationships. Medium-term studies bridge the gap between *in vitro* and *in vivo* screening methods for mutagenicity and genotoxicity and the long-term carcinogenicity study, with their inherent disadvantages (Ito *et al.*, 1992). Various medium-term systems including multiorgan systems have been introduced, using as test organs skin, liver, lung, mammary gland, stomach, kidney, thyroid, pancreas, intestines and urinary bladder either separately or in certain combinations in rats, mice and/or hamsters (Ward & Ito, 1988; Ito *et al.*, 1989; Ogiso *et al.*, 1990; Ito *et al.*, 1992). The emphasis here will be on mouse skin and liver systems, because these have been used most widely for quantitative purposes.

5.2.2.1 Mouse skin

The two-stage (multistage) model of mouse skin is one of the oldest experimental systems of carcinogenesis. The terms "initiation" and "promotion" were defined in this system by Friedwald & Rous (1944) and an experimental "initiation–promotion" protocol was developed shortly thereafter (Mottram, 1944; Berenblum & Shubik, 1947) which is still used today with only minor modifications. Studies in mouse skin were, from the very beginning, primarily directed towards mechanistic aspects of carcinogenesis. Today, carcinogenic polycyclic aromatic hydrocarbons, and in particular 7,8-dimethyl-benz[a]anthracene (DMBA), are primarily used for initiation, while a large variety of different agents of quite diverse chemical nature are used as "promoters" in mouse skin. These include diterpene (phorbol)-ester type compounds, e.g. 12-O-tetradecanoylphorbol-13-acetate (TPA), alkaloids such as teleocidine and staurosporine, reactive oxygen-producing agents such as benzoyl peroxide, phenols and certain carcinogens, such as 7-bromomethylbenzo[a]anthracene (for a review see Slaga, 1984). The vast majority of studies were performed with TPA. Various strains of mice have been used that differ markedly in their responsiveness to TPA promotion. The most sensitive are Sencar mice, while C57BL/6 mice, for example, are comparatively insensitive (Slaga, 1986). The experimental end-point is generally the benign tumour (papilloma) of the skin. Time-dependent increases in the fraction of papilloma-bearing animals (tumour rate) and the average number of tumours per mouse (tumour yield) are recorded as quantitative response parameters. Data on carcinomas of the skin, which develop later during the experiment, are less frequently recorded. In the "standard inititation–promotion protocol", a carcinogen is administered topically on the shaved back of the mouse at a dose which is low enough not to produce significant numbers of tumours by itself. The promoting agent (e.g. TPA dissolved in acetone) is subsequently administered by chronic (often biweekly) topical painting on the mouse back skin. The first papillomas are observable at about six weeks after the start of TPA treatment. Hennings (1989) concluded that the frequency of papilloma occurrence and the relative rate of malignant conversion to carcinomas is dependent on the duration of TPA treatment (Table 5.1). In the study by Hennings et al., (1983), the rate of malignant conversion of papillomas to carcinomas was increased by treating papilloma-bearing mice with a second application of an "initiating" carcinogen - according to the initiation–promotion–initiation (IPI) protocol.

Mutational activation of the c-Ha-*ras* proto-oncogene appears to play an important role during initiation of mouse skin carcinogenesis:

Table 5.1. Papilloma and carcinoma development in Sencar mice[a]

Group[b]	Duration of promotion	Total no. of papillomas per group	Total no. of carcinomas per group	Percentage conversion
1	5	189	25	13.2
2	10	582	24	4.1
3	20	748	24	3.2
4	40	734	20	2.7

[a] Source: Hennings (1989).
[b] Groups of 30 Sencar mice underwent tumour-initiating treatment with 20 mg dimethylbenz[a]anthracene (DMBA) and weekly promoting treatments with 2 mg 12-O-tetradecanoylphorbol-13-acetate (TBA) for the indicated periods of time. The experiment was terminated at week 52.

100% (48/48) of mouse skin papillomas induced by DMBA were demonstrated to carry *ras* mutations (Brown *et al.*, 1990). Different carcinogens produce distinctly different mutational spectra, suggesting that *ras* mutations represent an initiating event in two-stage skin carcinogenesis (Balmain & Brown, 1988; Brown *et al.*, 1990). Mutations of the *p53* tumour–suppressor gene may represent a later genetic alteration occurring at the papilloma/carcinoma transition (Ruggeri *et al.*, 1991; Kress *et al.*, 1992).

All potent tumour promoters in mouse skin induce epidermal hyperplasia, which is brought about by quite diverse mechanisms: agents of the phorbol ester group interact with intracellular signal transduction pathways, in that they mimic the stimulatory action of the second messenger, diacylglycerol, on enzymes of the protein kinase C family (Nishizuka, 1988); the Ca^{2+} ionophor A 23187 acts by changing intracellular Ca^{2+} concentration (Slaga *et al.*, 1982); and okadaic acid elicits its effects by inhibiting phosphoprotein phosphatases (Suganuma *et al.*, 1988). The appearance and persistence of papillomas in the initiation–promotion experiment in mouse skin depends on permanent mitogenic stimulation (Burns *et al.*, 1976). Upon discontinuation of treatment, more than 80% of papillomas may disappear. Not all skin mitogens are epidermal tumour promoters (Marks *et al.*, 1982). This led Boutwell (1964) to the assumption that promotion may consist of two separate events, which he called "conversion" and "propagation". Experimental results in support of this concept include those of Slaga *et al.* (1980), using TPA as a "converting" agent and mezerein as a "propagating" agent, and of Fürstenberger *et al.* (1981), who used TPA and its retinoyl derivative RPA. While "propagation" reflects the chronic mitogenic component, and may be better termed "promotion" (Marks & Fürstenberger, 1990), "conversion" appears to be mechanistically different. A single treatment with a "converting" agent (e.g. TPA) is sufficient, when combined with a subsequent chronic treatment with a "non-converting" but hyperplasiogenic agent (e.g. mezerein or RPA), for promotion of papilloma formation, and the initiation–conversion sequence (but not the initiation-promotion sequence) can be inverted (Fürstenberger *et al.*, 1985; for a review see Marks & Fürstenberger, 1990). Although the mouse skin principally represents an excellent model for quantitative analyses of carcinogenesis (because both the formation and the growth of tumours are readily visible and can be analysed at different time points for one and the same animal), the number of relevant studies is comparatively limited. Detailed quantitative analyses of the carcinogenic process in mouse skin were performed by Burns (1989). Recently, birth and death rates of papillomas in initiation–promotion experiments in mouse skin have been modelled (Kopp-Schneider & Portier, 1992).

5.2.2.2 Liver

Hepatocarcinogenesis in rodents is a very useful tool for use in studying critical changes occurring during the carcinogenic process in liver. Exposure of experimental animals to hepatocarcinogens leads to the formation of altered hepatic foci (AHF) characterized by increases or decreases in certain cellular substrates such as glycogen and in the activity and/or level of a large variety of different enzymes which can be used as markers for their identification. Among many others, these include the enzymes γ-glutamyl transpeptidase, canalicular adenosine triphosphate, glucose-6-phosphatase, various cytochromes P-450, epoxide hydrolase, glucuronosyl transferase and the placental form of glutathione transferase (GST-P), which may be used to detect even single enzyme-altered cells (for a recent review, see Pitot, 1990). AHF have been shown to be monoclonal in origin (Rabes *et al.*, 1982; Williams *et al.*, 1983; Weinberg *et al.*, 1987) and to display, in comparison with their surrounding normal hepatocytes, an increase in cell proliferation rates (Rabes *et al.*, 1972; Emmelot & Scherer 1980; Rotstein *et al.*, 1986; Bannasch & Zerban, 1990; Schulte-Hermann *et al.*, 1990; Bannasch & Zerban, 1992) or a decrease in the rate of apoptosis (Schulte-Hermann *et al.*, 1990). There is accumulating evidence to suggest that at least some of the AHF represent precursor lesions causally related to the carcinogenic process in liver. This is substantiated by the sequential appearance of AHF and tumours, the similarity of many marker enzyme changes in both types of lesions (Goldfarb & Pugh, 1981), the observation of "foci within foci" (Potter, 1984; Scherer *et al.*, 1984) and the observation of quantitative relationships between the development of AHF and the later manifestation of hepatic tumours (Emmelot & Scherer, 1980; Kunz et al., 1983; Vesselinovitch & Mihailovitch, 1983; Schwarz et al., 1989b; Pitot et al., 1990). The fact that AHF occur in much larger numbers than liver neoplasms makes their detection easier and increases the power of their statistical evaluation. In addition, since they precede the occurrence of the neoplasms, they have been used to detect carcinogenic effects at dose levels that would not be expected to lead to neoplasms within the lifetime of the animals (Kunz et al., 1983; Zerban et al., 1988; Schwarz et al., 1989a,b).

Experimental protocols. A large number of different experimental protocols exist which use the evolution of AHF as a medium-term end-point of hepatocarcinogenesis (for reviews, see Goldsworthy & Hanigan, 1987; Bannasch & Zerban 1992). Of these, the most "simplistic" employs chronic treatment with a single test agent and one or more sacrifice time points. More often, initiation–promotion protocols are used which can essentially be subdivided into two general categories (Pitot, 1990). In the first, a single dose of an initiating carcinogen is administered in combination with a mitotic stimulus; this can be physiological in the neonate or can be brought about by a partial hepatectomy in the adult or the administration of a single high necrogenic dose of a carcinogen. Short continuous carcinogen feeding periods have also been used for the initiation of hepatocarcinogenesis. Subsequently, test agents with presumed promoting activity are administered chronically for various periods of time. These protocols allow the analysis of the dose–response of the initiating carcinogen as well as the dose– and time–response of the "promoting" agents. In the second category of protocols, the "resistent hepatocyte model" developed by Farber and colleagues (Solt & Farber, 1976; Farber & Cameron, 1980) is used. In this model, initiated liver cells are generated by brief exposure of rats to a carcinogen such as N-nitrosodiethylamine (NDEA). Subsequently, selection to proliferation resulting in the rapid formation of AHF or hyperplastic nodules is accomplished by exposure to dietary 2-acetylaminofluorene in combination with a stimulus for hepatocyte proliferation such as partial hepatectomy or carbon tetrachloride

administration. The selective toxicity of 2-acetylaminofluorene for normal hepatocytes observed in this system may be explained both by a decrease in metabolic toxification of the carcinogen in the initiated cells and a decreased level of uptake of this agent by initiated hepatocytes. Thus, resistance appears to provide the initiated cells with a selective growth advantage in a toxic environment. Quantitative studies employing systems including selection procedures of the above types are particularly suited to the study of the effects of initiators. However because the selection procedure itself causes intense "promotion", the identification of "promoting agents" by means of these protocols is less effective (Pitot, 1990). The most extensive study, covering a total of 179 test chemicals, has been published by Ito and associates (Ito et al., 1988b, 1992). In their protocol, rats are given a single dose of NDEA for initiation, followed by chronic administration of the test agent after a two-week recovery period. One week after the start of chronic treatment, animals are subjected to a partial hepatectomy to maximize any interactions between proliferation and the effects of the test agent. On week 8 after NDEA administration, all animals are sacrificed and AHF are quantified in their livers using GST-P as a marker for their identification.

Stereological procedures in quantitative analyses of AHF. The relevant parameters for quantitative analyses are the number of AHF per liver and the volume fraction occupied in liver by enzyme-altered tissue. The latter can be estimated directly from data on the areal fraction of focal transections in the two-dimensional space which directly corresponds to the volume fraction in the three-dimensional space (Delesse, 1848). The volume fraction of AHF gives a rough measure of the total number of enzyme-altered cells per liver. The number of AHF in the three-dimensional space, however, can only be estimated indirectly on the basis of data on the number and size distribution of two-dimensional transections from AHF observed within tissue sections. Stereological procedures have to be used here (for a review, see Campbell et al., 1982). Albeit unfortunately not generally recognized, the omission of stereological procedures for evaluating the (three-dimensional) number of foci from the number and size of their (two-dimensional) transections can generate false-positive results (Campbell *et al.*, 1982). This is because any increase in the mean size of AHF—which is a hallmark of the activity of promoting agents—will, for simple statistical reasons, increase proportionally the frequency of countable focal transections, often referred to as "foci/cm^2".

Potency ranking of agents using AHF. The quantitative analysis of AHF makes it possible to study the initiating and promoting potencies of liver cancer risk factors. Since AHF are of monoclonal origin, the number of foci can serve as a rough estimate of the initiating potency of a test agent, while promoter-mediated clonal expansion of cells within AHF leads to changes in their size distribution (Pitot *et al.*, 1987; Schwarz *et al.*, 1989a,b; Pitot *et al.*, 1990). On the basis of these considerations, Pitot and co-workers have recently defined indices that may be used to rank test chemicals according to their initiating and/or promoting activities (Pitot *et al.*, 1987, 1990), as follows:

Initiation index (for single-dose experiments) = (total number of AHF - number of spontaneous AHF) × liver^{-1} × (mmol/kg body weight)$^{-1}$.

Promotion index (determined in initiation–promotion experiments) = (volume fraction (%) of liver occupied by AHF in test animals)/(volume fraction (%) of liver occupied by AHF in animals initiated but not receiving test agents) × mmol^{-1} × weeks^{-1}.

The authors (Pitot *et al.*, 1987) recognize that these expressions are probably oversimplifications. With respect to the "initiation index" it must be remembered that the number of single initiated cells produced by a given carcinogen in liver will most probably exceed the number of AHF clonally derived from these cells. This is due to the fact that not all AHF may exhibit the enzyme change used as marker for their identification, and that AHF can only be counted if their size exceeds a certain detection limit. In addition, there is a non-zero probability that initiated cells or small foci will become extinct by natural death, as shown by analyses of the size distribution of AHF, which demonstrated that a major fraction of initiated cells may never develop into

visible AHF (Moolgavkar *et al.*, 1990; Luebeck *et al.*, 1991), and by the observation of a rapid decline in carcinogen-induced single GST-P-positive hepatocytes in liver shortly after carcinogen exposure (Satoh *et al.*, 1989). The "promotion index" is also influenced by various factors. Effects mediated on AHF growth by promoting agents are often not linearly related to dose and time of treatment. In addition, the strain and sex of test animals, as well as differences in the initiation–promotion protocols used in different laboratories, may well affect the experimental outcome. Initiating and promoting potencies can also be defined by modelling liver foci data. In this way, initiating and promoting indices for *N*-nitrosomorpholine in rat liver have been determined (Moolgavkar *et al.*, 1990; see also section 6.4), and a potency ranking for the promoting activity of different polyhalogenated biphenyls in rat liver has also been established (Luebeck *et al.*, 1991).

5.2.2.3 Other organs

Lungs of strain A mice. Strain A mice are prone to develop lung tumours (mainly adenomas originating from type II pneumocytes). This bioassay has been used to test over 400 chemicals (Stoner & Shimkin, 1985; Maronpot *et al.*, 1986). Since too many known carcinogens were negative in this assay, a negative result is not very meaningful and must be verified by means of other carcinogenicity bioassays (Ito *et al.*, 1992).

Sprague–Dawley rat mammary glands. Female Sprague–Dawley rats are sensitive to the development of mammary tumours after treatment with carcinogens such as *N*-methyl-*N*-nitrosourea (MNU), 3-methylcholanthrene, benzo[*a*]pyrene and, in particular, DMBA. Other rat strains may also be used. In the two-stage model of this assay, DMBA is usually used as the initiator (McCormick & Moon, 1985). The general applicability of this assay is rather limited (Ito *et al.*, 1992).

Stomach. The stomach models are used for initiation–promotion studies using *N*-methyl-*N*-nitro-*N*-nitrosoguanidine (MNNG) as the initiator. The end-point is neoplasia (Takahashi *et al.*, 1986). Later, an assay was developed using pepsinogen isozyme 1-altered pyloric glands as early end-point markers (Tatematsu *et al.*, 1988).

To enhance the sensitivity of the gastric mucosa to any carcinogenic action, a saturated solution of sodium chloride is given by stomach tube. This model is currently being validated for use as a medium-term bioassay (Ito *et al.*, 1992).

Kidney. Tsuda *et al.* (1985) developed an initiation–promotion assay for the rat kidney, using *N*-ethyl-*N*-hydroxyethylnitrosamine as the initiator and glutathione-S-transferase, glucose-6-phosphate dehydrogenase and γ-glutamyltranspeptidase as markers of preneoplastic and neoplastic renal changes. More studies are needed to evaluate the usefulness of this system (Ito *et al.*, 1992).

Thyroid. Two-stage models for thyroid carcinogenesis have been studied mainly in rats after initiation with *N*-nitrosobis(2-hydroxypropyl)-amine (NDHPA) given by the intraperitoneal, subcutaneous or oral route. The promoting effect of compounds such as 3-amino-1,2,3-triazole, 4,4-diaminodiphenylmethane and phenobarbital on thyroid carcinogenesis have been demonstrated using this model (Hiasa *et al.*, 1984, 1985). A disadvantage of this bioassay is that thyroid carcinogenesis is affected by hormonal conditions, so that levels of serum iodine, thyroxine and thyroid-stimulating hormone (TSH) must be controlled (Ito *et al.*, 1992).

Pancreas. Two medium-term pancreas models are widely used, one in Syrian golden hamsters and one in rats (Pour *et al.*, 1981; Longnecker, 1986). The initiators used are *N*-nitrosobis(2-oxopropyl)amine and azaserine for hamsters and rats, respectively. Tumours and preneoplastic lesions in hamsters are of ductular origin and are histologically similar to human pancreatic cancer. Pancreatic lesions in rats are of acinar origin. The use of both models in a comparative way has appeared to be a successful approach in studies on the role of lifestyle factors (fat, coffee, alcohol, vitamins) in pancreatic carcinogenesis (Woutersen & Van Garderen-Hoetmer, 1988; Woutersen *et al.*, 1989a,b). Since it is well known that pancreatic carcinogenesis is markedly affected by dietary fat and protein (Birt & Pour, 1985; Longnecker, 1986; Appel *et al.*, 1990, 1991), these factors must be carefully controlled in studies using these bioassays.

Intestines. Initiation–promotion models for the rat intestines have been developed but the available information is not yet sufficient to evaluate their significance as a medium-term bioassay (Ito *et al.*, 1992). Shirai *et al.* (1985) studied the modifying effects of antioxidants on 1,2-dimethylhydrazine-induced colon carcinogenesis in F344 rats.

Urinary bladder. Hicks *et al.* (1975) developed a two-stage model for the rat urinary bladder. Initiation was achieved by direct injection of MNU into the bladder or by dietary administration of *N*-[4-(5-nitro-2-furyl)-2-thiazolyl]formamide (FANFT). Using this model, promoting activity has been detected for sodium saccharin, sodium cyclamate, tryptophane and several other chemicals (Cohen *et al.*, 1979; Fukushima *et al.*, 1981). However, injection of MNU is technically difficult, and FANFT is not sufficiently potent to initiate carcinogenesis effectively (Ito *et al.*, 1992). A simpler rat bladder model of shorter duration, using *N*-nitrosobutyl(4-hydroxybutyl)amine in drinking-water for four weeks as the initiating step, has been developed by Fukushima *et al.* (1983). Preneoplastic lesions and tumours can be quantified simply. With this system, the mechanisms underlying bladder carcinogenesis have been extensively studied (Fukushima, 1991). To increase the sensitivity of the model and to shorten the experimental period, epithelial proliferation was induced by unilateral ligation (Miyata *et al.*, 1985) or ingestion of uracil (Shirai *et al.*, 1986; Masui *et al.*, 1988).

Multiple organs. In order to develop a system for the detection of carcinogenicity in a variety of organs, two different medium-term assays in rats involving multiorgan, wide-spectrum initiation have been introduced (Ito *et al.*, 1992). In one model, MNU is used as an initiating agent. With this model, Uwagawa *et al.* (1991) showed that all of six carcinogens investigated in the MNU model induced organ-specific effects within 20 weeks. Thus, if many organs and tissues are appropriately initiated, the organ-specific carcinogenic potential of a chemical applied subsequently can be assessed in the intact animal. The two major disadvantages of this model are the early death of 10–20% of the animals due to lymphoma or leukaemia, and weak initiation of liver and several other main organs (Ito *et al.*, 1992).

In the NDEA–MNU–NDHPA rat model, sequential treatment with three potent carcinogens that have different spectra of carcinogenic activity is used as the initiation step. NDEA is a hepatocarcinogen, MNU is a wide-spectrum carcinogen and NDHPA induces neoplastic changes in the thyroid, lung, kidneys and urinary bladder. The results obtained so far with this model have been satisfactory (Ito *et al.*, 1992). Several other combinations of carcinogens have been used in attempts to establish appropriate initiation (Ito *et al.*, 1988a; Jang *et al.*, 1991; Hagiwara *et al.*, 1993; Hirose *et al.*, 1993). Further investigations are necessary to optimize the experimental period, and the dose and type of pretreatment carcinogens. In addition, more appropriate marker lesions for each organ and more sensitive evaluation methods are required to improve this multiorgan, medium-term bioassay.

5.3 Transgenic animals

A number of reviews of the use of transgenic animals in cancer research have been published (Adams & Cory, 1991; Griesemer & Tennant, 1992; Fowlis & Balmain, 1993). Many cloned oncogenes and some tumour-suppressor genes have been introduced in the germ line of mice. In addition to the coding sequence, promoter regions or some tissue-specific promoter elements have also been introduced. In the case of tissue-specific promoters, expression in specific tissues can be induced and tumours in these tissues studied (Table 5.2). Altogether, it is estimated that by 1992 more than 10 000 transgenic animals had been produced (Griesemer & Tennant, 1992).

Table 5.2. Tissue-specific tumour development in transgenic mice[a]

Regulatory element used	Expressed gene	Phenotype
Haematopoietic system:		
IgEµ	c-*myc*	B- or pre-B-cell lymphoma
IgEµ	*pim*-1	T-cell lymphoma
IgEµ	*bcl*-2	Extended B-cell survival/ follicular proliferation
bcr	*bcr/abl*	Acute leukaemia (myeloid or lymphoid)
GP91 p Hox	SV40 T Ag	Histiocytic lymphoma
Skin:		
Keratin 10	Ha-*ras*	Papilloma
Zeta-globin	v-Ha-*ras*	Papilloma/carcinoma
Polyoma virus	BNFL-1	Epidermal hyperplasia
Keratin 14	TGF-α	Epidermal hyperplasia/ papilloma
Keratin 6	HPV-1 early region	Epidermal hyperplasia
H2K MHC	v-*jun*	Epidermal hyperplasia Dermal fibrosarcoma
BPV-1	BPV-1	Fibrosarcoma
Tyrosinase	SV40 T Ag	Melanocytic hyperproliferation Malignant melanoma
Mammary gland:		
MMTV LTR	c-*myc*	Mammary carcinoma
MMTV LTR	v-Ha-*ras*	Mammary carcinoma Harderian gland tumour
MMTV LTR	N-*ras*	Mammary carcinoma Harderian gland tumour Male infertility

Table 5.2. (Contd) Tissue-specific tumour development in transgenic mice[a]		
Regulatory element used	**Expressed gene**	**Phenotype**
MMTV LTR	int-1	Mammary carcinoma
		Salivary gland tumour
MMTV LTR	int-2	Mammary carcinoma
		Prostate gland tumour
MMTV LTR	TGF-a	Mammary carcinoma
MMTV LTR	c-neu	Mammary carcinoma
Whey acidic protein	c-myc + Ha-ras	Mammary carcinoma
Brain:		
SV40 or metallothionine	SV40 T Ag	Choroid plexus tumours
Polyoma virus early region	Polyoma virus T Ag	Pituitary tumours
Liver:		
α-1-Anti-trypsin	SV40 T Ag	Liver carcinoma
Metallothionine	TGF-α	Liver carcinoma
Albumin	Hepatitis B virus	Liver carcinoma
Bone:		
Protamine 1	SV40 T Ag	Bone tumour
		Heart tumour
Various	c-fos	Bone tumour
Small intestine:		
Intestinal fatty acid binding protein	SV40 T Ag	Crypt proliferation
Large intestine:		
Glucagon	SV40 T Ag	Colon carcinoma
Lung:		
IgEμ + SV40 promoter	ras	Lung adenomas
Albumin	H-ras	Lung adenocarcinomas
Thyroid:		
Thyroglobulin	SV40 T Ag	Adenocarcinoma
Moloney LTR	mos	C-cell thyroid tumours/ phaeochromocytomas (MEN II)
Kidney:		
Renin	SV40 T Ag	Vascular hyperplasia
Pancreas:		
Insulin	SV40 T Ag	Pancreatic carcinoma

a   Adapted from Fowlis & Balmain (1993). IgEμ: immunoglobulin heavy chain enhancer; GP91 p Hox: cytochrome b sequence; BPV-1: bovine papilloma virus type 1; HPV-1: human papilloma virus type 1; MMTV LTR: mouse mammary tumour virus long terminal repeat; BNFL-1: gene in Epstein-Barr virus; TGF-α: transforming growth factor α; Moloney: Moloney murine sarcoma virus; MEN II: multiple endocrine neoplasia II.

Transgenic animals offer at least three unique opportunities to study carcinogenesis. Of these, the first is in mechanistic research, where the effects of transgene expression reveal the functions of the particular gene concerned, and the second is in the testing of carcinogens and modifiers of carcinogenicity, as discussed below. Finally, transgenic mice can be used as models of *in vivo* mutagenesis.

Several carcinogenicity studies have been conducted in transgenic lines of mice, higher tumour incidences and shorter tumour latency periods being found in transgenic than in non-transgenic mice (Rao *et al.*, 1991). These studies indicate that carcinogenicity testing in transgenic mice is a feasible and promising approach. Validation will require considerably more research; trangenic models still require standardization, replication and application to a far wider range of substances than the few known carcinogens evaluated so far. However, eventually a battery of transgenic mouse lines might conceivably be used in long- and medium-term screening assays for carcinogens *in vivo* (Griesemer & Tennant, 1992).

Statistical analysis of the transgenic mouse assay has recently been discussed by Carr & Gorelick (1995) and Fung *et al.* (1997). Methods for testing for trend in mutation rates and modelling dose–reponse relationships are described, allowing for overdispersion (extrabinomial variation) in mutation frequencies.

5.4 Use of biomarkers

All the biomarkers used in human studies, ranging from DNA and protein adducts to mutations and cytogenetic changes, have also been studied in animal models. They offer the advantage that large doses can be administered in a single exposure under controlled conditions. It is, however, disappointing that only a few biomarker studies have been incorporated into long-term carcinogenicity bioassays to enable conclusions to be drawn about the predictive value of a particular biomarker. In ethylnitrosourea-treated rats, sister chromatid exchanges, scored at one and seven days after treatment, were elevated in the group of animals diagnosed with cancer at sacrifice (Aitio *et al.*, 1988). Of the many types of biomarkers, only DNA adducts and cytogenetic changes are discussed below.

DNA adducts of over 200 chemicals have been identified chemically *in vitro* (Hemminki *et al.*, 1994). About one-third of these have been identified in experimental animals using well characterized standards. The adducts of only five compounds have been measured in chronic carcinogenicity studies, either as part of the bioassay or in a simulated long-term experiment (reviewed by Poirier & Beland, 1992). The studies covered liver and bladder adducts of 2-acetylaminofluorene and 4-aminobiphenyl, liver adducts of aflatoxin B_1 and NDEA and lung adducts of a tobacco-specific nitrosamine, 4-(N-methyl-N-nitrosoamino)-1-(3-pyridyl)-1-butanone. In all cases, the adduct levels increased linearly with dose at low doses. For most of the compounds, they were correlated with tumour yields. Poirier & Beland (1992) conclude that "Taken together, these data suggest that when extrapolating from high doses to low doses within an animal model, the extent of DNA adduct formation will most often correlate with the extent of tumorigenesis. However, in animal model experiments where the number of animals is limited, tumor incidences may not be measurable when DNA adduct levels are low or in the absence of toxicity and/or cell proliferation".

In the case of 4-aminobiphenyl, adducts have been measured in urinary bladder DNA both in experimental animals and in humans. Poirier & Beland (1992) calculated that the 50% tumour incidence equalled 156 fmol adducts/µg of DNA in mice as compared with 0.815 fmol/µg in humans. The levels refer to the main 4-aminobiphenyl adduct at the C8 position of guanine. Even when corrected for lifespan, higher levels of adducts were still required in the mouse than in humans to induce tumours. Although such calculations rely on a number of assumptions (Poirier & Beland, 1992), they show that the new technologies allow such comparisons. The conclusion in the case of 4-aminobiphenyl was that, per unit dose, humans appeared to be more sensitive than mice to the induction of bladder tumours. 4-Aminobiphenyl has also been detected in the haemoglobin of both smokers and non-smokers, the levels found being 150 pg/g haemoglobin among smokers and 30 ng/g among non-smokers (Bryant *et al.*, 1987).

Cytogenetic studies on carcinogenic chemicals in humans and animals have been reviewed by

Sorsa *et al.* (1992). For the known human carcinogens, 19/27 human and 15/27 animal studies were positive for at least one cytogenetic endpoint, namely chromosomal aberration, sister chromatid exchange or micronucleus. For the probable and possible human carcinogens, an equal number of human and animal studies were positive, namely 6/10 and 5/15, respectively. For some of the carcinogens, no tests have been carried out. Among the 31 carcinogens that caused chromosomal aberrations in humans, all but five compounds were also positive in animals (15 compounds tested). The results were often reproduced in *in vitro* tests (Sorsa *et al.*, 1992). Among the 16 carcinogens causing sister chromatid exchanges, all but one were positive in the animals tested (five compounds positive). Among the six carcinogens causing micronuclei, all of the four tested were positive in experimental animals. The authors concluded that there was a reasonable correlation between the cytogenetic findings in animals and humans. The apparent discrepancies were often thought to be due to the differences in levels of exposure.

Proto-oncogenes and tumour-suppressor genes are mutational targets for carcinogens. In a variety of cases, "carcinogen-specific" mutational patterns have been demonstrated in one of these genes in animal tumours. This is particularly true for *ras* gene mutations, which have been studied in great detail (for a review, see Balmain & Brown, 1988; Harris, 1992). Mutations in one of the three *ras* oncogenes represent one of the very early, probably initial, events in chemically induced mouse skin, mouse liver, rat mammary gland and hamster buccal pouch epithelium carcinogenesis (Wiseman *et al.*, 1986; Kumar *et al.*, 1990; Buchmann *et al.*, 1991; Kwong *et al.*, 1992).

Well studied examples of carcinogen-specific differences in the patterns of *ras* mutations are rat mammary carcinomas induced by MNU and DMBA-induced mouse skin papillomas where the former contain C:G to A:T transitions (Zarbl *et al.*, 1985) and the latter A:T to T:A transversions in the Ha-*ras* gene (Quintanilla *et al.*, 1986). Both types of mutations were predicted on the basis of the types of DNA adducts produced by these carcinogens and their mutational patterns *in vitro*. Carcinogen-specific differences in the types of *ras* single-base substitutions were also well characterized in mouse liver (Wiseman *et al.*, 1986). The expected type of *ras* mutations, namely, AT transitions, was also detected in various tumours from rats exposed to aristolochic acid (Schmeiser *et al.*, 1990). More recently, carcinogen-specific mutations in the *p53* tumour-suppressor gene have been described in various animal tumours induced by agents including benzo[*a*]pyrene, alkylating N-nitroso compounds and ultraviolet radiation (Kress *et al.*, 1992; Ohgaki *et al.*, 1992; Ruggeri *et al.*, 1993).

5.5 Short-term tests

Short-term tests have been the subject of intensive research in the past two decades. Large numbers of chemicals were evaluated in the existing test systems and new systems were devised. The total number of systems ranging from DNA binding to *in vivo* studies in animals and humans exceeds 100. Examples of large data sets can be found in several IARC Monographs, (International Agency for Research on Cancer, 1987). Genetic activity profiles were used in the presentation of the data (Waters *et al.*, 1988). Several national and international validation studies have been carried out.

Based on two data sets, namely the chemicals evaluated by IARC and those tested by the US National Toxicology Program, it was established that most carcinogens were detected in mutation tests (Ashby & Tennant, 1988; Ashby *et al.*, 1989; Bartsch & Malaveille, 1990; Ashby & Tennant, 1991; McGregor, 1992a). However, the predictivity varied markedly between different chemical classes. The National Toxicology Program database showed that the *Salmonella* assay was essentially sufficient to detect the positive compounds. When supplemented with the bone-marrow micronucleus test, the combination detected the vast majority of the known human carcinogens (Shelby & Zeiger, 1990).

Using the human carcinogens identified by IARC, Swierenga & Yamasaki (1992) calculated that, of the 27 chemicals or mixtures, 19 were positive in bacterial tests and some were not tested; the main negative results were obtained for metals and benzene. However, when all mutagenic end-points, including chromosomal aberrations, were covered, practically all agents were positive in at least one test system. A similar analysis by Ashby (1992) gave results in agreement with those of Swierenga & Yamasaki (1991), and the author points out that, by scoring mutagenicity in *Salmonella* and aberrations or micronuclei in rodent bone marrow, only the fibres asbestos and erionite remain negative.

The IARC database was examined in an attempt to correlate carcinogenicity in animals with genotoxicity and acute mammalian toxicity. Only those agents for which carcinogenic potency information was available were studied. For both mice and rats, more chemicals were potent carcinogens if they had been categorized in Group 1 (human carcinogens) than if they had been assigned to one of the other categories (McGregor, 1992a). Predictive assays for carcinogenicity considered to be of high specificity included *in vivo* cytogenetic, hepatocyte unscheduled DNA synthesis, *Salmonella* (five commonly used strains), and mammalian cell *hprt* locus mutation assays. None of the relationships was strong enough to form the basis of a simple categorization process, but they could serve to alert investigators to chemicals of special toxicological interest and importance (McGregor, 1992a,b). The human carcinogens were active in those genotoxicity tests with higher specificity for identifying rodent carcinogens. Interestingly, the genotoxic carcinogens did not appear to differ in their potency from non-genotoxic carcinogens.

Ashby & Tennant (1988) have pointed out that, if one applies structural judgement to divide the test compounds into those that resemble known electrophiles (structurally alerting) and those unlikely to form electrophiles, the predictivity of the *Salmonella* test is particularly good. The chemical judgement together with the *Salmonella* assay make a combination that is not essentially strengthened by additional tests (Ashby & Tennant, 1991).

Results of *Salmonella* mutagenicity data have been correlated with the TD_{50} values obtained from the National Cancer Institute–National Toxicology Program databases. The correlation between mutagenic and carcinogenic potencies was 0.41 for the 80 chemicals tested (McCann *et al.*, 1988). If only three chemicals, at extreme ends of the potency scale, were removed from the analysis, the correlation decreased to 0.24. However, the correlations obtained would probably depend on the chemical class studied, and bacterial mutagenicity studies cannot be considered a general predictor of carcinogenic potency.

Two commonly used tests assaying for non-mutational end-points are cell transformation and gap-junction intercellular communication assays (Swierenga & Yamasaki, 1992). Overall, the cell transformation test predicts human carcinogens better than the *Salmonella* assay, and is positive for a number of carcinogens that do not induce mutations. The predictivity of the intercellular communication assay is considered to be reasonable for human carcinogens (Swierenga & Yamasaki, 1992). Correlations with carcinogenic potency have not been attempted with these two systems.

A new area of *in vivo* mutagenesis testing is provided by transgenic animals. The animals are constructed with suitable marker vectors. Integrated shuttle vectors, mutated *in vivo*, are rescued and analysed *in vitro* (Gossen *et al.*, 1989; Kohler *et al.*, 1990).

5.6 Conclusions

In this chapter, the use of long- and medium term carcinogenicity studies in animals to identify carcinogenic hazards has been discussed. In the absence of epidemiological data, such animal studies remain the most widely accepted means of identifying agents with carcinogenic potential. The long-term rodent bioassay is now well developed, and excellent guidelines on experimental protocols are now available. Although the use of high doses such as the maximum tolerated dose in animal experiments has been criticized with respect to relevance to humans, such doses are used to provide adequate statistical power with experiments of practical size. Animal cancer tests employing a series of increasing dose levels are useful in identifying carcinogenic hazards and in estimating carcinogenic risks.

The statistical analysis of cancer bioassay data is also well developed, but can require the use of sophisticated methodologies if appropriate inferences are to be made. Particular difficulties arise when the time of tumour onset is not readily determined, since an end-point that is not directly observable must be inferred. Methods for the analysis of interval-censored data can then be employed.

Because of the time and expense associated with two-year rodent bioassays, medium-term assays for obtaining information on carcinogenic hazards have been developed. These assays are available for a number of organ systems, including multiorgan systems. The mouse skin is one of the oldest experimental systems of carcinogenesis, dating back to the initiation–promotion protocols of Berenblum and Shubik. Medium-term assays in mouse skin focus on papillomas as an indicator of carcinogenic potential. The rodent liver provides a useful organ system for the study of hepatocarcinogenesis. Experimental protocols focus on hepatic foci in exposed animals as an indicator of potential cancer risk. Stereological methods can be used to rank the potency of agents with respect to their ability to alter liver foci.

As in molecular epidemiology, biomarkers can be exploited in toxicological studies. DNA adducts formed by over 200 chemicals have been identified in experimental animals, although few adducts have yet been measured in long-term bioassays. Cytogenic end-points, including chromosome aberration, sister chromatid exchange, and micronucleus, are being investigated. A review of the cytogenetic studies done to date indicates that over half of the animal and human carcinogens examined tested positive for at least one of these end-points. Proto-oncogenes and tumour-supressor genes provide an array of identified targets for carcinogenic agents. The identification of specific mutations serves to establish the molecular basis for carcinogenesis, and provides a means of identifying carcinogenic hazards.

Short-term tests have been vigorously developed over the last two or three decades, to the point where well over 100 such tests are now available. Although bacterial mutagenicity tests are insufficient to identify human carcinogens with precision, the use of an expanded battery, including tests for chromosomal aberrations, offers promise as a tool for carcinogen identification. Non-genotoxic end-points focusing on cell transformation and cell-to-cell communication may also prove useful in identifying carcinogens that are not DNA-reactive.

References

Adams, J.M & Cory, S. (1991) Transgenic models of tumor development. *Science*, **254**, 1161-1173

Aitio, A., Cabral, J.R.P., Camus, A.-M., Galendo, D., Bartsch, H., Aitio, M.-L., Norppa, H., Salomaa, S., Sorsa, M., Husgafvel-Pursianen, K. & Nurminen, M. (1988) Evaluation of sister chromatid exchange as an indicator of sensitivity to N-ethyl-N-nitrosourea-induced carcinogenesis in rats. *Teratog. Carcinog. Mutag.*, **8**, 273-286

Appel, M.J., van Garderen-Hoetmer, A. & Woutersen, R.A. (1990) Azaserine-induced pancreatic carcinogenesis in rats: promotion by a diet rich in saturated fat and inhibition by a standard laboratory chow. *Cancer Lett.*, **55**, 239-248

Appel, M.J., Roverts, W.G. & Woutersen, R.A. (1991) Inhibitory effects of micronutrients on dietary fat promoted pancreatic carcinogenesis in rats. *Carcinogenesis*, **12**, 2157-2161

Archer, L.E. & Ryan, L.M. (1989) On the role of cause-of-death data in the analysis of rodent tumorigenicity experiments. *Appl. Stat.*, **38**, 81-95

Arnold, D.L., Faber, E. & Krewski, D. (1988) Carcinogenicity testing: Histopathology and the blind method. *Comments Toxicol.*, **2**, 67-80

Ashby, J. (1992) Use of short-term tests in determining the genotoxicity or nongenotoxicity of chemicals. In: Vaino, H., Magee, P., McGregor, D. & McMichael, A.J., eds, *Mechanisms of Carcinogenesis in Risk Identification* (IARC Scientific Publications No. 116), Lyon, International Agency for Research on Cancer, pp. 135-164

Ashby, J. & Morrod, R.S. (1991) Detection of human carcinogens. *Nature*, **352**, 185-186.

Ashby, J. & Tennant, R.W. (1988) Chemical structure, Salmonella mutagenicity and extent of carcinogenicity as indicators of genotoxic carcinogenesis among 222 chemicals tested in rodents by the USNCI/NTP. *Mutat. Res.*, **204**, 17-115

Ashby, J. & Tennant, R.W. (1991) Definitive relationships among chemical structure, carcinogenicity and mutagenicity for 301 chemicals tested by the US NTP. *Mutat. Res.*, **257**, 229-306

Ashby, J., Tennant, R.W., Zeiger, E. & Stasiewics, S. (1989) Classification according to chemical structure, mutagenicity to Salmonella and level of carcinogenicity of a further 42 chemicals. *Mutat. Res.*, **223**, 73-103

Balmain, A. & Brown, K. (1988) Oncogene activation in chemical carcinogenesis. *Adv. Cancer Res.*, 51, 147-182

Bannasch, P. & Zerban, H. (1990) Tumours of the liver. In: Turusov, V.S. & Mohr, U., eds. *Pathology of Tumours in Laboratory Animals*, Vol. 1., *Tumours of the Rat*, 2nd ed. (IARC Scientific Publications No. 99), Lyon, International Agency for Research on Cancer, pp. 199-240

Bannasch, P. & Zerban, H. (1992) Predictive value of hepatic preneoplastic lesions as indicators of carcinogenic response. In: Vainio, H., Magee, P.N., McGregor, D.B. & McMichael A.J., eds, *Mechanisms of Carcinogenesis in Risk Identification* (IARC Scientific Publications No. 116), Lyon, International Agency for Research on Cancer, pp. 389-427

Bartsch, H. & Malaveille, C. (1990) Screening assays for carcinogenic agents and mixtures: an appraisal based on data in the IARC Monograph series. In: Vainio, H., Sorsa, M. & McMichael, A.J., eds, *Complex Mixtures and Cancer Risk* (IARC Scientific Publications No. 104), Lyon, International Agency for Research on Cancer, pp. 65-74

Berenblum, I. & Shubik, P. (1947) A new quantitative approach to the study of stages of chemical carcinogenesis in the mouse's skin. *Br. J. Cancer*, i, 383-391

Bickis, M & Krewski, D. (1985) Statistical design and analysis of the long-term carcinogenicity bioassay. In: Clayson, D., Krewski, D., Munro, I.C., eds, *Toxicological Risk Assessment*, Vol. I, *Biological and Statistical Criteria*, Boca Raton, FL, CRC Press, pp 125-147

Bickis, M. & Krewski, D. (1989) Statistical issues in the analysis of the long-term rodent carcinogenicity bioassay: an empirical evaluation of statistical decision rules. *Fundam. Appl. Toxicol.*, 12, 202-221

Birt, D.F. & Pour, P.M. (1985) Interaction of dietary fat and protein in spontaneous diseases of Syrian golden hamsters. *J. Natl Cancer Inst.*, 75, 127-133

Boutwell, R.K. (1964) Some biological effects of skin carcinogenesis. *Prog. Exp. Tumour Res.*, 4, 207-250

Brown, K., Buchmann, A. & Balmain, A. (1990) Carcinogen-induced mutations in the mouse c-Ha-*ras* gene provide evidence for multiple pathways for tumour progression. *Proc. Natl Acad. Sci. USA*, 87, 538-542

Bryant, M.S., Skipper, P.L., Tannenbaum, S.R. & Maclure, M. (1987) Hemoglobin adducts of 4-aminobiphenyl in smokers and nonsmokers. *Cancer Res.*, 47, 602-608

Buchmann, A., Bauer-Hofmann, R., Mahr, J., Drinkwater, N.R., Luz, A. & Schwarz, M. (1991) Mutational activation of the c-Ha-*ras* gene in liver tumors of different rodent strains: correlation with susceptibility to hepatocarcinogenesis. *Proc. Natl Acad. Sci. USA*, 88, 911-915

Burnett, R., Krewski, D. & Bleuer, S. (1989) Efficiency robust tests for rodent tumourgenicity experiments. *Biometrika*, 76, 317-324

Burns, F.J. (1989) Mouse skin papillomas as a stage in cancer progression. In: Slaga, T.J., Klein-Szanto, A.J.P., Boutwell, R.K., Stevenson, D.E., Spitzer, H.L. & D'Motto, B, eds, *Skin Carcinogenesis: Mechanisms and Human Relevance*, New York, NY, Alan R. Liss, pp. 81-93

Burns, F.J., Vanderlaan, M., Snyder, E. & Albert, R. (1976) Regression kinetics of mouse skin papillomas. *Cancer Res.*, 36, 1422-1426

Campbell, H.A., Pitot, H.C., Potter, V.R. & Laishes, B.A. (1982) Application of quantitative stereology to the evaluation of enzyme-altered foci in rat liver. *Cancer Res.*, 42, 465-472

Carr, G.J. & Gorelick, N.J. (1995) Statistical design and analysis of mutation studies in transgenic mice. *Environ. Mol. Mutagen.*, 25, 246-255.

Carr, C.J. & Kolbye, A.C. Jr (1991) A critique of the use of the maximum tolerated dose in bioassays to assess cancer risks from chemicals. *Reg. Toxicol. Pharmacol.*, 14, 78-87

Chen, J.J. (1996) Global test for analysis of multiple tumour data from animal carcinogenicity experiments. *Stat. Med.*, **15**, 1217-1225.

Clayson, D.B., Iverson, F. & Mueller, R. (1991) An appreciation of the maximum tolerated dose: an inadequately precise decision point in designing a carcinogenesis bioassay. *Teratog. Carcinog. Mutag.*, **11**, 279-296

Cohen, S.M., Arai, M., Jacobs, J.B. & Friedell, G.H. (1979) Promoting effect of saccharin and DL-tryptophan in urinary bladder carcinogenesis. *Cancer Res.*, **39**, 1207-1217

Crump, K.S., Krewski, D. & Wong, Y. (1998). Meta-analytic estimates of the proportion of liver carcinogens in screening bioassays conducted under the National Toxicology Program. *Risk Anal.* (in press)

Delesse, A. (1848) Pour déterminer la composition des roches. *Ann. Mines*, **13**, 379-388

Dewanji, A. & Kalbfleisch, J. D. (1986) Nonparametric methods for survival/sacrifice experiments. *Biometrics*, **42**, 325-341

Dewanji, A. & Krewski, D. & Goddard, M.J. (1993) A Weibull model for the estimation of tumorigenic potency. *Biometrics*, **49**, 367-377

Dinse, G.E. (1988) A prevalence analysis that adjusts for survival and tumour lethality. *Appl. Statist.*, **37**(3), 435-445

Dinse, G.E. & Haseman, J. K. (1986) Logistic regression analysis of incidental-tumor data from animal carcinogenicity experiments. *Fundam. Appl. Toxicol.*, **6**, 44-52

Emmelot, P. & Scherer, E. (1980) The first relevant cell stage in rat liver carcinogenesis: a quantitative approach. *Biochim. Biophys. Acta*, **605**, 247-304

Faccini, J.M., Butler, W.R., Friedmann, J.-C., Hess, R., Reznik, G.K., Ito, N., Hayashi, Y. & Williams, G.M. (1992) IFSTP guidelines for the design and interpretation of the chronic rodent carcinogenicity bioassay. *Exp. Toxicol. Pathol.*, **44**, 443-456

Farber, E. & Cameron, R. (1980) The sequential analysis of cancer development. *Adv. Cancer Res.*, **31**, 125-226

Farrar, D.B. & Crump, K.S. (1988) Exact statistical tests for any carcinogenic effect in animal bioassays. *Fundam. Appl. Toxicol.*, **11**, 652-663

Farrar, D.B. & Crump, K.S. (1990) Exact statistical tests for any carcinogenic effect in animal bioassays. *Fundam. Appl. Toxicol.*, **15**, 710-721

Feron, V.J. & Kroes, R. (1986) The long-term study in rodents for identifying carcinogens: some controversies and suggestions for improvements. *J. Appl. Toxicol.*, **6**, 307-311

Finkelstein, D.M. (1986) A proportional hazards model for interval-censored failure time data. *Biometrics*, **42**, 845-854

Fowlis D.J. & Balmain, A. (1993) Oncogenes and tumour suppressor genes in transgenic mouse models of neoplasia. *Eur. J. Cancer*, **29A**, 638-645

Friedwald, W.F. & Rous, P. (1944) The initiating and promoting elements in tumor production: an analysis of the effect of tar, benzpyrene and methylcholanthrene on rabbit skin. *J. Exp. Med.*, **80**, 101-125

Fukushima, S. (1991) Modification of tumor development in the urinary bladder. In: Ito, N. & Sugano, H., eds, *Modification of Tumor Development in Rodents*, Basel, Karger, pp. 154-174

Fukushima, S., Friedell, G.H., Jacobs, J.B. & Cohen, S.M. (1981) Effect of l-tryptophan and sodium saccharin on urinary tract carcinogenesis initiated by N-[4-(5-nitro-2-furyl)-2-thiazolyl]formamide. *Cancer Res.*, **41**, 3100-3103.

Fukushima, S., Hagiwara, A., Ogiso, T., Shibata, M. & Ito, N. (1983) Promoting effects of various chemicals in rat urinary bladder carcinogenesis initiated by N-nitroso-n-butyl(4-hydroxybutyl)amine. *Food Chem. Toxicol.*, **21**, 59-68

Fung, K.Y., Krewski, D. & Smythe, R.T. (1996) A comparison of tests for trend with historical controls in carcinogen bioassay. *Can. J. Stat.*, **24**, 431-454

Fung, K.Y., Krewski, D., Zhu, Y., Shephard, S. & Lutz, W. (1997). Statistical analysis of the *lacI* transgenic mouse mutagenicity assay. *Mutat. Res.*, **374**, 21-40

Fürstenberger, G., Berry, D.L., Sorg, B. & Marks, F. (1981) Skin tumour promotion by phorbol esters is a two-stage process. *Proc. Natl Acad. Sci. USA*, **78**, 7722-7726

Fürstenberger, G., Kinzel, V., Schwarz, M. & Marks, F. (1985) Partial inversion of the initiation–promotion sequence of multistage tumourigenesis in the skin of NMRI mice. *Science*, **230**, 76-78

Gart, J.J., Chu, V & Tarone, R. E. (1979) Statistical issues in interpretation of chronic bioassay tests for carcinogenicity. *J. Natl Cancer Inst.*, **62**(4), 957-974

Gart, J.J., Krewski, D., Lee, P.N., Tarone, R.E. & Wahrendorf, J., eds (1986) *Statistical Methods in Cancer Research*, Vol. III, *The Design and Analysis of Long-term Animal Experiments* (IARC Scientific Publications No. 79), Lyon, International Agency for Research on Cancer

Gart, J.J. & Tarone, R.E. (1987) On the efficiency of age-adjusted tests in animal carcinogenicity experiments. *Biometrics*, **43**, 235-244

Gaylor, D.W., Chen, J.J. & Kodell, R.L. (1985) Experimental design of bioassays due for screening and low dose extrapolation. *Risk Anal.*, **5**, 9-16

Gold, L.S., Sawyer, C.B., Magaw, R., Backman, G.M., de Veciana, M., Levinson, R., Hooper, N.K., Havender, W.R., Bernstein, L., Peto, R., Pike, M.C., & Ames, B.N. (1984). A carcinogenic potency database of the standardized results of animal bioassays. *Environ. Health Perspect.*, **59**, 9-319

Gold, L.S., Manley, N.B., Slone, T.H., Garfinkel, G.B., Rohrbach, L., & Ames, B.N. (1993) Fifth plot of the carcinogenic potency database: results of animal bioassays published in the general literature through 1988 and by the National Toxicology Program through 1989. *Environ. Health Perspect.*, **100**, 65-135.

Goldfarb, S. & Pugh, T.D. (1981) Enzyme histochemical phenotypes in primary hepatocellular carcinomas. *Cancer Res.*, **41**, 2092-2095

Goldworthy, T.L. & Hanigan, M. (1987) Models of hepatocarcinogenesis in the rat–contrasts and comparisons. *CRC Crit. Rev. Toxicol.*, **17**, 61-89

Gossen, J.A., De Leeuw, W.J.F., Tan, C.H.T., Zwarthoff, E.C., Berends, F., Lohman, P.H.M., Knook, D.L. & Vijg, J. (1989) Efficient rescue of integrated shuttle vectors from transgenic mice: a model for studying mutations *in vivo*. *Proc. Natl Acad. Sci. USA*, **86**, 7971-7975

Griesemer, R.A. (1992) Dose selection for animal carcinogenicity studies: a practitioner's perspective. *Chem. Res. Toxicol.*, **5**, 737-741

Griesemer, R. & Tennant, R. (1992) Transgenic mice in carcinogenicity testing. In: Vaino, H., Magee, P., McGregor, D. & McMichael, A.J., eds, *Mechanisms of Carcinogenesis in Risk Identification* (IARC Scientific Publications No. 116), Lyon, International Agency for Research on Cancer, pp. 429-436

Hagiwara, A., Tanaka, H., Imaida, K., Tamano, S., Fukushima, S. & Ito, N. (1993) Correlation between medium-term multi-organ carcinogenesis bioassay data and long-term observation results in rats. *Jpn. J. Cancer Res.*, **84**, 237-245

Harris, C.C. (1992) Tumour suppressor genes, multistage carcinogenesis and molecular epidemiology. In: Vaino, H., Magee, P., McGregor, D. & McMichael, A.J., eds, *Mechanisms of Carcinogenesis in Risk Identification* (IARC Scientific Publications No. 116), Lyon, International Agency for Research on Cancer, pp. 67-85

Haseman, J.K. & Lockhart, A. (1994) The relationship between use of the maximum tolerated dose and study sensitivity for detecting rodent carcinogenicity. *Fundam. Appl. Toxicol.*, **22**, 382-391

Haseman, J.K., Huff, J. & Boorman, G.A. (1984) Use of historical control data in carcinogenicity studies in rodents. *Toxicol. Pathol.*, **12(2)**, 126-135

Hemminki, K., Dipple, A., Shuker, D.E.G., Kodlubar, F.F., Segerbäck, D. & Bartsch, H. (1994) *DNA Adducts: Identification and Biological Significance* (IARC Scientific Publications No. 125), Lyon, International Agency for Research on Cancer

Hennings, H. (1989) Malignant conversion: the first stage in progression from benign to malignant tumours. In: Slaga, T.J., Klein-Szanto, A.J.P., Boutwell, R.K., Stevenson, D.E., Spitzer, H.L. & D'Motto, B., eds, *Skin Carcinogenesis: Mechanisms and Human Relevance*, New York, NY, Alan R. Liss, pp. 81-93

Hennings, H., Shores, M., Wenk, M.L., Spangler, E.F., Tarone, R. & Yuspa, S.H. (1983) Malignant conversion of mouse skin tumours is increased by tumour initiators and unaffected by tumour promoters. *Nature*, **304**, 67-69

Hiasa, Y., Kitahori, Y., Enoki, N., Konishi, N. & Shimoyama, T. (1984) 4,4-Diaminodiphenyl-methane: promoting effect on development of thyroid tumors in rats treated with N-bis (2-hydroxypropyl)nitrosamine. *J. Natl Cancer Inst.*, **72**, 471-476.

Hiasa, Y., Kitahori, Y., Konishi, N., Shimoyama, T. & Lin, J.-C. (1985) Sex differential and dose dependence of phenobarbital promoting activity in N-bis-(2-hydroxypropyl)nitrosamine-initiated thyroid tumorigenesis in rats. *Cancer Res.*, **45**, 4087-4090

Hicks, R.M., Wakefield, J.St.J. & Chowaniec, J. (1975) Evaluation of a new model to detect bladder carcinogens or co-carcinogens: results obtained with saccharin, cyclamate and cyclophosphamide. *Chem.-Biol. Interactions*, **11**, 225-253

Hirose, M., Tanaka, H., Takahashi, S., Futakuchi, M., Fukushima, S. & Ito, N. (1993) Effects of sodium nitrite, catechol, 3-methoxycatechol, or butylated hydroxyanisole in combination in a rat multiorgan carcinogenesis model. *Cancer Res.*, **53**, 32-37

International Agency for Research on Cancer (1980) *IARC Monographs on the Evaluation of the Carcinogenic Risk of Chemicals to Humans*, Suppl. 2, *Long-term and Short-term Screening Assays for Carcinogens: a Critical Appraisal*, Lyon

International Agency for Research on Cancer (1987) *IARC Monographs on the Evaluation of Carcinogenic Risks to Humans*, Suppl. 6, *Genetic and Related Effects: An Updating of Selected IARC Monographs from Volumes 1 to 42*, Lyon

Ito, N., Imaida, K., Tsuda, H., Shibata, M., Aoki, T., de Camargo, J.L.V. & Fukushima, S. (1988a) Wide-spectrum initiation models: possible applications to medium-term multiple organ bioassays for carcinogenesis modifiers. *Jpn. J. Cancer Res.*, **79**, 413-417

Ito, N., Tsuda, H., Tatematsu, M., Inoue, T., Tagawa, Y., Aoki, T., Uwagawa, S., Kagawa, M., Osigo, T., Masui, T., Imaida, K., Fukushima, S. & Asamoto, M. (1988b) Enhancing effect of various hepatocarcinogens on induction of preneoplastic glutathione s-transferase placental form positive foci in rats–an approach for a new medium-term bioassay system. *Carcinogenesis*, **9**, 387-394

Ito, N., Imaida, K., Hasegawa, R. & Tsuda, H. (1989) Rapid bioassay methods for carcinogens and modifiers of hepatocarcinogens. *CRC Crit. Rev. Toxicol.*, **19**, 386-415

Ito, N., Shirai, T. & Hasegawa, R. (1992) Medium-term bioassays for carcinogens. In: Vainio, H., Magee, P.N., McGregor D.B. & McMichael, A.J., eds, *Mechanisms of Carcinogenesis in Risk Identification* (IARC Scientific Publications No. 116), Lyon, International Agency for Research on Cancer, pp. 353-388

Jang, J.J., Cho, K.J., Lee, Y.S. & Bae, J.H. (1991) Modifying response of allyl sulfide, indole-3-carbinol and germanium in a rat multi-organ carcinogenesis model. *Carcinogenesis*, **12**, 691-695

Kodell, R.L. & Ahn, H. (1997). An age-adjusted trend test for the tumor incident rate for multiple sacrifice experiemnts. *Biometrics*, **53**, 75-82.

Kohler, S.W., Provost, G.S., Kretz, P.L., Dycaico, M.J., Sorge, J.A. & Short, J.M. (1990) Development of a short-term, *in vivo* mutagenesis assay: the effects of methylation on the recovery of a lambda phage shuttle vector from transgenic mice. *Nucleic Acids Res.*, **18**, 3007-3013

Kopp-Schneider, A. & Portier, C.J. (1992) Birth and death/differentiation rates of papillomas in mouse skin. *Carcinogenesis*, **13**, 973-978

Kress, S., Sutter, C., Strickland, P.T., Mukhtar, H., Schweizer, J. & Schwarz, M. (1992) Carcinogen-specific mutational pattern in the *p53* gene in UVB-radiation induced squamous cell carcinomas of the mouse skin. *Cancer Res.*, **52**, 6400-6403

Krewski, D., Kovar, J. & Bickis, M. (1984) Optimal experimental designs for low dose extrapolation II. The case of nonzero background. In: Dwivedi, T.D. & Chaubey, Y.P., eds.., *Topics in Applied Statistics*, Montreal, Concordia University, pp. 167-191

Krewski, D., Kovar, J., Bickis, M. & Arnold, D.L. (1986) Optimal experimental designs for low dose extraopolation I. The case of zero background. *Utilitas Mathematica*, **29**, 245-262

Krewski, D., Smythe, R.T., Dewanji, A. & Colin, D. (1988) *Statistical tests with historical controls (with discussion)*. In: Grice H.C. & Ciminera, J.L., eds, *Carcinogenicity: The Design, Analysis and Interpretation of Long-Term Animal Studies*, New York, NY, Springer-Verlag, pp. 23-38

Krewski, D., Goddard, M.J. & Zielinski, J.M. (1992). Dose–response relationships in carcinogenesis. In: Vainio, H., McGee, P.N., McGregor, D.B. & McMichael, A.J., eds, *Mechanisms of Carcinogenesis in Risk Identification*. (IARC Scientific Publications No. 116), Lyon, International Agency for Research on Cancer, pp. 579-599

Kumar, R., Sukumar, S. & Barbacid, M. (1990) Activation of *ras* oncogens preceding the onset of neoplasia. *Science*, **248**, 1101-1104

Kunz, H.W., Tennekes, H.A., Port, R.E., Schwarz, M., Lorke, D. & Schaude, G. (1983) Quantitative aspects of chemical carcinogenesis and tumor promotion in liver. *Environ. Health Perspect.*, **50**, 113-122

Kwong, Y,.Y., Husain, Z. & Biswas, D.k. (1992) c-Ha-*ras* gene mutation and activation precede pathological changes in DMBA-induced *in vivo* carcinogenesis. *Oncogene*, **7**, 1481-1489

Lagakos, S.W. & Louis, T.A. (1988) Use of tumour lethality to interpret tumorigenicity experiments lacking cause-of-death data. *Appl. Stat.*, **37**, 169-180

Leroux, B.G., Krewski, D. & Wei, L.J. (1992) Score tests for interval-censored data with applications to carcinogenicity experiments. In: Saleh, E. ed., *Nonparametric Statistics and Related Topics*, Amsterdam, Elsevier, pp. 59-74

Littlefield, N.A., Farmer, J.H., Gaylor, D.W. & Sheldon, W.G. (1980) Effects of dose and time in a long-term, low-dose carcinogenic study. *J. Environ. Pathol. Toxicol.*, **3**, 17-34

Longnecker, D.S. (1986) Experimental pancreatic cancer: role of species, age, sex and diet. In: Rozen, P., ed., *Frontiers of Gastrointestinal Research*, Basel, Karger, pp. 8-92

Luebeck, E.G., Moolgavkar, S.H., Buchmann, A. & Schwarz, M. (1991) Effects of polychlorinated biphenyls in rat liver: quantitative analysis of enzyme altered foci. *Toxicol. Appl. Pharmacol.*, **111**, 469-484

Malani, H.M. & Van Ryzin, J. (1988) Comparison of two treatments in animal carcinogenicity experiments. *J. Am. Stat. Assoc.*, **83**(404), 1171

Marks, F. & Fürstenberger, G. (1990) The conversion stage of skin carcinogenesis. *Carcinogenesis*, **11**, 2085-2092

Marks, F., Berry, D.L., Bertsch, S., Fürstenberger, G & Richter, H. (1982) On the relationship between epidermal hyperproliferation and skin tumour promotion. In: Hecker, E., Fusenig, N.E., Kunz, W., Marks, F. & Thielmann, H.W., eds, *Carcinogenesis: A Comprehensive Survey*, Vol. 7, New York, NY, Raven Press, pp. 331-346

Maronpot, R.R. (1985) Considerations in the evaluation and interpretation of long-term animal bioassays for carcinogenicity. In: Milman, H.A. & Weisburger, E.K., eds, *Handbook of Carcinogen Testing*, Park Ridge, IL, Noyes Publications, pp. 372-382

Maronpot, R.R., Shimkin, M.B., Witschi, H.P., Smith, L.H. & Cline, J.M. (1986) Strain A mouse pulmonary tumor test results for chemicals previously tested in National Cancer Institute carcinogenicity tests. *J. Natl Cancer Inst.*, **76**, 1101-1112

Masui, T., Shirai, T., Takahashi, S., Mutai, M. & Fukushima, S. (1988) Summation effect of uracil on the two-stage and multistage models of urinary bladder carcinogenesis in F344 rats initiated with N-butyl-N-(4-hydroxybutyl)nitrosamine. *Carcinogenesis*, **9**, 1981-1985

McCann, J., Gold, L.S., Horn, L., McGill, R., Graedel, T.E. & Kaldor, J. (1988) Statistical analysis of salmonella test data and comparisons to results of animal cancer tests. *Mutat. Res.*, **205**, 183-195

McCormick, D.L. & Moon, R.C. (1985) Tumorigenesis of the rat mammary gland. In: Milman, H. & Weisburger, E.K., eds, *Handbook of Carcinogen Testing*, Park Ridge, IL, Noyes Publications, pp. 215-229

McGregor, D.B. (1992a) Chemicals classified by IARC: their potency in tests for carcinogenicity in rodents and their genotoxicity and acute toxicity. In: Vainio, H., Magee, P.N., McGregor, D.B. & McMichael, A.J., eds, *Mechanisms of Carcinogenesis in Risk Identification* (IARC Scientific Publications No. 116), Lyon, International Agency for Research on Cancer, pp. 323-352

McGregor, D.B. (1992b) Chemicals classified by IARC: an investigation of some of their toxicological characteristics. *Toxicol. Lett.*, **64/65**, 637-642

McKnight, B. (1988) A guide to the statistical analysis of long-term carcinogenicity assays. *Fundam. Appl. Toxicol.*, **10**, 355-364

McKnight, B. & Crowley, J. (1984). Tests for differences in tumor incidence based on animal carcinogenesis experiments. *J. Am. Stat. Assoc.*, **79**, 639-648

McKnight, B. & Wahrendorf, J. (1992) Tumour incidence rate alternatives and the cause-of-death test for carcinogenicity. *Biometrika*, **79**, 131-138

Miyata, Y., Fukushima, S., Hirose, M., Masui, T. & Ito, N. (1985) Short-term screening of promoters of bladder carcinogenesis in N-butyl-N-(4-hydroxybutyl)-nitrosamine-initiated, unilaterally ureter-ligated rats. *Jpn. J. Cancer Res.*, **76**, 828-834

Montesano, R., Bartsch, H., Vainio, H., Wilbourn, J. & Yamasaki, H, eds (1986) *Long-term and Short-term Assays for Carcinogenesis: A Critical Appraisal* (IARC Scientific Publications No. 83), Lyon, International Agency for Research on Cancer

Monticello, T.M., Renne, R. & Morgan, K.T. (1991) Chemically induced cell proliferation in upper respiratory tract carcinogenesis. In: Butterworth, B.E., Slaga, T.S., Farland, W & McClain, M., eds, *Chemically Induced Cell Proliferation: Implications for Risk Assessment*, New York, NY, Wiley-Liss, pp. 323-335

Moolgavkar, S.H., Luebeck, E.G., DeGunst, M., Port, R.E. & Schwarz, M. (1990) Quantitative analysis of enzyme-altered foci in rat hepatocarcinogenesis experiments. I. Single agent regimen. *Carcinogenesis*, **11**, 1271-1278

Mottram, J.C. (1944) A developing factor in epidermal blastogenesis. *J. Pathol. Bacteriol.*, **56**, 181-187

Nishizuka, Y. (1988) The molecular heterogeneity of protein kinase C and its implication for cellular regulation. *Nature*, **334**, 662-665

Ogiso, T., Tatematsu, M., Tamano, S., Hasegawa, R & Ito, N. (1990) Correlation between medium-term liver bioassay system data and results of long-term testing in rats. *Carcinogenesis*, **11**, 561-566

Ohgaki, H., Hard, G., Hirota, N., Maekawa, A., Takahashi, M. & Kleihues, P. (1992) Selective mutation of codon 204 and 213 of the *p53* gene in rat tumors induced by alkylating N-nitroso compounds. *Cancer Res.*, 52, 2995-2998

Peto, R. (1974) Guidelines on the analysis of tumour rates and death rates in experimental animals. *Br. J. Cancer*, 29, 101-105

Peto, R., Gray, R., Brantom, P. & Grasso, P. (1984) Nitrosamine carcinogenesis in 5170 rodents: chronic administration of sixteen different concentrations of NDEA, NDMA, NPYR and NPIP in the water of 4440 inbred rats, with parallel studies on NDEA alone of the effects of age at starting (3, 6 or 20 weeks) and of species (rats, mice or hamsters) In: O'Neill, I.K., von Borstel, R.C., Miller, C.T., Long, J. & Bartsch, H. eds., *N-Nitroso Compounds: Occurrence, Biological Effects and Relevance To Human Cancer* (IARC Scientific Publications No. 57), Lyon, International Agency for Research on Cancer, pp. 627-665

Peto, R., Pike, M.C., Day, N.E., Lee, R.G., Parish, S., Peto, J., Richards, R. & Wahrendorf, J. (1980) Guidelines for simple, sensitive signifcance tests for carcinogenic effects in long-term animal experiments. In: *IARC Monographs on the Evaluation of the Carcinogenic Risk of Chemicals to Humans*, Suppl. 2, *Long-term and Short-term Assays for Carcinogens: A Critical Appraisal*, Lyon, International Agency for Research on Cancer, pp. 311-346

Peto, R., Gray, R., Brantom, P. & Grasso, P. (1991) Effects on 4080 rats of chronic ingestion of N-nitrosodiethylamine or N-nitrosodimethylamine: a detailed dose–response study. *Cancer Res.*, 51, 6415-6451

Pitot, H.C. (1990) Altered hepatic foci: their role in murine hepatocarcinogenesis. *Ann. Rev. Pharmacol. Toxicol.*, 30, 465-500

Pitot, H.C., Goldsworthy, T.L., Moran, S., Kennan, W., Glauert, H.P., Maronpot, R.R. & Campbell, H.A. (1987) A method to quantitate the relative initiating and promoting potencies of hepatocarcinogenic agents in their dose–response relationships to altered hepatic foci. *Carcinogenesis*, 8, 1491-1499

Pitot, H.C., Neveu, M.J., Hully, J.R., Rizvi, T.A. & Campbell, H. (1990) Multistage hepatocarcinogenesis in the rat as a basis for models of risk assessment of carcinogenesis. In: Moolgavkar, S.H., ed., *Scientific Issues in Quantitative Cancer Risk Assessment*, Boston, Basel, Berlin, Birkhaüser, pp. 69-95

Poirier, M.C. & Beland, F.A. (1992) DNA adduct measurements and tumor incidence during chronic carcinogen exposure in animal models: implications for DNA adduct-based human cancer risk assessment. *Chem. Res. Toxicol.*, 5, 749-755

Portier, C.J. (1991) Design of two-year carcinogenicity experiments: dose allocation, animal allocation and sacrifice times. In: Krewski, D. & Franklin, C.A., eds, *Statistics in Toxicology*, New York, NY, Gordon and Breach, pp. 457–469

Portier, C.J. & Bailer, A. J. (1989) Testing for increased carcinogenicity using a survival-adjusted quantal response test. *Fundam. Appl. Toxicol.*, 12, 731-737

Portier, C. & Hoel, D. (1983) Optimal design of the chronic animal bioassay. *J. Toxicol. Environ. Health*, 12, 1-9

Potter, V.R. (1984) Use of two sequential applications of initiators in the production of hepatomas in the rat: an examination of the Solt–Farber protocol. *Cancer Res.*, 44, 2733-2736

Pour, P.M., Runge, R.G., Birt, D., Gingell, R.M., Lawson, T., Nagel, D., Wallcare, L. & Salmasi, S.Z. (1981) Current knowledge of pancreatic carcinogenesis in the hamster and its relevance to the human disease. *Cancer*, 47, 1573-1587

Prentice, R.L., Smythe, R.T., Krewski, D., Mason, M. (1992) On the use of historical control data to estimate dose response trends in quantal bioassay. *Biometrics*, 48, 459-478

Purchase, I.F.H., Stafford, J. & Paddle, G.M. (1985) Vinyl chloride—a cancer case study. In: Clayson, D.B., Krewski, D. & Munro, J., eds, *Toxicological Risk Assessment*, Vol. II, *General Criteria and Case Studies*, Boca Raton, FL, CRC Press, pp. 167-194

Quintanilla, M., Brown, K., Ramsden, M., & Balmain, A. (1986) Carcinogen-specific mutation and amplification of Ha-*ras* during mouse skin carcinogenesis. *Nature*, 322, 78-80

Rabes, H.M., Scholze, P. & Jantsch, B. (1972) Growth kinetics of diethylnitrosamine-induced enzyme-deficient "preneoplastic" liver cell populations *in vivo* and *in vitro*. *Cancer Res.*, 32, 2577-2586

Rabes, H.M., Bücher, T., Hartmann, A., Linke, I. & Dünnwald, M. (1982) Clonal growth of carcinogen-induced enzyme deficient preneoplastic cell population in mouse liver. *Cancer Res.*, 42, 3220-3227

Rao, G.N., Tennant, R.W., Braun, A.G., Russfield, A. & Leder, P. (1991) Transgenic mouse models for assessment of carcinogenic potential of chemicals. In: *Transgenic Mice in Developmental Biology and Toxicology*, Research Triangle Park, NC, National Institute of Environmental Health Sciences, pp. 46-58

Rotstein, J., Sarma, D.S.R. & Farber, E. (1986) Sequential alterations in growth control and cell dynamics of hepatocytes in early precancerous steps in hepatocarcinogenesis. *Cancer Res.*, 46, 2377-2385

Ruggeri, B., Caamano, J., Goodrow, T., DiRado, M., Bianchi, A., Tono, D., Conti, C.J. & Klein-Szanto, A.J.P. (1991) Alterations of the *p53* tumor suppressor gene during mouse skin tumor progression. *Cancer Res.*, 51, 6615-6621

Ruggeri, B., Dirado, M., Zhang, S.Y., Bauer, B., Goodrow, T. & Klein-Szanto, A.J.P. (1993) Benzo[*a*]pyrene-induced murine skin tumors exhibit frequent and characteristic G to T mutations in the *p53* gene. *Proc. Natl Acad. Sci. USA.*, 90, 1013-1017

Satoh, K., Hatayama, I., Tateoka, N., Tamai, K., Shimizu, T., Tatematsu, M., Ho, N. & Sato, K. (1989) Transient induction of GST-P positive hepatocytes by DEN. *Carcinogenesis*, 10, 2107-2111

Scherer, E., Feringa, A.W. & Emmelot, P. (1984) Initiation–promotion–initiation. Induction of neoplastic foci within islands of precancerous liver cells in the rat. In: Börzsönyi, M., Laps, K., Day, N.E. & Yamasaki, H., eds, *Models, Mechanisms and Etiology of Tumour Promotion* (IARC Scientific Publications No. 56), Lyon, International Agency for Research on Cancer, pp. 57-66

Schmeiser, H.H., Janssen, J.W.G., Lyons, J., Scherf, H.R., Pfau, W., Buchmann, A., Bartram, C.R. & Wiessler, M. (1990) Aristolochic acid activates *ras* genes in rat tumours at deoxyadenosine residues. *Cancer Res.*, 50, 5464-5469

Schulte-Herman, R., Timmermann-Troisiener, I., Barthel, G. & Bursch, W.(1990) DNA synthesis, apoptosis, and phenotypic expression as determinants of growth of altered foci in rat liver during phenobarbital promotion. *Cancer Res.*, 50, 5127-5135

Schwarz, M. Buchmann, A., Schulte, M., Pearson D. & Kunz, W. (1989a) Heterogeneity of enzyme-altered foci in rat liver. *Toxicol. Lett.*, 49, 297-317

Schwarz, M., Pearson, D., Buchmann, A. & Kunz, W. (1989b) The use of enzyme-altered foci for risk assessment of hepatocarcinogens. In: Travis, C., ed., *Biologically Based Methods for Cancer Risk Assessment* (NATO ASI Series), New York, NY, Plenum, pp. 31-39

Shelby, M.D. & Zeiger, E. (1990) Activity of human carcinogens in the Salmonella and rodent bone marrow cytogenetic tests. *Mutat. Res.*, 234, 257-261

Shirai, T., Ikawa, E., Hirose, M., Thamavit, W. & Ito, N. (1985) Modification by five antioxidants of 1,2-dimethyl-hydrazine-initiated colon carcinogenesis in F344 rats. *Carcinogenesis*, 6, 637-639

Shirai, T., Ikawa, E., Fukushima, S., Masui, T. & Ito, N. (1986) Uracil-induced urolithiasis and the development of reversible papillomatosis in the urinary bladder of F344 rats. *Cancer Res.*, 46, 2062-2067

Slaga, T.J., ed. (1984) *Mechanisms of Tumour Promotion*, Vol. 2., *Tumour Promotion and Skin Carcinogenesis*, Boca Raton, FL, CRC Press

Slaga, T. (1986) SENCAR mouse skin tumorigenesis model versus other strains and stocks of mice. *Environ. Health Perspect.*, **68**, 27-32

Slaga, T.J., Fischer, S.M., Nelson, K. & Gleason, G.L. (1980) Studies on the mechanism of skin tumour promotion: evidence for several stages of promotion. *Proc. Natl Acad. Sci. USA*, **77**, 3659-3663

Slaga, T.J., Fischer, S.M., Weeks, C.E., Klein-Szanto, A.J.P. & Reiners, J.J. (1982) Studies on the mechanisms involved in multistage carcinogenesis in mouse skin. *J. Cell Biol.*, **18**, 99-119

Solt, D. & Farber, E. (1976) New principle for the analysis of chemical carcinogenesis. *Nature*, **263**, 701-703

Sorsa, M., Wilbourn, J. & Vainio, H (1992) Human cytogenetic damage as a predictor of cancer risk. In: Vainio, H., Magee, P.N., MaGregor, D.B. & McMichael, A.J., eds, *Mechanisms of Carcinogenesis in Risk Identification* (IARC Scientific Publications No. 116), Lyon, International Agency for Research on Cancer, pp. 543-554

Stich, H. (1984) The selection of doses in chronic toxicity/carcinogenicity studies. In: Grice, H., ed., *Current Issues in Toxicology*, New York, NY, Springer Verlag, pp. 9-49

Stoner, G.D. & Shimkin, M.B. (1985) Lung tumors in strain A mice as a bioassay for carcinogenicity. In: Milman, H. & Weisburger, E.K., eds, *Handbook of Carcinogen Testing*, Park Ridge, IL, Noyes Publications, pp. 179-214

Suganuma, M., Fujiki, H., Suguri, S., Yoshizawa, M., Hirota, M., Nakayasu, M. Ojika, M., Wakamatsu, K., Yamada, K. & Sugimura, T. (1988) Okadaic acid: an additional non-phorbol-12-tetradecanoate-13-acetate-type tumour promoter. *Proc. Natl Acad. Sci. USA*, **85**, 1768-1771

Swenberg, J.A., Hoel, D.G. & Magee, P.N. (1991) Mechanistic and statistical insight into the large carcinogenesis bioassays on *N*-nitrosodiethylamine and *N*-nitrosodimethylamine. *Cancer Res.*, **51**, 6409-6414

Swierenga, S.H.H. & Yamasaki, H. (1992) Performance of tests for cell transformation and gap-junction intercellular communication for detecting nongenotoxic carcinogenic activity. In: Vainio, H., Magee, P.N., McGregor, D.B. & McMichael, A.J., eds, *Mechanisms of Carcinogenesis in Risk Identification* (IARC Scientific Publications No. 116), Lyon, International Agency for Research on Cancer, pp. 165-193

Takahashi, M., Hasegawa, R., Furukawa, F., Toyoda, K., Sato, H. & Hayashi, Y. (1986) Effects of ethanol, potassium metabisulfite, formaldehyde and hydrogen peroxide on gastric carcinogenesis in rats after initiation with *N*-methyl-*N*-nitro-*N*-nitrosoguanidine. *Jpn. J. Cancer Res.*, **77**, 118-124

Tarone, R.E. (1982) The use of historical control information in testing for a trend in proportions. *Biometrics*, **38**(1), 215-220

Tatematsu, M., Aoki, T., Asamoto, M., Furikata, C. & Ito, N. (1988) Coefficient induction of pepsinogen 1-decreased pyloric glands and gastric cancer in five different strains of rats treated with N-methyl-N'-nitro-N-nitrosoguanidine. *Carcinogenesis*, **9**, 495-498

Tsuda, H., Moore, M.A., Asamato, M., Satoh, K., Tsuchida, S., Sato, K., Ichihara, A. & Ito, N. (1985) Comparison of the various forms of glutathione S-transferase with glucose-6-phosphate dehydrogenase and γ-glutamyltranspeptidase as markers of preneoplastic and neoplastic lesions in rat kidney induced by *N*-ethyl-*N*-hydroxyethylnitrosamine. *Jpn. J. Cancer Res.*, **76**, 919-929

US National Research Council (1993) Use of the maximum tolerated dose in animal bioassays for carcinogenicity. In: *Issues in Risk Assessment.*, Washington, DC, National Academy Press, pp. 1–183

Uwagawa, S., Tsuda, H., Inoue, T., Tagawa, Y., Aoki, T., Kagawa, M., Ogiso, T. & Ito, N. (1991) Enhancing potential of 6 different carcinogens on multi-organ tumorigenesis after initial treatment with *N*-methyl-*N*-nitrosourea in rats. *Jpn. J. Cancer Res.*, **82**, 1397-1405

Vainio, H., Magee, P., McGregor, D. & McMichael, A.J., eds (1992) *Mechanisms of Carcinogenesis in Risk Identification* (IARC Scientific Publications No. 116), Lyon, International Agency for Research on Cancer

Vesselinovitch, S.D. & Mihailovitch, N. (1983) Kinetics of diethylnitrosamine hepatocarcinogenesis in the infant mouse. *Cancer Res.*, **43**, 4253-4259

Ward, J.M. & Ito, N. (1988) Development of new medium-term bioassays for carcinogens. *Cancer Res.*, **48**, 5051-5054

Ward, J.M. & Reznik, G. (1983) Refinements of rodent pathology and the pathologist's contribution to evaluation of carcinogenesis bioassays. *Prog. Exp. Tumor Res.*, **26**, 266-291

Waters, M.D., Stack, H.F., Brady, A.L., Lohman, P.H.M., Haroun, L. & Vainio, H. (1988) Use of computerized data listings and activity profiles of genetic and related effects in the review of 195 compounds. *Mutat. Res.*, **205**, 295-312

Weinberg, W.C., Berkwits, L. & Iannacone, P.M. (1987) The clonal nature of gamma-glutamyl transpeptidase positive hepatic lesions induced by initiation promotion in ornithine carbamoyltransferase mosaic mice. *Carcinogenesis*, **8**, 565-570

Williams, E.D., Wareham, K.A. & Wovell, S. (1983) Direct evidence for the single cell origin of mouse liver cell tumors. *Br. J. Cancer*, **47**, 723-726

World Health Organization (1989) *Formaldehyde* (Environmental Health Criteria 89), Geneva

Wiseman, R.W., Stowers, S.J., Miller, E., Anderson, M.W. & Miller, J.A. (1986) Activating mutations of the c-Ha-*ras* protooncogene in chemically induced hepatomas of the male B6C3 F1 mouse. *Proc. Natl Acad. Sci. USA*, **83**, 5825-5829

Woutersen, R.A. & van Garderen-Hoetmer, A. (1988) Inhibition of dietary fat-promoted development of (pre)neoplastic lesions in exocrine pancreas of rats and hamsters by supplemental vitamins A, C and E. *Cancer Lett.*, **41**, 179-189

Woutersen, R.A., van Garderen-Hoetmer, A., Bax, J. & Scherer, E. (1989a) Modulation of dietary fat-promoted pancreatic carcinogenesis in rats and hamsters by chronic ethanol consumption. *Carcinogenesis*, **10**, 453-459

Woutersen, R.A., van Garderen-Hoetmer, A., Bax, J. & Scherer, E. (1989b) Modulation of dietary fat-promoted pancreatic carcinogenesis in rats and hamsters by chronic coffee consumption. *Carcinogenesis*, **10**, 179-189

Zarbl, H., Sukumar, S., Arthur, A.V., Martin-Zanca, D. & Barbacid, M. (1985) Direct mutagenesis of Ha-*ras*-1 oncogenes by *N*-nitroso-*N*-methylurea during initiation of mammary carcinogenesis in rats. *Nature*, **315**, 382-385

Zerban, H., Preussmann, R. & Iannasch, P. (1988) Dose–time relationship of the development of preneoplastic lesions induced in rats with low doses of *N*-nitrosodiethanolamine. *Carcinogenesis*, **9**, 607-610

Quantitative Estimation and Prediction of Human Cancer Risks
S. Moolgavkar, D. Krewski, L. Zeise, E. Cardis and H. Møller
IARC Scientific Publications No. 131
International Agency for Research on Cancer, Lyon, 1999

6: Empirical Approaches to Risk Estimation and Prediction

Daniel Krewski, Elisabeth Cardis, Lauren Zeise and Victor J. Feron

6.1 Introduction

The quantitative estimation and prediction (QEP) of human cancer risk is facilitated by the establishment of a functional relationship between dose and response. Dose is measured in terms of the reactive metabolite or proximate carcinogen reaching the target tissue, and response in terms of the risk of tumour occurrence at that dose. In the absence of information on tissue dose, the level of exposure may be used as a surrogate for dose.

Epidemiologists often express risk as the increase in the age-specific tumour incidence rate at a given level of exposure. For risk assessment applications, however, the lifetime probability of a particular tumour occurring is often of more interest. Estimates of risk may be adjusted for intercurrent mortality or standardized in terms of the mortality experience of a specified population. When direct information on tumour incidence is unavailable, it is sometimes possible to make inferences about the tumour incidence rate based on tumour mortality data. (This requires reliable information on tumour lethality or cause-of-death.)

Modelling dose–response relationships is central to the QEP of cancer risks. Once a dose–response model characterizing the relationship between dose and response has been developed, estimates of risk at any dose within the range of the original data can be obtained. If necessary, the model may also be used to predict risks outside the range of the original data, although extrapolations well beyond the original data range are subject to considerable uncertainty.

This chapter focuses on empirical dose–response models that may be used for the quantitative estimation and prediction of cancer risk. Although such models may fit the available data well and provide reasonable estimates of risk, they are essentially statistical in nature.

Consequently, direct biological interpretations of the model parameters or inferences about the underlying mechanisms of carcinogenesis are usually not possible. Biologically based dose–response models are discussed in section 7.5.

Despite their limited biological basis, empirical dose–response models enjoy certain advantages. Because such models do not attempt to describe the complex mechanisms by which tumours are induced, they retain an element of simplicity. Flexible statistical models with as few as three or four parameters are capable of describing a wide variety of dose–response patterns observed in toxicological and epidemiological studies of carcinogenesis. In general, the database needed to fit an empirical dose–response model is less extensive than that required to develop a biologically based dose–response model. Consequently, the application of statistical dose–response models for the quantitative estimation and prediction of cancer risks is comparatively straightforward.

To date, most applications of QEP have been based on models fitted to data derived from a single epidemiological or toxicological study. In recent years, risk models have also been derived through combined analyses of data from different studies. For example, Lubin *et al.* (1994) conducted a combined analysis of 11 cohorts of underground miners to estimate the excess lung cancer risk due to inhalation of radon gas. Similarly, the International Agency for Research on Cancer conducted a combined analysis of nuclear workers in Canada, the United Kingdom and the United States to estimate the cancer risks of occupational exposure to ionizing radiation (IARC Working Group, 1994).

In section 6.2, we describe a number of empirical models that have been used to describe dose–response relationships observed in epidemiological studies. Examples include logistic regression models widely employed in the analysis of case–control studies, and relative risk regression models used in the analysis of cohort studies. Statistical dose–response models that have been used in long-term laboratory studies of carcinogenicity are described in section 6.3. These include purely empirical models such as the logistic and Weibull models, as well as models that have a limited biological basis such as the Armitage–Doll multistage model. We note that this distinction between empirical models that can be used to describe dose–response relationships observed in epidemiological and toxicological studies is based on past practice rather than limited applicability: there is no compelling reason why models traditionally used in epidemiological studies could not be applied to laboratory data and vice versa.

Although the doses used in laboratory studies of carcinogenicity are generally held constant throughout the study period, human exposure to carcinogenic substances present in the environment can vary substantially over time. The implications of time-dependent exposure patterns for the quantitative estimation and prediction of risk are examined in section 6.4. In particular, the use of cumulative lifetime exposure as an approximate indicator of lifetime risk is evaluated.

The potency of carcinogenic agents can be expressed in different ways. In section 6.5, quantitative measures of carcinogenicity are reviewed, including the TD_{50}, which is defined as the dose causing a 50% tumour response rate in an exposed population with appropriate adjustments for background response. TD_{50} values for rodent carcinogens are known to vary widely, spanning some seven orders of magnitude, and are also known to be highly correlated with the maximum tolerated dose used in long-term laboratory studies of carcinogenicity. The slope of the dose–response curve in the low-dose region has also been used as a measure of carcinogenic potency, and is strongly correlated with TD_{50}.

Because humans may be exposed to more than one carcinogenic agent simultaneously, there is a need to consider risk assessment methods for joint exposures and mixtures. Of particular concern is the possibility of synergistic effects, in which the risk associated with joint exposure to two or more agents exceeds the sum of the risks

for each agent alone. In section 6.6, measures of interaction are discussed, along with theoretical and empirical evidence of both synergistic and antagonistic effects.

The distinction between the *estimation* and *prediction* of risk was emphasized in Chapter 1, the essential difference being that prediction of risk requires extrapolation outside the original data range. In section 6.7, we discuss extrapolations that are often required in the quantitative prediction of risk. These include extrapolation from occupationally exposed populations to the general population, extrapolation from high to low doses, and extrapolation from one temporal exposure pattern to another. Inferences about human cancer risks based on laboratory tests also raise the difficult problem of interspecies extrapolation.

Uncertainty and sensitivity analysis, useful tools in the quantitative estimation and prediction of cancer risk, are discussed in section 6.8. There are many sources of uncertainty in risk estimation and prediction which need to be examined to determine the reliability of the results obtained. Sensitivity analysis is a useful tool for identifying key parameters which, if altered only slightly, can have a marked impact on risk predictions.

6.2 Modelling epidemiological data

In epidemiological studies, modelling is carried out to estimate the risk of cancer as a function of the exposure of interest and of the host and environmental factors which may modify risk. Epidemiological studies used for quantitative estimation of risk should generally encompass a range of exposure levels to permit characterization of the relationship between exposure and risk. The two main types of studies which provide data for this purpose are: (i) *cohort studies*, in which a group of persons with a range of exposure levels is followed, for mortality or morbidity, from a particular disease; and (ii) *case–control studies*, in which the exposure history of all cases and appropriate controls is reconstructed.

The most common measures of risk used in QEP are the age- and time-specific "absolute" and "relative" risk. Both of these measures can be expressed as a function of the level of the exposure of interest as described below. Absolute risk (AR) cannot be estimated from case–control studies without supplementary information on the level of risk in unexposed individuals. Relative risk (RR) can, however, be estimated from both case–control and cohort studies. Most of the developments in empirical QEP models for the analysis of epidemiological data have focused on RR models.

6.2.1 Cohort studies

Data from cohort studies are often analysed using methods developed for grouped, rather than individual, data. The data are summarized in tabular form, with the number of events and person-years of follow-up allocated to cells, defined by the relevant level $k = 1, ..., K$ of the exposure variable and $j = 1, ..., J$ of a set of relevant covariates such as age and sex. As an example, Tables 6.1 and 6.2 present, respectively, the distribution of lung cancers and person–years of follow-up by $K = 9$ levels of smoking and $J = 8$ age groups from the prospective follow-up of over 34 000 British doctors (Doll & Peto, 1981)

The parameter of interest is the rate λ_{jk} of mortality or morbidity from the disease under study in stratum jk. The observed rate is obtained as the ratio of events o_{jk} (deaths or disease occurrences) and person–years of observation n_{jk} in the stratum $\hat{\lambda} = q_{jk}/n_{jk}$. For example, the observed rate of lung cancer among non-smokers aged 55–59 among the British doctors in Tables 6.1 and 6.2 was $2/8905 = 0.22$ per 1000, compared with $6/4357 = 1.38$ per 1000 among smokers of 20–24 cigarettes per day of the same age.

The numbers of events in each cell are considered to be independent Poisson random variables with means and variances $E(o_{jk}) = \mathrm{Var}(o_{jk}) = \lambda_{jk} n_{jk}$. The denominators, n_{jk}'s, are assumed to be fixed. For a technical justification for the use of the Poisson model see Breslow & Day (1987).

Table 6.1. Distribution of cancer cases by age and amount smoked[a]

Age group	Never smoked	Average number of cigarettes per day							
		1–4	5–9	10–14	15–19	20–24	25–29	30–34	35–40
40–44	0	0	0	1	0	0	0	1	0
45–49	0	0	0	0	1	0	2	2	0
50–54	1	0	0	2	3	5	3	3	3
55–59	2	1	0	1	0	6	4	5	3
60–64	0	1	1	1	2	7	3	5	6
65–69	0	0	1	1	0	9	3	5	3
70–74	0	1	1	2	2	3	4	0	2
75–79	0	0	0	1	3	3	2	2	0

[a] Source: Doll & Peto (1981)

Table 6.2. Distribution of person–years by age and amount smoked[a]

Age group	Never smoked	Average number of cigarettes per day							
		1–4	5–9	10–14	15–19	20–24	25–29	30–34	35–40
40–44	17 846	1 216	2 041	3 795	4 824	7 046	2 523	1 715	892
45-49	15 832	1 000	1 745	3 205	3 995	6 460	2 565	2 123	1 150
50-54	12 226	853	1 562	2 727	3 278	5 583	2 620	2 226	1 281
55-59	8 905	625	1 355	2 288	2 466	4 357	2 108	1 923	1 063
60-64	6 248	509	1 068	1 714	1 829	2 863	1 508	1 362	826
65-69	4 351	392	843	1 214	1 237	1 930	974	763	515
70-74	2 723	242	696	862	683	1 053	527	317	233
75-79	1 772	208	517	547	370	512	209	130	88

[a] Source: Doll & Peto (1981)

Different models for the rate λ_{jk} can be postulated and parameters estimated using maximum likelihood. The most commonly used model in epidemiological applications is the relative risk (RR) model, in which the effect of the exposure k is to multiply the background rate λ_{j0} (the rate in stratum j in the absence of the exposure) as follows:

$$\lambda_{jk} = \lambda_{j0} \, f(x_k).$$

Here, f is a function of the (mean or median) level of exposure x_k λ_{jk} in category k. This function may depend on other factors, such as age or time since exposure, sex, and smoking history. To simplify fitting, this model is often expressed as:

$$\log \lambda_{jk} = \alpha_j + \beta_k,$$

where $\alpha_j = \log \lambda_{j0}$ and $\beta_k = \log f(x_k)$.

An often used parametrization of the RR model is the *constant linear excess relative risk* model:

$$\lambda_{jk} = \lambda_{j0} \, [1+ \beta_{xk}].$$

Here, the parameter β is referred to as the excess relative risk (ERR) per unit of exposure. The RR at a given exposure x, a more commonly used measure of risk in epidemiology, can be obtained by multiplying the ERR by the exposure x and adding 1. Whereas βx is a linear function of the exposure x, non-linear functions may also be worth exploring.

The constant linear ERR model is widely used for estimating radiation risks (US National Academy of Sciences/National Research Council, Committee on the Biological Effects of Ionizing Radiation, 1988, 1990; United Nations Scientific Committee on the Effects of Atomic Radiation, 1988, 1994). In particular, it has been fitted to data on approximately 80 000 survivors of the atomic bombs in Hiroshima and Nagasaki to obtain estimates of the ERR per Sv of dying or being diagnosed with cancer (Shimizu *et al.*, 1992). These estimates provide one of the foundations of current radiation protection recommendations (International Commission on Radiological Protection, 1991). As these estimates are derived from a population having received relatively high exposures in a very short time, how-

ever, the International Commission on Radiological Protection (ICRP) has recommended that they be divided by a dose–dose-rate effectiveness factor (DDREF) of 2 to extrapolate risks to the low dose–rate chronic exposure circumstances of interest in usual environmental and occupational settings (International Commission on Radiological Protection, 1991). It is acknowledged that this value of the DDREF is subject to uncertainty.

The constant linear ERR model has also been used in combined analyses of cancer mortality data on 96 000 nuclear industry workers from Canada, the United Kingdom and the USA (Cardis *et al.*, 1995) in order to obtain the most precise *direct* estimate of the carcinogenic risk of protracted low-dose exposure to external ionizing radiation, and thus test the adequacy of the extrapolations from data on atomic bomb survivors. In that study, estimates of individual annual occupational radiation doses were available for each worker included in the study population. The exposure x_k in stratum j_k was taken to be the mean cumulative occupational radiation dose (in Sv). The ERR for all cancers excluding leukaemia, and leukaemia excluding chronic lymphatic leukaemia (CLL), the two main groupings of causes of death for which risk estimates have been derived from high-dose studies, were estimated to be 0.07 per Sv (90% confidence interval (CI): -0.4–0.3) and 2.18 per Sv (90% CI: 0.1–5.7), respectively. These values can be used to predict risks at different dose levels; they correspond, for example, to a relative risk of 0.99 for all cancers excluding leukaemia for a cumulative protracted dose of 100 mSv. For leukaemia excluding CLL, the corresponding value of the relative risk is 1.22, implying a 22% increased risk of dying from leukaemia for a cumulative protracted dose of 100 mSv. Although these estimates are lower than the corresponding estimates obtained from studies of atomic bomb survivors, they are compatible with a range of possibilities, from a reduction of risk at low doses, to risks twice those on which current radiation protection recommendations are based (Cardis *et al.* 1995; IARC Working Group, 1994).

Variations of this model in which the parameter β is allowed to vary over time (with, for example, time since exposure, age at exposure, or attained age) have also been fitted to data on atomic bomb survivors, nuclear industry workers and uranium miners (US National Academy of Sciences/National Research Council, Committee on the Biological Effects of Ionizing Radiation, 1988, 1990; Cardis *et al.*, 1995; Lubin *et al.*, 1995).

Relative risk models are the most generally used models in epidemiology for several reasons. For many exposures they appear to describe the relationship between exposure and the age-specific risk of cancer better than absolute risk models. Using such models, risk estimates can be obtained without imposing any assumptions on the baseline rates of disease, λ_{j0}. They also provide a convenient framework for communicating information about radiation risks.

In some cases, relative risk models may not adequately describe the relation between exposure and cancer risk. *Absolute risk models*

$$\lambda_{jk} = \alpha_j + \beta_k$$

in which the exposure is postulated to add to the background risk, are then more appropriate. While a relative risk model appears to be a good description of risk for solid cancers following radiation exposure in adulthood in the atomic bomb survivors, the risk of leukaemia may be better described by a time-dependent absolute risk model (Shimizu *et al.*, 1992). It should be noted that fitting additive risk models to epidemiological data is computationally more difficult in practice than fitting relative risk models.

Much attention has been given in recent years to methods for discriminating between additive and multiplicative risk models, particularly in the area of radiation risk estimation (US National Academy of Sciences/National Research Council, Committee on the Biological Effects of Ionizing Radiation, 1990; International Commission on Radiation Protection, 1991). Unless the data are quite extensive, however, reasonably good fits of both absolute and relative risk models to the same data are usually possible, and it is rarely feasible to distinguish between models on statistical terms alone (Pierce & Preston, 1984). The leukaemia risk model of the US National Research Council Vth Committee on the Biological Effects of Ionizing Radiations (BEIR V) represents a case in point:

essentially comparable fits could be obtained using either additive or relative risk models, provided risk was allowed to vary with time. However, somewhat different modifying effects were required in the two models, and the relative risk model generally provided a more parsimonious description of the data (US National Academy of Sciences/National Research Council, Committee on the Biological Effects of Ionizing Radiation, 1990).

Even when they fit equally well in the range of data used for analyses, relative and absolute risk models may lead to quite different predictions of risk outside of the range of data. For example, the United Nations Scientific Committee on the Effects of Atomic Radiation (UNSCEAR) in its 1988 report predicted the excess lifetime mortality and loss of life expectancy for all cancers except leukaemia for a Japanese population (United Nations Scientific Committee on the Effects of Atomic Radiation, 1988). For an organ dose of 1 Gy of low linear energy transfer (LET) radiation received at high dose rate, a relative risk projection model predicts 61 extra deaths (90% CI: 48–75) compared with 36 (28–44) deaths with an absolute risk model. The projections of loss of life expectancy resulting from such an exposure using the two models are 0.73 years (0.57–0.90) and 0.91 years (0.71–1.10), respectively.

In practice, a cohort is rarely followed up until extinction, nor are all subjects followed until they experience the event under study. For example, in the atomic bomb survivors cohort, 65% of the population was still alive at the end of 1985, 40 years after exposure occurred (Shimizu *et al.*, 1992). An individual subject i in the cohort is then followed until t_i, the time of the event of interest, death from another cause, loss to follow-up (if follow-up is active), or the end of the study, whichever occurs first. Subjects who have not experienced the event of interest before the end of their follow-up may do so at a later time. Such a subject is said to be censored at time t_i.

In cohort studies, models may also be fitted to the original data before categorization. One of the most commonly used models for this purpose is the proportional hazards model:

$$\lambda(t; Z(t)) = \lambda_0(t) \exp(X(t) \beta)$$

introduced by Cox (1972). Here, $\lambda(t; Z(t))$ denotes the hazard function for the disease of interest at time t for an individual with covariate history $Z(t)$ and $\lambda_0(t)$ is the baseline hazard function. This is a semi-parametric relative risk model. The partial likelihood approach of Cox (1972) can be used to estimate the parameters β_j efficiently without specifying the baseline hazard $\lambda_{0j}(t)$. An important generalization of this model is to let the nuisance function $\lambda_0(t)$ vary within specific subsets of the data. This is useful, for example, if some confounding factors do not appear to have a multiplicative effect on the hazard function. More general relative risk regression models

$$\text{RR }(t; Z(t)) = r(X(t) \beta)$$

can also be used, where r is any positive function found to be consonant with the data.

Fitting of additive risk models to continuous data is also feasible but requires modelling the baseline risk parametrically. This is generally difficult because the parameters which determine baseline risks are not usually known.

6.2.2 Case–control studies

In case–control studies, actual rates of disease in exposed and non-exposed subjects cannot generally be estimated as the cases and controls are drawn with different sampling probabilities from the population under study. An immediate consequence is that the relative risk cannot be estimated from case–control studies. When the disease is relatively rare, however, the odds ratio (OR) is a good estimate of the relative risk. Since specific types of cancer are relatively rare, this approximation is of considerable use in cancer risk estimation with case–control data. OR is defined as follows:

$$\text{OR} = \frac{\text{number of exposed cases/}}{\text{number of unexposed cases}} \Big/ \frac{\text{number of exposed controls/}}{\text{number of unexposed controls}}$$

Analyses are generally based on multiplicative risk regression models in which OR is modelled as a function of exposure. In case–control studies, the numbers of cases in the stratum jk, defined by the level of the exposure variable k and of the set of covariates j, are assumed to be distributed as independent binomial observations with response probability p_{jk} and sample size n_{jk} (the total number of cases and controls in the stratum). The special case of the logistic regression model:

$$\text{logit }(p) = \log (p_{jk}/(1\text{-}p_{jk})) = \alpha_j + \beta_k$$

is widely used in the analysis of case–control studies. The OR for exposure at level k relative to no exposure is:

$$\text{OR}_k \text{ vs. } 0 = [p_{jk}/(1\text{-}p_{jk})] \big/ [p_{j0}/(1\text{-}p_{j0})] = \exp (\beta_k)$$

As with cohort analyses, covariate adjustment can be done by stratification. Different shapes of the dose–response relationship can be explored by using models other than the logistic. Inferences in case–control studies are generally based on large sample approximations (Breslow & Day, 1980). When the number of subjects in a study is small, hypothesis tests and estimation can be based on the exact binomial likelihood (Mehta et al., 1986); procedures are available in the statistical package EGRET (Statistics and Epidemiology Research Corporation, 1990).

Logistic regression has been used in the analysis of case–control studies of lung cancer risk following residential radon exposure (Blot et al., 1990; Schoenberg et al., 1990; Pershagen et al., 1993; Létourneau et al., 1994; Alavanja et al., 1995; Auvinen et al., 1996). These and other studies are described in more detail in Chapter 8. In a combined analysis of three of these studies, Lubin et al. (1994) applied an ERR model of the form:

$$\text{logit }(p_{xr}) = \alpha x + \exp [1+\beta r]$$

where x is a vector of covariates, including study location, age, smoking status, and cigarette consumption. The level of radon exposure r was modelled as a continuous variable (specifically, the time-weighted mean radon concentration in the houses occupied by each study subject). The regression coefficients α and β are estimated based on the study data. The estimated ERR was 0.00 per pCi/l (95% CI: -0.05–0.07). This estimate is consistent with the null hypothesis of no risk, as well as the small risk predicted by downward extrapolation of the data from 11 cohorts of underground miners exposed to higher levels of radon than those generally found in homes (Lubin *et al.*, 1995; US National Academy of Sciences/National Research Council, Committee on the Health Risks of Exposure to Radon, 1998).

6.2.3 Generalized linear models

The empirical models used for risk estimation in epidemiological studies are mostly relative risk models, fitted using logistic regression in case–control studies or Poisson or proportional hazards regression in cohort studies. These models belong to the family of generalized linear models (McCullagh & Nelder, 1983) in which:

- the outcome of interest is represented by a vector y of length N, assumed to be the realization of a vector of random variables Y which are independently distributed with mean m;
- the distribution of Y is a member of an exponential family such as the normal, binomial or Poisson distributions;
- the explanatory variables enter as a linear sum of their effects, the linear predictor $\eta = X\beta$, where β is the vector of parameters
- the vector μ is the systematic part of the model and is linked to the linear predictor by a "link" function $g(.)$ such that $\eta = g(\mu)$

In logistic regression, the Ys (the number of cases) are independent binomial variates with response probability p and denominator N (the number of cases and controls in each stratum) and the logit of p is described as a linear function of exposure. In Poisson regression, the number of cases in each stratum are assumed to be independent Poisson random variables with means and variances λN, where N (the number of person–years at risk in each stratum) and the log of λ is written as a linear function of exposure.

Unlike the biologically based models discussed in Chapter 8, empirical models provide little biological insight into the mechanisms of carcinogen-

esis. Indeed, as shown in Chapter 8, empirical models are widely used in the analysis of data from epidemiological studies, and provide the basis for many current cancer risk estimates. Empirical models, and in particular generalized linear models, are highly flexible and can accommodate a wide range of exposure–response relationships, including the modifying effects of important covariates on risk. There are a number of convenient computer programs for fitting such models, including GLIM (Numerical Algoriths Group, 1978) used for fitting generalized linear models, SAS (SAS Institute, Inc., 1989), for logistic regression and survival models, EGRET (Statistics and Epidemiology Research Corporation, 1990) for logistic regression and survival analysis, EPICURE (Preston *et al.*, 1993), for Poisson regression and logistic regression, and GENSTAT (Numerical Algorithms Group, 1980), for logistic regression and survival analysis.

6.2.4 Choice of model form

Studies in which little quantitative information is available on exposure are usually analysed by testing for trends in risk across broad exposure categories and by estimating the relative risks in different categories with respect to a baseline (non-exposed or minimally exposed) exposure category.

In studies in which more detailed individual or group level information is available on exposure, it is possible to include continuous variables in the model to describe the effects of exposure, and derive risk estimates per unit exposure or dose. Commonly used dose–response relationships for radiation risk estimation include the linear relative risk model:

$$\lambda_{jk} = \lambda_{j0} (1 + \beta \, \alpha_k),$$

and the linear quadratic relative risk model:

$$\lambda_{jk} = \lambda_{j0} (1 + \beta \, \alpha k + \gamma \, \alpha k^2)$$

(US National Academy of Sciences/National Research Council, Committee on the Biological Effects of Ionizing Radiations, 1980). In the former case, the parameter β reflects the excess relative risk per unit dose α. Many other exposure–response relationships may be usefully explored (Wahrendorf, 1986).

It is well known that cancer risk can vary with a number of covariates in addition to the level of exposure, including age at exposure, duration of exposure, and time since exposure; variables that are inevitably correlated with one another. In particular, such effects have been observed with cancer risks due to exposure to ionizing radiation (US National Academy of Sciences/National Research Council, Committee on the Biological Effects of Ionizing Radiations, 1990) and smoking (International Agency for Research on Cancer, 1986).

The effects of factors modifying the association between exposure and disease (such as age, sex, or calendar year) can be accommodated through stratification, with different risk estimates derived within each stratum defined in terms of the effect modifiers. Another approach is to use a parametric model in order to describe the interactions between the exposure of interest and the modifying factors.

In empirical models, however, the choice of which of these variables to include in the model is somewhat ad hoc, since these variables can be highly correlated. In contrast, the biologically based models discussed in Chapter 7 provide a framework within which all temporal characteristics of risk can be naturally accommodated.

If a model is to be used for the estimation and prediction of cancer risks, it is important to assess whether it fits the observed data. However, the fact that a model fits the data well does not imply that the model is correct: as noted above, the BEIR V committee found that both absolute and relative risk models "fitted" the leukaemia data equally well (US National Academy of Sciences/National Research Council, Committee on the Biological Effects of Ionizing Radiations, 1990). While such models may provide comparable estimates of risk within the observable response range, predictions of risk outside this range may differ substantially.

Goodness of fit of generalized linear models can be assessed by examining the differences between observed and fitted values, called "residuals" (Belsley et al., 1980). In generalized linear models, the 'deviance' is defined as twice the log of the ratio of likelihoods of the model of interest and a fully parametrized or saturated model. For normal theory linear models, the deviance has a chi-square distribution, and asymptotic results are available for other models. In general, the deviance does not follow a chi-square distribution even asymptotically, although the difference of deviances of nested models has an asymptotic chi-square distribution and can thus be used to test for significance of parameters in nested models (McCullagh & Nelder, 1989).

In some cases, the assumption that observations are independently distributed random variables may not hold. Suppose, for example, we wish to study gene–environment interactions affecting the risk of cancer. Clusters of two or more cases occurring in the same family are collected (cf. Ghadirian et al., 1991), along with appropriate controls. The data collected in the study would be of the form:

$$Y_{ij} = \begin{cases} 1 \text{ for breast cancer} \\ 0 \text{ otherwise} \end{cases}$$

where ij denotes the ith individual in the jth family. The data can be analysed using a random effect model of the form:

$$\text{logit } p_{ij} = \log (p_{ij}/(1\text{-}p_{ij})) = a_j + b_1 x_{ij1} + ... + b_K x_{ijK}$$

where $x_{ij1}, ... x_{ijK}$ denote the covariates. Here, a_j, the family specific intercept, is random with a distribution $f(a)$ and $p_{ij} = P[Y_{ij} = 1| a_j, X_{ij}]$, where $X_{ij} = (X_{ij1} ..., X_{ijK})$. As the variance of the a_j is greater than zero, the variability of the observations exceeds the binomial variation which would be expected on the basis of a fixed-effect model. Various statistical packages such as EGRET (Statistical and Epidemiology Research Corporation, 1990) allow the fitting of random-effect models by introducing an extra parameter s to account for the random effects. Examples of random-effect models used for case–control analyses include the beta–binomial (Crowder, 1978), logistic–normal (Pierce & Sands, 1975) or logistic–binomial (Mauritsen, 1984) regression models. Random effects can also be used to accommodate extra-Poisson variation in cohort studies.

Random-effect models are also useful in combining data from different studies. For example, Wang et al. (1996) used a random-effects approach to fit a linear model to the data on lung cancer mortality in 11 cohorts of underground miners considered previously by Lubin *et al.* (1994). In this application, the random-effects approach represents a natural way to describe cohort heterogeneity, and provides a useful framework for the combined analysis of data from multiple sources. Wang *et al.* (1996) also illustrate how two-stage methods of analysis can be used for such combined analyses.

6.2.5 Other measures of risk

Epidemiological studies focus largely on the estimation of age and time-specific disease incidence rates as a measure of risk. For risk-assessment purposes, however, the probability of developing a tumour over the course of a lifetime is generally of greater interest. As few epidemiological studies cover the entire life span of a population under study, derivation of lifetime risk generally requires predictions outside the range of observation. Many QEPs are based on "lifetime risk", i.e. the probability of developing the event of interest during one's life, as a function of exposure. Extrapolation across population groups may also be required, such as the extrapolations of radiation-induced cancer mortality and morbidity that are carried out from the follow-up of atomic bomb survivors to members of the public in other countries for radiation protection purposes (United Nations Scientific Committee on the Effects of Atomic Radiation, 1994). In many cases, lifetime risk will also depend on the age at exposure and other modifying factors such as age and concomitant environmental exposures. Mortality from competing causes will also affect lifetime risk.

Various measures of lifetime risk have been proposed in the literature. The *excess lifetime risk* (ELR) (US National Academy of Sciences/National Research Council, Committee on the Biological Effects of Ionizing Radiations, 1988,1990) is defined as the increase in the lifetime risk experienced by an individual as a result of the specific exposure, estimated as the difference between the proportion of people dying of the lesion of interest in the exposed population and the proportion dying of the same cause in

an otherwise identical but non-exposed population. For an instantaneous exposure to a dose D at age e, the excess lifetime risk for cause c is given by:

$$\text{ELR}_c(D,e) = \int_e^\infty m_c(a|D,e)S(a|D,e)\mathrm{d}a - \int_e^\infty m_c(a)S(a|e)\mathrm{d}a$$

where $m_c(a|D,e)$ and $m_c(a)$ denote the death rates from cause c at age a with or without instantaneous exposure to total dose D at age e and $S(a|e)$ is the probability that an individual survives to age a given that he or she was alive at age e.

The *lifetime risk of exposure-induced* death or EID (United Nations Scientific Committee on the Effects of Atomic Radiation, 1988) is defined as an individual's risk of dying from a cancer attributable to the exposure in question. For an instantaneous exposure to a dose D at age e, the lifetime risk of exposure-induced death (REID) for cause c is given by:

$$\text{REID}_c(D,e) = \int_e^\infty [m_c(a|D,e) - m_c(a)]S(a|D,e)\mathrm{d}a$$

Neither of these measures provides any information about the time at which the cancer or death occurs. For risk-management purposes, however, it is important to distinguish between two exposures which may entail the same lifetime risk, but which may cause death at quite different ages. In some cases, therefore, predictions of *years of life lost* (United Nations Scientific Committee on the Effects of Atomic Radiation, 1988), defined as the difference between life expectancy in an unexposed individual and that in an individual exposed at age a, are derived. These will usually depend on a, the age at exposure. For an instantaneous exposure to a dose D at age e, the loss of life expectancy (LLE) is given by:

$$\text{LLE}(D,e) = \int_e^\infty S(a|e)\mathrm{d}a - \int_e^\infty S(a|D,e)\mathrm{d}a$$

It should be kept in mind that, although not all cancers result in death, many will affect the quality of life and that their impact will be greater for cancers occurring at a younger age. As an example, a large increase in the number of cases of papillary thyroid carcinoma has been reported in Belarus following the Chernobyl accident (Kazakov *et al.*, 1992; Demidchik *et al.*, 1994), and, more recently, in some areas of the Ukraine (Tronko *et al.*, 1994) and the Russian Federation (Tsyb *et al.*, 1994). Among more than 500 cases occurring in Belarus in the last six years, only two have died; all have been treated surgically, however, and a large proportion have undergone two or more operations on the thyroid (Demidchik, 1996, personal communication). Although predictions of years of life lost are increasingly being used in QEPs for agents such as ionizing radiation, little has been done to predict the "years of lowered quality of life", a much more subjective quantity associated with exposures.

6.3 Modelling toxicological data

Statistical models may also be used to summarize dose–response data derived from laboratory studies. For the most part, we focus on experiments involving a series of increasing dose levels, including an unexposed control group, the dose level being held constant throughout the duration of the experimental period (Krewski & Goddard, 1990). Most long-term animal experiments encompass the greater part of the expected lifespan of the test species, which is typically 2–3 years for rodents. In describing such models, it will be convenient to distinguish between models used to describe the lifetime probability of cancer and those which are used to describe the temporal patterns of tumour incidence. Note that the lifetime probability of cancer will be influenced by the survival rate of the animals in the experiment, early mortality reducing the opportunity for tumour occurrence.

6.3.1 Quantal-response models

Dose–response models used to describe the relationship between the lifetime probability of cancer and dose are referred to as quantal-response models since the response of interest (the presence or absence of a given tumour in a given animal during the course of the study) is a binary random variable. Krewski & Van Ryzin (1981) have published a detailed review of quantal-response models for toxicological data, including carcinogenicity data, and such models have also been discussed by Finney (1971), Govindarajarlu (1988), and Hubert (1992).

Tolerance-distribution models are based on the notion that each animal has its own tolerance to the test agent, and that a toxic response will occur whenever the dose d exceeds the tolerance t. If $G(\tau)$ ($0<\tau<\infty$) denotes the cumulative distribution of tolerances in the population of interest, the probability that an individual animal selected at random from among those exposed to dose d will respond is simply $P(d) = Pr\{\tau<d\} = G(d)$.

A general class of tolerance-distribution models is defined by $G(\tau) = F(\alpha+\beta\log\tau)$, where F denotes any cumulative distribution function standardized so as to be free of unknown parameters, and α and $\beta>0$ are unknown parameters to be estimated on the basis of the experimental data. Perhaps the best known model in this class is the probit model, for which F corresponds to the standard normal distribution function:

$$F(x) = (2\pi)^{-1/2} \int_e^\infty \exp(-u^2/2)\mathrm{d}u$$

In this case, the distribution of tolerances is lognormal. The logistic model with

$$F(x) = [1 + \exp(-x)]^{-1}$$

and the Weibull model with

$$F(x) = 1 - \exp\{-\exp(x)\}$$

are also used to describe quantal-response toxicity data. Prentice (1976) has described a more general parametric family of dose–response models that includes the above models as special cases.

Although these models generally provide similar fits to data from dose–response experiments within the observable response range, they can differ appreciably when extrapolated to very low doses. The shape of the dose–response curves for both the logistic and Weibull models is determined by the value of the shape parameter β: in the low-dose region, the dose–response curve may be linear ($\beta = 1$), sublinear ($\beta>1$) or supralinear ($\beta<1$). In contrast, the probit model exhibits a sublinear behaviour in the low-dose region regardless of the values of the model parameters.

As specified above, each of these models implies $P(0) = 0$, so that tumours cannot occur spontaneously in the absence of exposure to the test agent. To allow for the occurrence of tumours in the control group, spontaneous tumours may be assumed to occur independently of those induced by the test agent or in a dose-wise additive fashion (Hoel, 1980). On the assumption of independence, the probability $P^*(d)$ of observing either a spontaneously occurring or an induced tumour at dose d is given by:

$$P^*(d) = \gamma + (1-\gamma)P(d),$$

where $0<\gamma<1$ denotes the spontaneous response rate. For additivity, spontaneous tumours are associated with an effective background dose δ, with

$$P^*(d) = P(d+\delta).$$

These two methods of allowing for background response generally lead to comparable descriptions of the dose–response relationship within the observable response range. An important implication of the additive background model is that the dose–response curve will be linear at low doses for any smoothly increasing distribution function F, including the probit, logit, and Weibull models discussed previously (Crump et al., 1976). In contrast, the shape of the dose–response curve in the low-dose region for the independent background model corresponds to that of the function F as indicated above.

Other dose–response models have a limited biological basis, postulating the random occurrence of one or more biological events as being responsible for tumour induction. For example, Rai & Van Ryzin (1981) consider a multi-hit model based on the concept that a tumorigenic response will occur following the occurrence of k fundamental (and unspecified) biological events in the target tissue. If it is assumed that the rate of occurrence of these events follows a homogeneous Poisson process, the probability of a response at dose d is given by:

$$P(d) = \int_0^d [\Gamma(k)]^{-1} \lambda^k t^{k-1} \exp(-\lambda t) dt,$$

where $\Gamma(k)$ denotes the gamma function and λd denotes the expected number of events occurring

during the period of interest. This same model can also be developed by assuming a gamma tolerance distribution, thereby permitting an extension to non-integer values of k. Background response can be accommodated by assuming either independence or additivity. At low doses, the dose–response curve can be linear ($k = 1$), sublinear ($k>1$) or supralinear ($k<1$). The case of $k<1$, however, does not seem plausible in that it would correspond to an infinite slope at the origin and could lead to unrealistic predictions of risk at very low doses.

The special case of $k = 1$ is known as the one-hit model, with

$$P(d) = 1 - \exp(-\lambda d)$$

in the absence of background response. With either independent or additive background tumours, the one-hit model is of the form:

$$P(d) = 1 - \exp\{-(\lambda_0 + \lambda_1 d)\}, \qquad (1)$$

where $P(0) = 1 - \exp\{-\lambda_0\}$ and $\lambda_1 \equiv \lambda$.

A widely used generalization of the one-hit model is the Armitage–Doll multistage model (cf. Armitage, 1985), which is discussed in detail in Chapter 7. A simplified version of the model that is commonly used in QEP is as follows:

$$P(d) = 1 - \exp\{-(q_0+q_1 d+...q_k d^k)\}, \qquad (2)$$

where $q_i \geq 0$ ($i = 1,...,k$). As discussed in section 6.3.2, the multistage model does have a biological interpretation in terms of a sequence of $k \geq 1$ fundamental biological events required to transform a normal cell into a cancer cell. Statistically, the use of a polynomial function of dose in equation (2) rather than the linear function in equation (1) permits the description of non-linear dose–response relationships. At low doses, the dose–response curve for the multistage model is well approximated by a linear function with slope $q_1>0$. (Although $q_1 = 0$ is possible in equation (2), the original formulation requires the slope at the origin to be strictly positive.)

Any of these quantal-response models may be fitted to data derived from long-term animal carcinogenicity experiments, provided that the number of dose groups is greater than or equal to the number of unknown model parameters. Suppose that a total of n animals are used in an experiment involving $m+1$ dose levels $0 = d_0 < d_1 < ... < d_m$, and that x_i of the n_i animals at dose d_i ($i = 0,1,...,m$) develop the tumour of interest during the course of the study. If it is assumed that each animal responds independently of all other animals, the likelihood of the observed outcome for a given dose–response model $P^*(d|\theta)$ depending on the vector of parameters $\theta = (\theta_1,..., \theta_t)$ is given by:

$$L(\theta) = \prod_{i=0}^{m} \binom{n_i}{x_i} (P_i^*)^{x_i} (Q_i^*)^{n_i - x_i}$$

where $P_i^* = P^*(d)$ and $Q_i^* = Q^*(d)$. Maximizing this binomial likelihood function with respect to θ leads to the maximum likelihood estimators $\hat{\theta}$ of θ (Krewski & Van Ryzin, 1981). Maximum likelihood estimators generally enjoy desirable statistical properties, including consistency and asymptotic normality. Once the estimator $\hat{\theta}$ has been obtained, the fit of the dose–response model to the experimental data can be evaluated using a chi-square goodness-of-fit test.

Methods other than maximum likelihood can also be used in parameter estimation, including the method of generalized estimating equations (GEEs) described by Liang & Zeger (1986). The GEE method requires specification only of the first two moments of the data rather than the complete distribution, and can easily accommodate extrabinomial variation. GEEs have been used in modelling data on mutagenicity (Krewski et al., 1993b) and developmental toxicity (Zhu et al., 1994; Krewski & Zhu, 1994) where the distribution of the data is unclear, and where overdispersion relative to the Poisson and multinomial distributions is apparent. Krewski & Zhu (1995) show how the Rao–Scott transformation can be used to eliminate such overdispersion, thereby simplifying the analysis.

Non-parametric approaches to modelling quantal dose–response data are also available (Kuo, 1988; Morris, 1988; Muller & Schmitt, 1988). However, these methods focus on the estimation of response rates at the experimental dose levels, thereby avoiding the problem of predicting cancer risks at other dose levels.

6.3.2 Models of time to response

Although useful in summarizing lifetime tumour incidence data from long-term animal experiments, quantal dose–response models do not take into account the age at which tumours were observed. A more complete description of the data derived from such experiments may be achieved using time-to-tumour models.

Let T be a random variable denoting the tumour onset time. Although T could be precisely defined as the time at which the first cancer cell appears, this time is difficult if not impossible to measure. Consequently, a more practical definition, such as the earliest possible time that a cancerous lesion could be detected clinically or histologically, is usually adopted. The probability of a tumour occurring by time t at dose d is then given by $P(t;d) = Pr\{T < t; d\}$. The complement of the tumour onset distribution $Q(t;d) = 1 - P(t;d)$ is known as the survivor function. The hazard function:

$$\lambda(t;d) = \lim_{\Delta t \downarrow 0} \frac{Pr\{T \in (t, t+\Delta t) \mid T > t\}}{\Delta t}$$

denotes the instantaneous probability of a tumour developing at time t in a tumour-free individual, and is used to describe the age-specific tumour incidence rate. The survivor and hazard functions are related by:

$$Q(t;d) = \exp\{-\Lambda(t;d)\},$$

where $\Lambda(t) = \int_0^t \lambda(u;d)du$, is the cumulative hazard function. Thus, we may model the distribution of tumour-onset times either in terms of $P(t;d)$ or $\lambda(t;d)$. Note that at a fixed time $t = t_0$, $P(t_0;d)$ considered as a function of d alone represents the dose–response relationship in the absence of intercurrent mortality.

Kalbfleisch et al. (1983) reviewed a number of different models for the tumour-onset distribution $P(t;d)$. A general class of log–linear models can be defined by:

$$\log T = \alpha + \beta \log d + \sigma W,$$

where the error variable W follows some specified distribution. Choosing a log–normal, log–logistic or Weibull error distribution yields a time-to-tumour model which, when evaluated at a fixed time t_0, corresponds to the probit, logit, and Weibull models discussed in section 6.3.1. Other flexible parametric models that may be used to describe the distribution of tumour-onset times are discussed by Lawless (1982).

The Cox regression model, originally proposed by Cox (1972), is widely used in the analysis of failure time data, including time to tumour or death. The hazard function for the Cox regression model is given by:

$$\lambda(t;d) = \lambda_0(t)\exp\{z(t)^T\beta\},$$

where $\lambda_0(t)$ is an unspecified baseline hazard function independent of dose d, $\beta = (\beta_1,..., \beta_p)^T$ is a vector of regression parameters, and $z(t) = (z_1(t),...,z_p(t))^T$ is a vector of covariates that may depend on both time t and dose d. When z is independent of time (for example, $z = (d,\log(d))^T$, the hazards at different doses are proportional. With time-dependent covariates, however, the hazard ratios in different dose groups can vary with time. For example, $z = (d, d\log(t))^T$ corresponds to:

$$\lambda(t;d) = \lambda_0(t)e^{d\beta_1}t^{d\beta_2}$$

In its general form, the Cox regression model is sufficiently flexible to describe a wide variety of dose–response relationships (Prentice et al., 1982).

The Armitage–Doll model, introduced in its quantal form in section 6.3.1, was originally developed to describe tumour occurrence times (Armitage & Doll, 1954, 1961). The model is based on the premise that a malignant transformation requires the occurrence, in sequence, of $k>1$ fundamental biological events within a single cell, generally held to involve damage to DNA, such as mutations at specific gene loci. The rate of transition to the ith stage at time u is assumed to be of the form:

$$\lambda_i(u) = a_i + b_i d(u), \tag{3}$$

where $d(u)$ denotes the dose at time u, thereby allowing for time-dependent dosing (Crump & Howe, 1984). In this general case, the cumulative hazard is approximately of the form:

$$\Lambda(t) = \int_0^t \int_0^{u_k} K \int_0^{u_2} \prod_{i=1}^{k} [a_i + b_i d(u_i)] du_1 \, K \, du_k$$

which reduces to:

$$\lambda(t) = \frac{t^k}{k!} \prod_{i=1}^{k} (a_i + b_i d) \tag{4}$$

when the dose d is held constant. For statistical purposes, it is convenient to use the polynomial approximation:

$$\lambda(t) = \frac{t^k}{k!} \sum_{i=0}^{k} q_i d^i$$

(Crump et al., 1977; Hartley & Sielken, 1977). This represents a slight generalization of equation (4) which is simpler to apply in practice.

The multistage model predicts that age-specific cancer incidence rates should be roughly proportional to the $(k-1)$st power of age, where k is the number of stages in the model. By allowing for up to six stages, the model is able to provide a good description of age-specific cancer rates in humans (Cook et al., 1969). However, the model as described here fails to take into account important factors in carcinogenesis, including tissue growth and cell kinetics. For this reason, it is not treated in this publication as a comprehensive biologically motivated model of carcinogenesis as discussed in Chapter 7.

Application of these or other time-to-tumour models depends on the amount of information available on tumour-onset times, whether or not cause of death can be determined, and the relationship between tumour mortality and competing causes of death (Krewski et al., 1983). With visible, palpable, or rapidly lethal tumours, it may be possible to determine the time of tumour-onset with some degree of accuracy. With occult tumours, however, direct information on the tumour-onset time is unavailable; all that can be said about occult tumours observed at the time of death is that they occurred at some time between the start of the study and the time of death.

The general process of tumour onset and development over time can be conveniently described within the general framework shown in Figure 6.1. An animal may develop a tumour at some time during the study period; such animals

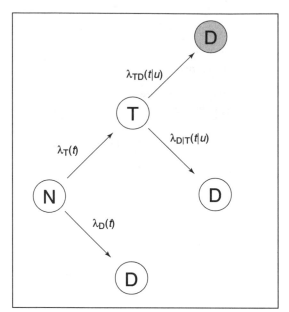

Figure 6.1. The states (N = normal, T = tumour, D = death) and transition rates, λ (*t* = time, *u* = time of tumour onset), for animals in a carcinogenicity experiment.

may then survive until the termination of the study, or die either as a consequence of the tumour or of some other competing cause prior to the end of the study. It is also possible that an animal may die during the course of the study from competing risks without developing a tumour. Finally, an animal may survive tumour-free until the end of the study period. By examining the tumour status and survival times of animals dying during the course of the study, it is possible to make certain inferences about the distribution of tumour-onset times in relation to dose.

The compartmental model in Figure 6.1 may be characterized in terms of the hazard function for tumour onset, $\lambda_T(u)$. Given the occurrence of a tumour at time *u*, the hazard functions for death due to the tumour or due to other causes are denoted by $\lambda_{TD}(t|u)$ and $\lambda_{D|T}(t|u)$, respectively. (Note that the cause of death must be determined in order to distinguish between λ_{TD} and λ_{TD}.) The hazard function for deaths due to competing risks prior to tumour occurrence is denoted by $\lambda_D(t)$. This compartmental model also provides a convenient basis for the development of statistical tools for the effects of the test agent on λ_T (Leroux *et al.*, 1992).

Maximum likelihood estimation with time-to-tumour data is more complex than with quantal-response data. As an illustration, suppose that observations (T_i, J_i, d_i) are available for each animal $i = 1,...,n$. Here, $J_i = 1$ if the *i*th individual is observed to have a tumour present at the time t_i of death or termination of the study; otherwise, $J_i = 0$. Exposure of the *i*th individual is at a constant level d_i. Consider first the case of rapidly lethal tumours, in which T_i will be approximately the time of tumour occurrence. If it is assumed that the time of tumour occurrence and the time of death due to competing risks are stochastically independent, the likelihood function is given by:

$$L = \prod_{i=1}^{n} \exp\{-\Lambda(T_i;d_i)\} \, |\, \lambda(T_i;d_i)]^{J_i}$$

Terms of the form $\{-\Lambda(T_i;d_i)\}\lambda(T_i;d_i)$ represent the contribution to the likelihood of animals developing tumours at time T; terms of the form $\exp\{-\Lambda(T_i;d_i)\} = Q(T_i;d_i)$ correspond to animals not developing tumours at the time of death due to competing risks or the termination of the study. Maximization of the likelihood function with respect to the unknown model parameters yields the fitted model.

With incidental tumours that are not life threatening, the likelihood function is of the form:

$$L = \prod_{i=1}^{n} [1-\exp\{-\Lambda(T_i;d_i)\}]^{J_i} [\exp\{-\Omega(T_i;d_i)\}]^{J_i}$$

assuming that the presence of a tumour does not affect the death rate from competing causes. Here, the terms $1-\exp\{-\Lambda(T_i;d_i)\}$ and $\exp\{-\Lambda(T_i;d_i)\} = Q(T_i;d_i)$ correspond to the probability of observing or not observing a tumour at the time *T* of death or study termination.

Likelihood construction with tumours of intermediate lethality is discussed by Kalbfleisch *et al.* (1983). One assumption that greatly simplifies the form of the likelihood and avoids certain identifiability issues is $\lambda_{D|T}(t|u) = \lambda_\tau(t)$ (McKnight & Crowley, 1984; McKnight, 1988). This is a strong assumption that asserts that the presence of a tumour does not affect the death rate due to competing risks. None the less, it is commonly invoked in applications of time-to-tumour models.

Non-parametric models for time-to-tumour data have been proposed by Dinse (1986) and Dewanji & Kalbfleisch (1986). These non-parametric models once again cannot be used to predict risks at doses other than those used in the original experimental protocol. Non-parametric models are also most useful with serial sacrifices, a design feature not included in most experimental protocols for long-term laboratory studies. This limitation may be circumvented by using the semi-parametric models proposed by Rai *et al.* (1999).

6.4 Patterns of exposure and risk

Long-term laboratory studies of carcinogenicity are, with some exceptions, conducted with exposure regimens in which the dose level is held constant for the duration of the study (Gart *et al.*, 1986). Because human exposure to carcinogenic substances can vary substantially over time, methods are required for the quantitative estimation and prediction of risks with time-dependent exposure patterns.

There are many sources of temporal variability in human exposures. Occupational exposures occur only in the workplace and for that part of a person's working lifetime during which he or she was employed at that workplace. Accidental exposures to carcinogenic substances can be of very short duration. Dietary exposures to pesticide residues that may possess carcinogenic potential are dependent on pesticide usage practices which may vary among geographical regions and on food consumption patterns that may change with age and the availability of food products. Long-term environmental trends, such as the thinning of the ozone layer, can also result in similar trends in exposure to environmental carcinogens, in this case to ultraviolet radiation.

A simple approach to dealing with time-dependent exposures is to base predictions of risk on the cumulative level of exposure, regardless of how the total dose was accumulated over time. The average daily exposure over the period of interest, calculated by dividing the total exposure by the number of days in that period, can also be used as the basis for risk estimation and prediction. The US Environmental Protection Agency (1986) suggests the use of average daily exposure in the quantitative estimation and prediction of risk as a default principle:

"Unless there is evidence to the contrary ... the cumulative dose received over a lifetime, expressed as the average daily exposure prorated over a lifetime, is recommended as an appropriate measure of exposure to a carcinogen. That is, the assumption is made that a high dose of a carcinogen received over a short period of time is equivalent to a corresponding low dose spread over a lifetime."

While this represents a reasonable default assumption, the lifetime average daily dose generally provides only an approximation to the actual lifetime risk. The accuracy of this approximation, explored later in this section, will depend on the existence and strength of any dose-rate effects.

Dose-rate effects have been documented in a number of cases. Moolgavkar *et al.* (1993) reported an inverse dose-rate effect with respect to radon-induced lung cancer among uranium miners. In this case, exposure to a fixed lifetime dose resulted in a greater risk when the exposure was experienced over a longer period of time. Lubin *et al.* (1995) have confirmed this effect in a combined analysis of 11 cohorts of underground miners exposed to radon.

The impact of dose-rate effects on predictions of risk based on the lifetime average daily dose in the multistage model has been considered by Kodell *et al.* (1987), Morrison (1987), Chen *et al.* (1988), Murdoch & Krewski (1988), Krewski & Murdoch (1990), and Murdoch *et al.* (1992). Goddard *et al.* (1995) have published a useful review of the literature on temporal aspects of risk characterization. These theoretical results take into account the effects of exposures occurring at different times for different forms of the multistage model and on the assumption that the susceptibility of the host does not change as a function of age. Following Crump & Howe (1984), suppose that the transition rate for the *i*th stage is as shown in equation (5) (p.146). In the special case when only one of the *k* transition rates ($1 \leq r \leq k$) depends on dose, Murdoch & Krewski (1988) show that the cumulative hazard is approximately:

$\Lambda(t) = a(t) + b(t)d_t^*.$

Here, $a(t) = (t^k/k!) \prod_{i=1}^{k} a_i$ denotes the cumulative hazard at time t in the absence of exposure, $b(t) = a(t)b_r/a_r$, and:

$$d_t = \frac{1}{t}\int_0^t d(u)R(u)du$$

where $R(u)$ denotes the relative effectiveness of dosing at time u. The quantity d_t^* represents an *equivalent constant dose* which, if administered up to time t, would lead to the same cumulative hazard $L(t)$ at time t as the time varying dose $d(u)$ ($0 \leq u \leq t$). Note that the cumulative risk

$$P(t) = 1 - \exp\{-\Lambda(t)\} \approx \Lambda(t) \qquad (5)$$

approximates the cumulative hazard for low to moderate risks, so that the equivalent constant dose also leads to approximately the same cumulative risk as the time varying dose.

It is clear from equation (5) that the equivalent dose is essentially a weighted average of the time varying dose, the relative effectiveness function being the weighting function. The properties of the relative effectiveness function are therefore important in determining the value of the equivalent constant dose d_t^*. For a multistage model consisting of k stages with stage r dose-dependent, the relative effectiveness functions are of the form:

$$R(u) = \frac{k!u^{r-1}(1-u)^{k-r}}{t^k(r-1)!(k-r)} \leq k \qquad (6)$$

The relative effectiveness functions for a multistage model with up to $k = 6$ stages and with stage r ($1 \leq r \leq k$) being dose-dependent are shown in Figure 6.2. When an early stage is dose-dependent, early exposures are more effective than late exposures. Conversely, when a late stage is dose-dependent, late exposures are more effective than early exposures. As indicated by equation (5), the relative effectiveness functions for the multistage model never exceed k, the number of stages in the model, and in fact achieve this upper bound only at time 0 when the first stage is dose-dependent or at time t when the last stage is dose-dependent. Note that the relative effectiveness function is

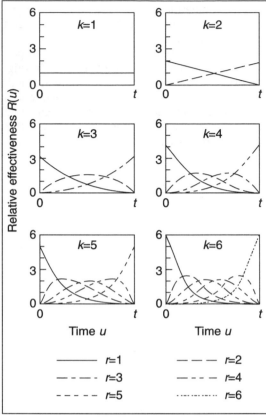

Figure 6.2. Relative effectiveness of dosing at different times in a k-stage model ($1 \leq k \leq 6$) with the rth stage dose-dependent. Source: Murdoch & Krewski (1988)

constant when $k = 1$, in which case early and late exposures are equally effective.

The lifetime average daily dose may be written as:

$$d_t = \frac{1}{t}\int_0^t d(u)du$$

where t denotes the expected lifespan of the population of interest. The ratio C = LECD/LADD of the lifetime equivalent constant dose (LECD) to the lifetime average daily dose (LADD) provides a measure of the accuracy of predictions of risk based on the LADD. In particular, the LADD will underestimate the cumulative hazard $\Lambda(t)$ (which approximates the lifetime risk $P(t)$) when C>1 and overestimate it when C<1. Note that C = 1 in the special case of a one-stage model since the relative effectiveness function is constant in this case.

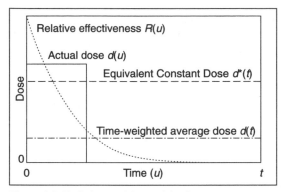

Figure 6.3. Equivalent and time-weighted average constant doses for a hypothetical time-dependent dose pattern in a six-stage model with the first stage dose-dependent ($R(.)$ not to scale).

To illustrate the application of this result, consider the hypothetical time-dependent exposure pattern illustrated in Figure 6.3 for a multistage model with $k=6$ and $r=1$. In this example, exposure to a dose d occurs during the first quarter of the lifetime and is zero thereafter:

$$d(u) = \begin{cases} d & 0 \le u \le t/4 \\ 0 & t/4 < u < t \end{cases}$$

In this case, the LECD $d_t^* = 0.82d$ exceeds the LADD $d_t^* = 0.25d$ by a factor of $C = 3.3$ since earlier exposures are more effective than later exposures. Thus, the use of the LADD would underestimate the actual lifetime risk by a factor of more than three.

Murdoch *et al.* (1992) evaluated the constant C in two specific applications in order to determine the extent to which the LADD might underestimate (or overestimate) the lifetime risk under conditions that might be expected to apply in practice. Their first example involved astronauts who might be assigned to work in a planned space station for periods of up to 180 days, during which time they might be exposed to trace levels of volatile organic compounds in a closed environment as well as to cosmic radiation (US National Research Council, 1992). The maximum value of C observed in this analysis was about 2, which occurred when $k = 6$ and $r = 4$. Thus, even though the relative effectiveness function could be as large as 6, the value of C was limited to about 2 in this case, largely because astronauts were assumed

to be 25–45 years of age at the start of their mission, thereby limiting the exposure period to one near the middle of their life span, and avoiding the extreme values of the relative effectiveness function, which occur early and late in life. The smallest value of C was 0.03, indicating that the LADD can substantially overestimate the actual risk as determined by the LECD.

The second example considered by Murdoch *et al.* (1992) involved dietary exposure to pesticide residues. The US National Research Council (1993b) was concerned about the possibility that infants and children might be at greater risk than adults, for three reasons. First, infants and children consume much greater quantities of certain foods, such as apple juice, than adults. Based on data from the 1977–1978 US Nation-wide Food Consumption Monitoring Survey, it was estimated that the average one-year-old consumed 30 times more apple juice each day than the average adult, on a body weight basis. Second, infants and children are exposed earlier in life, which would lead to higher relative effectiveness of exposure with an early-stage carcinogen. Finally, it is possible that perinatal tissues undergoing rapid growth and development may be more susceptible to carcinogenic stimuli than mature tissues. The mathematical analyses described above are based on the assumption that susceptibility is constant over time.

The values of C in this second example ranged from 0.27 to 3.74 for apple juice, and from 0.79 to 1.33 for three other foods (potato, tomato, and lettuce), reflecting different patterns of consumption in young people as compared with adults. The maximum value of $C = 3.74$ obtained with apple juice occurred when $k = 6$ and $r = 1$, reflecting the high relative effectiveness of exposure early in life in this case.

Similar analyses can be carried out for other models of carcinogenesis, including the more biologically based two-stage birth–death–mutation model discussed in section 7.5.3. Murdoch *et al.* (1992) calculated the values of C for these two examples and for this more biologically based model, making specific assumptions about the rate of tissue growth and the birth–death kinetics of initiated cells that had completed the first stage. The conclusions were broadly similar to those reported here, although the maximum values of C were found to be somewhat larger when initiated cells were assumed to proliferate rapidly. These findings are consistent with previous theoretical results reported by Chen *et al.* (1988) for the two-stage model. Murdoch (1992) noted that the relative effectiveness function for the multistage model can be scaled so as to be independent of the time t at which lifetime risk is evaluated, whereas the relative effectiveness function for the two-stage birth-death-mutation model is not scaleable.

6.5 Carcinogenic potency

The strength of agents with carcinogenic potential may be expressed in terms of quantitative measures of carcinogenic potency, first mentioned in the scientific literature in the 1930s. Twort & Twort (1930, 1933) examined the times at which tumours appeared during the course of animal experiments, and used the time at which 25% of the animals developed tumours as a measure of carcinogenic potency. Related measures of carcinogenic potency that took into account both the time of tumour appearance and intercurrent mortality in laboratory studies of carcinogenicity were later proposed by Iball (1939) and Irwin and Goodman (1946). Reviews of other measures of carcinogenic potency have been published by Barr (1985) and Goddard *et al.* (1993).

6.5.1 The TD_{50}

More recent developments in measuring carcinogenic potency are related to the TD_{50} index introduced by Peto *et al.* (1984) and Sawyer *et al.* (1984). Formally, TD_{50} is defined as the dose that will halve the proportion of tumour-free animals at a specified point in time. If $P(d)$ denotes the probability of a tumour occurring at dose d, TD_{50} is that dose d that satisfies the equation:

$$R(d) = [P(d)-P(0)]/[1-P(0)] = 0.5, \qquad (7)$$

where $R(d)$ is the extra risk over background at dose d. Thus, once the dose–response relationship $P(d)$ has been determined, TD_{50} may be estimated from equation (6).

Sawyer *et al.* (1984) used a hazard function of the form:

$$\lambda(t;d) = (1+bd)\lambda_0(t), \qquad (8)$$

where $\lambda_0(t)$ denotes the baseline hazard at time t in the absence of exposure. This leads to an essentially linear dose–response relationship

$$P(d;T) = 1-\exp\{-(1+bd)\Lambda_0(T)\} \qquad (9)$$

at a fixed time T, in the absence of mortality from causes other than tumour occurrence. Other hazard functions based on dose–response models discussed earlier in this chapter could also be used to accommodate non-linear dose–response relationships.

Ideally, the time of tumour occurrence would be used as the basis for statistical inference about the hazard function for tumour induction. Unfortunately, since most tumours in live animals are unobservable, the tumour-onset time is generally unknown. Sawyer *et al.* (1984) avoided this problem by using the time of death of those animals with tumours as a proxy for the time of tumour onset. Although this will be appropriate for tumours that are rapidly lethal, Portier & Hoel (1987) found that estimates of TD_{50} are quite sensitive to assumptions about tumour lethality.

Finkelstein & Ryan (1987) addressed this problem by using the methods of Peto *et al.* (1980) for combining tumour mortality and prevalence data to estimate TD_{50}. Bailar & Portier (1993) used survival-adjusted quantal-response data, as described by Bailar & Portier (1988), to estimate TD_{50}.

Dewanji *et al.* (1993) used Weibull models for the time of tumour onset, time to death due to tumour occurrence, and the time to death from competing risks to estimate TD_{50}. Specifically, the survivor functions for the time to tumour onset (X), the time to death from tumour (Y), and the time to death from competing risks are given by:

$$S_x(t,d) = \exp\{-(\alpha+\beta d^\delta)t^\eta\}$$
$$S_y(t,d) = \exp\{-(\alpha+\beta d^\delta)\rho t^\eta\}$$

and

$$S_z(t,d) = \exp\{-(\mu+\nu d^\delta)t^K\}$$

respectively, where, for example, $S_x(t,d) = Pr(X>t|d)$ denotes the probability that the time to tumour onset X exceeds t at dose d, and ρ is the

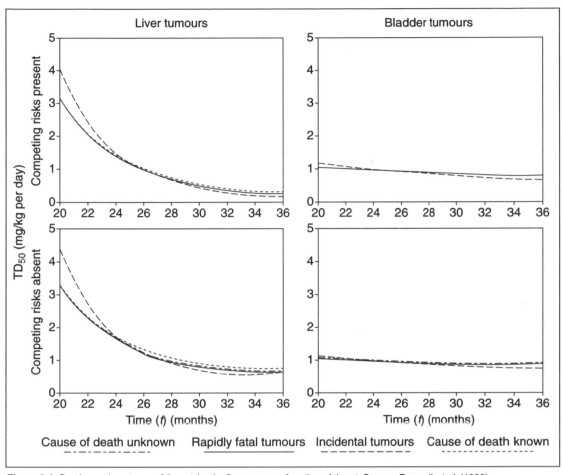

Figure 6.4. Carcinogenic potency of 2-acetylaminofluorene as a function of time *t*. Source: Dewanji *et al.* (1993)

tumour-lethality parameter, with $\rho = 0$ (and hence $S_y = 1$) corresponding to non-lethal or incidental tumours and $\rho = 1$ ($S_y = S_x$) rapidly lethal tumours. Intermediate values of ρ between zero and 1 represent tumours of intermediate lethality.

This Weibull model can be fitted to the data without direct information on the tumour-onset time X. Different forms of the model can be fitted depending on the availability of cause-of-death information, or the assumptions concerning tumour lethality. These include the following special cases: (i) cause of death and tumour lethality unknown; (ii) rapidly fatal tumours; (iii) incidental tumours; and (iv) cause of death known (death from tumour, death from competing risks with tumour, and death from competing risks without tumour).

The application of this model can be illustrated using the data reported by Littlefield *et al.* (1980) on liver and bladder tumours induced by 2-acetylaminofluorene (2-AAF). Since cause-of-death information was available in this study, TD_{50} can be estimated under conditions i–iv above. Estimates of TD_{50} can also be obtained in the presence or absence of competing risks, and as a function of time on test (Figure 6.4).

In this application, assumptions i–iv lead to similar estimates of TD_{50} for both liver and bladder tumours. Note that although TD_{50} values for bladder tumour change relatively little between 20 and 36 months on test, those for liver tumours drop markedly during this period. TD_{50} values in the presence of competing risks are only slightly lower than those in the absence of such risks.

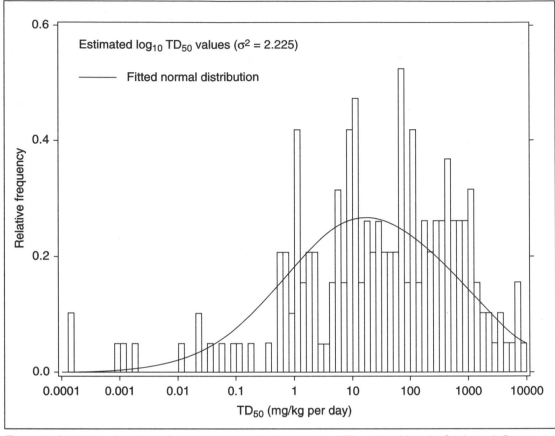

Figure 6.5. Distribution of carcinogenic potency for a sample of 191 values of TD_{50} selected from the Carcinogenic Potency Database. Source: Krewski *et al.* (1993a)

Other measures of carcinogenic potency have also been proposed, including measures based on the slope of the dose–response curve. In early work on interspecies correlation of carcinogenic potency described in section 6.7.2, Crouch & Wilson (1979) used the parameter in the reparametrized one-hit model

$$P(d) = 1 - (1-\alpha)\exp\{-\beta d/(1-\alpha)\}$$

to measure potency. Since $P(d) = \alpha+\beta$ at low doses, β represents the slope of this essentially linear dose–response model.

Another widely used measure of carcinogenic potency is the upper 95% confidence limit q_1^* on the parameter q_1 of the multistage model in equation 2 (cf. Anderson *et al.*, 1983). The linear term $q_1>0$ in the multistage model represents the slope

of the dose–response curve at low doses. Although the maximum likelihood estimate of q_1 can be zero, the upper confidence limit q_1^* is always strictly positive (Crump, 1984). Since

$$P(d) - P(0) = q_1 d,$$

q_1^* is sometimes referred to as a "unit risk factor".

6.5.2 Variation in carcinogenic potency

Gold *et al.* (1984, 1990) have tabulated the TD_{50} values for a large number of chemical carcinogens in their Carcinogenic Potency Database (CPDB). The TD_{50} values in the CPDB were calculated using the statistical methods developed by Sawyer *et al.* (1984). All TD_{50} values are expressed in common units of mg/kg body weight per day, and corrected for intercurrent mortality whenever individual animal survival times are available. The CPDB currently includes data on over 4000 experiments on more than 1000 different chemicals. The carcinogenic potency of these chemicals expressed in terms of TD_{50} varies by a factor of more than 10 million.

Krewski *et al.* (1990) examined the distribution of TD_{50} values for subsets of chemical carcinogens selected from the CPDB which appeared to be roughly lognormal. Goddard *et al.* (1993) used an empirical Bayes method proposed by Louis (1984) to adjust for the sampling error associated with individual TD_{50} values in order to obtain an estimate of the distribution of actual rather than estimated TD_{50} values. The application of this methodology is illustrated using a sample of 191 chemical carcinogens selected from the CPDB in Figure 6.5. The empirical Bayes estimator effectively shrinks the original distribution towards its centre, thereby eliminating variability due to sampling error in the TD_{50} values.

The distribution of carcinogenic potency is potentially applicable to the regulation of carcinogens (cf. Munro, 1990). Rulis (1986) and Flamm *et al.* (1987) proposed using this distribution to establish a level of toxicological insignificance below which a detailed assessment of risk would not be required. The essence of this proposal is the assumption that a new and as yet untested chemical would probably not be more potent than the most potent carcinogens comprising the lower tail of this distribution; exposure guidelines established for these carcinogens would then apply to the new compound. The principle advantage of this strategy is that it avoids the need for expensive toxicological testing of agents for which human exposure may be extremely low. A disadvantage is that the carcinogenicity of the untested chemical is not established until a long-term bioassay has been completed. Before this procedure is applied in practice, additional details such as the selection of an appropriate quantile of the potency distribution used to define toxicological insignificance, remain to be worked out (Woutersen *et al.*, 1984).

6.5.3 Correlation between TD_{50} and other measures of toxicity

Several investigators have noted a strong correlation between TD_{50} and the maximum tolerated dose (MTD) used in long-term animal cancer studies (Bernstein *et al.*, 1985; Gaylor, 1989; Krewski *et al.*, 1989b; Reith & Starr, 1989a,b). This correlation ($r = 0.294$) is illustrated in Figure 6.6 using a sample of 191 chemicals selected from the CPDB by Krewski *et al.* (1993a). Although the TD_{50} values used in this analysis are based on an essentially linear dose–response model as in equation (5), the correlation obtained with TD_{50} values estimated using the Armitage–Doll multistage model is equally high.

Bernstein *et al.* (1985) attributed this high correlation to the limited range of possible TD_{50} values relative to the MTD, and the large variation in MTDs for different chemicals. Subsequent analytical results reported by Kodell *et al.* (1990) and Krewski *et al.* (1993) support this argument.

The absence of points in the upper left-hand triangular region in Figure 6.6 is due to the lower limit on the number of tumours observed in the exposed groups in laboratory experiments required to demonstrate a significant increase in tumour occurrence. This implies that highly toxic chemicals of weak carcinogenic potency would probably go undetected in a standard bioassay, since such agents would not yield a measurable excess of tumours at the MTD. Crouch *et al.* (1987) attribute the absence of points in the lower right-hand triangular region to a lack of chemicals with extremely high potency relative to their MTDs. An informal search for such "supercarcinogens" conducted by the US National Research Council (1993a) failed to reveal any points clearly located in this region.

TD_{50}, which provides a measure of carcinogenic potency at high doses, is also highly correlated with the value of $q_1{}^*$ derived from the linearized multistage model (LMS), which provides a measure of carcinogenic potency at low doses on the assumption of low-dose linearity (Krewski *et al.*, 1993). Both measures of potency are correlated with the MTD. Gaylor (1989), and later Gaylor & Gold (1995), proposed exploiting the correlation between $q_1{}^*$ and the MTD in order to arrive at preliminary estimates of low-dose risk. As with the concept of toxicological insignificance introduced by Rulis (1986), this approach to obtaining preliminary estimates of low dose risk does not require toxicological data on the carcinogenic potential of the agent of interest. However, such preliminary estimates of

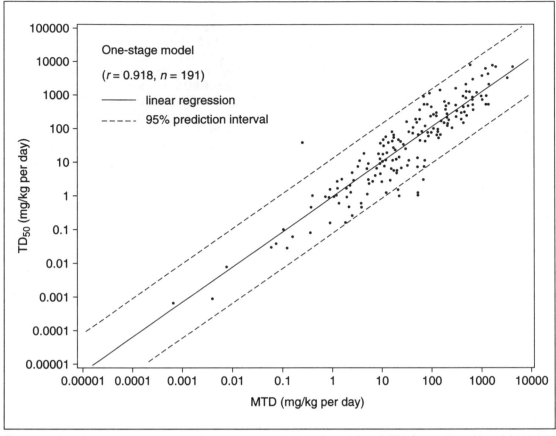

Figure 6.6. Associations between carcinogenic potency and maximium tolerated dose (MTD). Source: Krewski *et al.* (1993a)

risk are calculated on the *assumption* that the agent is potentially carcinogenic; long-term laboratory testing would still be required to confirm this assumption.

TD_{50} is also known to be correlated with other indicators of toxicity. Metzger *et al.* (1987) reported a correlation of $r = 0.6$ between TD_{50} and acute toxicity as measured by LD_{50}. McGregor (1992) calculated the correlation between TD_{50} and LD_{50} for different classes of carcinogens established by the International Agency for Research on Cancer. Although this analysis was based on a limited number of agents, the highest correlations were observed in Group 1 (known human carcinogens) with $r = 0.7$ for mice and $r = 0.9$ for rats.

Travis *et al.* (1990ab, 1991) reported a correlation of $r = 0.4$ between TD_{50} and mutagenic potency as determined by the Ames *Salmonella* assay. Higher correlations were also found between TD_{50} and composite indicators of mutation, acute and chronic toxicity, and reproductive anomalies. When the analysis was restricted to carcinogens affecting specific target organs (lung or liver), for example, correlation coefficients in the neighbourhood of $r = 0.9$ were obtained.

6.5.4 Numerical ranking systems

Numerical ranking schemes for carcinogenic potency (i.e. quantitative carcinogenic activity) have been developed as means of priority setting and regulation of carcinogens. Some authors (Gold *et al.*, 1984; Peto *et al.*, 1984; Sawyer *et al.*, 1984; Gold *et al.*, 1987) use TD_{50} as the only measure of carcinogenic potency (see above); others have proposed the use of a unit risk factor for risk estimation (US Environmental Protection Agency, 1986).

Some of the ranking systems used are entirely based on scores for parameters of carcinogenic activity (Squire, 1981, 1983; Theiss, 1983; Squire, 1984; Lutz, 1986), while the systems more recently proposed are based on dose potency (measured as TD_{50}) either in combination with human exposure estimates (Ames et al., 1987) or adjusted by weighting factors that describe other parameters of carcinogenicity (Nesnow, 1990; Willems et al., 1990; Nesnow, 1991).

Squire (1981, 1983, 1984) proposed a ranking system based on evidence from animal and geno-toxicity studies. Six factors are involved in this system, each factor being divided into subfactors to which scores are assigned, leading to total scores varying between 13 and 100. Two major criticisms are that dose potency is inadequately weighted (Crump, 1983) and that absence of a carcinogenic effect in one or more species is not taken into account at all (Willems et al., 1990). Theiss (1983) presented a ranking scheme based on a tier system; the results of short-term studies are assigned to tier 1, data from animal studies to tier 2 and evidence from epidemiological studies to tier 3 to differentiate between weak and strong carcinogens. Lutz (1986) also suggested distinguishing between weak and strong carcinogens using liver DNA binding as a measure of carcinogenic activity.

Ames et al. (1987) introduced the ratio of human exposure dose to rodent potency dose (HERP) as a measure of possible carcinogenic hazard to man. HERP is based on estimated lifelong daily exposure of humans and the TD_{50} values estimated from rodent studies. It is calculated by expressing human exposure (daily lifetime dose in mg/kg body weight) as a percentage of the rodent TD_{50} (in mg/kg body weight). According to the authors, HERP should not be used as a direct estimate of human hazard because: (a) at low-dose rates, human susceptibility may differ systematically from rodent susceptibility; (b) the general shape of the dose–response curve is not known and (c) the mechanism of action, i.e. genotoxic versus non-genotoxic activity, is not taken into account. Ames et al. (1987) calculated HERP indices for 36 compounds; they ranged from 0.0002% for chloroform in well-water to 140% for occupational exposure to ethylene dibromide.

Willems et al. (1990) developed a system for ranking genotoxic carcinogens occurring in the workplace which is based on dose potency (measured as TD_{50}) adjusted by six weighting factors. The final result is a potency index expressed as the estimated tumour incidence in humans at an exposure concentration of 1 mg/m^3 under occupational conditions of exposure (8 h per day, five days a week for 40 years). The six weighting factors are: (i) relevance of route of exposure; (ii) number of species with tumours versus number of species examined; (iii) malignancy of the tumours; (iv) presence or absence of a dose–response relationship; (v) metabolism; and (vi) epidemiological data not suitable for quantitative extrapolation. The proposed system, which can easily be adapted to non-occupational situations, makes it possible to use all relevant animal and human data for the ranking of carcinogens according to their estimated hazard in humans in a comprehensible and consistent manner. The authors stress that adjustment of dose potency by means of weighting factors is a subjective activity, heavily dependent on expert judgement.

Recently, Nesnow (1990, 1991) described a multifactorial ranking system based on TD_{50} and the highest average daily dose (HADD) administered in a chronic animal study that did not result in an increased tumour incidence. Both TD_{50} and HADD are converted to log decile units and are then adjusted by weighting factors that, in the case of TD_{50}, describe other parameters of carcinogenic activity and, in the case of HADD, lack of carcinogenic activity in both sexes or in more than one species. The usefulness of this ranking system was explored using data from 142 chemicals tested in the National Toxicology Program. The author considered this multifactorial carcinogen activity scheme to be an initial attempt to develop the methods needed to assess the potential cancer risk of chemicals, and concluded that no absolute measure of carcinogenic activity exists but only estimates that try to quantitate it.

6.6 Joint exposures and carcinogenic mixtures

Much of the literature on carcinogenic risk assessment focuses on the risks associated with exposure to a single agent. In reality, humans may be exposed to more than one carcinogenic substance at the same time. Siemiatycki (1991) has conducted a detailed population-based case–control study of the potential cancer risks associated with more than 300 substances found in the workplace in Montreal, Canada. This pioneering investigation involved constructing exposure profiles for each of these agents for nearly 4000 male cancer patients recruited in Montreal between 1979 and 1986. People are also exposed to complex carcinogenic mixtures, such as emissions from roofing tar and diesel exhaust (US National Research Council, 1988; Vainio *et al.*, 1990; Calabrese, 1991; Krewski & Thomas, 1992). In this section, we consider scientific approaches to estimating the risks associated with carcinogenic mixtures. Of particular concern is the possibility of interactive effects between two agents, in which the risk associated with joint exposure is greater than the sum of the risks due to exposure to each agent alone.

6.6.1 Modelling the risk of joint exposures

Different approaches have been proposed for measuring the interaction between two toxicants. Kaldor & L'Abbe (1990) noted that interaction depends on the scale used to measure risk. Whereas the age-specific relative risk is often used to describe cancer risk in epidemiological investigations, particularly in case–control studies, the cumulative risk, expressed as the probability of a tumour occurring by a specified time, is often of more interest in risk-assessment applications. Once the scale of measurement has been established, interaction can then be defined (Cox, 1984).

Kodell & Pounds (1991) discussed interaction in terms of departures from either *response additivity* or *dose additivity*. Dose additivity implies identical biological action of two chemicals in that one chemical is simply a dilution of the other, whereas response additivity implies both biological and statistical independence of action.

Let $P(d_1, d_2)$ denote the probability of a carcinogenic response given continuous exposure up to given age t to a dose d_1 of a first agent C_1 and a dose d_2 of a second agent C_2. Similarly, let $P_i(d_i)$ denote the probability of a tumour occurring following exposure to a dose d_i of chemical C_i alone ($i = 1,2$).

For dose additivity,

$$P(d_1, d_2) = P_1(d_1 + \rho\, d_2) = P_2(d_1/\rho + d_2),$$

where ρ is the relative potency of C_1 to C_2 (i.e., $d_1 = \rho\, d_2$). For response additivity,

$$\begin{aligned}
P(d_1, d_2) &= P_1(d_1) + [1 - P_1(d_1)]P_2(d_2) \\
&= P_1(d_2) + [1 - P_2(d_2)]P_1(d_1) \\
&= P_1(d_2) + P_2(d_2) - P_1(d_1)P_2(d_2).
\end{aligned}$$

Interaction is sometimes characterized in terms of departures from additivity of age-specific relative risks. Specifically, if $h(d_1, d_2)$ denotes the cancer incidence or cancer mortality rate at time t for exposure to doses d_1 and d_2 of carcinogens c_1 and c_2, the relative risk is given by:

$$RR(d_1, d_2) = h(d_1, d_2)/h(0,0),$$

where $h(d_1, d_2)$ denotes the age-specific incidence or mortality rate in the absence of exposure to either C_1 or C_2. Lack of interaction is then expressed in terms of the additive relative risk model:

$$RR(d_1, d_2) = RR(d_1, 0) + RR(0, d_2) - 1.$$

A supra-additive relative risk, such as the multiplicative relative risk:

$$RR(d_1, d_2) = RR(d_1, 0)RR(0, d_2),$$

then reflects a synergistic effect between d_1 and d_2.

Although the additive excess relative risk model provides a useful baseline for evaluating interaction, Kaldor & L'Abbe (1990) noted that, following a logarithmic transformation of the relative risk, the multiplicative model will become the baseline for evaluating interaction. Thomas & Whittemore (1988) and Greenland (1993) discussed the use of these two models in evaluating interaction. Steenland & Thun (1986) applied these models in evaluating the interaction between tobacco and occupational exposures in the causation of lung cancer.

Although age-specific relative risk is a widely used measure of cancer risk, the probability $P(d_1, d_2)$ of a tumour occurring by a certain age is also of interest in cancer risk assessment.

Zielinski *et al.* (unpublished data) attempted to relate the additive relative risk model to response additivity, with relative risk now defined by $RR(d_1,d_2)=P(d_1,d_2)/P(0,0)$. Given an additive relative risk model, it can be shown that:

$$P(d_1,d_2) = [P_1 \ (d_1)+P_2 \ (d_2) \ - \ P_1 \ (d_1)P_2 \ (d_2) \ - \ P(0,0)]/[1 - P(0,0)].$$

Thus, when the spontaneous tumour response rate $P(0,0)$ is small, the additive relative risk model implies that the response will also be additive.

6.6.2 Theoretical predictions of the risks of joint exposures

Brown & Chu (1989) conducted a systematic investigation of the type of interaction that might be expected following joint exposure to two carcinogens C_1 and C_2 with the Armitage–Doll multistage model of carcinogenesis. Interaction was measured in terms of the index of synergy

$$S = [R(d_1,d_2) - R+(d_1,d_2)]/[RR_*(d_1,d_2) - RR+(d_1,d_2)]$$

due to Thomas (1982). Here, RR+ and RR$_*$ denote the relative risk for the additive and multiplicative relative risk models respectively. Note that S = 0 corresponds to additive age-specific relative risk and S = 1 indicates multiplicative relative risk. Thus, values of $S>0$ reflect synergism whereas $S<0$ indicates antagonism.

For the approximate form of the multistage model, Brown & Chu (1989) showed that, if two

carcinogens affect the same stage, the result will be an additive relationship. When two carcinogens affect only the first and last stages, respectively, this will result in a multiplicative relative risk relationship (cf., Siemiatycki & Thomas, 1981). In general, however, two carcinogens that affect different stages of the model will not produce a multiplicative relative risk relationship. Short exposures that occur close together in time and not at very young or very old ages can produce an almost additive relative risk relationship. Brown & Chu (1989) concluded that a multiplicative relative relationship following exposure to two carcinogens provides evidence of action at two different stages. However, consideration needs to be given to the temporal pattern of exposure to the two agents when attempting to make such mechanistic inferences with an almost additive relative risk relationship.

Kodell *et al.* (1991) carried out a similar analysis for an approximate form of the two-stage clonal expansion model of carcinogenesis. This demonstrated that exposure to two carcinogens, each acting only as an initiator, promoter or completer, can lead to both additive and supra-additive relative risk, including multiplicative and supramultiplicative relative risk in certain cases (Table 6.3). For example, exposure either to two initiators or to two completers leads to additive relative risk, regardless of the temporal pattern of exposure. As is the case with two carcinogens affecting the first and last stages, respectively, in the Armitage–Doll multistage model, exposure to an initiator and a completer results in multiplica-

Table 6.3. Interaction between two carcinogens in the two-stage clonal expansion model of carcinogenesis[a]

Carcinogen C_1	Carcinogen C_2	Interaction
Initiator	Initiator	Additive
Completer	Completer	Additive
Initiator	Completer	Multiplicative
Promoter	Promoter	Supramultiplicative
Initiator	Promoter	Multiplicative, supramultiplicative
Initiator	Initiator and completer	Supra-additive, submultiplicative
Initiator	Initiator and promoter	Supra-additive, supramultiplicative
Promoter	Promoter and completer	Supramultiplicative

[a] Source: Kodell *et al.*, (1991).

tive relative risk, regardless of the temporal exposure patterns to these two agents. A supramultiplicative relative risk can occur with exposure to two promoters, or with exposure to an initiator followed by a promoter. This latter observation is consistent with the findings of laboratory initiation–promotion studies in which exposure to either the initiator or promoter alone produces little response, but initiation followed by promotion produces a marked response.

Kodell *et al.* (1991) also considered the joint effects of two agents that may affect more than one stage of the model (initiation, promotion, and completion). In general, the joint effects of two such agents will depend on the relative magnitude of the effects on the first- and second-stage mutation rates and on the rate of clonal expansion of initiated cells. For example, non-overlapping exposures to an initiator and an initiator–completer yields supra-additive but submultiplicative relative risk, the actual effect depending on the magnitude of the effects on the first- and second-stage mutation rates.

Zielinski *et al.* (unpublished data) extended the results of Brown & Chu (1989) and Kodell *et al.* (1991) in two ways. First, the exact rather than the approximate forms of both the multistage and two-stage models were used. Second, an alternative definition of relative risk in terms of the probability of a tumour occurring by a given age was also investigated. Although the exact forms of the multistage and two-stage models led to predictions of interaction that were somewhat similar to those based on the commonly used approximate forms of these two models, both quantitative and qualitative differences were noted in many of the cases considered. When lifetime tumour risks were considered, both models predicted departures from response additivity for a range of assumptions. More specific statements about interaction when using the exact forms of the multistage and two-stage models require specification of the temporal patterns of exposure to C_1 and C_2.

6.6.3 Empirical studies of the risks of joint exposures

Epidemiological studies have provided clear evidence of interactive effects between agents known to cause cancer in humans. Whittemore

& MacMillan (1983) demonstrated a supra-additive but submultiplicative relationship in the age-specific mortality rate for lung cancer among uranium miners exposed to radon and tobacco smoke. Although this result was confirmed in a reanalysis of these data by Moolgavkar *et al.* (1993) using the two-stage model of carcinogenesis discussed in detail in Chapter 7, it did not indicate a biological interaction between radon and tobacco smoking at the molecular level. Alcohol consumption and tobacco smoking have also been shown to interact synergistically in the induction of oral cancer (International Agency for Research on Cancer, 1986), the age-specific relative risks being approximately multiplicative. Other examples of interactive effects have been described by the US National Research Council (1988) and by Vainio *et al.* (1990). Interactions between tobacco and other agents have been reviewed in detail by Saracci (1987).

The effects of joint exposure to two carcinogenic substances have been examined in a number of laboratory investigations. Elashoff *et al.* (1987) and Fears *et al.* (1988, 1989) reported the results of a systematic study of binary combinations of chemicals selected from among 12 known or possible chemical carcinogens. A series of experiments with pairs of chemicals was conducted, in each of which there were four dose groups for each of the two chemicals involved (including a low dose of zero and a high dose approaching the maximum tolerated dose for that chemical), yielding 16 treatment groups for each binary combination. In this series of experiments, examples of synergism (such as the induction of liver tumours among animals exposed to lasiocarpine and cycasin), antagonism (such as the inhibition by nitrilotriacetic acid of stomach tumours induced by *N*-methyl-*N'*-nitro-*N*-nitrosoguanidine), and additivity were observed.

A comprehensive database of interactions between two chemical carcinogens observed in animal experiments has been established by Arcos *et al.* (1988). This database includes information on the route of exposure, dose levels, test species, and results obtained. Approximately 90% of the binary combinations involved a polycyclic aromatic hydrocarbon (PAH), an aromatic amine, a nitrosamine, a nitrosamide, or an azo dye. The skin was the target tissue in about half of all of the synergistic combinations in the database. For binary combinations involving PAHs, antagonism was the predominant interaction. A similar database of inhibitors of chemical carcinogenesis has been established by Bagheri et al. (1988-89).

Initiation–promotion experiments provide a rich collection of examples of interaction between two agents capable of influencing the process of carcinogenesis (Börzsönyi et al., 1984). In a typical initiation–promotion protocol, animals are exposed to a DNA-reactive initiator for a short period of time (sometimes only a single exposure) followed by prolonged exposure to a non-genotoxic promoting agent. Whereas exposure to either the initiator or promoter alone is insufficient to result in an appreciable increase in tumour occurrence rates, sequential exposure to the initiator and promoter results in a marked increase in tumour risk.

Rao et al. (1989) established a database on tumour promoting agents, which includes information on co-carcinogens. (A co-carcinogen is an agent which, when given simultaneously with another agent, results in an observable increase in tumour response.) Most of the initiating agents were aldehydes, acids, aliphatic hydrocarbons, or solvents. The promoting agents were much more diverse, although fatty acids and esters constituted the largest chemical class of promoters in the database.

6.6.4 Modelling joint exposures

The modelling of epidemiological and toxicological data with combined exposures has been discussed by Thomas & Whittemore (1988) and Krewski et al. (1990), respectively. Methods for discriminating between additive and multiplicative relative risk models based on epidemiological data are of particular interest in the modelling of combined exposures (cf. Thomas, 1981; Breslow & Storer, 1985). Combined exposures studied include exposure to tobacco and alcohol in relation to the risk of cancers of the upper respiratory and digestive tracts (Roy, 1991), and exposure to tobacco and radon in relation to lung cancer (Moolgavkar et al., 1993; Lubin et al., 1994).

A number of approaches have been proposed for fitting mixture models which describe risks as intermediate between additive and multiplicative. These models include the additive and the multiplicative relative risk models as special cases, and allow formal testing of the hypothesis of additivity or multiplicativity of risk through likelihood-ratio tests. Moolgavkar & Venzon (1987) have reviewed the three families of mixture models which have been proposed for model discrimination in case–control studies. If RR (x) denotes the relative risk for an individual with covariate vector x relative to the reference value $x = 0$, the models can be described as follows:

• The log-linear additive mixture model proposed by Thomas (1981):

$$\log R(x, \beta, \rho) = \rho \, \beta x + (1- \rho) \log (1+ \beta x).$$

Here, ρ is the mixture parameter, and β is the vector of regression parameters associated with the exposures. This model simplifies to an additive model when $\rho = 1$ and to a multiplicative model when $\rho = 0$.

• The power model proposed by Breslow & Storer (1985):

$$\log R(x, \beta, \rho) = \frac{(1+ \beta x)\rho - 1}{\rho} \quad \text{when } \rho \neq 0$$

$$\log R(x, \beta, \rho) = \log (1+ \beta x) \quad \text{when } \rho = 0.$$

This model also simplifies to an additive risk model when $\rho = 1$ and to a multiplicative model when $\rho = 0$.

• The model proposed by Guerrero & Johnson (1982):

$$\log R(x, \beta, \rho) = \frac{\log(1+ \rho \, \beta x)}{\rho} \quad \text{when } \rho \neq 0$$

$$\log R(x, \beta, \rho) = \beta x \quad \text{when } \rho = 0.$$

This simplifies to an additive risk model when $\rho = 0$ and to a multiplicative model when $\rho = 1$.

These models provide a useful basis for testing the hypotheses of additivity or multiplicativity of the relative risk using standard statistical tests such as the likelihood ratio test (Breslow & Storer, 1985). Interpretation of the results of analyses using such models is difficult, however, in particular since the models proposed by Thomas (1981) and by Breslow & Storer, 1985) are not invariant under different scaling of the covariate vector x (Moolgavkar & Venzon, 1987). In addition, inferences based on the asymptotic standard errors may be flawed when the relative risk is not multiplicative; likelihood-based procedures should therefore be used as the basis for statistical inference (Moolgavkar & Venzon, 1987).

6.7 Risk prediction

In many situations, direct estimates of carcinogenic risk are not possible, necessitating the prediction of risk by the extrapolation of results obtained under conditions different from those of immediate interest. Extrapolation may be required between occupationally exposed groups of workers and the general population, or between different exposure patterns, as discussed in section 6.4. Extrapolation from high to low doses is often required: occupationally, groups are generally subjected to higher levels of exposure than the general population, and laboratory studies of carcinogenicity are conducted at much higher doses than those experienced by humans. Predictions of human risk based on laboratory data require uncertain extrapolations between species. Laboratory studies may also be conducted using routes of exposure different from those predominant in human populations.

6.7.1 Extrapolation from high to low doses

Epidemiological or toxicological data may be extrapolated from high to low doses on the basis of a suitable mathematical model fitted to the experimental data. As discussed in section 6.2, many dose–response relationships observed in epidemiological investigations are adequately characterized by a linear dose–response model. In contrast, bioassay data often exhibit marked nonlinearity due to factors such as saturation of pharmacokinetic processes involved in metabolic activation of the parent compound or potentiation of a tumorigenic response by the induction of cellular proliferation at high doses. As indicated in section 6.3, a number of flexible statistical models are capable of describing such non-linear dose–response relationships.

It is well known that different statistical models may provide a good fit to experimental data within the observable response range, yet yield widely divergent results when extrapolated to very low doses (Krewski & Van Ryzin, 1981; Zeise et al., 1987). This occurs because many statistical models may exhibit either a sublinear or supralinear behaviour at low doses. When the constraint of low-dose linearity is imposed, predictions of low-dose risk obtained with different models are quite comparable (Krewski et al., 1991).

In regulatory applications of quantitative cancer risk assessment, there is a strong tendency to employ methods of prediction which assume that the dose–response curve for carcinogenesis is linear in the low-dose region. This view is reflected in the principles of risk assessment put forward by the US Office of Science and Technology Policy (1985), which stated that:

"When data and information are limited, and when much uncertainty exists regarding the mechanism of carcinogenic action, models or procedures which incorporate low-dose linearity are preferred when compatible with the limited information."

This view is also expressed in the cancer risk assessment guidelines proposed by the US Environmental Protection Agency (1986):

"In the absence of adequate information to the contrary, the linearized multistage procedure will be employed."

These guidelines should not be viewed as being incompatible with the existence of a threshold for chemical carcinogenesis. However, when clear information indicating the existence of such a mechanism does not exist, low-dose linearity has been proposed as a default assumption in the absence of evidence to the contrary. Even when this default assumption is incorrect, its use is likely to lead to an upper bound on the actual risk.

The assumption of low-dose linearity is supported to some extent by both theoretical and empirical considerations (Krewski et al., 1995a).

If the transition rates between different stages in the Armitage–Doll multistage model are assumed to be linearly related to dose, the model predicts that the dose–response curve will be linear in the low-dose region (Van Ryzin, 1982). Crump et al. (1976) showed that a linear approximation to the dose–response curve for the Armitage–Doll model will be quite accurate whenever the increase in risk does not exceed the background response rate. Crump et al. (1976) further argued that, if a carcinogenic agent acts by accelerating an already ongoing process, the dose–response curve will then, under quite general conditions, be linear at low doses. Hoel (1980) subsequently showed that this additive background model also applies even in the case of partial additivity. Schell & Leysieffer (1989) showed that the one-hit model, which is essentially linear at low to moderate doses, provides an upper bound on risk for any dose–response model satisfying an increasing failure rate condition in dose. At doses below those associated with saturation of activation or deactivation pathways, pharmacokinetic models for metabolic activation are typically characterized by first-order linear kinetic systems (Hoel et al., 1983; Whittemore et al., 1986; Krewski et al., 1987).

Empirical support for low dose linearity in the case of genotoxic carcinogens is provided by the observation that many DNA adducts are linearly related to dose, even at extremely low doses (Lutz, 1990, 1991; Beland et al., 1991). Although these adducts may play a role in tumour induction, this argument in support of low-dose linearity would be strengthened if similar results were available for adducts which had been fixed as mutations. Dose–response curves for mutations observed in the Ames Salmonella assay often appear linear at low to moderate doses (Krewski et al., 1992), non-linearity at high doses being attributed to cytotoxicity; these results may or may not be applicable to mammalian systems.

The ability of large-scale laboratory studies to resolve the shape of the dose–response curve at low dose levels is limited (Clayson & Krewski, 1986; Krewski et al., 1989a). The largest bioassay ever conducted was the ED01 study with 2-acetylaminofluorene at the US National Center for Toxicological Research (Staffa & Mehlman, 1979). This study, which involved over 24 000 mice, pro-

duced an almost linear dose–response curve for liver tumours, and a highly non-linear "hockey stick" dose–response curve with an apparent no-effect level for bladder tumours. Brown & Hoel (1983) noted that the apparently linear liver tumour data were also consistent with a model which included a threshold in the low-dose region. Conversely, Gaylor et al. (1985) reported that the bladder tumour data exhibited a slight but detectable linear trend at doses below the apparent no-effect level.

A subsequent study conducted by the British Industrial Biological Research Foundation examined the tumorigenic effects of a number of nitroso compounds in over 5000 rats, mice, and hamsters (Peto et al., 1991a,b). The main experiment involved 16 doses of N-nitrosodimethylamine (NDMA) and N-nitrosodiethylamine (NDEA) and over 4000 inbred rats. Carcinogenic effects were observed primarily in the liver (NDMA and NDEA) and oesophagus (NDEA only). These effects were observed at doses of only 0.01 mg/kg per day, and appeared to be linear at the lowest doses tested.

Different statistical methods have been proposed for low-dose extrapolation of bioassay data under the constraint of linearity at low doses. The most widely used method is based on the LMS model as implemented by Crump (1984). Van Ryzin (1980) suggested that any model that fitted the data could be used to estimate the dose producing an excess lifetime risk of 1%, followed by simple linear extrapolation to lower doses. Similar procedures have been implemented by Gaylor & Kodell (1980) and Farmer et al. (1982). Gross et al. (1970) suggested that data at the upper end of the dose range should be discarded until a linear model provided an adequate description of the remaining data. A variation on this approach based on a series of linearized upper bounds on risk in the low-dose region has been developed by Krewski et al. (1991). All of these methods generally yield comparable estimates of risk at low doses.

6.7.2 Interspecies extrapolation

Extrapolation of experimental data on carcinogenic risks obtained in animals to humans is based on the premise that mammalian species respond in a similar fashion to toxic agents. All agents classified as human carcinogens by the International Agency for Research on Cancer have also been shown to produce a carcinogenic response in one or more animal species (McGregor, 1992). Chemicals that cause cancer in rats or mice also tend to cause cancer in mice or rats, respectively, with an observed overall concordance in the bioassay of about 75% (Haseman & Huff, 1987; Gold *et al.*, 1989). Lave *et al.* (1988) suggested that this level of concordance might represent an upper bound on the degree of concordance between rodents and humans. Piegorsch *et al.* (1992) pointed out that species concordance depends on carcinogenic potency, and estimated that, for carcinogens of moderate potency, the maximum possible species concordance may be limited to about 80%. This imperfect qualitative agreement between species suggests a cautious approach in quantitative interspecies extrapolation.

The approach to quantitative interspecies extrapolation can be considered in terms of the allometric equation:

$$P = a \times BW^b,$$

where P represents a measure of carcinogenic potency in a given species, BW denotes a typical body weight in that species, a is a constant related to the carcinogenicity of a particular agent and b is the empirically determined scaling constant, assumed to hold for a variety of species and agents (Watanabe *et al.*, 1992). The US Food and Drug Administration has used a value of $b = 1$, corresponding to interspecies extrapolation on the basis of body weight, whereas the US Environmental Protection Agency has employed $b = 2/3$, corresponding roughly to extrapolation on the basis of body surface area (Watanabe *et al.* 1992). Predictions of human risk based on the results of tests on rats and mice are approximately 6 and 13 times higher, respectively, based on surface area as compared with body weight. Several governmental agencies in the USA, including those mentioned above, have recently endorsed a recommendation to use $b = 3/4$ (US Environmental Protection Agency, 1992; US Agency for Toxic Substances and Disease Registry, 1993).

In assessing possible empirical scaling constants (b), across-species comparisons have been made for three types of data: acute and subchron-

ic toxicity data for cancer chemotherapeutic agents in a variety of mammalian species, including humans (Freireich *et al.*, 1966; Schein *et al.*, 1979; Collins *et al.*, 1986, 1990); cancer potencies in mice and rats derived from long-term cancer bioassays of the National Cancer Institute or National Toxicology Program or compiled in the Cancer Potency Database; and cancer potencies in rodents and humans of primarily occupational carcinogens (Allen *et al.*, 1988; Crouch & Wilson, 1979; Goodman & Wilson, 1991a) or chemotherapeutic agents (Dedrick & Morrison, 1992; Kaldor *et al.*, 1988).

Freireich *et al.* (1966) compiled values of LD_{10} (the dose resulting in 10% mortality) or MTDs in humans and several other mammalian species for 18 cancer chemotherapeutic agents. They found that scaling the animal dose on the basis of surface area provided a reasonably good prediction of human dose, but that body-weight scaling from animals underpredicted human toxicity. Collins *et al.* (1986, 1990) similarly found for 16 cancer chemotherapeutic agents that mouse LD_{10} values scaled on the basis of surface area provided a good estimate of the maximum tolerated dose in humans. Travis & White (1988) analysed the combined data of Freireich *et al.* (1966) and Schein *et al.* (1979) on additional chemotherapeutic agents. They found the best estimate of b to be 0.74, with 95 % confidence limits that excluded $b = 1$, and barely excluded $b = 0.67$. On the basis of this analysis, they proposed that $b = 3/4$ should be used to extrapolate cancer potencies from rodents to humans. Watanabe *et al.* (1992), after reanalysing the same data set, noted that surface area scaling is consistent with the data if non-homogeneity of variances is taken into account. They also noted that, if one assumes that different chemicals can scale differently across species, the maximum tolerated doses in humans of the chemicals in the databases considered by Freireich *et al.* (1966) and Schein *et al.* (1979) are consistent with scaling constants ranging from 0.42 to 0.97.

A number of empirical studies of the carcinogenic potency of agents that are effective in two species have been conducted. Crouch & Wilson (1979) demonstrated a positive correlation in carcinogenic potency in rats and mice in terms of the slope of the one-hit model. Crouch (1983) subsequently suggested that interspecies extrapolation of carcinogenic potency should be accurate to within a factor of less than five. Gaylor & Chen (1986) later compared TD_{50} values for 190 chemical carcinogens selected from the CPDB. Metzger *et al.* (1989) compared TD_{50} values for 264 agents in the CPDB and found the best fit for scaling falling between surface-area and body-weight scaling. Although the median ratio of TD_{50} values in these two species was close to 1, there were a number of cases in which they differed by a factor of more than 100. McGregor (1992) subsequently reported that amides and halides exhibit disparate TD_{50} values in rats and mice.

Bernstein *et al.* (1985) and Reith & Starr (1989b) suggested that the interspecies correlation in carcinogen potency observed in these investigations is due to the corresponding correlation in the MTDs for rats and mice. (It will be remembered that TD_{50} is highly correlated with the MTD in rodent carcinogenicity studies.) However, Monte Carlo-based analyses by Crouch *et al.* (1987) and Zeise *et al.* (1986) indicate that interspecies correlations of cancer potency cannot be entirely explained as an artifactual result of the correlation between cancer potency and MTD. Shlyakhter *et al.* (1992) and Freedman *et al.* (1992) found similar results for the correlation between TD_{50} and MTD.

Allen *et al.* (1988) compared the carcinogenic potency of 23 chemicals in animals and humans for which data were available in the relevant species. A number of different methods of interspecies extrapolation were considered, including the choice of the interspecies scaling factor *b*, and tumour morphology (benign and malignant tumours combined or malignant tumours only). Most methods yielded evidence of an animal–human correlation in carcinogenic potency, with rank correlation coefficients of up to 0.9 reported. Despite this high correlation, the error associated with predictions of carcinogenic potency in humans based on animal data was substantial, as was the uncertainty in the estimates of cancer potency derived from human data.

Kaldor *et al.* (1988) compared the TD_{50} values of 15 chemotherapeutic agents that increase the risk of secondary tumours (acute non-lymphocyt-

ic leukaemia) in humans; the TD_{50} values were calculated on the basis of animal experiments. The authors found these results encouraging in terms of predicting potency rankings, but cautioned against the quantitative prediction of human carcinogenic potency on the basis of these data. In their comparisons of cancer potencies for cancer chemotherapeutic agents, Kaldor *et al.* (1988) as well as Dedrick & Morrison (1992), found the best correspondence when dose was expressed as cumulative mg/kg over the lifetime. Raabe *et al.* (1983) noted a similar finding in cross-species comparisons of bone cancer risk from radium exposure for watch dial painters and beagle dogs.

Goodman & Wilson (1991a) compared predictions of cancer risks based on TD_{50} values in the CPDB against epidemiological data on 29 chemicals for which the evidence of carcinogenicity in humans was somewhat equivocal. Many of these compounds, in fact, fall in Group 3 (not classifiable with respect to human carcinogenicity) in the categorization scheme used by the International Agency for Research on Cancer; none were in Group 1. The authors concluded that the excess risks observed in the epidemiological investigations (which may or may not have been statistically significant) were roughly compatible with predictions based on the animal data. Following a review of interspecies comparisons of carcinogenic potency, Goodman & Wilson (1991b) concluded that "there is a good correlation of the carcinogenic potencies between rats and mice, and the upper limits on potencies in humans are consistent with rodent potencies for those chemicals for which human exposure data are available".

Because selection of an interspecies scaling constant is an inherently uncertain exercise, it has been argued that a distribution of plausible values, rather than a point estimate, of the scaling constant should be used (Crouch, 1983). This notion is explored more generally in the next section.

6.8 Variability, uncertainty and sensitivity analyses

Carcinogenic risks will vary in accordance with a number of factors. The level of risk depends on the potency of the carcinogen, the level of exposure, and the susceptibility of the host. The potency of chemical carcinogens varies greatly, with the TD_{50} values derived from long-term laboratory studies spanning some seven orders of magnitude. Exposure levels also vary markedly, from trace amounts of chemical contaminants present in air, water, soil, or food to somewhat higher levels encountered in certain occupational settings and extremely high levels associated with accidental exposures. Individual susceptibility is determined by a number of variables including pharmacokinetic factors governing the uptake, distribution, and metabolism of xenobiotics; the immunological competence of the host; and pharmacodynamic factors including DNA damage and repair. These issues are discussed in Chapter 7.

In addition to variation in the level of risk posed by different carcinogens under different conditions of exposure, there is generally some uncertainty as to the level of risk experienced by an individual due to his or her unique susceptibility to a given agent under well defined conditions of exposure. Estimates of risk based on either epidemiological or toxicological data are always subject to some degree of sampling error. This error can be reduced, but not entirely eliminated, through the use of larger studies. Risk estimates based on epidemiological studies can be subject to other random errors, such as measurement errors in exposure ascertainment, as well as systematic biases (see Chapter 4), such as recall bias in questionnaire-based studies. Predictions of risk requiring extrapolation from one set of conditions to another are also subject to uncertainty. As discussed in section 6.7, predictions of human risks based on toxicological data require uncertain extrapolations from high to low doses, from one route of exposure to another, and from animals to humans.

Sensitivity analysis seeks to identify key factors which have a strong influence on estimates of risk. Predictions of risk based on the Armitage–Doll multistage model were seen to be particularly sensitive to the value of the first order term (q_1) in the model. Sensitivity analyses of complex physiologically based pharmacokinetic models (see Chapter 7) involving 20 or more parameters have been conducted in an attempt to identify those which have the greatest influence on model-based predictions of tissue dose. Once sensitive parameters have been identified, uncertainty can be reduced by obtaining the best possible estimates of the parameter values.

6.8.1 Sources and characterizations of variability

The cancer risks faced by individuals within a given population will vary depending on the level of exposure to a carcinogenic agent as well as the degree of susceptibility to that agent. Human exposure to carcinogenic agents in the environment can vary substantially. For example, ingestion of pesticide residues present on food in accordance with the tolerances established by regulatory agencies are determined both by application practices and food consumption patterns. The US National Research Council (1993b) recently proposed methods for characterizing exposure to dietary residues of pesticides, taking into account both variation in residue levels in food and variation in food patterns within and among individuals. The distribution of residue levels in food can be estimated from the results of residue monitoring. Food consumption distributions reflecting differences in consumption among individuals and within individuals on different days can be estimated from food consumption surveys. These two distributions can be combined to obtain an estimate of the distribution of the average daily intake of a particular pesticide that has been approved for use on one or more crops.

The data on which to assess interindividual variability in cancer risk due to differences in human susceptibility are limited. Differences in cancer risk in identifiable subpopulations can sometimes be distinguished epidemiologically, as in the case of different lung cancer risks experienced by smokers and non-smokers. The risk of liver cancer due to aflatoxin exposure is much higher in individuals infected with the hepatitis B virus than in individuals without the virus.

Information on interindividual differences in susceptibility to exposure to carcinogenic agents can be obtained by examining the variation of pharmacokinetic and genetic factors known to influence carcinogenesis. Hattis & Barlow (1996) have recently reviewed the literature on interindividual variability in such factors as metabolic activation, detoxification, and DNA repair. The results showed that interindividual variation was limited in most cases to about an order of magnitude.

Analytical methods have been developed for characterizing variability in carcinogenic risk, particularly those based on Monte Carlo techniques (Morgan & Henrion, 1990; Fiering et al., 1984; Crouch, 1983; Portier & Kaplan, 1989; Bois et al., 1990). If the distributions of each of the factors affecting carcinogenic risk are specified, Monte Carlo simulation can be used to explore the extent of overall variability in risk. Bois et al. (1995) modelled the variability in the physiological and pharmacokinetic processes involved in 4-aminobiphenyl (ABP) carcinogenesis, and used the fraction of ABP bound to DNA as a surrogate indicator of cancer risk. A pharmacokinetic model was used to describe activation and deactivation processes as well as physiological risk factors such as urinary pH, and interindividual variability in risk assessed by Monte Carlo simulation. In this analysis, the underlying distributions of the relevant variables were derived from published studies, most of which were in vitro studies of enzymatic activity. Low- and high-risk subgroups were characterized using plausible extremes for parameter values corresponding to low and high variability respectively. A difference in DNA binding by roughly a factor of 1×10^6 was found between the least susceptible individuals (with high urinary pH, high N-acetylation, and low oxidation) and the most susceptible (with low urinary pH, low N-acetylation, and high N-oxidation). The simulation fraction of ABP bound to DNA varied considerably.

In the absence of direct information on interindividual variation in susceptibility, default assumptions may be used as a guide to the likely degree of variation (US National Research Council, 1994). In general, a default assumption for the degree of human variability in cancer risk may be difficult to establish due to a lack of data (US National Research Council, 1994). Based on preliminary work by Hattis et al. (1986) and Finkel (1987), roughly 10% of the population differs from the median individual by more than a factor of 25–50. Since the available data are limited with respect to sample size, it is difficult to determine the overall shape of the distribution of interindividual variability, including the tails of the distribution, which reflect highly susceptible or resistant population subgroups.

6.8.2 Sources and characterizations of uncertainty

There are many sources of uncertainty in risk estimation based on either epidemiological or toxicological data, particularly when predictions of risk are made by extrapolating from one set of conditions to another. For example, there is uncertainty in extrapolating from the high doses used in laboratory studies to the lower levels of exposure experienced by humans (Olin et al., 1995). Additional uncertainty exists when laboratory animal data are translated to humans, when extrapolating from one route of exposure to another, or when results of a toxicological subchronic study are used to estimate thresholds for chronic studies (Allen et al., 1988). In epidemiological studies, exposure ascertainment and disease diagnosis may be highly uncertain. In studies using computerized record linkage to link exposure data from one database to data on health status in another database, even vital status can be in error (Bartlett et al., 1993).

Finkel (1995) used uncertainty analysis techniques to compare the carcinogenic risks of the mycotoxin aflatoxin, which occurs naturally in many nut products, and the pesticide alar used on apples in the United States. The best single estimates of risk for these two agents suggested that aflatoxin would pose a risk approximately 18 times greater than that of alar. Finkel (1995) evaluated the uncertainty in these estimates, including the uncertainty in extrapolating laboratory data on alar to humans. When all of the uncertainties associated with the estimates of the carcinogenic risks of these two substances are taken into account, it does not appear possible to establish which of these two substances poses a greater risk.

Population pharmacokinetics has been used in pharmaceutical applications to study drug kinetics in non-homogeneous human populations and to define relationships between drug kinetics and identifiable patient features, such as liver function, sex, age and weight (Whiting et al., 1986; Beal & Sheiner, 1982; Sheiner & Ludden, 1992; Beal & Sheiner, 1998). Bayesian procedures have been developed for dose adjustment based on feedback responses. A fully Bayesian method has been developed for analysing population pharmacokinetic models with complex multiparameter structures using Gibbs sampling (Racine-Poon & Smith, 1992; Wakefield et al., 1994). Bois et al. (1994) have used these techniques to describe both uncertainty and interindividual variability in tetrachloroethylene metabolism, the fraction metabolized being used as a surrogate for the carcinogenic metabolite. They also fitted a hierarchical population model to human kinetic data reported by Monster et al. (1979) using Bayesian methods. At an inhalation exposure level of 50 ppm, the median fraction of tetrachlorethylene metabolized was estimated to be 1.5% using iterative simulation, with 95% confidence limits of 0.52% and 4.1%; at 0.001 ppm, the median was 36%, with confidence limits of 15% and 58%.

In this analysis, the reported confidence limits include both uncertainty and variability within the population studied (young adult males), the degree of variability being comparable to the degree of uncertainty. General methods for the analysis of uncertainty and variability which allow for the disaggregation of these two factors as well as the decomposition of uncertainty and variability into their different components have been proposed by Rai et al. (1996). This general approach simplifies when the risk is a multiplicative function of the variables affecting risk (Rai & Krewski, 1998).

6.8.3 Sensitivity analysis

Sensitivity analyses can be used to identify factors which have a particularly strong influence on cancer risk. Formal methods of sensitivity analysis have been developed for use in systems analysis, in which the output of a particular system is related to a number of inputs (Saltelli & Homma, 1992). In cancer risk assessment applications, the system may be represented as a biologically based model involving a number of factors affecting exposure or susceptibility. Sensitivity is expressed in terms of the degree of change in the model output relative to the degree of change in a particular model parameter. Krewski et al. (1995b) have applied sensitivity analysis methods to identify physiological, biochemical, or metabolic parameters in physiological pharmacokinetic models used to describe the metabolic activation of xenobiotics.

6.9 Summary and conclusions

In this chapter, we have discussed empirical approaches to the quantitative estimation and prediction of human cancer risk. In assessing cancer risk, it is important to distinguish between estimates of risk derived from direct observation of human populations of interest under relevant conditions of exposure, and predictions of risk that require the extrapolation of results obtained under circumstances different from those of immediate interest. In most cases, estimates of risk will be more reliable than predictions of risk. Because regulatory applications of carcinogenic risk assessment seek to control the cumulative risk experienced during the course of a lifetime, our emphasis is on the estimation and prediction of lifetime rather than age-specific risks.

The two primary sources of information for the quantitative estimation and prediction of human cancer risk are epidemiological studies of human populations and toxicological experiments conducted on animal models. For purposes of risk estimation, analytical epidemiological studies are preferred; ecological studies are to be avoided because of the potential for serious bias. Although laboratory studies can be conducted under specified conditions of exposure and with a much greater degree of control over potential sources of bias, this increased precision is achieved at the expense of requiring uncertain extrapolation from animals to humans.

The quantitative estimation and prediction of risk is facilitated by the development of a model relating exposure and risk. Once such a model has been developed, it is possible to predict risk at levels of exposure different from those in the original study. When information on temporal aspects of risk is available, predictions of risk under other patterns of exposure may also be made.

A number of empirical models exist that can be used to describe dose–response relationships observed in epidemiological investigations. Although sophisticated relative risk regression models can be fitted to data from both case–control and cohort studies, dose–response relationships observed in epidemiological investigations are often adequately characterized by a linear model.

Although providing limited biological insight into the mechanisms of carcinogenesis, empirical models are very useful in cancer risk assessment. Reasonable estimates of risk can be obtained within the range of observed data, using a number of flexible empirical models involving a manageable number of parameters, although predictions of risk outside this range may differ substantially. Models may be evaluated for goodness of fit, although discrimination among competing models is difficult, particularly with sparse data. Empirical models can provide useful information on the covariates affecting risk, such as attained age, age at first exposure, time since first exposure, and duration of exposure. Direct or inverse exposure rate effects have also been described.

In contrast to epidemiological investigations, non-linear dose–response relationships are frequently observed in long-term animal experiments. Non-linearity can occur as a consequence of saturation of metabolic activation or detoxification pathways, or of cell proliferation induced by high-dose toxicity. It can described using any one of a number of flexible statistical models that have little or no biological basis. For example, a simple three-parameter Weibull model can describe a range of dose–response relationships, including concave, convex, linear, and possibly sigmoid relationships. Weibull models are also capable of describing temporal patterns in which risk is related to a power of time.

In this chapter, we have included the Armitage–Doll multistage model within the class of statistical models that can be used for the quantitative estimation and prediction of risk. This model does have a limited biological basis in terms of describing malignant transformation as the consequence of a normal stem cell passing through a number of different stages to become a cancer cell. However, the model remains an incomplete description of the process of carcinogenesis, ignoring important factors such as tissue growth and cell kinetics. Biologically based dose–response models are discussed in detail in Chapter 7.

Although modelling crude lifetime tumour incidence rates or tumour mortality rates unadjusted for competing risks is relatively straightforward in statistical terms, modelling tumour incidence rates when the tumour-onset times are unobservable is more difficult. Given relatively strong assumptions about the relationship between death rates in the presence and absence of incident tumours, it is possible to make inferences about tumour-onset times based on mortality data. Such analyses are considerably simplified with either non-lethal tumours that are unlikely to result in the death of the host, or with rapidly lethal tumours for which the time of death serves as a reasonable proxy for the tumour-onset time. With tumours of intermediate lethality, information on the cause of death of individuals in the study is of value in modelling tumour incidence.

Daily doses in laboratory studies of carcinogenicity are generally held constant throughout the course of an experiment, whereas humans are subjected to levels of exposure which vary over time. A simple approach to the analysis of studies with time-dependent exposures is to base estimates on cumulative lifetime exposure or, equivalently, on the average daily exposure. Given an estimate of carcinogenic potency, the lifetime risk can be estimated by multiplying the average daily dose by the carcinogenic potency. This approach to risk estimation is only approximate in the presence of dose-rate effects. Theoretical results obtained using relative effectiveness functions for the Armitage–Doll model suggest that the use of the average daily dose may underestimate the actual lifetime risk by a factor of only 2–3. However, overestimation of risk can be much greater. More direct estimates of risk based on the actual temporal patterns of exposure are not possible with many statistical models. Accommodation of time-dependent exposures in model fitting is more readily done within the context of the biologically based models discussed in Chapter 7.

The strength of agents with carcinogenic properties may be expressed in terms of quantitative measures of carcinogenic potency. Although a number of different indices have been proposed in the literature, TD_{50}, defined as the dose resulting in an induced tumour response rate of 50%, with appropriate adjustment for background response, has come to be widely used as an indicator of carcinogenic potency. The Carcinogenic Potency Database established and maintained by Lois Gold and colleagues at the University of

California at Berkeley now contains potency information on approximately 1000 chemicals that have been shown to induce tumours in rodents. The potency of these agents varies tremendously, spanning some seven orders of magnitude.

TD_{50} has been shown to be highly correlated with the maximum tolerated dose used in long-term animal studies, and to a lesser extent with other measures of toxicity including LD_{50} and mutagenic potency expressed in the Ames *Salmonella* assay. TD_{50}, which reflects carcinogenic potency at high dose levels, is also highly correlated with measures of potency at low doses, such as the value of $q1^*$ derived from the linearized multistage model. The strong correlation between TD_{50} and the MTD has raised questions concerning its interpretation as an indicator of carcinogenicity or toxicity. This same correlation has been exploited in predicting TD_{50} on the basis of the MTD, and to obtain preliminary estimates of cancer risk in advance of long-term animal testing.

Although the focus of this chapter is on the estimation and prediction of carcinogenic risks associated with exposure to a single agent, humans may be exposed to more than one agent simultaneously or sequentially, and to complex carcinogenic mixtures. Of particular concern with such joint exposures is the potential for synergistic effects in which the joint risk is in some sense greater than the sum of the component risks. There now exists a relatively large body of epidemiological and toxicological data confirming the existence of both synergistic and antagonistic effects. However, theoretical arguments also suggest that such effects will be predominant at relatively high levels of exposure, low exposures leading to approximately additive risks.

When direct estimates of risk are not possible, predictions of risk may be attempted by extrapolating results obtained under other conditions. Since laboratory experiments are generally conducted at relatively high doses, often within an order of magnitude of the MTD, there is a need for downward extrapolation to lower doses. It is well known that different statistical models, all of which may fit the data equally well in the experimentally observable response range, can lead to widely divergent results when extrapolated to very low doses. This occurs because different models

may exhibit varying degrees of non-linearity in the low-dose region. In the absence of clear evidence to the contrary, it is often assumed that excess cancer risk is directly proportional to dose in the low-dose region. This should be viewed as a default assumption that can be challenged in the presence of sufficient knowledge about the mechanism of carcinogenic action of the agent of interest, particularly those that act by non-genotoxic mechanisms (International Expert Panel on Carcinogen Risk Assessment, 1996). The hypothesis of low-dose linearity may be appropriate for genotoxic carcinogens, and is supported by the linearity of DNA adducts observed even at very low doses. Attempts to resolve the shape of the dose–response curve at low doses by direct experimentation using large sample sizes have been unsuccessful to date.

Quantitative extrapolation of results obtained in animal cancer tests to humans is subject to considerable uncertainty. Although all known human carcinogens are also effective in animals, the converse relationship cannot be fully evaluated because of a lack of adequate human data on most rodent carcinogens. Qualitative concordance between rats and mice is limited to about 75%, without regard for tissue specificity. Allometric considerations have prompted suggestions that quantitative estimates of carcinogenic potency may be scaled between species on the basis of surface area or body weight, or on an intermediate scale such as body weight raised to the 3/4 power, assuming that the agent of interest is effective in both species. Comparisons of the carcinogenic potencies of agents that are effective in both rats and mice, or in both rodents and humans, have indicated a relative high correlation in potency in different species, although interspecies predictions of potency can easily be subject to errors of 100-fold or greater.

A complete characterization of carcinogenic risk requires the consideration of variability, uncertainty, and sensitivity. Variability in risk can occur because of differences in individual sensitivity and in different levels and patterns of exposure. There are many sources of uncertainty in the quantitative estimation and prediction of human cancer risks, including well recognized factors such as sampling error and potential biases in both epidemiological and toxicological studies. However, uncertainties due to extrapolation between doses, routes of exposure, and species are generally of greater importance. With model-based predictions of risk, it may be possible to identify critical parameters to which the resulting estimates are most sensitive. Overall uncertainty may then be reduced by obtaining estimates of those parameters that are as accurate and precise as possible. If a comprehensive analysis of variability, uncertainty, and sensitivity is conducted, the results may be summarized in terms of a distribution of plausible values of risk rather than of a single estimate without an adequate statement of the uncertainty of that estimate.

References

Alavanja, M.C., Brownson, R.C., Benichou, J., Swanson, C. & Boice, J.D. (1995) Attributable risk of lung cancer in lifetime nonsmokers and long-term ex-smokers (Missouri, United States). *Cancer Causes Control*, 6, 209-216.

Allen, B.C., Crump, K.S. & Shipp, A. (1988) Correlation between carcinogenic potency of chemicals in animals and humans. *Risk Anal.*, 8 531-544.

Ames, B.N., Magaw, R. & Gold, L.S. (1987) Ranking possible carcinogenic hazards. *Science*, 236, 271-280

Anderson, E. L. and the Carcinogen Assessment Group of the US Environmental Protection Agency (1983) Quantitative approaches in use to assess cancer risk. *Risk Anal.*, 3, 277-295

Arcos, J.C., Woo, Y.-T. & Lai, D.Y. (1988) Database of binary combinations of effects of chemical carcinogens. *Environ. Carcinog. Rev.*, C6, 1-150

Armitage, P. (1985) Multistage models of carcinogenesis. *Environ. Health Perspect.*, 63, 195-201

Armitage, P. & Doll, R. (1954) The age distribution of cancer and a multistage theory of carcinogenesis. *Br. J. Cancer*, 8, 1-12

Armitage, P. & Doll, R. (1961) Stochastic models for carcinogenesis. In: Neymann, G., ed., *Proceedings of the Fourth Berkeley Symposium on Mathematical Statistics and Probability*, Berkeley, CA, University of California Press, pp. 19-37

Auvinen, A., Makelainen, I., Hakama, M., Castren, O., Pukkala, E., Reisbacka, H. & Rytomaa, T. (1996) Indoor radon exposure and risk of lung cancer: a nested case–control study in Finland. *J. Natl Cancer Inst.*, 88, 14, 966-972

Bailar, A.J. & Portier, C.J. (1988) Effects of treatment-induced mortality and tumor induced mortality on tests for carcinogenicity. *Biometrics*, 44, 417-431

Bailar, A.J. & Portier, C.J. (1993) An index of tumorigenic potency. *Biometrics*, 44, 417-431

Barr, J.T. (1985) The calculation and use of carcinogenic potency. *Reg. Toxicol. Pharmacol.*, 5, 432-459

Bartlett, S., Krewski, D., Wang., Y. & Zielinski, J.M. (1993) Evaluation of error rates in large scale computerized record linkage studies. *Surv. Methodol.*, 19, 3-12.

Beal, S.L. & Sheiner, L.B., (1982) Estimating population kinetics. CRC *Crit. Rev. Biomed.Eng.*, 8(3), 195-222

Beal, S.L. & Sheiner, L.B., (1998) Heteroscedastic nonlinear regression. *Technometrics*, 30, 327

Beland, F.A., Fullerton, N.F., Smith, B.A. & Poirier, M.C. (1991) DNA adduct formation and aromatic amine tumorigenesis. In: D'Amato, R., Slaga, T.J., Farland, W. & Henry, C., eds, *Relevance of Animal Studies to the Evaluation of Human Cancer Risk*, Wiley, New York, NY, pp. 79-92

Belsley, D.A., Kuh, E., & Welsch, R.E. (1980) *Regression diagnostics: Identifying Influential Data and Sources of Collinearity*, New York, NY, Wiley

Bernstein, L., Gold, L.S., Ames, B.N., Pike, M.C. & Hoel, D.G. (1985) Some tautologous aspects of the comparison of carcinogenic potency in rats and mice. *Fundam. Appl. Toxicol.*, 5, 79-87

Bhageri, D., Doeltz, M.K., Fay, J.R., Helmes, C.T., Monasmith, L.A. & Sigman, C.C. (1989) Database of inhibitors of carcinogenesis. *Environ. Carcinog. Rev.*, C6, vii-xviii, 1-159

Blot, W.J., Xu, Z.Y., Boice, J.D.,Jr., Zhao, D.Z., Stone, B.J., Sun, J., Jing, L.B. & Fraumeni, J.F.,Jr (1990) Indoor radon and lung cancer in China. *J.Natl Cancer Inst.*, **82**, 1025-1030

Bois, F.Y., Zeise, L., & Tozer, T.N. (1990) Precision and sensitivity of pharmacokinetic models for cancer risk assessment: tetrachloroethylene in mice, rats and humans. *Toxicol. Appl. Pharmacol.*, **102**, 300-315

Bois, F.Y., Gelman, A., Jiang, J. & Maszle, D.R. (1994) *A Toxicokinetic Analysis of Tetrachloroethylene Metabolism in Humans*, Berkeley, CA, California Environmental Protection Agency, Office of Environmental Health Hazard Assessment

Bois, F.Y., Krowech, G. & Zeise, L. (1995) Modelling human interindividual variability in metabolism and risk: the example of 4-aminobiphenyl. *Risk Anal.*, **15**, 205-213

Börzsönyi, M., Day, N.E., Lapis, K. & Yamasaki, H., eds (1984) *Models, Mechanisms and Etiology of Tumour Promotion* (IARC Scientific Publications No. 56), Lyon, International Agency for Research on Cancer

Breslow, N.E. & Day, N.E. (1980) *Statistical Methods in Cancer Research*, Vol. I, *The Analysis of Case–control Studies* (IARC Scientific Publications No. 32), Lyon, International Agency for Research on Cancer

Breslow, N.E. & Day, N.E. (1987) *Statistical Methods in Cancer Research*, Vol. II *The Design and Analysis of Case–control Studies* (IARC Scientific Publications No. 82), Lyon, International Agency for Research on Cancer

Breslow, N.E. & Storer B.E. (1985) General relative risk functions for case–control studies. *Am. J. Epidemiol.*, **122**, 149-62

Brown, C.C. & Chu, K.C. (1989) Additive and multiplicative models and multistage carcinogenesis theory. *Risk Anal.*, **9**, 99-105

Brown, K.G. & Hoel, D.G. (1983) Modelling time-to-tumor data: Analysis of the ED01 study. *Fundam. Appl. Toxicol.*, **3**, 458-469.

Calabrese, E. (1991) *Multiple Chemical Interactions*, Chelsea, MI, Lewis Publishers

Cardis, E., Gilbert, E.S., Carpenter, L., Howe, G.R., Kato, I., Armstrong, B.K., Beral, V., Cowper, G., Douglas, A.J., Fix, J.J., Fry, S.A., Kaldor, J., Lavé, C., Salmon, L., Smith, P.G., Voelz, G.L. & Wiggs, L.D. (1995) Effects of low doses and low dose-rates of external ionizing radiation: Cancer mortality among nuclear industry workers in three countries. *Radiat.Res.*, **142**, 117-132

Chen, J.J., Kodell, R.L. & Gaylor, D.W. (1988) Using the biological two-stage model to assess risk from short-term exposures. *Risk Anal.*, **6**, 223-230

Clayson, D.B. & Krewski, D. (1986) The concept of negativity in experimental carcinogenesis. *Mutat. Res.*, **167**, 233-240

Collins, J.M., Zaharko, D.S., Dedrick, R.L. & Chabner, B.A. (1986) Potential role for preclinical pharmcology in phase I clinical trials. *Cancer Treat. Rep.* **70**, 73-80

Collins, J.M., Grieshaber, C.K., & Chabner, B.A. (1990) Pharmacologically guided phase I clinical trials based upon preclinical drug development. *J. Natl Cancer Inst.*, **82**, 1321-1326

Cook, P.J., Doll, R. & Fellingham, S.A. (1969). A mathematical model for the age distribution of cancer in man. *Int. J. Cancer*, **4**, 93-112

Cox, D.R. (1972) Regression models with life-tables. *J. R. Stat. Soc.* B34, 187-220

Cox, D.R. (1984) Interaction. *Int. Stat. Rev.*, **52**, 1-31.

Crouch, E.A.C. (1983) Uncertainties in inter-species extrapolation of carcinogenicity. *Environ. Health Perspect.*, **50**, 321-327

Crouch, E.A.C. & Wilson, R. (1979) Interspecies comparison of carcinogenic potency. *J. Toxicol. Environ. Health*, **5**, 1095-1118

Crouch, E.A.C., Wilson, R. & Zeise, L. (1987) Tautology or not tautology? *J. Toxicol. Environ. Health,* **20**, 1-10

Crowder, M.J. (1978) Beta-binomial ANOVA for proportions. *Appl. Stat.* **27**, 34-37

Crump, K.S. (1983) Ranking carcinogens for regulation. *Science,* **219**, 236-238

Crump, K.S. (1984) An improved procedure for low-dose carcinogenic risk assessment for animal data. *J. Environ. Pathol. Toxicol. Oncol.,* **5**, 339-348

Crump, K.S. (1990) *Toxicological Risk Assessment Programme (TOXRISK),* Version 3.1, Ruston, LA, Clement International Corporation, K.S. Crump Division

Crump, K.S. & Howe, R.B. (1984) The multistage model with a time-dependent dose pattern: applicaions to carcinogenic risk assessment. *Risk Anal.,* **4**, 163-176

Crump, K.S., Hoel, D.G., Langley, C.H. & Peto. R. (1976) Fundamental carcinogenic processes and their implications for low dose risk assessment. *Cancer Res.,* **36**, 2973-2979

Crump, K.S., Guess, H.A. & Deal, K.L. (1977) Confidence intervals and tests of hypotheses concerning dose–response relations inferred from animal carcinogenicity data. *Biometrics,* **50**, 437-451

Dedrick, R.L. & Morrison, P. (1992) Carcinogenic potency of alkylating agents in rodents and humans. *Cancer Res.,* **52**, 2464-2467

Demidchik, E.P., Kazakov, V.S., Astakhova, L.N., Okeanov, A.E. & Demidchik, Y.E. (1994) Thyroid cancer in children after the Chernobyl accident: clinical and epidemiological evaluation of 251 cases in the Republic of Belarus. In: Nagataki, S., ed., *Nagasaki Symposium on Chernobyl: Update and Future,* Amsterdam, Elsevier Science, pp. 21-30

Dewanji, A. & Kalbfleisch, J.D. (1986). Nonparametric methods for survival/sacrifice experiments. *Biometrics,* **42**, 325-341.

Dewanji, A., Krewski, D. & Goddard, M.J. (1993) A Weibull model for the estimation of tumorigenic potency. *Biometrics,* **49**, 367-377

Dinse, G.E. (1986) Nonparametric prevalence and mortality estimators for animal experiments with incomplete cause-of-death data. *J. Am. Stat. Assoc.,* **81**, 328-336

Doll, R. & Peto, R. (1981) *The Causes of Cancer. Quantitative Estimates of Avoidable Risks of Cancer in the United States Today,* Oxford, Oxford University Press

Elashoff, R.M., Fears, T.R. & Schniederman, M.A. (1987) Statistical analysis of a carcinogen mixture experiment. *J. Natl Cancer Inst.,* **79**, 509-526

Farmer, J.H., Kodell, R.L. & Gaylor, D.W. (1982). Estimation and extrapolation of tumor probabilities from a mouse bioassay with survival/sacrifice components. *Risk Anal.,* **2**, 27-34

Fears, T.R., Elashoff, R.M. & Schneiderman, M.A. (1988) The statistical analysis of a carcinogen mixture experiment. II. Carcinogens with different target organs, N-methyl-N-nitro-N-nitrosoguanidine, N-butyl-N-(4-hydroxybutyl)nitrosamine, dipentylnitrosamine and nitrilotriacetic acid. *Toxicol. Ind. Health,* **4**, 221-255

Fears, T.R., Elashoff, R.M. & Schniederman, M.A. (1989) The statistical analysis of a carcinogen mixture experiment. III. Carcinogens with different target systems, aflatoxin B1, N-butyl-N-(4-hydroxybutly)-nitrosamine, lead acetate and thiouracil. *Toxicol. Ind. Health,* **5**, 1-23

Fiering, R., Wilson, E. & Zeise, L. 1984) Statistical distributions of health risks. *Civil Eng. Syst.,* **1**, 129-138

Finkel, A.M. (1987) *Uncertainty, Variability and the Value of Information in Cancer Risk Assessment,* PhD thesis, Boston, MA, Harvard School of Public Health

Finkel, A. (1995) Toward less misleading comparisons of uncertain risks: the example of aflatoxin and alar. *Environ. Health Perspect.,* **103**, 376-385

Finkelstein, D.M. & Ryan, L.M. (1987) Estimating carcinogenic potency from a rodent tumorigenicity experiment. *Appl. Stat.*, **36**, 121-133

Finney, D.J. (1971) *Probit Analysis*, 3rd ed., London, Cambridge University Press

Flamm, W.G., Lake, L.R., Lorentzen, R.J., Rulis, A.M., Schwartz, P.S. & Troxell, T.C. (1987). Carcinogenic potencies and the establishment of a threshold of regulation for food contact substances. In: Whipple, C., ed., *De Minimis Risk*, New York, NY, Plenum Press, pp. 87-92

Freedman, D.A., Gold, L.S. & Stone, T.H. (1992) *How Tautological are Inter-species Correlations of Carcinogenic Potencies?* (Technical Report No. 334), Berkeley, CA, Department of Statistics, University of California,

Freireich, Gehan, E.A., Rall, D.P., Schmidt, L.H. & Skipper, H.E. (1966) Quantitative comparison of toxicity of anticancer agents in the mouse, rat, hamster, dog, monkey, and man. *Cancer Chemother. Rep.*, 50(4), 219-244

Gart, J.J., Krewski, D., Lee, P.N., Tarone, R.E. & Wahrendorf, J. (1986) *Statistical Methods in Cancer Research*, Vol. III, *The Design and Analysis of Long-Term Animal Experiments* (IARC Scientific Publications No. 79), Lyon, International Agency for Research on Cancer

Gaylor, D.W. (1989) Preliminary estimates of the virtually safe dose for tumors obtained from the maximum tolerated dose. *Reg. Toxicol. Pharmacol.*, 9, 1-18

Gaylor, D.W. & Chen, J.J. (1986) Relative potency of chemical carcinogens in rodents. *Risk Anal.*, 6, 283-290

Gaylor, D.W. & Gold, L.S. (1995) Quick estimate of the regulatory virtually safe dose based on the maximum tolerated dose for rodent bioassays. *Reg. Toxicol. Pharm.*, 22, 57-63

Gaylor, D.W. & Kodell, R.L. (1980). Linear interpolation algorithm for low dose risk assessment of toxic substances. *J. Environ. Pathol. Toxicol*,. 4, 305-312

Gaylor, D.W., Greenman, D.L. & Frith, C.H. (1985) Urinary bladder neoplasms induced in Balb/C female mice with low doses of 2-acetylaminofluorene. *J. Environ. Pathol. Toxicol.*, 6, 127-136

Ghadirian, P., Boyle, P., Simard, A., Baillargean, J. Maisonneuve, P. & Perret, C. (1991) Reported family aggregation of pancreatic cancer within a population-based case–control study in the Francophone community in Montreal, Canada. *Int. J. Pancreatol.*, 10, 183-195

Goddard, M.J., Krewski, D. & Zhu, Y. (1993) Measuring carcinogenic potency. In: Cothern, C.R. & Ross, N.P., eds, *Environmental Statistics, Assessment, and Forecasting*, Boca Raton, FL, Lewis, pp. 193-208

Goddard, M.J., Murdoch, D.J. & Krewski, D. (1995) Temporal aspects of risk characterization. *Inhalation Toxicol.*, 7, 1005-1018

Gold, L.S., Sawyer, C.B., Magaw, R., Backman, G.M., de Veciana, M., Levinson, R., Hooper, N.K., Havender, W.R., Bernstein, L., Peto, R., Pike, M.C. & Ames, B.N. (1984) A carcinogenic potency database of the standardized results of animal bioassays. *Environ. Health Perspect.*, **58**, 9-319

Gold, L.S., Slone, T.H., Backman, G.M., Magaw, R., Da Costa, M., Lopipero, P., Blumenthal, M. & Ames, B.N. (1987) Second chronological supplement to the carcinogenic potency database: standardized results of animal bioassays published through December 1984 and by the National Toxicology Program through May 1986. *Environ. Health Perspect.*, **74**, 237-329

Gold, L.S., Slone, T.H. & Bernstein, L. (1989) Summary of carcinogenic potency and positivity for 492 rodent carcinogens in the carcinogenic potency database. *Environ. Health Perspect.*, **79**, 259-272

Gold, L.S., Slone, T.H., Backman, G.M., Eisenberg, S., Da Costa, M., Wong, M., Manley, N.B., Rohrback, L. & Ames, B.N. (1990) Third chronological supplement to the Carcinogenic Potency Database: standardized results of animal bioassays published through December 1986 and by the National Toxicology Program through June 1987. *Environ. Health Perspect.*, **84**, 215-286

Goodman, G. & Wilson, R. (1991a) Quantitative prediction of human cancer risk from rodent carcinogenic potencies: a closer look at the epidemiological evidence for some chemicals not definitively carcinogenic in humans. *Reg. Toxicol. Pharmacol.*, **14**, 118-146

Goodman, G. & Wilson, R. (1991b) Predicting the carcinogenicity of chemicals in humans from rodent bioassay data. *Environ. Health Perspect.*, **94**, 195-218

Govindarajarlu, Z. (1988) *Statistical Techniques in Bioassay*, Basel, Karger

Greenland, S. (1993) Basis problems in interaction assessment. *Environ. Health Perspect.*, **101**, Suppl. 4, 59-65

Gross, M.A., Fitzhugh, O.G. & Mantel, N. (1970) Evaluation of safety for food additives: an illustration involving the influence of methyl salicylate on rat reproduction. *Biometrics*, **26**, 181-194

Guerrero, V.M. & Johnson, R.A. (1982) Use of the Box–Cox transformation with binary response models. *Biometrika*, **69**, 309-314

Hartley, H.O. & Sielken, R.L., Jr (1977) Estimation of "safe doses" in carcinogenic experiments. *Biometrics*, **33**, 1-30

Haseman, J.K. & Huff, J.E. (1987) Species correlation in longterm carcinogenicity studies. *Cancer Lett.*, **37**, 125-132

Hattis, D. & Barlow, K. (1996) Human interindividual variability in cancer risks—technical and management challenges. *Hum. Ecol. Risk Assess.*, 2(1), 194-220

Hattis, D., Erdreich, L., & DiMauro, T. (1986) *Human Variability in Parameters that are Potentially Related to Susceptibility to Carcinogenesis—I. Preliminary Observations, Report to the Environmental Criteria and Assessment Office* (Report No. CTPID 86-4), Cambridge, MA, MIT Center for Technology, Policy and Industrial Development

Hoel, D.G. (1980) Incorporation of background in dose–response models. *Fed. Proc.*, **39**, 73-75

Hoel, D.G., Kaplan, N.L. & Andersen, M.W. (1983). Implication of nonlinear kinetics on risk estimation in carcinogenesis. *Science*, **219**, 1032-1037

Hubert, J.J. (1992) *Bioassay*, Dubuque, IA, Kendall/Hunt

IARC Working Group (1994) Direct estimates of cancer mortality due to low doses of ionising radiation: an international study. *Lancet*, **344**, 1039-1043

Iball, J. (1939) The relative potency of carcinogenic compounds. *Am. J. Cancer*, **35**, 188-190

International Agency for Research on Cancer (1986) *IARC Monographs on the Evaluation of Carcinogenic Risks to Man*, Vol. 38, *Tobacco Smoking*, Lyon

International Commission on Radiological Protection (1991) *Recommendations of the International Commission on Radiological Protection*, Oxford, Pergamon Press

International Expert Panel on Carcinogen Risk Assessment (1996) The use of mechanistic data in the risk assessments of ten chemicals: an introduction to chemical-specific reviews. *Pharmacol. Ther.*, **71**, 1-5

Irwin, J.O. & Goodman, N. (1946) The statistical treatment of the carcinogenic properties of tars (Part I) and mineral oils (Part II). *J. Hyg.*, **44**, 362-420

Kalbfleisch, J.D., Krewski, D. & Van Ryzin, J. (1983) dose–response models for time-to-response toxicity data. *Can. J. Stat.*, **11**, 25-49

Kaldor, J.M. & L'Abbe, K.A. (1990) Interaction between human carcinogens. In: Vainio, H., Sorsa, M. & McMichael, A.J., eds, *Complex Mixtures and Cancer Risk* (IARC Scientific Publications No. 104), Lyon, International Agency for Research on Cancer, pp. 35-43

Kaldor, J.M., Day, N.E. & Hemminki, K. (1988) Quantifying the carcinogenicity of antineoplastic agents. *Eur. J. Cancer,* **24**, 703-711

Kazakov, V.S., Demidchik, E.P. & Astakhova, L.N. (1992) Thyroid cancer after Chernobyl *Nature,* **359**, 21

Kodell, R.L. & Pounds, J.G. (1991) Assessing the toxicity of chemical mixtures. In: *Statistics in Toxicology* Krewski, D. & Franklin, C.A., eds., New York, NY, Gordon & Breach, pp. 557-589

Kodell, R.L., Gaylor, D. & Chen, J. (1987) Using average lifetime dose rate for intermittent exposures to carcinogens. *Risk Anal.,* **7**, 339-345

Kodell, R.L., Gaylor, D.W. & Chen, J.J. (1990) Carcinogenic potency correlations: real or artifactual? *J. Toxicol. Ind. Health,* **21**, 1-9

Kodell, R.L., Krewski, D. & Zielinski, J. (1991) Additive and multiplicative relative risk in the two-stage clonal expansion model of carcinogenesis. *Risk Anal.,* **11**, 483-490

Krewski, D. & Goddard, M.J. (1990) Principles of bioassay design. *Drugs Inf. J.,* **24**, 381-394

Krewski, D. & Murdoch, D.J. (1990) Cancer modelling with intermittent exposures. In: Moolgavkar, S.H., ed., *Scientific Issues in Quantitative Cancer Risk Assessment,* Boston, New York, Birkhäuser, pp. 196-214

Krewski, D. & Thomas, R.D. (1992). Carcinogenic mixtures. *Risk Anal.,* **12**, 105-113

Krewski, D. & Van Ryzin, J. (1981) Dose response models for quantal response toxicity data. In: Csorgo, M., Dawson, D.A., Rao, J.N.K. & Saleh, E., eds, *Statistics and Related Topics*, Amsterdam, North-Holland, pp. 201-231

Krewski, D. & Zhu, Y. (1994) Applications of multinomial dose–response models in developmental toxicity risk assessment. *Risk Anal.,* **14**, 595-609

Krewski, D. & Zhu, Y. (1995) A simple data transformation for estimating benchmark doses in developmental toxicity experiments. *Risk Anal.,* **15**, 29-39

Krewski, D., Crump, K. S., Farmer, J., Gaylor, D. W., Howe, R., Portier, C., Salsburg, D., Sielken, R. L., and Van Ryzin, J. (1983) A comparison of statistical methods for low dose extrapolation utilizing time-to-tumor data. *Fundam. Appl. Toxicol.,* **3**, 140-156

Krewski, D., Murdoch, D.J. & Withey, J.R. (1987) The application of pharmacokinetic data in carcinogenic risk assessment. In: *Pharmacokinetics in Risk Assessment, Drinking Water and Health*, Vol. 8, Washington, DC, National Academy Press, pp. 441-468

Krewski, D., Goddard, M.J. & Murdoch, D. (1989a) Statistical considerations in the interpretation of negative carcinogencity data. *Reg. Toxicol. Pharmacol.,* **9**, 5-22

Krewski, D., Murdoch, D.J. & Withey, J. (1989b) Recent developments in carcinogenic risk assessment (with discussion). *Health Phys.,* **57** (Suppl. 1), 313-326

Krewski, D., Szyszkowicz, M. & Rosenkranz, H. (1990) Quantitative factors in chemical carcinogenesis. *Reg. Toxicol. Pharmacol.,* **12**, 13-29

Krewski, D., Gaylor, D.W. & Szyszkowicz, M. (1991) A model-free approach to low dose extrapolation. *Environ. Health Perspect.,* **90**, 279-285

Krewski, D., Leroux, B.G., Creason, J. & Claxton, L. (1992). Sources of variation in the mutagenic potency of complex chemical mixtures based on the *Salmonella*/microsome assay. *Mutat. Res.,* **276**, 33-59

Krewski, D., Gaylor, D.W., Soms, A.P. & Szyszkowicz, M. (1993a) Correlation between carcinogenic potency and the maximum tolerated dose: implications for risk assessment. In: Committee on Risk Assessment, National Research Council, *Issues in Risk Assessment*, Washington, DC, National Academy Press, pp. 111-171

Krewski, D., Leroux, B.G., Bleuer, S.R. & Claxton, L. (1993b) Modelling the Ames *Salmonella*/microsome assay. *Biometrics*, **49**, 499-510

Krewski, D., Gaylor, D.W. & Lutz, W.K. (1995a) Additivity to background and linear extrapolation. In: Olin, S., Farland, W., Park, C., Rhomberg, L., Scheuplein, R., Starr, T. & Wilson, J., eds, *Low Dose Extrapolation of Cancer Risks: Issues and Perspectives*, Washington, DC, ILSI Press, pp. 105-121

Krewski, D., Wang, Y., Bartlett, S. & Krishnan, K. (1995b) Uncertainty, variability, and sensitivity analysis in physiologic pharmacokinetic models. *Biopharm. Stat.*, **5**, 245-271

Kuo, L. (1988) Linear Bayes estimators of the potency curve in bioassay. *Biometrika*, **75**, 91-97

Lave, L.B., Ennever, F.K., Rosenkranz, H.S. & Omenn, G.S. (1988) Information value of the rodent bioassay. *Nature*, **336**, 631-633

Lawless, J.F. (1982) *Statistical Models and Methods for Lifetime Data*, New York, NY, Wiley

Leroux, B.G., Krewski, D. & Wei, L.J. (1992) Score tests for interval-censored data with applications to carcinogenicity data. In: Saleh, A.K.M.E., ed., *Nonparametric Statistics and Related Topics*, Amsterdam, Elsevier, pp.59-74

Létourneau, E.G., Krewski, D., Choi, N.W., Goddard, M.J., McGregor, R.G., Zielinski, J.M. & Du, J. (1994) Case–control study of residential radon and lung cancer in Winnipeg, Manitoba, Canada. *Am. J. Epidemiol.* **140**, 310-322

Liang, K.-Y. & Zeger, S.L. (1986) Longitudinal data analysis using generalized linear models. *Biometrika*, **73**, 13-22

Littlefield, N.A., Farmer, J.H., Gaylor, D.W. & Sheldon, W.G. (1980) Effects of dose and time in a long-term, low-dose carcinogenic study. *J. Environ. Pathol. Toxicol.*, **3**, 17-35

Louis, T.A. (1984) Estimating a population of parameter values using Bayes and empirical Bayes methods. *J. Am. Stat. Assoc.*, **79**, 393-398

Lubin, J.H., Boice, J.D.J., Edling, C., Hornung, R.W., Howe, G., Kunz, E., Kusiak, R.A., Morrison, H.I., Radford, E.P., Samet, J.M., Tirmarche, M., Woodward, A., Xiang, Y.S. & Pierce, D.A. (1994) *Radon and Lung Cancer Risk: A Joint Analysis of 11 Underground Miners Studies*, Bethesda, MD, National Institutes of Health

Lubin, J.H., Boice, J.D. Jr & Edling, C. (1995) Lung cancer in radon-exposed miners and estimation of risk from indoor exposure, *J. Natl Cancer Inst.*, **87**, 817-827

Lutz, W.K. (1986) Quantitative evaluation of DNA binding data for risk estimation and for classification of direct and indirect carcinogens. *J. Cancer Res. Clin. Oncol.*, **112**, 85-91

Lutz, W.K. (1990) Dose–response relationship and low dose extrapolation in chemical carcinogenesis. *Carcinogenesis*, **11**, 1243-11247

Lutz, W.K. (1991) Dose–response relationship for chemical carcinogenesis by genotoxic agents. *Soz. Praev. Med.*, **36**, 243-248

Mauritsen, R.H. (1984) *Logistic Regression with Random Effects*, Seattle, WA, Department of Biostatistics, University of Washington

McCullagh, P. & Nelder, J.A. (1983) *Generalized Linear Models* (Monographs on Statistics and Probability), London, New York, Chapman and Hall

McCullagh, P. & Nelder, J.A. (1989) *Generalized Linear Models*, London, Chapman and Hall

McGregor, D.B. (1992) Chemicals classifed by the IARC: their potency in rodent carcinogenicity tests, genotoxicity and acute toxcity. In: Vainio, H., Magee, P.N., McGregor, D.B. & McMichael, A.J., eds, *Mechanisms of Carcinogenesis in Risk Identification* (IARC Scientific Publications No. 104) International Agency for Research on Cancer, Lyon, pp. 323-352

McKnight, B. (1988) A guide to the statistical analysis of long-term carcinogenicity assays. *Fundam. Appl. Toxicol.*, **10**, 355-364

McKnight, B. & Crowley, J. (1984) Tests for differences in tumour incidence based on animal carcinogenesis experiments. *J. Am. Stat. Assoc.*, **79**, 639-648.

Mehta, C.R., Patel, N.R. & Gray, R. (1986) Computing an exact confidence interval for the common odds ratio in several 2×2 contingency tables. *J. Am. Stat. Assoc.*, **80**(392), 969-973

Metzger, B., Crouch, E. & Wilson, R. (1987) On the relationship between carcinogenicity and acute toxicity. *Risk Anal.*, **9**,169-177

Monster, A.C., Boersma, G., & Steenweg, H. (1979) Kinetics of tetrachloroethylene in volunteers: influence of exposure concentrations and work load. *Int. Arch. Occup. Environ. Health*, **42**, 303-309

Moolgavkar, S.H. & Venzon, D.J. (1987) General relative risk regression models for epidemiologic studies. *Am. J. Epidemiol.*, **126**(5), 949-961

Moolgavkar, S.H., Luebeck, G., Krewski, D. & Zielinski, J.M. (1993) Radon, cigarette smoke, and lung cancer: a reanalysis of the Colorado uranium miners' data. *Epidemiology*, **4**, 204-217

Morgan, M.G. & Henrion, M. (1990) *Uncertainty: A Guide to Dealing with Uncertainty in Quantitative Risks and Policy Analysis*, Cambridge, Cambridge University Press

Morris, M.D. (1988) Small-sample confidence limits for parameters under inequality constraints with application to quantal bioassay. *Biometrics*, **44**, 1083-1092

Morrison, P.F. (1987) Effects of time-variant exposure on toxic substance response. *Environ. Health Perspect.*, **76**, 133-140

Muller, H.G. & Schmitt, T. (1988) Kernel and probit estimates in quantal bioassay. *J. Am. Stat. Assoc.*, **83**, 750-760

Munro, I.C. (1990) Safety assessment procedures for indirect food additives: an overview. Report of a workshop. *Reg. Toxicol. Pharmacol.*, **12**, 2-12

Murdoch, D.J. (1992) Scalable relative effectiveness models. *Stat. Probab. Lett.*, **13**, 321-324

Murdoch, D.J. & Krewski, D. (1988) Carcinogenic risk assessment with time dependent exposure patterns. *Risk Anal.*, **8**, 521-530

Murdoch, D.J., Krewski, D. & Wargo, J. (1992) Cancer risk assessment with intermittent exposure. *Risk Anal.*, **12**, 569-577

Nesnow, S. (1990) A multi-factor ranking scheme for comparing the carcinogenic activity of chemicals. *Mutat. Res.*, **239**, 83-115

Nesnow, S. (1991) Multifactor potency scheme for comparing the carcinogenic activity of chemicals. *Environ. Health Perspect.*, **96**, 17-21

Numerical Algorithms Group (1978) *GLIM. User's Manual*, Release 3, Revision 6, Oxford

Numerical Algorithms Group (1980) *GENSTAT. User's Manual*, Release 4.04, Oxford

Olin, S., Farland, W., Park, C., Rhomberg, L., Scheuplein, Starr, T., & Wilson, J. (1995) *Low-dose Extrapolation of Cancer Risks: Issues and Perspectives*, Washington, DC, International Life Sciences Institute

Pershagen, G., Axelson, O. & Clavensjo, B. (1993) *Radon in Dwellings and Cancer. A Country-wide Epidemiological Investigation* (IMM report 2/93), Stockholm, Institute of Environmental Medicine, Karolinska Institute

Peto, R., Pike, M., Day, N., Gray, R., Lee, P., Parish, S., Peto, J., Richards, S. & Wahrendorf, J. (1980) Guidelines for simple, sensitive significance tests for carcinogenic effects in long term animal experiments. In: *IARC Monographs on the Evaluation of the Carcinogenic Risk of Chemicals to Humans*, Suppl. 2, *Long-Term and Short-Term Screening Assays for Carcinogens: A Critical Appraisal*, Lyon, International Agency for Research on Cancer, pp. 331-425

Peto, R., Pike, M.C., Bernstein, L., Swirsky, L. & Ames, B.N. (1984) The TD_{50}: A proposed general convention for the numerical description of the carcinogenic potency of chemicals in chronic-exposure animal experiments. *Environ. Health Perspect.*, **58**, 1-8

Peto, R., Gray, R., Brantom, P. & Grasso, P. (1991a) Effects on 4080 rats of chronic ingestion of *N*-nitrosodiethylamine or *N*-nitrosodimethylamine: a detailed dose–response study. *Cancer Res.*, **51**, 6415-6451

Peto, R., Gray, R., Brantom, P. & Grasso, P. (1991b) Dose and time relationships for tumour induction in the liver and esophagus of 4080 inbred rats by chronic ingestion of *N*-nitrosodiethylamine or *N*-nitrosodimethylamine. *Cancer Res.*, **51**, 6452-6469

Piegorsch, W.W., Carr, G.J., Portier, C.J. & Hoel, D.G. (1992) Concordance of carcinogenic response between rodent species: Potency dependence and potential underestimation. *Risk Anal.*, **12**, 115-121.

Pierce, D.A. & Preston, D.L. (1984) Hazard function modelling for dose–response analysis of cancer incidence in the A-bomb survivor data. In: Prentice, R.L. & Thompson, D.J., eds, *A-bomb Survivor Data: Utilization and Analysis*, Philadelphia, PA, Society for Applied and Industrial Mathematics, pp. 51-66

Pierce, D.A. & Sands, B.R. (1975) *Extra-Bernouilli Variation in Binary Data* (Technical Report 46), Corvallis, OR, Department of Statistics, Oregon State University

Portier, C.J. & Hoel, D.G. (1987) Issues concerning the estimation of the TD_{50}. *Risk Anal.*, **7**, 437-447

Portier, C.J. & Kaplan, N.L. (1989) Variability of safe dose estimates when using complicated models of the carcinogenic process. *Fundam. Appl. Toxicol.*, **13**, 533-544

Prentice, R.L. (1976) A generalization of the probit and logit methods for dose response curves. *Biometrics*, **32**, 761-768

Prentice, R.L., Peterson, A.V. & Marek, P. (1982) Dose mortality relationships in RFM mice following ^{137}Cs gamma ray irradiation. *Radiat. Res.*, **90**, 57-76

Preston, D.L., Lubin, J.H. & Pierce, D.A. (1993) *EPICURE risk regression and data analysis software*, Seattle, WA, Hisusoft International Corporation

Raabe, O.G., Book, S.A. & Parks, N.J. (1983) Lifetime bone cancer dose–resonse relationships in beagles and people from skeletal burdens of 226Ra and 90Sr. *Health Phys.*, **44**(Suppl. 1), 33-48

Racine-Poon, A. & Smith, A.F. (1992) Population models. In: Berry, D.A., ed., *Statistical Methodology in the Pharmaceutical Sciences*, New York, NY, Marcel Dekker, pp. 139-162

Rai, K. & Van Ryzin, J. (1981) A generalized multihit dose–response model for low-dose extrapolation. *Biometrics*, **37**, 341-352

Rai, S.N. & Krewski, D. (1998) Analysis of uncertainty and variability in multiplicative models. *Risk Anal.*, **18**, 37-45

Rai, S.N., Krewski, D. & Bartlett, S. (1996) A general framework for the analysis of uncertainty and variability in risk assessment. *Health and Ecol. Risk Assess.*, **2**, 972-989

Rai, S.N., Matthews, D.E. & Krewski, D. (1999) Mixed scale models for survival/sacrifice experiments. *Can. J. Stat.*, (in press)

Rao, V.R., Woo, Y.-T., Lai, D.Y. & Arcos, J.C. (1989) Database on promoters of chemical carcinogenesis. *Environ. Carcinog. Rev.*, **C7**, ix-xxxvi, 145-386

Reith, J.P. & Starr, T.B. (1989a) Experimental dosing constraints on carcinogenic potency estimates. *J. Toxicol. Environ. Health*, **27**, 287-296

Reith, J.P. & Starr, T.B. (1989b). Chronic bioassays: relevance to quantitative risk assessment of carcinogens. *Reg.Toxicol. Pharmacol.*, **10**, 160-173

Roy, P. (1991) *Synergie Entre les Facteurs de Risque Tabac et Alcool dans les Cancers des Voies Aéro-digestives Supérieures*, Lyon, Université Claude Bernard

Rulis, A.M. (1986) *De minimis* and the threshold of regulation. In: Felix, C.W., ed., *Food Protection Technology*, Chelsea, MI, Lewis, pp. 29-37

Saltelli, A. & Homma, T. (1992) Sensitivity analysis for model output: performance of black box techniques on three international benchmark exercises. *Comput. Stat. Data Anal.*, **13**, 73-94

Saracci, R. (1987) The interactions of tobacco smoking and other agents in cancer etiology. *Epidemiol. Rev.*, **9**, 175-193

SAS Institute, Inc. (1989) *SAS/STAT user's guide*, version 6, 4th ed., Cary, NC

Sawyer, C., Peto, R., Bernstein, L. & Pike, M.C. (1984) Calculation of carcinogenic potency from long-term animal carcinogenesis experiments. *Biometrics*, **40**, 27-40

Schein, P.S., Davis, R.D., Carter, S., Newman, J., Schein, D.R. & Rall, D.P. (1979) The evaluation of anticancer drugs in dogs and monkeys for the prediction of qualitative toxicities in man. *Clin. Pharmacol. Ther.*, **11**, 3-40

Sheiner, L.B. & Ludden, T.M. (1992) Population pharmacokinetics/dynamics. *Ann. Rev. Pharmacol. Toxicol.*, **32**,185-209

Schell, M.J. & Leysieffer, F.W. (1989) An increasing failure rate approach to low dose extrapolation. *Biometrics*, **45**, 1117-1123

Schoenberg, J.B., Klotz, J.B., Wilcox, H.B., Nicholls, G.P., Gil del Real, M.T., Stemhagen, A. & Mason, T.J. (1990) Case–control study of residential radon and lung cancer among New Jersey women. *Cancer Res.*, **50**, 6520-6524

Shimizu, Y., Kato, H., Schull, W.J. & Hoel, D.G. (1992) Studies of the mortality of A-bomb survivors. 9. Mortality, 1950–1985: Part 3. Noncancer mortality based on the revised doses (DS86). *Radiat. Res.*, **130**, 249-266

Shlyakhter, A., Goodman, G. & Wilson, R. (1992) Monte Carlo simulation of animal bioassays. *Risk Anal.*, **12**, 73-82

Siemiatycki, J. (1991) *Risk Factors for Cancer in the Workplace*, Boca Raton, FL, CRC Press

Siemiatcyki, J. & Thomas, D.C. (1981) Biological models and statistical interactions: an example from multistage carcinogenesis. *Int. J. Epidemiol.*, **10**, 383-387

Squire, R.A. (1981) Ranking animal carcinogens: a proposed regulatory approach. *Science*, **214**, 877-880

Squire, R.A. (1983) Ranking carcinogens for regulation. *Science*, **219**, 238

Squire, R.A. (1984) Carcinogenic potency and risk assessment. *Food Addit. Contam.*, **1**, 221-231

Staffa, J. & Mehlman, M.A. (eds.). (1979) *Innovations in Cancer Risk Assessment: ED01 Study*, Park Forest South, IL, Pathotox Publishers

Statistics and Epidemiology Research Corporation (1990) *EGRET, Reference Manual*, Seattle, WA

Steenland, K. & Thun, M. (1986) Interaction between tobacco smoking and occupational exposures in the causation of lung cancer. *J. Occup. Med.*, **28**, 110-118

Theiss, J.C. (1983) The ranking of chemicals for carcinogenic potency. *Reg. Toxicol. Pharmacol.*, **3**, 320-328

Thomas, D.C. (1981) General relative risk models for survival time and matched case–control studies. *Biometrics*, **37**, 673-86

Thomas, D.C. (1982) Temporal effects and interactions in carcinogenesis. In: Prentice, R.L. & Whittemore, A.S., eds, *Environmental Epidemiology: Risk Assessment*, Philadelphia, PA, Society for Industrial and Applied Mathematics, pp. 107-121

Thomas, D.C. & Whittemore, A.S. (1988) Methods for testing interactions, with applications to occupational exposures, smoking, and lung cancer. *Am. J. Ind. Med.*, **13**, 131-147.

Travis, C.C. & White, R.K. (1988) Interspecies scaling of toxicity data. *Risk Anal.*, **8**, 119-125

Travis, C.C., Richter Pack, S.A., Saulsbury, A.W. & Yambert, M.W. (1990a) Prediction of carcinogenic potency from toxicology data. *Mutat. Res.*, **241**, 21-36

Travis, C.C., Saulsbury, A.W. & Richter Pack, S.A. (1990b) Prediction of cancer potency using a battery of mutation and toxicity data. *Mutagenesis*, **5**, 213-219

Travis, C.C., Wang, L.A. & Waehner, M.J. (1991) Quantitative correlation of carcinogenic potency with four different classes of short-term test data. *Mutagenesis*, **6**, 353-360

Tronko, N.D., Epstein, Y., Oleinik, V., Bogdanova, T., Likhtarev, I., Gulko, G., Kairo, I. & Sobolev, B. (1994) Thyroid gland in children after the Chernobyl accident (yesterday and today). In: Nagataki, S., ed., *Nagasaki Symposium on Chernobyl: Update and Future*, Amsterdam, Elsevier Science, pp. 31-46

Tsyb, A.F., Parshkov, E.M., Ivanov, V.K., Stepanenko, V.F., Matveenko, E.G. & Skoropad, Y.D. (1994) Disease indices of thyroid and their dose dependence in children and adolescents affected as a result of the Chernobyl accident.In: Nagataki, S., ed., *Nagasaki Symposium on Chernobyl: Update and Future*, Amsterdam, Elsevier Science, pp. 9-19

Twort, C.C. & Twort, J.M. (1930) The relative potency of carcinogenic tars and oils. *J. Hyg.*, **29**, 373-379

Twort, C.C. & Twort, J.M. (1933) Suggested methods for the standardization of carcinogenic activity of different agents for the skin of mice. *Am. J. Cancer*, **17**, 293-320

United Nations Scientific Committee on the Effects of Atomic Radiation (1988) *Sources and Effects of Ionizing Radiation*, New York, NY, United Nations

United Nations Scientific Committee on the Effects of Atomic Radiation (1994) *Sources and Effects of Ionizing Radiation*, New York, NY, United Nations

US Agency for Toxic Substances and Disease Registry (1993) *Cancer Policy Framework*, Atlanta, GA, US Department of Health and Human Services, Public Health Service

US Environmental Protection Agency (1986) Guidelines for carcinogen risk assessment. *Fed. Regist.*, **51**, 33992-34003

US Environmental Protection Agency (1992) Draft report: A cross-species scaling factor for carcinogen risk assessment based on equivalence of $mg/kg^{3/4}/day$. Notice. *Fed. Regist.* **57**, 24152-24173

US National Academy of Sciences/National Research Council, Committee on the Biological Effects of Ionizing Radiations (1980) *The Effects on Populations of Exposure to Low Levels of Ionizing Radiation*, BEIR III, Washington, DC, National Academy Press

US National Academy of Sciences/National Research Council, Committee on the Biological Effects of Ionizing Radiations (1988), *Health Effects of Radon and Other Internally Deposited Alpha-Emitters*, BEIR IV, Washington, DC, National Academy Press

US National Academy of Sciences/National Research Council, Committee on the Biological Effects of Ionizing Radiations (1990), *Health Effects of Exposure to Low Levels of Ionizing Radiation*, BEIR V, Washington, DC, National Academy Press

US National Academy of Sciences/National Research Council, Committee on Health Risks of Exposure to Radon (1998), *Health Effects of Exposure to Radon*, BEIR VI, Washington, DC, National Academy Press

US National Research Council (1988) *Complex Mixtures: Methods for In Vivo Toxicity Testing*, Washington, DC, National Academy Press

US National Research Council (1992) *Spacecraft Maximum Allowable Concentration*, Washington, DC, National Academy Press

US National Research Council (1993a) *Issues in Risk Assessment*, Washington, DC, National Academy Press

US National Research Council (1993b) *Pesticides in the Diets of Infants and Children*, Washington, DC, National Academy Press.

US National Research Council (1994) *Science and Judgment in Risk Assessment*, Washington, DC, National Academy Press

US Office of Science and Technology Policy (1985) Chemical carcinogens: a review of the science and its associated principle. *Fed. Regist.*, **50**, 10371-10442

Vainio, H., Sorsa, M. & McMichael, A.J., eds (1990) *Complex Mixtures and Cancer Risk* (IARC Scientific Publications No. 104), Lyon, International Agency for Research on Cancer

Van Ryzin, J. (1980) Quantitative risk assessment. *J. Occup. Med.*, **22**, 321-326

Van Ryzin, J. (1982) Discussion: The assessment of low-dose carcinogenicity. *Biometrics*, 38(Suppl.), 130-139

Wahrendorf, J. (1986) The changing face of cancer epidemiology. *Stat. Med.*, **5**, 547-553

Wakefield, J.C., Smith, A.F.M., Racine-Poon, A. & Gelkland, A.E. (1994) Bayesian analysis of linear and non-linear population models using the Gibbs sampler. *Appl. Stat. J. R. Stat. Soc. Series C*, **43**, 201-221

Wang, Y., Krewski, D., Lubin, J.H. & Zielinski, J.M. (1996) Meta-analysis of multiple cohorts of underground miners exposed to radon. In: *Proceedings of Statistics Canada Symposium 95, From Data to Information—Methods and Systems*, Ottawa, Statistics Canada, pp. 21-28

Watanabe, K., Bois, F.Y. & Zeise, L. (1992) Interspecies extrapolation: A reexamination of acute toxicity data. *Risk Anal.*, **12**, 301-310

Whiting, B., Kelman, A.W., & Grevel, J. (1986) Population pharmacokinetics: theory and clinical application. *Clin. Pharmacokin et.*, **11**, 387-401

Whittemore, A.S. & MacMillan A. (1983) Lung cancer mortality among U.S. uranium miners: a reappraisal. *J. Natl Cancer Inst.*, **70**, 489-499

Whittemore, A.S., Grosser, S.C. & Silvers, A. (1986) Pharmacokinetics in low dose extrapolation using animal cancer data. *Fundam. Appl. Toxicol.*, **7**, 183-190

Willems, M.I., Blijleven, W.G.H., Splinter, A., Roelfzema, M. & Feron, V.J. (1990). *Classification of Occupational and Genotoxic Carcinogens on the Basis of Their Carcinogenic Potency* (Report No. S88), Voorburg, Directorate-General of Labour, Ministry of Social Affairs and Employment, p. 96.

Woutersen, R.A., Til, H.P. & Feron, V.J. (1984) Subacute versus subchronic oral toxicity study in rats: comparative study of 82 compounds. *J. Appl. Toxicol.*, **4**(5), 277-80

Zeise, L., Crouch, E.A.C. & Wilson, R. (1986) A possible relationship between toxicity and carcinogenicity. *J. Am. Coll. Toxicol.*, **5**, 137-151

Zeise, L., Wilson, R. & Crouch, E.A.C. (1987) Dose–response relationships for carcinogenesis: a review. *Environ. Health Perspect.*, **73**, 259-308

Zhu, Y., Krewski, D. & Ross, W.H. (1994) Dose–response models for correlated multinomial data from developmental toxicity studies. *Appl. Stat.*, **43**, 583-598

Quantitative Estimation and Prediction of Human Cancer Risks
S. Moolgavkar, D. Krewski, L. Zeise, E. Cardis and H. Møller
IARC Scientific Publications No. 131
International Agency for Research on Cancer, Lyon, 1999

7: Mechanisms of carcinogenesis and biologically based models for estimation and prediction of risk

Suresh Moolgavkar, Daniel Krewski and Michael Schwarz

7.1 Introduction

In contrast with the empirical approaches to risk estimation considered in Chapter 6, emphasis is placed in this chapter on methods of estimation that take into account current knowledge about the biological mechanisms by which cancerous lesions can develop. The use of biologically based cancer risk-assessment methods has several advantages over empirical methods. First, mechanistic models of carcinogenesis can be interpreted in biological terms, and the plausibility of key model parameters evaluated as such. Second, model lack of fit may suggest appropriate revisions to existing hypotheses about cancer mechanisms. Finally, the use of validated biologically based models will increase the confidence with which results obtained under one set of circumstances can be extrapolated to other conditions.

The development of a comprehensive biologically based approach to cancer risk estimation requires considerable information on the principal factors influencing carcinogenesis. It will be necessary to integrate information from different sources, including data on tissue growth, cell kinetics, mutation rates, and preneoplastic lesions. Early biological effects in the sequence of events leading to neoplastic transformation may also be considered. In addition to these pharmacodynamic data, pharmacokinetic data on the absorption, distribution, metabolism, and elimination of chemical substances to which humans are exposed may also be taken into account. Ideally, an integrated pharmacokinetic/pharmacodynamic model may be developed, validated and used to obtain biologically based estimates of cancer risk.

Clearly, we are not even close to developing such comprehensive models, and there is consid- erable scepticism in certain quarters regarding the use of "biologically based" models, such as multi- stage models, for QEP. Critics of the approach contend that there is much that we do not yet understand about the process of malignant trans- formation, and that the attempt to develop bio- logically based models is premature. Yet others contend that, unless some of the parameters of the models can be determined from ancillary experiments, the use of such models is nothing more than an exercise in "curve-fitting". To a large extent such criticism is based on unrealistic expectations and a general misunderstanding of the properties of these models. The modelling approaches described in this chapter make no claim to explicitly considering every single step in carcinogenesis. While, clearly, it is true that there is much to learn about the processes underlying malignancy, it is also true that there is much we already know. We know that carcinogenesis is a multistage process, and that the kinetics of cell division and cell death play important roles. It is these important features of the process that the models described here attempt to incorporate explicitly. The approach described can be thought of as a hybrid approach, one that combines some relevant biological considerations with rigorous statistical techniques for data analyses.

Biological factors involved in neoplastic trans- formation are discussed in section 7.2. Most human cancers occur as the result of a multistage process, usually requiring two or more heritable genetic alterations for neoplastic transformation, modulated by other factors such as DNA repair processes and cellular kinetics. Interindividual and interspecies variation in cancer susceptibility are discussed in sections 7.3 and 7.4, respectively. Biologically based dose–response models incorpo- rating the main determinants of carcinogenesis are described in section 7.5. Physiologically based pharmacokinetic models that can be used to describe the formation of reactive metabolites and the delivery of these metabolites to target tissues are outlined in section 7.6. Many carcinogens appear to act via mechanisms that are receptor-mediated. Mathematical models to describe receptor binding mechanisms are discussed in section 7.7. The application of such models in describing ligand/receptor binding by dioxin (TCDD) in liver tissue is discussed, and the implications of such models for low-dose risk assessment examined.

7.2 Mechanisms of carcinogenesis
7.2.1 Introduction

Our present understanding of carcinogenesis as a complex multistage process is based on observations from histopathological, epidemiological, biochemical and molecular biological studies (Vainio et al., 1992). Phenotypically altered cell populations that precede the development of benign and malignant neoplasms have been observed in a variety of epithelial tissues including the liver, pancreas, lung, kidney and urinary bladder of experimental animals and humans, and are generally believed to represent precursors of cancer in the respective organs (Bannasch, 1986 a,b). Clonal malignant cell populations have been demonstrated within preneoplastic lesions in liver, providing direct evidence of their precursor nature (Scherer et al., 1984). Similarly, malignant neoplasia have been described as emerging at low frequency from hyperplastic lesions such as papillomas of the skin (Hennings et al., 1983; Carter, 1984). Epidemiological evidence led to the formulation of the multistage model which relates cancer incidence to age, or to duration of exposure to specific agents (Armitage & Doll, 1954). Experimental findings, historically developed from results obtained in the mouse skin carcinogenesis system, led to the operational definition of the stages of *initiation, promotion* and *progression* (Berenblum, 1941; Boutwell, 1964). More recently, molecular biology has given support to the hypothesis that normal cells develop into cancer cells by the sequential acquisition of heritable alterations at the level of the DNA (Fearon & Vogelstein, 1990; Bishop, 1991). Knowledge about the number and frequency of

occurrence of heritable alterations in relevant target genes, such as proto-oncogenes and tumour suppressor genes, and about the kinetics of proliferation of affected cell populations is of importance for biologically based carcinogenesis models for quantitative estimation and prediction of risk.

7.2.2 Oncogenes and tumour-suppressor genes

Molecular analysis of human cancers commonly shows genetic alterations including chromosomal translocation, gene amplification and point mutations. In many cases proto-oncogenes and tumour-suppressor genes have been demonstrated to be targets of genetic damage within cancer cells. A large number of these genes have been identified and cloned (Bishop, 1991; Weinberg, 1991). Proto-oncogenes are normal cellular genes which, when inappropriately activated and converted into oncogenes, cause dysregulation of cellular growth and differentiation pathways. Oncogenes are dominantly acting transforming genes, i.e. mutation of one allele of a proto-oncogene is sufficient to induce an alteration in the phenotype of the cell. Genetic changes in tumour-suppressor genes, in contrast, are recessive in nature: inactivation of both cellular alleles is required to eliminate entirely gene products that negatively regulate cell proliferation. Oncogenes can immortalize primary cells in culture and cooperate with other oncoproteins in transformation (see, for example, Land et al., 1983). Introduction of wild-type tumour-suppressor genes into transformed cells often suppresses the transformed phenotype (Levine et al., 1991; Marshall, 1991).

Several human tumours, including the most common adult cancers of the lung, the colon and the breast, appear to develop through the sequential loss or inactivation of multiple tumour suppressor genes and/or the activation of proto-oncogenes. The number of genetic alterations required for expression of the fully malignant phenotype appears to vary from cancer to cancer. In the case of retinoblastoma, the best studied of the human childhood cancers, two mutations that inactivate both copies of the underlying susceptibility gene, the *RB* tumour-suppressor gene, suffice for tumour development. Both copies of the *RB* gene are inactivated by somatic mutation during the genesis of sporadic retinoblastoma and some other cancers including osteosarcoma, soft-tissue sarcoma and carcinomas of the breast, bladder and lung (Bishop, 1991; Weinberg, 1991).

Transmission of one of the *RB* mutations via the germline leads to an approximately 90% risk of developing retinoblastoma at an early age, and multiple bilateral tumours are often observed. This is due to the fact that the retinoblasts need to suffer only one instead of two *RB* mutations during malignant transformation (Knudson, 1971).

More than two genetic changes appear to be necessary in the case of other human cancers. The most thoroughly analysed example is that of the colon, where an accumulation of genetic alterations in three tumour-suppressor genes (*APC*, *p53* and *DCC*) and one proto-oncogene (*K-ras*) have been observed during progressive stages of tumour development (Fearon & Vogelstein, 1990). Moolgavkar & Luebeck (1992a) have shown that, given current estimates of locus-specific mutation rates, the incidence of colon cancer in the general population and among familial polyposis subjects is most consistent with a model involving three mutations on the pathway to malignancy, unless an early event increases the rates of subsequent mutations, i.e. confers a *mutator phenotype* on the cell, in which case a higher number of mutations would adequately describe the data. Evidence for this latter possibility is provided by the recent demonstration of genes on chromosomes 2, 3 and 7 (*hMSH2*, *MMLHI*, *hPMS1* and *hPMS2*), responsible for some fraction of familial colorectal cancer and associated with a strong increase in genomic instability in tumour cells (Aaltonen *et al.*, 1993; Peltomaki *et al.*, 1993). Similar genomic instability has also been reported in some cases of sporadic colon cancers (Lonov *et al.*, 1993; Thibodeau *et al.*, 1993).

Perhaps the most frequently detected genetic alterations in human cancers are point mutations in one allele of *p53* together with a deletion of the other (Hollstein *et al.*, 1991; Levine *et al.*, 1991; Greenblatt *et al.*, 1994). Germline mutations in *p53*, which are characteristic of the Li–Fraumeni syndrome, are associated with an increased risk for the development of numerous types of tumours with an early age of onset (Malkin *et al.*, 1990; Srivastava *et al.*, 1990). Wild-type *p53* serves as a cell cycle control gene, since progression from G1 to S-phase is often blocked in cells expressing high levels of the protein (Diller *et al.*, 1990: Mercer *et al.*, 1990). Induction of DNA damage in cells leads to an arrest in G1 mediated by wild-type *p53*, thus allowing the affected cells to repair their genetic material (Kastan *et al.*, 1991). This *p53*-dependent cell cycle checkpoint pathway is defective in the human autosomal recessive disorder ataxia telangiectasia (AT), in which hypersensitivity to radiation and a marked increase in cancer incidence occur (Kastan *et al.*, 1992). A candidate tumour-suppressor gene (*ATM*) mutated in AT patients was recently identified on chromosome 11q22-23 (Savitsky *et al.*, 1995). Its link to *p53* remains to be unravelled. Cells unable to repair DNA damage are driven into apoptosis. which is also mediated by *p53* (Yonish-Rouach *et al.*, 1991; Lane, 1992; Shaw *et al.*, 1992; Clarke *et al.*, 1993; Lowe *et al.*, 1993). Loss of wild-type *p53* from cells is associated with gene amplification of the mutated *p53*, which appears to represent a late stage of tumorigenesis (Livingstone *et al.*, 1992; Yin *et al.*, 1992). The reason for this is unclear. Very recently, it has been demonstrated that hypoxia induces apoptosis in wild-type *p53* but not in *p53*-mutated tumour cells. Thus, tumour cells with *p53* mutations have a selective proliferation advantage under conditions of low oxygen, which frequently occurs in more advanced solid tumours (Graeber *et al.*, 1996). Other mutated tumour-susceptibility genes in various cancers have been identified and cloned. These include *BRCA1*, a gene that confers susceptibility to early onset of ovarian and breast cancers (Futreal *et al.*, 1994), *p16/MTS1* which is mutated in a variety of different tumours (Kamb *et al.*, 1994), and *FHIT* which shows genetic aberrations in nearly all small-cell lung cancers and in a high proportion of non-small-cell lung cancers (Sozzi *et al.*, 1996). Thus, susceptibility genes for some of the most frequent human cancers have been identified.

As briefly described above, loss of function of both alleles of a tumour-suppressor gene is a prerequisite for phenotypic alteration. Inactivation of both alleles may be brought about by mechanisms other than direct mutation or deletion of the alleles. Thus, for example, the phenomenon of *dominant negative* action (Herskowitz, 1987) has been described for the *p53* gene, in which the mutant form of the p53 protein binds to and neutralizes the product of the wild-type gene (Gannon *et al.*, 1990) or even drives the wild-type p53 product into a mutant conformation (Milner & Medcalf, 1991).

7.2.3 Proliferation and terminal differentiation of cells

Disruption of normal cell proliferation and differentiation is the *sine qua non* of the malignant state. Conversely, there is accumulating evidence that the kinetics of cell proliferation and differentiation in normal and premalignant cells are important in the carcinogenic process. As discussed below, increases in cell division rates may lead to increases in the rate of critical mutational events, and an increase in cell division without a compensatory increase in differentiation or apoptosis leads to an increase in the size of critical target cell populations. These observations indicate that carcinogenesis involves successive genomic changes, each change resulting in further disruption of cellular kinetics, which, in turn, accelerates the acquisition of more mutations.

Cell proliferation is controlled by various intracellular and intercellular signal pathways. The control of cell proliferation and, in particular, the role of the various genes implicated in carcinogenesis is beginning to be better understood. Many proto-oncogenes play an important role within cellular networks involved in the transduction of signals that stimulate cells to proliferate (Bishop, 1991). Some tumour-suppressor genes, on the other hand, regulate cellular proliferation negatively (Weinberg, 1991).

Recent findings are clarifying the molecular control mechanisms during specific stages of the cell cycle and are beginning to reveal relationships between disturbances of cell cycle control and cancer development. It is now becoming clear that the onset of the cell cycle is regulated by a mechanism common to all eukaryotic cells (for review, see Murray & Kirschner, 1989; Nurse, 1990; Murray, 1994; Draetta, 1994). The decision as to whether a cell becomes quiescent or goes into division is triggered by extracellular factors via complex signal transduction pathways affecting regulatory factors that control the cell cycle. The most important factors are cyclin-dependent

kinases which regulate the activity of several proteins by phosphorylation. Cyclins are a family of protein kinases that accumulate during the cell cycle and are abruptly destroyed by proteolysis at mitosis (Draetta *et al.*, 1989; Draetta, 1994; Murray, 1994). Mathematical models for cell cycle control including interaction of p32cdc2 kinase and cyclins have been developed (Norel & Agur, 1990; Tyson, 1991).

The connection with cancer is becoming clearer. The gene product pRb of the retinoblastoma susceptibility gene *RB*, which is affected by mutation in retinoblastoma and other cancers (see above), functions as a negative regulator of cell proliferation. This can be prevented by phosphorylation of pRb by G1- and S-phase cyclins (Hinds *et al.*. 1992). Cyclins can become constitutively expressed in tumours, for example, by chromosomal rearrangement or hepatitis B virus integration (Wang *et al.*, 1990; Motukura *et al.*, 1991). Underphosphorylated pRb functions by forming a complex with, and thereby inactivating, the transcription factor E2F, which regulates the transcription of immediate early genes such as c-*fos*, c-*myc* and N-*myc*, thus limiting the progression of cells through the cell cycle (Robbins *et al.*, 1990; Chellappan *et al.*, 1991; Rustgi *et al.*, 1991; Weinberg, 1995).

Tissue homeostasis is controlled by proliferation and by terminal differentiation and death of cells. Physiologically unwanted cells are eliminated by apoptosis, a form of controlled cellular *suicide*. Thus, apoptosis may be a normal part of the terminal differentiation programme of somatic cells. By morphological criteria, apoptosis has been shown to proceed through several distinct stages, such as condensation of chromatin, fragmentation into membrane-bound apoptotic bodies, phagocytosis by neighbouring cells and degradation by lysosomes of the host cells (Bursch *et al.*, 1992). Although the molecular biology of apoptosis is far from understood, a variety of different genes have been implicated in the control of the apoptic programme, including, as mentioned above, the *p53* tumour-suppressor gene. Restoration of wild-type p53 protein expression in cells that normally lack p53 results in rapid induction of apoptosis (Yonish-Rouach *et al.*, 1991; Shaw *et al.*, 1992). Wild-type p53 is also required for initiation of apoptosis induced by agents that cause DNA strand breakage (Clarke *et al.*, 1993; Lowe *et al.*, 1993). A second gene identified in the control of apoptosis is the *bcl-2* oncogene. This gene is frequently translocated and juxtaposed to the immunoglobulin heavy-chain locus in follicular B-cell lymphomas. Translocation leads to constitutive expression of the *bcl-2* protein, Bcl-2, which is associated with a block in apoptosis and augmentation of cell survival (Hockenbery *et al.*, 1990. Strasser *et al.*, 1991).

A synergism has also been described for the two tumour-suppressor proteins p53 and Rb. Dysregulation of Rb leading to increased transcriptional activity of E2F is normally counterbalanced by p53-induced apoptosis of the affected cells. Abrogation of p53 and Rb wild-type function is required for sustained proliferation and escape from apoptosis (Quin *et al.*, 1994; Wu & Levine, 1994; White, 1994).

The discussion above has focused on the genetic control of cell proliferation and apoptosis. It is clear that this control may be modified by signals impinging on the cell and, in particular, by the local environment in which the cell finds itself. Thus, gap-junctional intercellular communication appears to play an important role in the control of cellular proliferation (Fitzgerald & Yamasaki, 1990; Trosko *et al.*, 1983).

7.2.4 Action of environmental agents

Environmental agents may affect either the rate at which heritable changes occur in target cells or the kinetics of cell proliferation and terminal differentiation, or both. Both *genotoxic* and *non-genotoxic* mechanisms are of importance here. Although there is no generally accepted definition of *genotoxicity*, the narrowest definition, namely *direct interaction with DNA*, will be used here. *Non-genotoxic* mechanisms will thus include alterations in DNA metabolism, DNA repair, DNA replication and other events that may be involved in the induction of heritable genomic changes, in addition to mechanisms that are usually labelled as *non-genotoxic*, such as modulation of cell proliferation, immune response and hormone actions.

7.2.4.1 Metabolic factors

Many chemical carcinogens act through electrophilic intermediates that are capable of binding covalently to cellular macromolecules including DNA (Miller, 1970). While some carcinogens function as directly DNA-damaging agents, the majority of DNA-reactive chemicals have to be activated to form the ultimate carcinogenic species via metabolic conversion in the body. Most of the enzymic reactions that convert chemically stable carcinogens to reactive intermediates are carried out by cytochrome P-450-dependent mono-oxygenases (Guengerich, 1988). A number of additional enzymes such as epoxide hydrolases, acetyltransferases, glutathione transferases, sulfotransferases and glucuronosyl transferases may be involved in metabolic activation and inactivation pathways.

Many of these enzymes, in particular of the cytochrome P-450 system, exist in polymorphic forms with differing substrate specificities and variation in expression levels among different cell types, organs, individuals and species. Organ- and species-specific effects of carcinogens are often correlated with the activities of certain isoenzymes, and polymorphic variation appears to be important for interindividual differences in cancer risk within the human population (Harris, 1989; Shields & Harris, 1991; for a recent review see Bartsch & Hietanen, 1996). Examples include polymorphic variation between individuals of cytochrome P-450 2D6, which metabolizes a variety of endogenous and exogenous compounds including the drug debrisoquine. When compared with poor metabolizers, extensive debrisoquine metabolizers show an increased lung cancer risk (Ayesh *et al.*, 1984; Caporaso *et al.*, 1990). Differences in lung cancer risk have been also correlated with interindividual differences in the activity of glutathione transferase-m. This enzyme is involved in the enzymic conjugation of reactive polycyclic hydrocarbon metabolites with glutathione resulting in their inactivation. Smokers are exposed to polycyclic hydrocarbons and individuals with glutathione-S-transferase-m activity are at lower risk for lung cancer than smokers without the enzyme (Seidegard *et al.*, 1986, 1990; Heckbert *et al.*, 1992; Nazar Stewart *et al.*, 1993). Interindividual differences in the activity of acetyltransferase, which is involved in the metabolism of certain carcinogenic aromatic amines, are correlated with bladder and lung cancer risks: slow acetylators are at higher risk for developing bladder cancer while rapid acetylation is correlated with increased risk for colon cancer (Mommsen et al., 1985; Hein, 1988; Vineis et al., 1990). Susceptibility to hepatocellular carcinoma may be associated with genetic variation in the enzymatic detoxification of aflatoxins, in particular by glutathione-S-transferase M1 (McGlynn et al., 1995; see also the discussion of the pharmacokinetics of aflatoxin in Chapter 8).

7.2.4.2 DNA binding

Nucleobase adduct patterns have been characterized in detail for a large variety of DNA-reactive carcinogens of various chemical classes including N-nitrosamines, polycyclic hydrocarbons, aromatic amines and aflatoxins. Overall binding of metabolites to DNA varies considerably between carcinogens as do the biological consequences of different DNA adducts. To allow a comparison, the covalent binding index has been introduced, which may span orders of magnitude between carcinogens (Lutz, 1979).

While some adducts possess miscoding or noncoding properties, which may eventually lead to the induction of mutations in DNA, others appear less relevant to mutagenesis and carcinogenesis (Topal, 1988; Balmain & Brown, 1989; Singer & Essigmann, 1991). The relative potency for formation of critical lesions in DNA is often better correlated with carcinogenic potential than overall binding of metabolites (Singer & Grunberger, 1983).

Adducts in DNA are eliminated both spontaneously (e.g. by loss of an adducted purine) and by enzymatic repair processes. Organ and cell type-specific differences in DNA repair capacity and site of tumour formation have been demonstrated to correlate well under a variety of experimental situations, where deficiency in the repair of certain promutagenic DNA adducts appear to be associated with increased risk of cancer initiation (Goth & Rajewsky, 1974; Kleihues & Margison, 1974; Swenberg et al., 1984). Persistence of modified bases in DNA, however, is not invariably predictive of cancer risk, e.g. certain aromatic amines are efficiently activated in hepatocytes leading to persistent adducts in their DNA but liver is not normally the target organ for carcinogenicity (Neumann, 1986).

A variety of biochemical methods are now available, including use of radioactive carcinogens, adduct-specific antibodies, fluorometrical determinations and DNA post-labelling, which all allow the detection of very low levels of carcinogen adducts in DNA. The concentrations of certain DNA adducts are often linearly related to external carcinogen dose with no indication of a threshold in the very low-dose range. Examples include N-nitrosodimethylamine (DMN), some aromatic amines, benzo[a]pyrene, 2-acetylaminofluorene and aflatoxin B_1 (Pegg & Balog, 1979; Neumann, 1983; Schwarz et al., 1985; Lutz, 1986; Beland et al., 1988).

DNA repair may alter otherwise linear dose–response characteristics: the formation of 7-methylguanine but not of O_6-methylguanine is related linearly to the external dose of DMN; the latter adducted base is eliminated from DNA by a methyltransferase protein which acts efficiently at low carcinogen doses but is overloaded at high dose levels (Pegg & Doland, 1987). DNA adducts can be monitored in both animals and humans, and may serve as a means of determining *internal* carcinogen doses. In humans, the doses in target *tissues* can be predicted from measurements of DNA adduct levels in surrogate tissues, such as white blood cells. Since constant chemical-specific proportions exist between DNA and protein binding, measurement of adducts in proteins such as haemoglobin may also be used to estimate tissue doses (European Chemical Industry, Ecology and Toxicology Centre, 1989; Hemminki, 1992).

The importance of base adducts resulting from endogenous processes is becoming increasingly recognized. For example, comparatively large concentrations of etheno- and other DNA adducts are formed from lipid peroxidation products. These can arise from reactive oxygen species generated during infectious diseases or degenerative processes such as liver cirrhosis (Ames et al., 1995; Nair et al., 1996).

7.2.4.3 Mutations in critical genes

Proto-oncogenes and tumour-suppressor genes are mutational targets for chemical carcinogens. In a variety of cases, the types of mutations induced are *carcinogen-specific*. The first line of evidence in favour of this concept came from the analysis of *ras* mutations in animal models (for a review, see Balmain & Brown, 1988). A linkage between exposure to certain cancer risk factors and certain patterns of *ras* mutations has also been proposed for some human cancers (Bos, 1989). More recently, the *p53* tumour-suppressor gene became the major target for studies in molecular epidemiology of both animal and human cancers. In animal systems, *carcinogen-specific p53* mutations have been described for benzo[*a*]pyrene, alkylating *N*-nitroso compounds and ultraviolet (UV) radiation (Kress *et al.*, 1992; Ohgaki *et al.*, 1992; Ruggeri *et al.*, 1993). Human squamous-cell carcinomas and basal-cell carcinomas show UV-typical mutational patterns (Brash *et al.*, 1991; Moles *et al.*, 1993). Hepatocellular carcinomas from patients living in geographical areas where aflatoxin B$_1$ and hepatitis B virus are major risk factors harbour G:C to T:A transversions at a mutational hotspot, whereas tumours from patients from other geographical regions do not (for a review, see Greenblatt *et al.*, 1994 and Chapter 8). Tobacco-related cancers are correlated with a high frequency of G:C to T:A transversions which might be due to polycyclic hydrocarbons present in cigarette smoke (Hollstein *et al.*, 1991; Caron de Fromentel & Soussi, 1992; Greenblatt *et al.*, 1994). Different mutational patterns have been observed in lung cancers from uranium miners exposed to radon (Vähäkangas *et al.*, 1992; Taylor *et al.*, 1994). C:G to T:A transitions at CpG sequences, which occur with comparatively high frequency in cancers of the colon, brain and in lymphoid malignancies (Hollstein *et al.*, 1991; Caron de Fromentel & Soussi, 1992), are assumed to result from deamination of 5-methylcytosine residues, and point to an important role of spontaneous events during tumorigenesis in these organs (Rideout *et al.*, 1990).

Chemically induced structural damage to DNA is used as the basis for a large variety of short-term tests for mutagenicity and carcinogenicity (Montesano *et al.*, 1986; Ashby & Tennant, 1988; Ashby, 1992).

7.2.4.4 Cell proliferation

Cell proliferation may affect the process of carcinogenesis in many different ways. Promutagenic lesions are *fixed* in DNA when cells undergo DNA synthesis before it can be repaired, and mutations are also induced spontaneously, by errors in DNA replication (Loeb, 1989).

Amplification, loss or rearrangement of genetic material may also occur during cell division. The rate of proliferation within a target cell population therefore appears to be a major factor governing the transition frequency between normal and initiated, and between initiated and tumour cells. Increased rates of proliferation, either physiologically or induced, are associated with elevated levels of initiation in many different systems. It has long been known that regenerative proliferation induced by surgical or chemical manipulation of the liver strongly increases the carcinogenic efficacy of DNA-reactive agents in this organ (Craddock, 1976). This effect is maximal when the carcinogens are administered shortly before or during the phase of active DNA synthesis (Craddock, 1971). The fact that DNA synthesis in liver occurs at highly elevated levels in very young animals is the basis for the use of neonates in single-dose carcinogen experiments (Vesselinovitch *et al.*, 1979; Peraino *et al.*, 1981). Stimulation of proliferation of mouse keratinocytes by administration of phorbol ester-type tumour promoters shortly before benzo[*a*]pyrene treatment is associated with enhancement of initiation by the polycyclic hydrocarbon (Goerttler & Loehrke, 1976). This co-carcinogenic effect (for definition, see Appel *et al.*, 1990) is mechanistically different from the promoting effects of the phorbol esters seen during the classical initiation–promotion protocol.

Compensatory or regenerative cell proliferation occurs at necrogenic doses of many different agents and may explain their *promoting* effects. Stimulation of the proliferation of bladder epithelial cells at higher doses of 2-acetylaminofluorene is likely to be responsible for the non-linearity of bladder tumour response in mice (Cohen & Ellwein, 1990). Other examples of agents believed to mediate their effects via the induction of regenerative hyperplasia include sodium saccharide in rat bladder and D-limonene in male rat kidney (Cohen & Ellwein, 1990; Swenberg *et al.*, 1992). Cytotoxicity is also the common denominator for those agents that mediate *promoting* effects by selection for toxin-resistant initiated cells. The phenomenon of selective toxicity has been most convincingly demonstrated in the rat liver system for hepatotoxins such as carbon tetrachloride or phalloidine, and hepatocarcinogens such as 2-acetylaminofluorene, certain *N*-nitrosamines and aromatic amines, and is related to a decrease in the uptake and/or the activation of these chemicals in enzyme-altered tumour precursor cells (Farber & Cameron, 1980).

Promotion of initiated target cells is also mediated by agents that act as direct mitogens. Their activity is best characterized in rodent liver and skin, and the discussion will therefore be focused on these two organs. Liver mitogens include certain drugs such as phenobarbital, several structurally unrelated pesticides, e.g. DDT and α-hexachlorocyclohexane, environmental contaminants such as dibenzo-*p*-dioxins and polyhalogenated biphenyls, sex hormones, e.g. ethinyl oestradiol and cyproterone acetate and peroxisome proliferators, e.g. chlofibrate, di(2-ethylhexyl)phthalate (DEHP) and Wy-14,643 (for a review see Schulte-Hermann, 1985). There is increasing evidence to suggest that the promoting activity of a variety of these agents is receptor-mediated. High-affinity receptors have been demonstrated for dibenzo-*p*-dioxins and related compounds, promoting steroids and peroxisome proliferators (Toft *et al.*, 1967; Poland *et al.*, 1976; Issemann & Green, 1990). A common feature of mitogenic liver tumour promoters is their ability to induce liver growth without showing overt hepatotoxicity (for a review, see Schulte-Hermann, 1985). This effect is assumed to represent an adaptive response of the organ to meet increased functional demands and is fully reversible upon withdrawal of the inducing agent (Schulte-Hermann, 1974).

Tumour-promoting phorbol esters are prototype mitogens in mouse skin (Hecker & Schmidt, 1974). Agents of this group interact with intracellular signal transduction pathways in that they mimic the stimulatory action of the second messenger diacylglycerol on enzymes of the protein kinase C family (Nishizuka, 1988).

Most tumour-promoting mitogens do not induce persistent increases in DNA synthesis in the target organs, even upon continuous administration. In normal liver, stimulatory effects are seen only during the first days of treatment until the liver mass has reached a new elevated plateau level (Schulte-Hermann, 1974). Similarly, phorbol ester-type tumour promoters produce a rapid but only transient hyperproliferative response in

mouse epidermis leading to chronic hyperplasia (Marks *et al.*, 1982). Exceptions in liver are certain peroxisome proliferators (Marsman *et al.*, 1988; Eacho *et al.*, 1991), ethinyl oestradiol (Mayol *et al.*, 1991) and 2,3,7,8-tetrachlorodibenzo-*p*-dioxin (TCDD) (Lucier *et al.*, 1991), which induce persistent increases in cell turnover probably associated with hepatotoxicity. Cells of enzyme-altered foci respond to single doses of tumour-promoting liver mitogens with accelerated proliferation (Schulte-Hermann *et al.*, 1981). Only a few agents, however, produce a sustained elevation in the number of DNA-synthesizing initiated hepatocytes as compared with the surrounding normal liver cells upon continuous treatment (Marsman & Popp, 1989; Schulte-Hermann *et al.*, 1990). The fact that enzyme-altered foci in liver respond to tumour promoters with accelerated enlargement even in the absence of sustained stimulation of proliferation points to an important role of apoptosis during the promotional phase in liver (Schulte-Hermann *et al.*, 1990). Enzyme-altered liver cells show a higher apoptotic rate than normal hepatocytes (Bursch *et al.*, 1984). Since administration of liver tumour promoters is associated with inhibition of apoptosis, increases in the net growth rate of enzyme-altered foci during chronic promoter treatment may be primarily driven by a decrease in the rate of elimination of initiated cells (Bursch *et al.*, 1984; Schulte-Hermann *et al.*, 1990; Stinchcombe *et al.*, 1995). The important impact of dietary factors on cancer is well documented (for a recent review see Willett, 1994). In experimental animals and presumably also in humans, caloric restriction reduces cancer formation. Interestingly, food restriction eliminates preneoplastic cells in rodent liver through apoptosis thus antagonizing the carcinogenic process in this organ (Grasl-Kraupp *et al.*, 1994).

7.2.5 Classification of carcinogenic agents

Cohen & Ellwein (1990) recently proposed a decision tree for the classification of carcinogenic agents based on their mechanism of action. According to their scheme, chemical carcinogens are first divided into those that interact directly with DNA ("genotoxic" mechanism) and those which do not ("non-genotoxic" mechanism). Chemical carcinogens that do not interact with DNA are assumed to exert their effects by increasing cell proliferation. These latter agents are divided into those that act via cellular receptors and those that act through a non-receptor mechanism, often by inducing cytotoxicity. This categorization recognizes that agents, no matter what their molecular mechanism of action, can influence cancer risk in one or both of two ways: by affecting the rate of heritable changes in the cell or by affecting cell proliferation kinetics. As pointed out above, "classical" promoting agents may well have major effects on the rate of apoptosis of initiated cells, and although Cohen and Ellwein's scheme does not explicitly allow for this effect, it could easily be extended to do so. This categorization of environmental carcinogens has important implications for the prediction of cancer risk at low exposure levels. Another advantage of such a classification scheme is that it moves us firmly away from earlier schemes in which agents are classified as "initiators", "promotors", and "complete carcinogens". Although such a classification scheme is often said to be based on mechanistic considerations, the terms "initiator", and "promoter" were originally operationally defined, and there is no general consensus on how they should be translated into the concepts of initiation and promotion. In fact it is probably desirable to jettison the terms "initiator" and "promoter" entirely, except when used in the original operational sense. They are, however, too well entrenched in the literature for us to attempt to do so in this publication.

7.3 Interindividual variation

7.3.1 Genetic predisposition

Reviewing the catalogue of dominant and recessive phenotypes (McKusick, 1975), Mulvihill (1977) counted 200 monogenic conditions in which the occurrence of neoplasia was a regular or occasional feature (McKusick, 1988). In approximately one-third of the conditions, the mode of inheritance was considered definitively proven (Mulvihill, 1977). Some dominant autosomal syndromes where the risk of cancer is elevated include adenomatous familial polyposis, basal-cell naevus syndrome, neurofibromatosis, thyroid carcinoma syndrome, multiple endocrine neoplasia and bilateral retinoblastoma (Emery, 1979; McKusick, 1988; Tomatis et al., 1990). Autosomal recessive conditions include albinism, ataxia

telangiectasia, Bloom's syndrome, Fanconi's anaemia and xeroderma pigmentosum.

The molecular basis for several of these diseases is currently being unravelled (Tomatis et al., 1990; Bishop, 1991; Vainio et al., 1992). Tumour-suppressor genes have been associated with many of the dominant conditions, while DNA repair and immunological deficiencies have been linked to the recessive conditions. It should be emphasized, however, that the classical Mendelian terms dominant and recessive may have complex interpretations in molecular terms (see, e.g. Weinberg, 1991).

In all of the above cancers, the hereditary forms represent a small fraction of those at the particular site concerned; the only exception is retinoblastoma, where the bilateral form accounts for almost half of all retinoblastomas (Tomatis et al., 1990). However, familial aggregations are also observed in common cancers, such as those of the breast, lung and colon, suggesting an inherited susceptibility. The salient features of familial aggregates often include cancers affecting bilateral organs, multifocal sites in the same organ or multiple primary sites, cancers occurring at an early age or in the sex not usually affected; rare cancers or cancers occurring as a feature of a disease syndrome (Berg, 1991).

It has been estimated that hereditary nonpolyposis colorectal cancer accounts for 4–13% of all colorectal cancer in the industrialized countries (Peltomaki et al., 1993). Individuals carrying the defect on chromosome 2 also had other types of tumours. This defect was shown to lead to short inserts in several chromosomes (Aaltonen et al., 1993; Thibodeau et al., 1993). It is estimated that one person in 200 is a carrier of this gene, so that the defect will be one of the most common inherited diseases known.

Mechanisms involved in genetic predisposition to cancer, some of which have been briefly discussed above, are currently the focus of considerable research, and may involve the regulation of cell growth, the metabolism of carcinogens, DNA repair and immune surveillance (Harris, 1991).

7.3.2 Interindividual and interspecies variation in carcinogen metabolism

A majority of chemical carcinogens require metabolism to a reactive intermediate in order to exert their effects on the cell. Interindividual variation in carcinogen metabolism is therefore likely to be one factor determining the consequences of exposure to a given chemical. Among important enzymes for such metabolism are the cytochromes P-450 and glutathione-S-transferases (GST), which are predominantly associated with carcinogen activation (by oxidation) and detoxification (by conjugation to glutathione), respectively. However, many other enzymes are involved in metabolism, including epoxide hydrolases, N-acetyltransferases, UDP-glucoronosyltransferases, alcohol dehydrogenases, prostaglandin synthase, etc. Thus, carcinogen metabolism in humans is complex, being mediated by a large group of enzymes of differing substrate specificity each of which can exhibit a large degree of interindividual variation in expression (see below).

To date, the human cytochromes P-450 comprise more than 25 identified genes coding for proteins with different, although often somewhat overlapping, substrate specificities (Wrighton & Stevens, 1992; Gonzalez, 1988). P-450 expression is similarly complex in animals, and the following observations regarding interspecies differences have been made: (i) different P-450s in different species can metabolize the same compound, or conversely a highly structurally related P-450 in two different species may have a different substrate specificity; (ii) the regulation of expression of related P-450s can vary across species; and (iii) there are species-specific P-450s (Gonzalez et al., 1991; Wrighton & Stevens, 1992). Similarly, GSTs are coded for by multigene families in humans and rats, and the isoenzymes have somewhat overlapping substrate specificities. While the isoenzymes in the rat and in humans appear to be similar, i.e. the same multigene families are present and there is considerable identity in primary structure across the two species (Ketterer, 1988), nevertheless the same interspecies considerations as for P-450 (points i–iii above) need to be taken into account.

Quantitative and qualitative differences in the tissue and cell specific expression of P-450, GST and other carcinogen-metabolizing enzymes across species can lead to different target organs for carcinogenesis with a given chemical. Interspecies differences in carcinogen metabolism

are therefore important for understanding the species specificity and organospecificity of chemical carcinogenesis, and in making valid extrapolations of carcinogenicity data from experimental animals to humans.

In addition to the above interspecies differences in carcinogen metabolism, interindividual variations in carcinogen metabolism in humans must also be considered. Such interindividual variation can be of genetic origin (inherited), e.g. in the case of genetic polymorphisms in a specific gene, or can be the result of alterations in gene expression due to induction by environmental exposures or through post-translational events such as mRNA or protein stabilization (acquired). The range of variation in expression in the enzyme activity of P-450 and GST has been assessed using specific antibodies in Western blots, specific substrates in in vitro assays or in vivo, and, more recently, rapid progress has been made as the relevant human genes have been cloned. The results in general suggest large variation between individuals. For example, in human liver, interindividual variations of between one and two orders of magnitude for the expression of some isoenzymes, including CYP1A2, CYP2A6, CYP3A4 and CYP2E1, have been reported (Camus et al., 1993). Some isoenzymes, mainly expressed extrahepatically, also show high interindividual variability, e.g. CYP1A1 in lung and placenta varied by several orders of magnitude (Fujino et al., 1984; Bartsch et al., 1992). The above-mentioned P-450s are all inducible, as are GST, by medicinal drugs, tobacco smoke, alcohol, dietary factors, etc., which could explain some of the variability in expression and activity. The inducible nature of these enzymes also raises the question of intraindividual variability in expression, which has not been extensively investigated for many metabolizing enzymes to date. However, genetic polymorphisms in some of these enzymes have also been described, e.g. for CYP1A1 (Kawajiri et al., 1991) and CYP2E1 (Uematsu et al., 1991), although their significance in terms of enzyme activity has not been determined. For other enzymes, phenotypic polymorphisms were observed, which subsequently resulted in the identification of the genetic polymorphisms responsible for the expressed phenotype. Examples include CYP2C18 and CYP2D6 (Gough *et al.*, 1990; Kagimoto *et al.*, 1990). Among the GSTs, the *GSTMI* gene has a deletion in a variable percentage of individuals in different populations, with significant differences in the frequency of the deletion between ethnic groups (Seidegaard *et al.*, 1985). As noted above, susceptibility to hepatocellular carcinoma may be associated with genetic variation in the detoxification of aflatoxin by GSTM1 (McGlynn *et al.*, 1995). Other enzymes involved in the detoxification, e.g. of benzo[*a*]pyrene, similarly show large interindividual variation (Petruzzelli *et al.*, 1988). Another enzyme for which genetic polymorphism has been described is *N*-acetyltransferase (NAT), which catalyses the acetylation of arylamines and hydrazines (Blum *et al.*, 1990; Ohsako & Deguchi, 1990). In general, there does not appear to be any coordinate regulation between carcinogen-metabolizing enzymes in humans (Ketterer *et al.*, 1991).

As described briefly above, there is wide interindividual variation, of at least up to two orders of magnitude, in carcinogen metabolism, reflecting both genetic and environmental factors. The impact of this variation needs to be evaluated in terms of the resulting biological effects involved in the carcinogenic process, including DNA-adduct formation, mutation and cell proliferation. A few studies in humans have examined interindividual variability in DNA and/or protein-adduct formation for a precisely measured exposure to a chemical carcinogen. These include studies of cancer patients treated with chemotherapeutic agents (e.g. procarbazine, dacarbazine), of individuals consuming a diet contaminated with aflatoxin, and of occupational exposures to polycyclic aromatic hydrocarbons. In these studies, there are considerable differences in the degree of interindividual variation. In the cancer patients treated with procarbazine or dacarbazine, the interindividual variation has been observed to be less than 10-fold (Souliotis *et al.*, 1990, 1992; Van Delft *et al.*, 1992). However, in studies of workers occupationally exposed to polycyclic aromatic hydrocarbons (Hemminki, 1991), or individuals exposed to aflatoxin through their diet (Wild *et al.*, 1992), the interindividual variation in carcinogen-DNA or -protein adduct formation was found to be of up to two orders of magnitude. Overall, this degree

of variation is similar to that seen in the metabolism of chemical carcinogens by human tissue explants, where interindividual variations in DNA-adduct formation were of one to two orders of magnitude (Vähäkangas *et al.*, 1984).

Several studies have examined the associations between genetic and phenotypic polymorphisms and the risk of specific cancers, including, *inter alia*, CYP2D6 and lung, colon, breast, liver, etc. cancer, CYPIA1 and CYP2E1 and lung cancer, GSTM1 and lung, bladder and liver cancer, NAT and bladder and lung cancer. A number of these have reported an increased risk associated with a specific geno- or phenotype. This association between carcinogen metabolism and disease therefore further suggests that interindividual variations in this parameter need to be considered in the quantitative estimation and prediction of human risk from exposure either to single chemicals or to complex mixtures of chemicals. The latter type of exposure raises the question of carcinogen interactions as competing substrates for one specific enzyme, a subject which requires further attention.

7.3.3 Interindividual variation in DNA repair

Rates of DNA alkylation and repair are major determinants of cancer initiation. As noted above, there are interindividual differences in the activities of enzymes that activate and detoxify procarcinogenic agents. Efficiency of DNA repair has also been found to vary among individuals. A number of hereditary DNA repair-deficiency syndromes are known which are related to the increased incidence of certain cancers, such as cancer of the skin (e.g. xeroderma pigmentosum), or the haemopoietic system (e.g. Bloom's syndrome and Fanconi's anaemia) (for recent reviews, see Bohr *et al.*, 1989; Stewart, 1992). Significantly reduced levels of DNA repair activity, as measured by unscheduled DNA synthesis in N-acetoxy-2-acetylaminofluorene-exposed mononuclear leukocytes, have been reported in individuals with a family history of cancer when compared with a group with no family history (Pero *et al.*, 1989). The activity of O_6-methylguanine-DNA methyltransferase, the repair enzyme responsible for the removal of O_6-methylguanine adducts in DNA, was significantly reduced in fibroblast cultures from lung cancer patients when compared with matched healthy controls (Ruediger *et al.*, 1989). Reduced capacity to repair photochemical damage in DNA has been demonstrated to be an important risk factor for basal-cell carcinoma in young individuals and in individuals with a family history of skin cancer (Wei *et al.*, 1993). Three- to five-fold differences in DNA repair in ultraviolet light- or *N*-acetoxy-2-acetylaminofluorene-exposed fibroblast cultures from normal control individuals were observed by Thielmann *et al.*(1991). More than 10-fold differences in the repair of DNA adducts of benzo[*a*]pyrene-7-8-dihydrodiol 9,10,-epoxide were observed in freshly isolated lymphocytes from apparently healthy individuals, while in a small fraction of individuals there was no detectable removal of adducts of this carcinogen at all (Oesch *et al.*, 1987). These interindividual differences in DNA repair may contribute in part to interindividual variations in cancer risk.

7.4 Interspecies variation

Many carcinogens exhibit more or less pronounced differences in carcinogenic potency and target organ selectivity between different species (Gold *et al.*, 1989; McGregor, 1992a). Much of the preceding discussion of interindividual variation in susceptibility to carcinogenesis also applies to interspecies variation. In fact, interspecies differences in activating and detoxifying enzymes and in the efficiency of DNA repair would be expected to be larger than interindividual variations.

Differences in the metabolism or covalent binding of carcinogen metabolites to cellular macromolecules, in particular DNA, have been correlated with interspecies differences in carcinogen susceptibility. Measurements have been performed *in vivo* and in cultured tissue systems (e.g. bladder explants or trancheobranchial systems), organ slices (e.g. from liver), isolated cells (e.g. hepatocytes in primary culture) and subcellular fractions (e.g. liver microsomes) from different species, including humans. A well studied example is aflatoxin B_1, which is a potent liver carcinogen in rats, but less potent in hamsters and essentially non-carcinogenic in mice (Wogan, 1973; Herrold, 1969; Adamson *et al.*, 1976). These species differences in aflatoxin B_1 carcinogenicity are well correlated with the extent of covalent binding of aflatoxin B_1 metabolites to DNA in

liver slices and isolated hepatocytes from these species (Booth *et al.*, 1981; Hsu *et al.*, 1987). The binding of aflatoxin B_1 to liver DNA differed about 1000-fold in rats and mice in one study (Croy & Wogan, 1981). Binding of aflatoxin B_1 metabolites to DNA of human liver cells occurs at a rate intermediate between those in rats and mice (Hsu *et al.*, 1987).

The calculated DNA adduct levels of 4-aminobiphenyl that would induce the same frequency of bladder tumours in humans and mice suggested that humans were more sensitive than mice (Poirier & Beland, 1992).

Marked differences are also observed in the susceptibility of different species to tumour-promoting agents. Phenobarbital is a potent liver tumour promoter in rats and mice, but not in the hamster (Stenbeck *et al.*, 1986). This is correlated with the induction of cytochrome P-450b by phenobarbital in these species (Lubet *et al.*, 1989). Certain hypolipidaemic drugs and industrial phthalate ester plasticizers are effective liver carcinogens in rats and mice. The carcinogenic activity of these agents has been linked to induction of proliferation of peroxisomes in these species (Reddy & Lalwani, 1983). Peroxisomal proliferation is much less pronounced in Syrian hamsters, guinea-pigs and marmosets (Lake *et al.*, 1989), suggesting that peroxisome proliferators may only be weakly hepatocarcinogenic in these species, or not at all. There is disagreement in the literature with respect to the induction of peroxisome proliferation in non-human primates and humans (Reddy & Lalwani, 1983).

7.5 Biologically based dose–response models
7.5.1 Introduction

The discussion of the processes underlying malignant transformation in the preceding sections indicates that carcinogenesis is a complex multistage process modulated by genetic and environmental influences. It is obviously impossible to take explicit account of all the factors involved in carcinogenesis in any model. In fact, since any model is an abstraction that incorporates (in the opinion of the modeller) the most important features of the process, any attempt to take explicit account of the myriad factors involved in carcinogenesis would defeat the whole purpose of modelling. The models described here acknowledge the multistage nature of carcinogenesis, and the importance of cell proliferation kinetics in the process. Modulating genetic and environmental factors affect carcinogenesis by affecting rates of mutation and cell proliferation.

The concept of multistage carcinogenesis was formalized in mathematical models some 40 years ago (Nordling, 1953; Armitage & Doll, 1954). Originally, these models were proposed in order to explain the observation that the age-specific incidence curves of many common carcinomas increase roughly with a power of age. The central thesis of the models — that a malignant tumour arises from a single cell that has sustained a small number of critical insults to its genetic apparatus — is supported by modern laboratory observations. The Armitage–Doll model, often called the multistage model, has proved to be enormously successful, and continues to be used today, both for data analysis and QEP, yet some of the fundamental features of this model are widely misunderstood, as discussed below.

Knudson (1971) proposed a two-mutation model for embryonal tumours based on a statistical study of retinoblastoma, a rare tumour of the retina in children. This occurs in both sporadic and dominantly inherited forms in the population, and Knudson's model provided an attractive biological explanation for the genesis of these two forms of the tumour. According to the model, retinoblastoma results from two critical mutations, both of which are somatic in sporadic cases. In inherited cases, however, the first mutation has occurred in the germ cell of an ancestor, while the second mutation is somatic. A child who inherits the first mutation from the germ cell of one of his parents is born with all the cells of his or her retina requiring only one more mutation (the second) for malignant transformation. Thus, the probability that at least one of the retinoblasts will acquire the second mutation is very high, and the child almost inevitably develops retinoblastoma. The salient features of Knudson's model for retinoblastoma have been shown to be correct (Cavanee et al., 1983; Godbout et al., 1983). Retinoblastoma is but one example of a neoplasm that occurs both sporadically and in heritable form; genetic predisposition to other neoplasia was briefly discussed earlier in this chapter. As a model tumour, retinoblastoma is particularly interesting because it illustrates one paradigm for the mechanism whereby genetic susceptibility is conferred: inheritance of the retinoblastoma gene is equivalent to the inheritance of one of the necessary steps in the genesis of the neoplasm. The mechanism whereby susceptibility is inherited in other heritable cancers is not so clear. There are suggestions that the susceptibility gene affects cell proliferation kinetics (Moolgavkar & Luebeck, 1992a) or that it confers a mutator phenotype on target cells (Aaltonen et al., 1993; Peltomaki et al., 1993).

Recent research suggests that sex-of-parent-specific phenomena such as genomic imprinting may play an important role in some forms of cancer, e.g. Wilms' tumour, rhabdomyosarcoma (Scrable et al., 1989; Sapienza, 1992) and retinoblastoma (Sapienza, personal communication). Mathematical models of carcinogenesis have not heretofore taken such considerations into account.

A crucial difference between the models proposed in the 1950s (Nordling, 1953; Armitage & Doll, 1954), and that proposed by Knudson (1971) is that the latter model took explicit account of the kinetics of cell division of the target cells (stem cells; in the case of the retina, these are retinoblasts). As discussed in the previous section, there is now considerable evidence that the kinetics of cell division and differentiation play an important role in carcinogenesis, and may indeed provide the key to understanding the role of promotion in the process (Moolgavkar & Knudson, 1981; Ames & Gold, 1990; Cohen & Ellwein, 1990; Preston-Martin et al., 1990). Thus, it is important that carcinogenesis models explicitly consider cell replication kinetics. In fact, when they are explicitly considered, a two-mutation model is the most parsimonious model consistent with both the epidemiological and experimental data (Moolgavkar & Knudson, 1981; Moolgavkar & Luebeck, 1990). However, recent laboratory work, especially in colon cancer, suggests that many mutations are associated with the process of malignant transformation (see, e.g. Fearon & Vogelstein, 1990). Thus, although two rate-limiting mutations are consistent with the incidence of malignant tumours in human and animal populations, in reality more than two mutations may be involved in the genesis of many tumours, so that models postulating more than two mutations must be considered. However, unlike the Armitage–Doll model, these models must explicitly incorporate cell proliferation kinetics. One serious problem is that such models very quickly become overparametrized. A good practical strategy, therefore, is to use the two-mutation model unless there is compelling biological evidence against it. It can be shown, moreover, that, using the mathematical formulation in the Appendix with information only on incidence of cancer, a two-mutation model with time-dependent second mutation rate cannot be distinguished (statistically) from a model with multiple mutations. Thus, without ancillary information, which is generally not available, there is not much point in fitting models with more than two mutations to incidence data.

Mathematical models of carcinogenesis are important for several reasons. First, they provide a framework within which the process of carcinogenesis can be viewed and questions about it asked. Thus, for example, various models of carcinogenesis have been used for the analysis of epidemiological and experimental data, and biological interpretations of the observations have been sought (see, e.g. Moolgavkar & Luebeck (1990) for a brief review of such applications). Second, from the statistical point of view, carcinogenesis models provide a rich class of hazard functions for the analysis of time-to-tumour data. Although the statistical properties of these models are not as well understood as those of the more commonly used models based on survival analysis, carcinogenesis models provide a very natural setting for the incorporation of time- and age-dependent exposure patterns into an analysis. Such time-dependent factors are rather difficult to study using the conventional methods of survival analysis. Furthermore, analysis of epidemiological data using conventional statistical methods often requires rather artificial assumptions, such as multiplicativity of relative risk or additivity of excess risk (see, e.g. US National Research Council, 1990). There is little biological reason to believe that risk should behave in this fashion, and such models are simply convenient descriptions of the data. Third, the analysis of intermediate lesions on the pathway to malignancy is

also greatly, facilitated by the use of stochastic carcinogenesis models (Moolgavkar et al., 1990b; Luebeck et al., 1991; Kopp-Schneider & Portier, 1992). In fact, much of the quantitative biological information in these data remained unexploited until quite recently, when methods based on mechanistic models were developed for analysis of the data. Fourth, use of cancer models leads naturally, to methods for joint analyses of premalignant and malignant lesions (Dewanji et al., 1991), which have not been possible with more traditional methodology. Finally, cancer models have been widely used in quantitative cancer risk assessment and, with increasing knowledge of cancer mechanisms, their use for this purpose is likely to increase.

In summary, stochastic cancer models offer a flexible class of functions for the analysis of data from epidemiological and experimental studies. The parameters of such models can be directly interpreted in biological terms. Although versions of these models have been in use for almost four decades, it is only recently that models explicitly incorporating cell replication kinetics have been considered. In view of the increasing evidence that cell proliferation plays a vital role in carcinogenesis, the investigation of such models is of great importance.

The purpose of this section is to give a brief account of carcinogenesis models and their use in QEP. Much of the mathematical material is relegated to the Appendix. Although we have made no attempt to give complete proofs and derivations, or to treat the most general cases, we hope that we have provided enough information for the mathematically mature reader to be able to fill in the blanks. The reader who feels uncomfortable with the mathematics may take the results on faith. For such a reader, we hope that the applications to data analysis will prove to be useful. Often, carcinogenesis models have been fitted to data without proper regard for statistical considerations. One of our goals is to introduce rigorous statistical methods for the analysis of data using cancer models.

Data to which carcinogenesis models can be fitted are generally derived from two sources. As stated earlier, the first models were derived in order to explain cancer incidence data, and much of the early model fitting was to incidence and mortality data from various population-based cancer registries. More recently, models have been fitted to other types of epidemiological data, such as cohort and case–control data (for a brief review see Moolgavkar & Luebeck (1990)). The analysis of cohort data is relatively straightforward; that of case–control data leads to some difficult methodological issues,which need to be addressed. Quantitative data available from animal carcinogenesis experiments, including those from initiation–promotion experiments, have also been analysed within the framework of cancer models.

A crucial difference between human and animal data is that, in human populations, specific cancer types are rare, whereas animal experiments are often conducted under conditions such that a large proportion of animals develop a certain type of tumour and many animals develop multiple tumours at the same site. Analyses using carcinogenesis models can be greatly simplified by making a mathematical approximation to the hazard (incidence) function. This approximation may occasionally be adequate for the analysis of some epidemiological data on tumours that are sufficiently rare, although we believe that the exact hazard function should be routinely used. The approximation is most emphatically not valid in the experimental situation in which tumours cannot be assumed to be rare, and there are strong indications that its use is misleading even in the analysis of epidemiological data. Nevertheless, this approximation continues to be widely used for analyses. This issue will be discussed in greater detail below.

The following fundamental assumptions underlie the models considered here: (1) cancers are clonal, i.e. malignant tumours arise from a single malignant progenitor cell; (2) each susceptible (stem) cell in a tissue is as likely to become malignant as any other; (3) the process of malignant transformation in a cell is independent of that in any other cell; and (4) once a malignant cell is generated, it gives rise to a detectable tumour with probability 1 after a constant lag time. The last two assumptions are clearly false, and are made for mathematical convenience. Methods for relaxing these assumptions are currently being investigated (Yang & Chen, 1991; Luebeck & Moolgavkar, 1994). A mathematical

review of some carcinogenesis models can be found in the book by Tan (1991).

7.5.2 The Armitage–Doll multistage model

The Armitage–Doll model, which has been used extensively in the last four decades, was first proposed to explain the observation that, in many human carcinomas, age-specific incidence rates increase roughly with a power of age. The age-specific incidence rate is a measure of the rate of appearance of tumours in a previously tumour-free tissue. The appropriate statistical concept is that of the hazard function.

For the tissue of interest, let T be a random variable representing time to appearance of a malignant tumour, and let

$$P(t) = \text{Prob}\{T \le t\}. \tag{1}$$

Then the hazard function $H(t)$ is defined by:

$$h(t) = \lim_{\Delta t \to 0} \frac{1}{\Delta t} \text{Prob}\{t < T \le t + \Delta t \mid T > t\}$$

$$= P'(t)/(1 - P(t)), \tag{2}$$

where $P'(t)$ denotes the derivative of $P(t)$. Suppose that there are N cells susceptible to malignant transformation in the tissue of interest, and that $T_1, T_2, \ldots, T_N$ are independent identically distributed random variables representing the time to transformation of the individual cells. Then, $T = \min \{T_1, T_2, \ldots, T_N\}$, i.e. T is a minimum order statistic. For a given susceptible cell, let $p(t)$ be the probability of malignant transformation by time t. An easy computation shows that the hazard function for the tissue is given by the expression:

$$h(t) = Np'(t)/(1 - p(t)). \tag{3}$$

The Armitage–Doll model postulates that a malignant tumour arises in a tissue when a single susceptible cell in that tissue undergoes malignant transformation via a finite sequence of intermediate stages, the waiting time between any stage and the subsequent one being exponentially distributed. Schematically, the model may be represented as follows:

$$E_0 \overset{\lambda_0}{\to} E_1 \overset{\lambda_1}{\to} E_2 \overset{\lambda_2}{\to} \ldots \overset{\lambda_{n-1}}{\to} E_n. \tag{4}$$

Here E_O represents the normal cell, E_n, represents the malignant cell, and the λ_j represent the parameters of the (exponential) waiting time distributions.

Let $p_j(t)$ represent the probability that a given cell is in stage E_j by time t. Then, $p_n(t) = p(t)$ is the probability that the cell is malignantly transformed by time t, and the expression for the hazard, $h(t)$, can be rewritten as:

$$h(t) = Np'_n(t)/(1 - p_n(t)). \tag{5}$$

In the usual treatment of the multistage model, two approximations are usually made at this point. First, at the level of the single cell, malignancy is a very rare phenomenon. Thus, for any cell, $p_n(t)$ is very close to zero during the life span of an individual, and $h(t)$ is approximately equal to $Np'_n(t)$.

An explicit expression for $Np'_n(t)$ in terms of the transition rates λ_i is presented in the Appendix (see also Moolgavkar 1978, 1991). It is shown that:

$$h(t) \approx Np'_n(t) = \frac{N\lambda_0\lambda_1\ldots\lambda_{n-1}}{(n-1)!}t^{n-1}\{1-\lambda t+f(\lambda, t)\}, \tag{6}$$

where $\lambda = n - 1 \sum_{\lambda=0}^{n-1} \lambda_i$ is the mean of the transition rates, and $f(\lambda, t)$ involves second and higher order moments of the transition rates,

Retention of only the first non-zero term (this is the second approximation) in this series expansion leads to the Armitage–Doll expression, namely:

$$h(t) \approx \frac{N\lambda_0\lambda_1\ldots\lambda_{n-1}t^{n-1}}{(n-1)!}. \tag{7}$$

Thus, with the two approximations made, this model predicts an age-specific incidence curve that increases with a power of age that is one less than the number of distinct stages involved in malignant transformation.

It is immediately obvious from the model that, given sufficient time, any susceptible cell eventually becomes malignant. Furthermore, since the waiting time distribution to malignant transformation is the sum of n exponential waiting time distributions, it follows that $h(t)$ is a monotone increasing function. Moreover, using equation (5) of this section and equation (A.2) of the

Appendix, computation shows that $h(t)$ has a finite asymptote: $\lim_{t\to\infty}h(t) = N\lambda_{min}$ where λ_{min} is the minimum of the transition rates. By contrast, the Armitage–Doll approximation increases without bound, and thus becomes progressively worse with increasing age.

A simple example serves to show that the Armitage–Doll approximation can be inadequate if the transition rates are not small enough. Consider a hypothetical malignant tumour that requires seven stages for its genesis, and suppose that the transition rates (per cell per year) are 1×10^{-4}, 2×10^{-4}, 34×10^{-4}, 7×10^{-3}, 8×10^{-3} and 9×10^{-3}, respectively, and that the number of susceptible cells in the tissue is 10^9. Table 7.1 compares the age-specific incidence rates predicted by the Armitage–Doll approximation with those obtained from the exact solution. A second example, more typical of the experimental situation, in which the majority of animals develop tumours by the end of the study, is shown in Figure 7.1

For future reference, we note here that the hazard function can be viewed as follows. Let $X_i(t)$, $i = 1, 2, \ldots, n$ be a sequence of random variables associated with each cell, with $X_i(t) = 1$ if the cell is in stage i at time t and 0 otherwise. The Kolmogorov equations in the Appendix imply that:

$$h(t)=Np'_n(t)/(1-p_n(t))=N\lambda_{n-1}E[X_{n-1}(t)\,|\,X_n(t)=0], \tag{8}$$

where E denotes the expectation. In other words, the hazard or incidence is proportional to the expected (or mean) number of cells in the penultimate stage, conditional on there being no cells that are malignant. When $p_n(t)$ is close to zero, or equivalently the transition rates are small enough, the conditional expectation may be approximated by the unconditional expectation, and:

$$h(t) \approx Np'_n(t) = N\lambda_{n-1}E[X_{n-1}(t)]. \tag{9}$$

Thus the Armitage–Doll approximation consists of replacing the conditional expectation of X_{n-1} by the unconditional expectation and then retaining only the first non-zero term in the Taylor series expansion of the unconditional expectation. Expressions similar to equations (8)

Table 7.1. Comparison of the age-specific incidence rates predicted by the Armitage–Doll approximation and the exact solution to the multistage model			
Age (years)	Age-specific incidence rates (per million)		Difference as a percentage of the Armitage–Doll approximation
	Armitage–Doll approximation	Exact solution	
25	3	3	0.0
30	10	9	10.0
35	26	23	11.5
40	58	50	13.8
45	119	99	16.8
50	223	183	17.9
55	395	318	19.5
60	666	526	21.0
65	1077	833	22.7
70	1680	1275	24.1
75	2542	1892	25.6
80	3743	2733	27.0

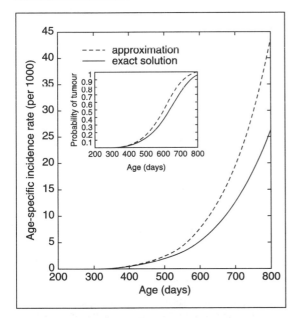

Figure 7.1. Age-specific incidence rate and probability of tumour as functions of age: hypothetical curves based on the Armitage–Doll model. A seven stage tumour was assumed in a tissue with 5×10^7 susceptible cells, and with transition rates of 10^{-3}, 2×10^{-3}, 10^{-4}, 2×10^{-4}, 10^{-5}, 1×10^{-5} and 5×10^{-5} (per cell per day), respectively. Note that the approximate solution overestimates both the incidence and the probability

and (9) can be written for the hazard function of the two-mutation model, as discussed later. Some implications of these expressions will be discussed in the section on the two-mutation model.

In order to model the action of environmental carcinogens, one or more of the transition rates can be made functions of the dose of the agent in question, where dose is to be thought of as the effective dose at the target tissue. Usually, the transition rates are modelled as linear functions of the dose, so that $\lambda_i = a_i + b_i d$ for one or more i. The assumption of first-order kinetics may be justified, at least for carcinogens that interact directly with DNA to produce mutations. Then, using the Armitage–Doll approximation (equation 7), the hazard function at age t and dose d can be written as $h(t, d) = g(d)t^{n-1}$, where $g(d) = \frac{N}{(n-1)!} \prod_i (a_i + b_i d)$, and the probability of tumour is approximately given by $P(t, d) = 1 - \exp[-\tilde{g}(d)t^n]$, with $\tilde{g}(d) = g(d)/n$. Note that $\tilde{g}(d)$ is a product of linear terms. It is in this form, called the linearized multistage model, that the Armitage–Doll model is applied to the problem of low-dose extrapolation. The proportion of animals developing tumours at a specified fixed age at each of three different dose levels is generally known. The, linearized multistage model is fitted to the data and the estimated parameters used to extrapolate risk to lower doses. There are formally at least two problems with this procedure. First, as noted above, the Armitage–Doll approximation may be poor when the probability of tumour is high, as is the case in the usual animal experiments used for risk assessment. Second, in statistical fitting of the linearized multistage model, $\tilde{g}(d)$ is treated as a general polynomial whereas it is really a product of linear terms.

The general expressions given above apply only when exposure to a carcinogenic agent starts at birth or very early in life, and continues at the same constant level throughout the period of observation, i.e. when the parameters of the model are constant. With time-dependent exposures, a starting point for the mathematical development is the set of Kolmogorov equations (Appendix, equation (A.I)), which hold even when the transition rates are time-dependent. However, the published papers use the approximation of equation (7) as their starting point (see, e.g. Whittemore, 1977; Day & Brown, 1980; Crump & Howe, 1984; Brown & Chu, 1987; Freedman & Navidi, 1989). As noted above, this approximation is inappropriate unless one has reason to believe that each of the transition rates is small enough. The approximation is almost certainly inappropriate when applied to experimental data.

7.5.3 The two-mutation model[1]

The version of the two-mutation model discussed here has been widely used for the analysis of data. Similar models were considered by Neyman & Scott (1967), Kendall (1960) and Kopp-Schneider & Portier (1992). The development here follows that in Moolgavkar & Luebeck (1990) and uses the same notation. The model assumes that

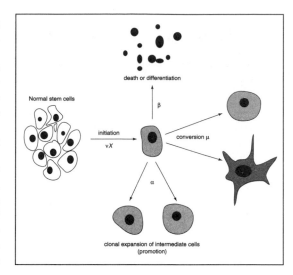

Figure 7.2. Pictorial representation of the two-mutation clonal expansion model

malignant transformation of a susceptible cell is the result of two specific, rate-limiting, hereditary (at the level of the cell) and irreversible events. Within this model, the first rate-limiting event can be identified with initiation, the second with malignant conversion, and the clonal expansion of intermediate cells with promotion (Figure 7.2).

Increased cell division rates and decreased cell death rates have both been implicated in promotion (Schulte-Hermann et al., 1990). After malignant transformation, relatively rapid changes lead to tumour progression. These are not explicitly modelled.

Within the framework of this model, environmental agents or genetic influences could affect the risk of cancer by directly affecting the rates of the first or second critical mutations, or by affecting the cell proliferation kinetics of normal or intermediate cells. Since mutation rates may

---

[1] This model should more properly be called the two-stage clonal expansion model. We emphasize here that we do not consider carcinogenesis to result from two rate-limiting mutations. Indeed, for most cancers, the number of rate-limiting mutations is not known. Rather, as emphasized in the text, this model should be thought of as a mathematical formulation of the initiation–promotion–progression paradigm. Initiation, which confers a growth advantage on the cell, is a rare event and the appearance of initiated cells in a tissue can reasonably be modelled by a time-dependent Poisson process. Thus, the two-stage clonal expansion model posits that the arrival of cells into the initiated compartment follows a Poisson process, and that promotion consists of the clonal expansion of these initiated cells by a birth and death process. Finally, one of the initiated cells may be converted into a malignant cell. This step may involve more than a single mutation, as well. From the mathematical point of view, incorporating more than one mutation in the progression of initiated to malignant cells, is equivalent to having a time-dependent second mutation rate in the two-stage model. This can be explicitly tested in the data. When more biological information (on the number of stem cells or on intermediate lesions on the pathway to malignancy, for example) is available, the model can be extended to include this information (e.g. Moolgavkar & Luebeck, 1992a).

depend upon rates of cell division, an agent that increases the rate of cell division may indirectly increase one or both mutation rates. An increase in cell division rate, without a compensatory increase in the rates of cell differentiation or cell death, will lead to an increase in the mean size of the population of susceptible cells and thus to an increase in cancer risk. For further details, see Moolgavkar & Knudson (1981) or Moolgavkar (1986).

In the mathematical development of the model briefly discussed below and described in detail in the Appendix, the growth of the population of normal cells is described deterministically, whereas the intermediate (initiated) cells are treated stochastically. This is appropriate because the number of normal cells is large and under tight homoeostatic control. In contrast, the number of initiated cells is small and under much looser homoeostatic control. The stochastic nature of intermediate cell growth has interesting consequences, which will be discussed in a later section. However, one consequence of particular interest was highlighted in a recent paper by Kopp-Schneider & Portier (1992) analysing papilloma counts in a mouse skin initiation–promotion experiment. They showed that the rate of cell division was equal to or slightly less than that of death (differentiation) during the promotion phase. Although this result is counterintuitive, it can be understood by considering the stochastic nature of intermediate cell growth: A large number of initiated cells is generated during initiation. A large fraction dies off, but a few papillomas arise because of stochastic fluctuations. Thus, clonal expansion of initiated cells can be brought about without increasing the net proliferation rate (i.e. the difference between the rates of cell division and cell death) of initiated cells. The original definition of promotion within the framework of the two-mutation model (Moolgavkar & Knudson, 1981; Moolgavkar, 1986) required an increase in the net proliferation rate of initiated cells. In view of the comments made above, this definition should probably be jettisoned.

Finally. the distinction between the concepts of initiation, promotion and the action of specific environmental agents must be kept clearly in focus. For example, while promotion is defined within the framework of the model as the clonal expansion of initiated cells, an agent deemed to be a promoter may have other effects as well. It could cause hyperplasia of the normal tissue and also, as pointed out above, indirectly increase the mutation rates.

The following assumptions are used in the mathematical development; for technical details see Moolgavkar & Luebeck (1990). Let $X(s)$ represent the number of normal susceptible cells in the tissue of interest at time (age) s, and suppose that intermediate cells, i.e. cells that have sustained the first rate-limiting event on the pathway to malignancy, arise from normal cells as a non-homogeneous Poisson process of intensity $v(s)X(s)$, where $v(s)$ is the first event rate. Note that v and X are not separately identifiable. However, information on one or the other may be available from independent sources. In a small interval of time s, an intermediate cell divides into two intermediate cells with probability $\alpha(s)$; it dies or differentiates with probability $\beta(s)$ (note that death and differentiation are equivalent events for carcinogenesis because both events remove the cell from the pool of susceptible cells); it divides into one intermediate cell and one cell that has sustained the second event (malignant cell) with probability $\mu(s)$. In many applications, the parameters are assumed to be constant or piecewise constant. In particular, this implies that the waiting times to cell division and cell death are assumed to be exponential.

Some comments on these mathematical assumptions are in order. The cell kinetics of intermediate cells are modelled in primitive fashion. There are whole volumes on the mathematical modelling of the cell cycle, and it is clear that cells do not divide or die with exponential waiting times (see, e.g. Jagers, 1983). Nevertheless, in the context of carcinogenesis modelling these simplifications appear to be entirely appropriate as a first approximation. However, more realistic cell cycle models need to be investigated. Once a malignant cell is generated it is assumed to give rise to a detectable tumour after a suitable lag time. This assumption is clearly false and there is clearly a time-to-detection distribution. Furthermore, malignant cells undoubtedly go through a birth–death process and as a consequence become extinct with non-zero probability. Incorporation of such considerations into the model would hopelessly overparametrize it; however, if information on the growth kinetics of malignant cells of the appropriate type is available from independent sources, the model could quite easily be extended to incorporate it. The requisite mathematics is being developed (e.g. Dewanji *et al.*, 1991; DeGunst & Luebeck. 1994; Luebeck & Moolgavkar, 1994; see also the papers by Chen & Farland, 1991; Yang & Chen, 1991).

In order to fit the model to epidemiological or experimental data in which the end-point of interest is the appearance of malignant tumours, the crucial quantity is the hazard function. In many initiation–promotion experiments, particularly on the mouse skin and the rodent liver, however, quantitative data are available on the number and size distribution of intermediate lesions, and, in fitting the model to these data, expressions for these quantities need to be derived from the model. We note here that, because the two-mutation model takes explicit account of the growth kinetics of intermediate lesions, the relevant quantities can be derived from this model. This is not possible with the Armitage–Doll model. Furthermore, the assumed stochasticity in the growth of intermediate lesions leads to a distribution of the sizes of the intermediate lesions. Mathematical details are provided in the Appendix.

7.5.4 The hazard function: analysis of incidence data

Suppose that $Y(t)$ and $Z(t)$ represent, respectively, the number of intermediate and malignant cells at age t. Then, as shown in the Appendix, the hazard function is given by the expression:

$$h(t) = \mu (t)E[Y(t)|Z(t) = 0], \qquad (10)$$

where E denotes the expectation. Note the similarity of this expression to the exact hazard function for the multistage model (equation (8)). Replacing the conditional expectation by the unconditional expectation leads to the approximate hazard function:

$$h(t) \approx \mu (t)E[Y(t)]. \qquad (11)$$

The differential equation for $E[Y(t)]$ can be solved to yield:

$$h(t) \approx \mu (t) \int_0^t \left\{ v(s)X(s) \exp \int_s^t [\alpha(u) - \beta(u)]du \right\} ds. \qquad (12)$$

If $\alpha \geq \beta$, then the approximate hazard function (equation (12)) increases continuously and without bound with age, whereas it can be shown (Moolgavkar. & Luebeck, 1990) that the exact hazard function (equation (10)) approaches a finite asymptote, as in the case of the exact hazard function of the multistage model. Some other observations regarding the qualitative differences between the exact and approximate solutions are worth emphasizing here. Although these comments are made about the two-mutation model, similar observations apply to the Armitage–Doll multistage model.

Consider first the effect of an environmental agent on the hazard function. Within the framework of the model, an environmental agent acts by affecting one or more of its parameters. When exposure to the agent ceases, the parameters revert to background levels. The subsequent behaviour of the hazard function can be quite complicated. It can be shown, however, that the exact hazard function approaches the background hazard (i.e. the hazard in the unexposed) asymptotically. This return to the background hazard may not be of practical importance because, depending upon the actual parameter values, it may occur well beyond the life span of the animal under study. Nonetheless, it is important to note that this is an important qualitative difference from the behaviour of the approximate hazard function, which returns (instantaneously) to background levels after exposure to an environmental agent ceases if and only if the agent affects only the second mutation rate. In all other cases, the approximate hazard function remains higher than the background level after exposure to an agent stops. Intuitively, the reason for the behaviour of the exact hazard function is as follows. When a population of individuals is exposed to an environmental agent, there is a distribution over the individuals in the population of the number of intermediate cells. The subsequent behaviour of the hazard function depends upon this distribution. Soon after exposure stops, the hazard is high because there are individuals in the population with large numbers of intermediate cells. With the passage of time, the population of exposed individuals who have not developed cancer becomes similar to that of unexposed individuals. The exact hazard function captures the stochastic nature of the size of the intermediate cell pool.

The approximate hazard function does not. The return of the hazard function to background levels has been observed in epidemiological studies, for example, in the study of leukaemia in atom bomb survivors. The important point to keep in mind is that this is predicted by any multistage model of carcinogenesis, provided that one does not allow oneself to be misled by inappropriate approximations (see also Little (1995)).

By analogy with the hazard function for the first malignant tumour (equation (10)), the hazard function for the second malignant tumour (i.e. the rate at which second malignant tumours occur at time t given that exactly one had occurred prior to time t) is given by the expression (Dewanji et al., 1991):

$$h_2(t) = \mu(t)E[Y(t) \mid Z(t) = 1]. \tag{13}$$

It can be shown that $h_2(t) > h(t)$, i.e. the incidence rate of a second malignant tumour, once the first has occurred, is higher than that of the first malignant tumour. The approximate hazard function, on the other hand, predicts exactly the same incidence rate for the second tumour as for the first. Intuitively, the incidence rate for the second malignant tumour should be higher than that of the first for the following reason. In a population of individuals all of whom have developed one malignant tumour, the mean number of intermediate cells is higher than in a population all the individuals of which have not developed a malignant tumour. So, here again, the approximate solution is unable to capture the inherent stochasticity of the situation.

In a recent paper, Little (1995) has developed general expressions for the hazard functions of models with an arbitrary number of stages, and with cell division and death allowed at each of the stages. Heidenreich (1996) has shown that, although the hazard function of the two-mutation model is couched in terms of four parameters (i.e. νX, α, β and μ), only three are identifiable. Thus, in fitting the hazard function to data, one constraint must be imposed on the biological parameters. A commonly used constraint is to assume a fixed value for X and to set $\nu = \mu$. Heidenreich (1996) explicitly constructs identifiable parameters when the parameters are constant. These results have been extended by Heidenreich et al. (1997a) to time-dependent parameters, e.g. with time-dependent exposure to environmental agents.

The hazard function derived from the two-mutation model has been used for the analysis of both experimental and epidemiological data (for a review, see Moolgavkar & Luebeck, 1990). When the approximate solution (equation (12)) is used, the hazard function is of the proportional hazards form if only the second mutation rate is a function of the covariates of interest. We believe now that the exact solution should always be used, and we describe briefly the analyses of two data sets, one experimental, the other epidemiological.

7.5.5 Radon and lung cancer in rats

The data included in the analysis were those obtained in rat experiments conducted under carefully controlled conditions by Dr F. Cross at the Battelle Pacific Northwest Laboratories at Richland, WA, USA. The experiments were conducted under radon-daughter exposure conditions that resulted in a dose at the cellular level of approximately 5mGy per working level month (WLM) of exposure. Data from 1797 animals exposed to radon daughters over the approximate range 320–10 240 WLM (1.1–36 Jhm^{-3}) were included in the analysis. The following information was available on each animal in the data set: the exact age when exposure to radon was begun, the radon-daughter exposure rate in WLM/week (WLM/w), the age at which exposure was stopped, the age at death or sacrifice, and the presence or absence of malignant lung tumour. All animals were followed until sacrifice or death. The objectives of the analysis were to estimate the mutation rates and intermediate cell proliferation parameters as functions of the radon exposure rates. This was achieved by maximizing the likelihood of the data. Let $P(t)$ be the probability of tumour by age t for some particular exposure-rate regimen. The survivor function is then $S(t) = 1 - P(t)$ and the hazard function $h(t) = S'(t)/S(t)$. The expressions for these quantities derived from the two-mutation model are discussed in the Appendix. In the opinion of the pathologist, the lung tumours were incidental, i.e. they did not cause the death of the animal. Thus, the likelihood of the data was constructed as follows. Because the tumours were incidental, the contribution to the likelihood by an animal that died (or was sacrificed) at age t is $P(t)$ if it had a tumour, or $S(t)$ if it was free of tumour, The full likelihood is the product of these terms over all the animals; the exact expressions and other details can be found in the relevant publication (Moolgavkar *et al.*, 1990a). Maximum likelihood estimates of the parameters were obtained. A comparison of observed and expected numbers of tumours in various exposure-rate categories indicated that the model described the data well. Radon was found to increase the first mutation rate and the net proliferation of intermediate cells, but had little effect on the second mutation rate, suggesting that the two mutational events differ in nature. The analysis also confirmed an inverse exposure-rate effect, i.e. fractionation of a given total exposure to radon increased the risk of lung cancer. Furthermore, this inverse exposure-rate effect could be attributed to the effect of radon on intermediate cell kinetics, i.e. on the promotional effect of radon.

The analysis was extended by Luebeck *et al.* (1996) to include 3750 rats exposed to varying radon regimens. New to this analysis was the parameterization of the two-mutation model such that cell killing by α particles could be explicitly considered. As in the previous analysis, the rate of the first mutation was found to be dependent on radon and consistent with *in vitro* rates measured experimentally, whereas the rate of the second mutation was not dependent on radon. An initial sharp rise in the net proliferation rate of intermediate cells was found with increasing exposure rate (model I). This model yielded an unrealistically high cell-killing coefficient. A second model (model II) was studied, in which the initial rise was attributed to promotion via a step function, implying that it was not due to radon but to the uranium ore dust that was used as a carrier aerosol. This model resulted in values for the cell-killing coefficient consistent with those found for *in vitro* cells. An inverse exposure-rate effect was seen, attributable, as in the previous analysis, to promotion of intermediate lesions. Since model II is preferable on biological grounds (it yields a plausible cell-killing coefficient), one conclusion of this analysis is that an inverse exposure-rate effect would not be seen in the absence of an irritant such as uranium ore dust.

7.5.6 Reanalysis of the Colorado Plateau uranium miners' data

Much of our knowledge regarding the interaction of radon and tobacco smoke in the aetiology of human lung cancer, derives from studies of uranium miners. We describe briefly a reanalysis of the lung cancer mortality in the Colorado Plateau uranium miners' cohort within the framework of the two-mutation model. This example is discussed in greater detail in Chapter 9. The analysis takes explicit account of the patterns of exposure to both radon and cigarette smoke experienced by individuals in the cohort. In contrast to the rat lung malignancies, which were incidental, human lung cancers are rapidly fatal. Thus, individuals who develop lung cancer contribute the probability density function for the time to tumour to the likelihood function. Individuals who do not develop lung cancer contribute the survivor function, as in the case of the experimental data. The parameters were estimated by maximizing the likelihood. As judged by a comparison of observed and expected number of lung cancers in various categories, the model described the data well. In addition, a comparison of theoretical and empirical Kaplan–Meier plots indicated that the model described the temporal pattern of failures well. A simultaneous reanalysis of the British doctors' cohort indicated that those model parameters relating to the effect of tobacco were similar in the two data sets. No evidence of interaction between radon and cigarette smoke was found with respect to their joint effect on the first or second mutation rates, or on the proliferation of intermediate cells. However, the age-specific relative risks associated with joint exposure to radon and cigarette smoke were supra-additive but submultiplicative. The analysis also confirmed an inverse exposure-rate effect, i.e. that fractionation of radon exposure leads to higher lung cancer risks. It is interesting to note that the analyses of the experimental and epidemiological data yielded consistent results despite the different likelihoods maximized. Thus, as in the case of the experimental data, analysis of the epidemiological data indicated that radon strongly affected the first mutation rate and the proliferation rate of intermediate cells. It was to the latter effect of radon that the inverse exposure-rate effect could be attributed. If the promotion of intermediate lesions is due to chronic irritation by dust in the mining environment, as the analysis of experimental data suggests (see section 7.5.5), then the inverse exposure-rate effect would not be expected with exposure to residential radon. In both epidemiological and experimental data, the second mutation rate was little affected. For details, see Moolgavkar et al.(1993).

Radon daughters are α-emitters, but the model has also been applied to γ-radiation. Little (1995, 1.996) has carried out detailed analyses of the Japanese atomic bomb survivor data using the two-mutation model and extensions of it. He concludes that "without some extra stochastic 'stage' appended (such as might be provided by consideration of the process of development of a malignant clone from a single malignant cell) the two-mutations model is perhaps not well able to describe the pattern of excess risk for solid cancers that is often seen after exposure to radiation." He prefers a three-mutation model for the atomic bomb survivor data. Little's analysis is based on consideration of mortality rather than incidence, however. For cancers that are not rapidly fatal, mortality data are a poor surrogate for incidence. The extra stochastic "stage" that Little deems necessary for a satisfactory description of the data could be construed to represent the time between occurrence of the malignant tumour and death. Little et al.(1996) analysed the incidence of acute lymphocytic leukaemia and of chronic lymphocytic leukaemia in England and Wales over the period 1971–1988, and concluded that the two-mutation model described the incidence of these leukaemias well.

Kai et al.(1997) presented analyses of the incidence of three solid cancers — lung, stomach and colon — among the cohort of atomic bomb survivors, using the two-mutation model. These analyses showed that the temporal evolution of risk following the (essentially) instantaneous exposure to radiation could be explained entirely by the hypothesis that the exposure resulted in the creation of a (dose-dependent) pool of initiated cells that was added to the pool of spontaneously initiated cells. The dose dependence of initiation was consistent with linearity down to the lowest doses in the cohort. There was no evidence of an age dependence of radiation-induced initiation, suggesting that the high excess relative risk seen in those irradiated as children is not due to an inherently higher susceptibility to radiation. Moolgavkar (1997) discussed some implications of these analyses for the assessment of radiation risks in other populations and with protraction of exposure. Heidenreich et al.(1997b) analysed the incidence of all solid cancers combined in the cohort of atomic bomb survivors, using both exact and approximate solutions of the two-mutation model, as well as two empirical models, the "age-at-exposure" model and the "age-attained" model. They concluded that these models, in which four parameters were estimated for each, described the data well, although the exact two-mutation model described some features of the data better than the other models.

7.5.7 Analysis of intermediate lesions

Many carcinogenesis experiments, and in particular initiation–promotion experiments, are characterized by the appearance of intermediate lesions, at least some of which are believed to be clones of initiated cells. Examples are provided by papillomas in mouse skin painting experiments and enzyme-altered foci in rodent hepatocarcinogenesis experiments. Because the two-mutation model explicitly considers the cell division and cell death (apoptosis) of initiated cells, it is possible to use it for the analyses of such lesions. The data are well quantified, particularly in the liver system, in which information is available on the number and size distribution of altered foci. In order to analyse these data, expressions for the number of intermediate clones together with their sizes, were derived from the two-mutation model (Dewanji et al., 1989; Luebeck & Moolgavkar, 1991). Likelihood-based methods can be used to fit the model to the data. We describe briefly the mathematical development in the Appendix; here, before doing so, we consider the consequences of explicitly considering cell division and cell death, rather than just the net rate of cell proliferation, i.e. the difference between division rate and death rate (Moolgavkar & Luebeck, 1992c):

• An important property of populations of cells undergoing cell division and cell death is that the population may become extinct. Thus, if the rate of apoptosis is greater than zero, an initiated cell will die without giving rise to a detectable lesion, such as a papilloma on the skin or an altered focus in the liver, with probability greater than zero. This conclusion may come as a surprise because the irreversibility of initiation appears to be current dogma. However, we are not asserting here that individual initiated cells revert to normal, but rather that, because initiated cells may die, initiation may be partially reversible at the level of the organ.

• If the rates of cell division and apoptosis are constant (independent of time), then the probability that an initiated cell and all its progeny will die is given (asymptotically) by the ratio of the rate of apoptosis to the rate of cell division. If the rate of apoptosis is higher than the cell division rate, then the (asymptotic) probability of extinction is 1. However, some foci may still be visible because of the stochastic nature of the process. In recent analyses of altered hepatic foci in rodent hepatocarcinogenesis experiments, it was concluded that most initiated cells (perhaps up to 90%) die without giving rise to altered foci (Moolgavkar *et al.*, 1990b; Luebeck *et al.*, 1991). Some preliminary data on cells positive for the placental form of glutathione-s-transterase (GST-P) appear to support this estimate (Satoh *et al.*, 1989; Schulte-Hermann, personal communication).

• The mean number of initiated cells at any time depends upon the rate of initiation and the net rate of intermediate cell division, $\alpha - \beta$. However, there is considerable stochastic variation around this mean number, and the actual number depends upon α and β individually, and not just upon their difference. Further, the distribution of altered cells in foci also depends upon α and β individually. Thus, for a given value of $\alpha - \beta$, large values of α and β lead to small numbers of large foci, and small values of α and β lead to large numbers of small foci. In a hypothetical example, suppose $\alpha - \beta = 0.01$ per cell per day, and suppose that one has the following two combinations of parameters: $\alpha = 0.5$, $\beta = 0.49$ and $\alpha = 0.1$, $\beta = 0.09$. Both these combinations of parameters lead to $\alpha - \beta = 0.01$ and thus to the same mean number of initiated cells, provided that the rates of initiation are identical. However, the first set of parameters

will lead to a small number of large foci, whereas the second set will lead to a large number of small foci. All other things being equal, the first combination of parameters carries a higher risk of malignant transformation than the second, because a high cell division rate implies a high mutation rate. Examples of the phenomenon described here are provided by promoters such as 4-diacetyoxyaminobenzene and the peroxisome proliferators, which lead to a small number of large foci, and others, such as *N*-nitrosodiethanolamine and phenobarbital, which lead to a large number of small foci. By measuring labelling indices, it should be possible to confirm that division rates in foci associated with the former compounds are higher than the division rates in foci associated with the latter compounds, when the doses are titrated to yield approximately the same volume fractions for the intermediate foci.

• The incidence of malignant tumours depends upon both α and β, and not just on their difference. One (biological) reason for this was pointed out above: a large cell division rate implies a large mutation rate. However, even if the mutation rates are assumed to be independent of cell division rates, the incidence function depends upon both α and β individually, as can be seen from the expression for the exact hazard function in the Appendix. This is a simple mathematical consequence of the model. Thus, simulations that take into account only the mean behaviour of cells in the intermediate compartment lead to erroneous results for the incidence of malignant tumours.

7.5.8 Rodent hepatocarcinogenesis

The mathematical expressions developed in the Appendix were used for the analysis of intermediate lesions in the rat liver model system. In a typical experiment, rats are briefly exposed to an initiator followed by long-term exposure to a promoter. Sometimes, a single agent is administered over a long period of time; this latter protocol is easier to handle mathematically. Figure 7.3 is a pictorial representation of the development of foci under an initiation–promotion regimen. The model system is characterized by the appearance in the liver of so-called enzyme-altered foci, which are clonal outgrowths, presumably of intermediate cells expressing a particular aberrant enzyme phenotype. These lesions are visible under the microscope when appropriately stained. Groups of rats exposed to varying doses of either initiator or promoter or both are sacrificed at various times, and their livers are sectioned and examined for enzyme-altered foci. The data consist of information on the number of (two-dimensional) foci seen per unit area in the liver cross-section and the sizes (radii in microns) of each of the two-dimensional sections of foci. Thus, the observation on each rat is a vector with the first entry being the number of two-dimensional sections of foci observed and the remaining entries consisting of the radii in microns of these observed sections. Since the rats are exposed to different doses of the agents under study and are sacrificed at different times, the observed vectors are functions of both dose and time. The objectives of the analysis are to estimate the parameters of the mathematical model as functions of the dose of the agent under study, and thus to quantitate the initiating and promoting actions of the agent. Two complications arise in the analysis. The first arises from stereological considerations: although the foci in the liver are three-dimensional, they are observed on cross-section in two dimensions. The second complication arises from the fact that the mathematical model yields the size of the foci in terms of the number of cells in them, whereas the observed measurement is in microns. The first complication is addressed by using a well known formula in stereology due to Wicksell (1925). A similar approach was used by Keiding *et al.* (1972). In order to address the second, information is required about the size of the altered hepatocyte. Some data are available in the literature (Jack *et al.*, 1990). Details on likelihood construction and maximization are omitted in the interests of space; they are described by Moolgavkar *et al.* (1990b), Luebeck *et al.*(1991), and Moolgavkar *et al.*(1996). A summary is given in the Appendix. In the first paper, a single-agent regimen was analysed. Rats were chronically exposed to *N*-nitrosomorpholine (NNM) in their drinking-water. The objective of the analysis was to characterize the action of NNM in terms of its initiating and promoting activities. In the other two papers, initiation–promotion (two-agent) protocols were analysed. The objective was to investigate the pro-

moting activities of various polychlorinated biphenyls (PCBs) and dioxin. One of the interesting conclusions of the analyses was that a large number, perhaps 90%, of initiated cells never develop into foci but become extinct. The dioxin example is discussed in Chapter 8.

A fundamental stereological assumption has heretofore been made in all analyses of altered hepatic foci, namely, that these foci are perfectly spherical. The classical methods employed by experimentalists use a "binning" procedure introduced by Saltykov to estimate the number of three-dimensional spheres in certain predetermined size classes from information on two-dimensional discs (see, e.g. Campbell *et al.*, (1986)). These methods are based on the explicit assumption that the foci are spherical. More recently, Nychka and colleagues (1984) used smoothing techniques to estimate the size distribution of foci from the size distribution of two-dimensional sections of foci. Their approach makes crucial use of a formula due to Wicksell (1925), which applies only to spheres. Moreover, their smoothing technique requires more data than are usually available in the typical experiment. The approach used by Moolgavkar and colleagues is different. Instead of using a stereological procedure to reconstruct the three-dimensional picture in the liver, they used stereology to translate the mathematical expressions for the three-dimensional quantities (e.g. number and size of foci) derived from the stochastic model into two-dimensional expressions that can then be fitted directly to the data. Keiding *et al.* (1972) used a similar approach to study the size distribution of nuclei in sections of the liver. However, both in Keiding's work and in that of Moolgavkar *et al.*, the Wicksell formula plays a prominent role, i.e. the assumption of spherical foci is crucial. Some preliminary attempts (Imaida *et al.*, 1989) have been made to study the bias in the Saltykov procedure that may be introduced by departures from sphericity; no systematic study has been undertaken, however. There is clear evidence that many hepatic foci are not spherical. Moreover, foci in other organs such as the kidney are far from spherical. Thus, there is a clear need for stereological methods that do not depend upon the assumption that foci are spherical. An approach to this problem has recently been proposed by Dewanji *et al.* (1996).

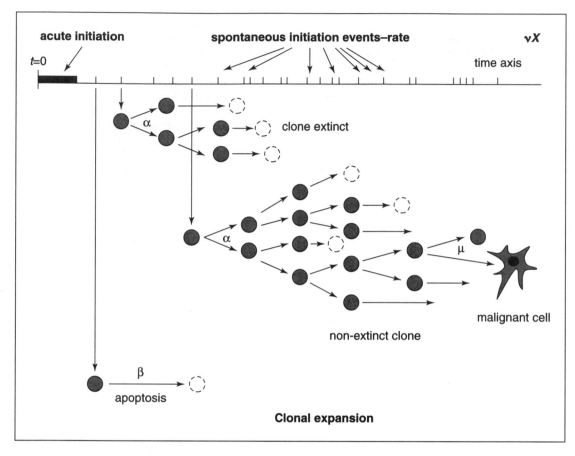

Figure 7.3. Schematic representation of clonal expansion processes. Altered cells are initiated during acute initiation at time $t = 0$ and spontaneously thereafter. Initiated cells (dark) may either divide or undergo apoptosis. If all cells in a clone undergo apoptosis, the clone becomes extinct. The probability of this occurring is high when the clone is small.

The methods discussed above cannot be applied to the analyses of very small foci. There is currently great interest in the analyses of foci with a single cell or a few cells, and statistical methods for the analyses of such small foci are now under development (deGunst & Luebeck, 1997).

7.5.9 Initiation–promotion in mouse skin

In a recent paper, Kopp-Schneider & Portier (1992) have applied similar methods to the analysis of papilloma counts in initiation–promotion experiments on mouse skin. The experiments consisted of a single application of 7,8-dimethylbenz[*a*]anthracene (DMBA) followed by repeated applications of a phorbol ester. Because papillomas are directly observable, the stereological

problems that arise in the analyses of the liver foci data are not encountered in the analyses of these data. However, there are other problems. Whereas the cells in an altered hepatic focus are generally considered to be homogeneous, the papillomas consist of cells of many different types. Thus the number of "initiated" cells in a papilloma is not known, and a parameter representing a threshold number of "initiated" cells above which papillomas become visible must be estimated from the data. In addition, since the papillomas are counted on the same animals followed forward in time, the counts at different times are not independent. Special care must be exercised when drawing inferences from such correlated longitudinal data; for details, see the paper by Kopp-Schneider & Portier (1992), who concluded that DMBA initiated a large number of cells, most of which did not give rise to visible papillomas. Furthermore, promoter treatment increased both the cell division rate and the rate of apoptosis. Perhaps most surprising is their finding that, during promotion, the rate of apoptosis was higher than that of cell division. This explains why a large number of initiated cells did not give rise to visible papillomas. Their analyses lead to some interesting conclusions, e.g. even when the rate of cell death of initiated cells is higher than that of cell division, stochastic fluctuations may lead to clonal growth of a few of these cells and to visible papillomas. They also predict that, unless either the growth kinetics of the papillomas change over time or one of the initiated cells in a papilloma becomes malignant, all papillomas will eventually become extinct.

7.5.10 Joint analyses of premalignant and malignant lesions

In many experimental data sets, information is available both on malignant and benign tumours. If the benign tumours are known to lie on the pathway to malignancy, it is important that they be considered in any analysis of the data. Currently, either the premalignant lesions are ignored or they are included in the malignant lesions. Both these procedures have obvious deficiencies. The first discards valuable information, and the second gives equal weight to premalignant and malignant lesions, which is clearly inappropriate. Recently, attempts have been made to quantify the appearance of foci within foci, i.e. the appearance of small islands, presumably clonal, of cells within altered hepatic foci, characterized by a second phenotypic change. These foci within foci may represent the earliest stage of malignancy. The mathematical tools required for analyses of data in which information on both premalignant and malignant lesions is available are currently being developed (Dewanji et al., 1991; de Gunst & Luebeck, 1994). Considerations of space preclude further consideration of this topic here.

7.5.11 Limitations of biologically based models

We have given examples here of the use of biologically based models for the analyses of epidemiological and experimental data. These models provide a flexible family of hazard functions for the analyses of time-to-tumour data. Time-and-age-dependent covariates are particularly easy to incorporate into these hazard functions. The models also provide mathematical expressions that can be used for analyses of data on intermediate lesions on the pathway to cancer. The parameters of the models can be directly interpreted in biological terms. It should he noted, however, that whether these interpretations are meaningful or not will depend upon how faithfully the model describes the underlying biological processes. Any model is an abstraction of reality. It is not possible to incorporate explicitly all that is known about carcinogenesis into any model, and there is an element of personal judgement in deciding which features of the carcinogenic process are essential in a model. Thus, the conclusions derived from fitting biological models to data should be viewed, not as statements of biological truth, but as hypotheses to be tested in future epidemiological or experimental studies. For example, analyses of both experimental and epidemiological data on radon-induced lung cancer confirms the inverse exposure-rate effect, and suggest that this effect is attributable to the promotional effect of radon. This hypothesis could be tested in future experimental studies.

A good statistical fit of a particular model to experimental or observational data does not validate the model. Any flexible model with as few as three disposable parameters is likely to be capable of describing a wide variety of outcomes. It follows that most data sets can be adequately described by statistical models without any biological basis, and that two different biologically based models may provide equally good fits to the data simply because of their statistical flexibility.

True model validation requires more than statistical goodness of fit. Ideally, the model should be developed using data from a number of different sources dealing with specific aspects of the model. For example, direct measures of tissue growth, key rate-limiting mutation rates, and the birth and death rates of intermediate cells could be used to accurately identify specific model components, and avoid the "overfitting" that is possible with multiparametric models applied to summary data on tumour occurrence rates. This does not appear to be currently feasible. Estimates of parameters obtained by fitting the two-mutation model to data suggest that the rates of cell division and death are closely linked, as is to be expected. Small perturbations in one of these rates without a compensatory change in the other can lead to very large changes in the incidence rates generated by the model. Currently available experimental methods yield measures of cell division and cell death that are too imprecise to be used directly in it. The best that can be done is to assess whether estimates of these quantities obtained by fitting the model to data are broadly consonant with experimental measurements.

The two-mutation model, which is the central focus of the modelling efforts described here, assumes that two rate-limiting events are involved in the carcinogenic process, and that cell division and cell death are important, although these are explicitly considered only for cells in the intermediate stage. A number of assumptions, both biological, and in the translation of biology into mathematical form, are therefore made in this model. An example of the latter type is that the lifetime of cells has an exponential distribution. Each of these types of assumption is open to question and may affect the conclusions drawn from the model. For example, there is now laboratory evidence suggesting that more than two rate-limiting events may be involved in the carcinogenic process. Little (1995, 1996) has suggested that, although a two-mutation model describes the epidemiological data on atomic bomb survivors quite well, some subtle features of the data are better described by a three-mutation model.

In summary, biologically based models provide a useful complement to the usual statistical models for the analyses of data. Generally, these models describe the data as well as statistical models, while allowing individual-level time- and age-dependent covariates to be incorporated into the analyses fairly easily. Conclusions of a biological nature, e.g. regarding the mechanism of action of the agent under investigation, must be considered as tentative and needing to be tested in future studies. A more detailed discussion of some of the issues raised here is given in Chapter 9.

7.5.12 Data requirements

It should be evident from the discussion of biologically based models that, in order to exploit

the full potential of these models, fundamental biological information is required. This topic is discussed in Chapter 9. It is quite clear that the usual bioassay with a control group and three different dose groups sacrificed at the same time will not provide the kind of information required for dose–response modelling.

An example of the application of the two-mutation model to quantitative cancer risk assessment (US National Research Council, 1993) has recently been presented. The data consisted of information on the number of animals with liver tumours at 78 weeks of age in each of four groups of mice: a control group and groups of mice exposed to chlordane, a termiticide, at 5, 25 and 50 ppm in the diet. For the purposes of risk assessment, chlordane was assumed to be a promoter, i.e. to increase the net rate of proliferation $(\alpha - \beta)$ of intermediate cells. Two parametric forms for $\alpha - \beta$ as a function of dose were assumed, and the probability of tumour at 78 weeks as a function of dose was fitted to the data using each of these dose–response functions and both the exact and approximate forms of the two-mutation model. The resulting four curves are shown in Figure 2, p. 209, of the National Research Council report. It was noted that, for a given dose–response function for $\alpha - \beta$, both the exact and approximate solutions fitted the data equally well, and gave similar results for extrapolation of risk (probability of tumour at 78 weeks) to low doses. It was further noted that, for a given solution to the model (exact or approximate), extrapolation to low doses was strongly dependent upon the form of the dose–response function for the net rate of proliferation of intermediate cells. Thus, one form of the dose–response curve for net proliferation yielded risks at low levels of exposure that were several orders of magnitude higher than those derived from the other form of the dose–response curve.

The conclusions of this analysis were that the shape of the dose–response curve for probability of tumour at low doses is very sensitive to assumptions regarding the dose–response of the parameters of the model, and that the exact and approximate solutions yielded essentially identical results. Some comments on these conclusions are in order. It is indeed true that the particular functional form assumed for the parameters of the model is a critical determinant of the behaviour of the dose–response function at low doses. A simple Taylor series argument, described in the US National Research Council report, shows this. However, it would be a mistake to conclude that the approximate solution may be used in place of the exact solution for analyses. With typical bioassay data (a control group, three dose groups and only one time of observation), it may be true that the approximate solution fits the data as well as the exact solution. With richer data, for example, with serial sacrifice or epidemiological cohort data, the approximate solution can yield results that are very different from those obtained by using the exact solution. Moreover, the important issues have to do not only with fit, but also with parameter estimates and inferences drawn from the model. Even with the sparse data set analysed in the above-mentioned report, the parameter estimates obtained by fitting the approximate model are quite different from those obtained by fitting the exact model. Furthermore, the inferences drawn from the analyses can be quite different as well. For example, cigarette smoking and lung cancer mortality were studied in a cohort of British doctors using both the approximate solution (Moolgavkar et al., 1989) and the exact one (Moolgavkar et al., 1993) to the two-mutation model. The former analysis suggested that the proliferation kinetics of the intermediate cells were little affected by cigarette smoke, whereas the latter indicated that cigarette smoke was a strong promoter. Finally, as noted above, the qualitative behaviour of the exact and approximate hazard functions is quite different. With time–dependent exposures, in particular, use of the approximate hazard function could be quite misleading.

One further point must be emphasized about the chlordane bioassay data analysed in the US National Research Council (1993) report. Even for a bioassay, this is a particularly poor data set. As can be seen from Figure 2 on page 209 of that report, the dose–response curve for the probability of tumour at 78 weeks is S-shaped. The actual data consist of tumour counts at 0, 5, 25 and 50 ppm. The first two data points lie on the lower leg of the S, before the curve has begun to rise, the other two on the upper leg of the S, i.e. after the curve has reached the point of saturation. Thus, there are no data in the most critical part of the dose–response curve, i.e. when it is rising. With a few data points in this critical range, it might have been possible to discriminate between the two postulated functional forms for $\alpha - \beta$.

7.6 Pharmacokinetic modelling

Pharmacokinetics is the study of the absorption, distribution, metabolism and elimination of xenobiotics in biological systems. By studying the fate of chemicals entering the body, it is possible to obtain information on the amount of either the parent compound or its metabolites reaching tissues that may be targets for the induction of cancerous lesions. Pharmacokinetics thus affords an opportunity to incorporate information on tissue dose in cancer risk assessment. Pharmacokinetic models permit an evaluation of the relationship between tissue dose and toxic response under different conditions of exposure. They also offer considerable insight into non-linear relationships that may exist between the level of exposure to environmental carcinogens and the dose of toxic metabolites reaching target tissues. In such cases, the use of tissue doses rather then environmental exposure levels will lead to more accurate estimates of potential cancer risk.

The development of physiologically based pharmacokinetic (PBPK) models has provided a powerful tool for tissue dosimetry. Such models attempt to describe the processes that regulate chemical disposition, taking into account the physiological characteristics of the biological system under study. In PBPK modelling, a biological system is envisaged as consisting of a small number of physiologically relevant compartments. The model is characterized by actual physiological parameters such as body weight, cardiac output, breathing rates, blood flow rates and tissue volumes. Biochemical parameters are used to describe the partitioning of the parent chemical or its metabolites among target tissues. Pharmacokinetic constants are also used to describe removal processes such as hepatic metabolism.

PBPK models offer a number of advantages over the compartmental models used previously in classical pharmacokinetic analyses. A physiologically based model can be interpreted in biological terms, and lead to an understanding of the actual pharmacokinetic processes governing chemical disposition in the body. Lack of fit of a particular model may suggest alternative hypotheses about pharmacokinetic processes involved in the distribution and metabolism of xenobiotics. PBPK models also offer a powerful tool for predicting target tissue dose from one route of exposure to another and between species. Once a PBPK model has been established for inhalation exposure, the same model can be used to predict doses in internal tissues following dermal exposure after modifying only those model parameters governing uptake by the body into the circulatory system. Similarly, a PBPK model established on the basis of studies in non-human mammalian species can be applied to humans after substituting the appropriate allometric, biochemical, and pharmacokinetic parameters for humans. Finally, by providing a means of estimating the dose of reactive metabolites reaching target tissues, PBPK models may lead to more accurate predictions of risk than can be obtained using environmental exposure levels, particularly when saturation effects lead to a non-linear relationship between environmental exposures and tissue doses.

7.6.1 Development of a PBPK model

A PBPK model envisages the body, as consisting of a small number of physiological compartments. Each compartment represents a relatively homogeneous group of organs or tissues, linked to the central blood compartment by arterial and venous blood flow. The model is characterized by physiological parameters such as tissue volumes and blood flow rates, biochemical parameters such as partition coefficients, and kinetic parameters for metabolism and removal.

7.6.1.1 Mathematical description of a PBPK model

A PBPK model is described mathematically by a system of non-linear partial differential equations that consist of a mass balance equation describing the entry and exit of xenobiotics in each compartment in the model. This system of equations can be solved simultaneously to predict the concentration of metabolites in each compartment as a function of time.

As an illustration, consider a single physiological compartment as shown in Figure 7.4. Here, $X(t)$ denotes the mass of the parent com-

pound or its metabolites in the compartment at time t. The concentration of this substance is then $C(t) = X(t)/U$, where U denotes the volume of the tissue in that compartment. The arterial and venous blood concentrations, denoted by $A(t)$ and $V(t)$ respectively, reflect the entry of the substance to the compartment and its exit from it via the circulatory system. (To maintain continuity of blood flow, the rates of arterial and venous blood flow are assumed to be equal.) In some cases, the compound of interest may enter or leave the compartment by pathways other than blood. The rates of the substance entering and leaving the compartment by non-circulatory pathways are denoted by $Y(t)$ and $Z(t)$, respectively.

With this notation, the mass balance equation for the compartment in Figure 7.4 is given by:

$$dX(t)/dt = Q[A(t) - V(t)] + Y(t) - Z(t), \qquad (14)$$

where Q denotes the rate of blood flow. If the solubility of the substance is the same in the tissue in this compartment as in blood, the concentration of the substance in the compartment is simply:

$$C(t) = V(t).$$

In the case of differential solubility in tissue and blood, we may write:

$$C(t) = V(t)P,$$

where P is the tissue-to-blood partition coefficient. Measurement of the partition coefficient P, which is greater than unity if the compound is more soluble in tissue than in blood and less than unity otherwise, is discussed later in this section.

More complex processes can also be described using extensions of the simple mass balance equation (14) above. Tissue solubility may change with dose if protein binding is saturable. Leung et al. (1990a) found it necessary to include a complex secondary binding mechanism to describe the metabolism of 2,3,7,8-tetrachlorodibenzo-p-dioxin (TCDD) in liver. Separate mass balance equations are needed for the blood compartment, or possibly a combined lung–blood compartment (Ramsay & Andersen, 1984).

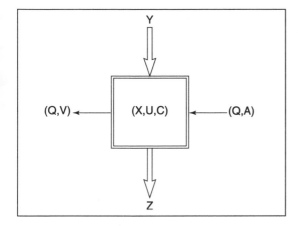

Figure 7.4. Schematic representation of a basic pharmacokinetic compartment (A = arterial blood concentration, V = venous blood concentration, Q = blood flow rate, X = mass of substance, C = compartmental concentration, U = compartmental volume, Y = input, Z = removal). Source: Krewski et al. (1991)

Separate equations are needed to describe direct input to, and removal from the body. In the case of intravenous injection of a dose d of a particular compound at time t_k directly into the blood compartment,

$$Y_b(t) = d\delta(t - t_k),$$

where $\delta(t)$ denotes the Dirac delta function and $Y_b(t)$ denotes the amount of the compound entering the blood supply at time t. Oral and dermal uptake can be described using first-order kinetics, or Michaelis–Menten kinetics (Michaelis & Menten, 1913; Gibaldi & Perrier, 1975) when uptake is saturable.

Removal can be accommodated in a similar manner. For water-soluble substances eliminated in urine, we have:

$$Z_k(t) = K_k U_k V_k(t),$$

where $Z_k(t)$ denotes the rate at which the substance is removed from the kidney, K_k is the removal coefficient, U_k is the volume of the kidney, and $V_k(t)$ is the venous concentration in the kidney. Implementation of this particular removal process is accomplished by isolating the kidney as a separate compartment attached to the liver (cf. Paustenbach et al., 1988).

Krewski et al. (1991) discuss the development of the mass balance equations to describe a general PBPK model in more detail. If all of the differential mass balance equations used to characterize the dynamics of individual compartments are linear, then a closed form solution of this system can be obtained by analytical means. In most cases, however, one or more processes involved in the system will be saturable, leading to a system of non-linear partial differential equations that must be solved using numerical methods. This can be done using computer software specifically designed for use in solving PBPK models (Mitchell & Gauthier, 1992; Steiner et al., 1989).

7.6.1.2 Selection of model compartments.

Physiological compartments should ideally be as homogeneous as possible. At the same time, the number of compartments should be kept small to simplify the analysis and interpretation of the results.

Fiserova-Bergerova (1983) suggests that tissues in which chemical concentrations increase or decrease at the same rate may be included in the same physiological compartment. Based on this criterion, richly perfused tissues such as the liver and kidneys could be combined to form a single class, and poorly perfused tissues such as skin and fat amalgamated to form another class. Since metabolism in the liver represents a function of particular importance in pharmacokinetics, the liver is usually treated as a special compartment. Furthermore, since fat will demonstrate a high partition coefficient for lipophilic compounds, fatty tissue is often considered as a separate compartment, particularly when studying fat-soluble substances. Blood is also considered as a single compartment because it provides chemical transport to all compartments in the body.

These considerations suggest the use of a PBPK model with the following five compartments: blood, liver, richly perfused tissue, poorly perfused tissue, and fat (Figure 7.5). With some variations, this basic five-compartment model has been widely used in PBPK modelling. With volatile compounds, for example, the blood compartment may be replaced by a blood/lung compartment. In other cases, unique target tissues such as mammary or foetal tissue may be explicitly defined as separate compartments (Fisher et al., 1988, 1989; O'Flaherty et al., 1992).

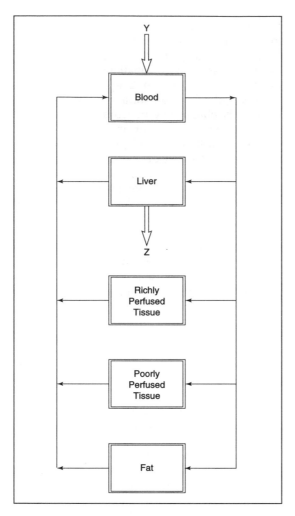

Figure 7.5. A five-compartment PBPK model. Source: Krewski *et al.* (1991)

7.6.2 Determination of physiological, biochemical and metabolic parameters

As was seen previously, the behaviour of a PBPK model is characterized by a system of differential equations that describe the flow, tissue binding, and metabolism of a chemical entering the body. These mass balance equations for the influx, efflux and removal of the chemical in each compartment are defined using relevant physiological, physicochemical, and biochemical parameters. Depending on the specific features incorporated, even a relatively simple five compartment model such as that illustrated in Figure 7.5

can involve more than 20 different parameters. Estimates of the values of all of these parameters are required before the model can be solved.

7.6.2.1 Physiological parameters

Physiological parameters of interest include tissue volumes, blood flow rates, cardiac output, and alveolar ventilation. Arms & Travis (1988) have compiled reference values for these and other physiological parameters for a generic 25-g mouse, a 250-g rat and a 70-kg man.

When such parameters are unavailable for an untested species, or parameter values are desired for individuals of different body weights, values can be estimated by scaling methods. Many of the physiological parameters required in PBPK models vary with body weight according to the power function:

$$Y = aW^b. \tag{15}$$

Here, Y is the physiological parameter of interest, W denotes body weight, and a and b are constants (Fiserova-Bergerova & Hughes, 1983). If $b = 1$, the parameter Y scales in direct proportion to body weight; if $b = 2/3$, Y is roughly proportional to body surface area. Tissue volume scales across species based on equation (15) with $0.70 < b < 0.99$, depending on the tissue considered (Aldolph, 1949). In interspecies scaling of cardiac output, a value of $b = 3/4$ appears to be more appropriate (Takezawa *et al.*, 1980).

7.6.2.2 Partition coefficients.

Partition coefficients are used to measure the affinity of a compound to tissues in the different compartments of a PBPK model. The partition coefficient P of a chemical between two media is defined as the ratio of the chemical concentration in the first medium to that in the second medium. A commonly used method for determining partition coefficients is the vial equilibration technique described by Sato & Nakajima (1979). With this approach, a known amount of the chemical in air, tissue, and blood is then measured. The inverse ratios of the concentration in air to the concentration in blood and the concentration in tissue are called the blood-to-air and tissue-to-air partition coefficients, respectively. The tissue-to-blood partition coefficient is then obtained by taking the ratio of the tissue-to-air and blood-to-air partition coefficients. Other approaches for measuring partition coefficients for non-volatile chemicals include *in vitro* equilibrium dialysis (Lin *et al.*, 1982) and *in vivo* constant infusion methods (Chen & Gros, 1979).

7.6.2.3 Metabolic parameters.

Biochemical constants governing metabolism have been estimated using different techniques, including measurement of the total amount of metabolites formed as a function of dose (Ghering *et al.*, 1978); examination of whole-body clearance (Andersen *et al.*, 1984); estimation of kinetic constants for metabolism *in vitro*; the study of clearance characteristics of isolated perfused livers (Rane *et al.*, 1977); or the use of non-invasive inhalation techniques (Gargas *et al.*, 1986; Gargas & Andersen, 1989).

If metabolism is mediated by an enzyme whose supply is limited with respect to the time of the reaction, the rate of metabolism will saturate as a function of time. This saturation effect is described by the Michaelis–Menten equation:

$$dM_m(t)/dt = V_{max}V(t)/[K_m + V(t)], \qquad (16)$$

where M_m is the amount of the metabolite formed, $V(t)$ is the concentration of the substrate in venous blood at time t, V_{max} is the maximum metabolic rate possible for the reaction, and K_m is the Michaelis constant defined as the venous blood concentration at which the metabolic rate is half V_{max}. When the rate of metabolism is not saturable, the rate of formation of the metabolite follows first-order kinetics with:

$$dM_m(t)/dt = kUV(t) \qquad (17)$$

Here, U is the volume of the tissue compartment (usually the liver) in which metabolism occurs, and k is the linear metabolic rate constant.

7.6.3 Tissue dosimetry

In the past, some measure of the exposure of the whole body has been used as a dose metameter for predicting carcinogenic risk. More accurate estimates of risk may be possible if some measure is used of the dose of reactive metabolites reaching target tissues. Moving closer to the site of pharmacodynamic action leads to more direct measures of exposure, transcending saturation efFects that can occur during metabolic activation. Although PBPK models provide a means of predicting tissue doses, consideration needs to be given to the most appropriate measure of dose to the target tissue.

Andersen (1981) suggested the use of an integrated measure of tissue dose based on the area under the concentration–time curve (AUC) for either the parent compound or its reactive metabolites in the tissue of interest. Specifically, the AUC for the parent compound in blood is defined by:

$$AUC_b = \int_0^\infty C_b(t)dt,$$

where $C_b(t)$ denotes the concentration in blood at time t. The AUC for serum can be determined by measuring the concentration of the parent compound in blood samples taken at frequent intervals. This cannot be done in most other compartments, however, since most tissue samples require destructive sampling. Once a PBPK model has been developed, however, it can be used to predict the concentration of metabolites in any of the tissue compartments included in the model.

For a linear PBPK model, the AUC of the parent compound in blood following intravenous administration of a single dose d can be expressed as:

$$AUC_b = d(1/Q_l + 1/k_l),$$

which involves only the blood flow rate Q_l to the liver and the rate of metabolism k_l in the liver. If the PBPK model has been well validated, this relationship can be used to estimate the AUC in blood without direct measurement of blood concentrations over time. The AUCs of the parent compound in other compartments are related to those in serum. For example, it can be shown that in liver:

$$AUC_l = P_l (AUC_b - d/Q_l).$$

Further data on the relationship between the AUC in target tissues and the AUC in blood are given by Pelekis *et al.* (1997).

7.6.4 Applications

Considerable experience with the development and application of PBPK models for toxic chemicals now exists. While PBPK models for volatile anaesthetics date back to Haggard (1924), these models were not widely applied to toxic chemicals until the 1970s. One of the earliest applications in toxicology was the development of a PBPK model for styrene by Ramsay & Andersen (1984). By analysing existing pharmacokinetic data, they deduced the partition coefficients and metabolic rates for styrene. The PBPK model used included compartments for the lung (as the site of uptake), fat (a storage depot), liver (the primary site of metabolism), richly perfused tissue (such as kidney and brain), and slowly perfused tissue (including muscle). Metabolism was saturable at inhalation exposures above 200 ppm for 6 h in mice and rats. The model was validated against other data from rats and humans, and used for dose-route, dose-level, and interspecies extrapolation.

One of the best known examples of PBPK modelling is its application to methylene chloride (Andersen et al., 1987). With methylene chloride, all model parameters except those governing metabolism were estimated without temporal observations on tissue concentrations (Gargas et al., 1990); metabolic constants were estimated from specialized gas-uptake studies utilizing a PBPK model for data analysis (Gargas et al., 1986).

The metabolism of methylene chloride proceeds via two pathways: oxidation by cytochrome P-450 enzyme systems, and conjugation by glutathione transferase enzymes. PBPK models for methylene chloride have focused on metabolism by these two pathways in the liver and lung, the two target sites for carcinogenicity in the mouse, and have implicated metabolites generated by the glutathione transferase pathway as being primarily responsible for tumour induction.

To date, more than 40 toxic chemicals have been subjected to PBPK modelling. Recent reviews have been provided by Andersen et al. (1993) and Krewski et al. (1993). This extensive experience with PBPK modelling has clearly established the feasibility of this methodology as a tool for tissue dosimetry.

7.6.5 Uncertainty, variability and sensitivity analyses

PBPK models require information on a number of parameters (including physiological, physicochemical, and biochemical constants) in order to simulate the kinetic behaviour of a chemical and its metabolites in the body. Uncertainty in the values of these parameters results in uncertainty in model-based predictions of tissue dose. Model parameters may also vary among individuals in a particular population, resulting in variability in the tissue doses received by different individuals in that population.

Predictions of tissue dose may be more sensitive to changes in certain model parameters than others. For example, the loss of a volatile chemical from within a closed chamber due to metabolism by study subjects within the chamber can be quite sensitive to the kinetic constants for metabolism, ventilation, or even blood flow (Gargas et al., 1990). Recently, Krewski et al.(1997) examined the uncertainty and sensitivity associated with parameters in PBPK models for three volatile organic compounds. Monte Carlo simulations indicated that the rate of cardiac output and fractional blood flow to richly perfused tissues and liver were the largest contributors to uncertainty in predicted tissue doses.

Uncertainty in the values of PBPK model parameters will lead to uncertainty in the estimates of cancer risk derived from model-based predictions of tissue dose. In a pioneering paper on this subject, Portier & Kaplan (1989) used a PBPK model for methylene chloride to evaluate uncertainty in predictions of lifetime risk arising as a consequence of uncertainty in the PBPK model parameters. In this analysis, a PBPK model was used to predict the concentrations of metabolites in lung and liver tissue, and a one-stage pharmacodynamic model to predict cancer risk in relation to tissue dose. Estimates of the uncertainty in the PBPK model parameters were based on published data, when available; otherwise, coefficients of variation for uncertainty in the model parameters were assigned values of 20–200%. This analysis demonstrated that allowing for uncertainty in the model parameters led to a relatively wide range of values for the corresponding range of cancer risk estimates. Although it did not allow for correlations among the model parameters and was based on a somewhat arbitrary assignment of variability to some of them, it is instructive in demonstrating how PBPK models can be used to evaluate at least part of the uncertainty in cancer risk estimates based on joint applications of pharmacokinetic and pharmacodynamic models. Krewski *et al.*(1995) have addressed the question of correlation among model parameters.

Other studies of the impact of the uncertainty in the parameters of PBPK models for tetrachloroethylene (Farrar *et al.*, 1989); benzene (Bois *et al.*, 1991), and styrene, methylchloroform and methylene chloride (Hetrick *et al.*, 1991) have also been conducted. This last study demonstrated that the extent of model sensitivity to parameter values may depend on the dose of the parent compound, the time at which tissue doses are predicted, and the species for which the PBPK model was developed.

It is important to recognize that, even though the uncertainty associated with cancer risk estimates for methylene chloride appeared to increase with the use of pharmacokinetic data, such estimates may well be more accurate than those based on external measures of exposure. Consideration thus needs to be given to risk estimation methods that optimize this gain in accuracy in relation to possible increased uncertainty. Statistically, it is desirable to minimize the mean squared error of estimates of risk, which takes into account both bias and precision.

7.6.6 Summary and conclusions

In this section, the development and application of PBPK models in cancer risk assessment has been discussed. In general terms, such models envisage a biological system as consisting of a small number of relatively homogeneous physiological compartments. They are characterized mathematically 'by systems of non-linear differential mass balance equations that can be readily solved using computer software developed specifically for this purpose.

The construction of appropriate PBPK models to describe the kinetic properties of specific chemicals is not a trivial undertaking. Model development requires information about the relevant physiological compartments and the physiological, physicochemical and biochemical parameters that characterize the model.

Once developed and tested, a PBPK model can be used to predict the dose of reactive metabolites reaching target tissues.

Substantial practical experience has now accumulated with PBPK models, and has demonstrated their utility as tools for describing the pharmacokinetic behaviour of toxic chemicals and predicting the dose of reactive metabolites reaching target tissues. In addition to providing a more relevant measure of exposure for risk-assessment applications, PBPK models facilitate extrapolations between different routes of exposure and between different species. To date, PBPK models have been developed for more than 40 different chemicals.

For applications in QEP, it is important to establish a clear linkage between the tissue doses predicted by the PBPK model and pharmacodynamic effects associated with tumour induction. Linkage of pharmacokinetic and pharmacodynamic effects provides a more complete description of the process of chemical carcinogenesis, and offers the promise of improved estimates of cancer risk. While the use of tissue dose rather than external measures of exposure may lead to more accurate estimates of risk, the uncertainty associated with PBPK-model-based predictions of tissue dose must not be overlooked. This uncertainty can be evaluated by considering the precision associated with each of the model parameters, and by identifying those parameters to which predictions of tissue dose are most sensitive.

7.7 Receptor-binding models

Receptor-mediated mechanisms are known to play an important role in chemical carcinogenesis (Lucier, 1992).

In basic ligand-receptor information theory, the term ligand is used to refer to drugs, toxic materials, antibodies, and other agents that act upon living cells (Denes *et al.*, 1996). The active site of the cell acted upon by the ligand L is the receptor R. Ligand–receptor interactions are presumed to satisfy the following assumptions: (1) the interaction between ligand and receptor is reversible; (2) the ligand can exist in two states: free or receptor bound; (3) the biological response is measured when the interaction between ligand and receptor has reached the state of equilibrium;

(4) the biological response is proportional to the number of occupied receptors.

The interaction between the ligand and its receptor is described by the stoichiometric equation:

$$L + R \overset{k_1}{\underset{k_{-1}}{=}} RL, \qquad (19)$$

where RL denotes the receptor–ligand complex and k_1 and k_{-1} are the forward and reverse reaction rates. The biological response is proportional to $[RL]$. By the law of mass action, we have:

$$\frac{[L]\,[R]}{[RL]} = \frac{k_{-1}}{k_1} = K \qquad (20)$$

at equilibrium, where K is the dissociation constant. Since a receptor may be either occupied or unoccupied, we have:

$$[R] + [RL] = [R_T] = r, \qquad (21)$$

where R_T is the total number of receptors. Hence:

$$[RL] = \frac{[L]}{[L] + K} \qquad (22)$$

Equation 22 can be generalized to:

$$[RL] = r\,\frac{[L]^n}{[L]^n + K} \qquad (23)$$

which is known as the Hill equation with exponent n (cf. Denes $et\ al.$, 1996).

More complex receptor-binding models of this type have been used to describe the toxic effects of 2,3,7,8-tetrachlorodibenzo-p-dioxin (TCDD). This is a persistent environmental contaminant that induces a broad spectrum of toxicological effects, including thymic atrophy, birth defects, and immunological effects (Silbergeld & Gasiewicz, 1989). It is also considered to be the most potent carcinogen among the halogenated aromatic hydrocarbons. Chronic treatment with as little as 10 µg/kg is sufficient to induce liver tumours in female rats (Kociba $et\ al.$, 1978; US National Toxicology Program, 1982).

TCDD is a potent, non-genotoxic tumour promoter (Pitot & Campbell, 1987; Kociba, 1984). In cells treated with TCDD, no DNA adducts could be detected, even using sensitive methods capable of detecting 1 adduct in 10^{11} nucleotides (Turtletaub $et\ al.$, 1991). Furthermore, TCDD is inactive in assays for genotoxic activity (Wassom $et\ al.$, 1977). The biological effects of TCDD are believed to be mediated by the binding of TCDD to a cytosolic receptor, the Ah receptor which sets off a complex cascade of events ultimately resulting in altered gene transcription.

Kohn & Portier (1993) developed a model for describing the action of TCDD and other halogenated aromatic hydrocarbons. In this model, it is assumed that the xenobiotic acts through the excess production of a particular protein such as cytochrome P-450. This protein is produced thanks to the presence of a natural ligand with which the xenobiotic interacts competitively. It is also produced continually, regardless of the presence of the xenobiotic or the natural ligand. The ligand first binds to a receptor with multiple binding sites, and the ligand–receptor complex binds to a DNA site, inducing the protein. The xenobiotic now competes with the ligand for receptor sites, and the xenobiotic–receptor complex competes with the ligand–receptor complex for DNA binding sites according to Hill kinetics.

Kohn & Portier (1993) used this model to conduct a theoretical study of the shape of the dose–response curves of TCDD and related xenobiotics. The dose–response curve is consistent with linearity at low doses, but non-linearity cannot be ruled out. Values of the Hill exponent of less than 1 imply supralinearity at lower doses, and shift the inflection point of the overall sigmoidal curve to lower doses. Positive cooperation, characterized by Hill exponents greater than 1, is associated with sublinearity in the low-dose region and a shift of the inflection point of the sigmoid curve to higher doses. Further results are reported by Portier $et\ al.$ (1993) and Kohn $et\ al.$ (1993).

Receptor binding appears to play an important role in the induction of the toxic effects of TCDD. Considerable work has been done on the development of biologically based models for both receptor binding and the pharmacokinetics of TCDD. Pharmacodynamic models for tumour induction are also available (Thorslund & Charnley, 1988; Tritscher $et\ al.$, 1992; Moolgavkar $et\ al.$1996). Ultimately, these results can be combined to obtain an integrated biologically based model of TCDD carcinogenesis (Andersen $et\ al.$, 1993).

7.8 Summary and conclusions

In this chapter, we have considered biologically based models for the quantitative estimation and prediction of cancer risks. In biological terms, cancer is thought to be a multistage process in which a normal stem cell undergoes a series of genetic alterations including chromosomal translocation, gene amplification and point mutations leading to the production of a malignant cancer cell. Activated oncogenes may play an important role in carcinogenesis by deregulating cellular growth and differentiation pathways. Inactivation of tumour-supressor genes may eliminate gene products that regulate cellular proliferation. Childhood retinoblastoma involves two somatic mutations that inactivate both copies of the RB tumour-supressor gene. More than two mutations may be required to induce other lesions: colon cancer may involve the inactivation of three tumour-supressor genes and activation of the K-*ras* proto-oncogene. It is not clear, however, which of these mutations are rate-limiting.

The rate of cell division also plays an important role in malignant transformation. Increases in cell division rates may lead to increased mutation frequency, as well as an increase in the pool of cells at risk of malignant transformation. Agents affecting the intracellular and intercellular pathways that control cellular proliferation can thus indirectly affect cancer risk.

The two-stage clonal expansion model of carcinogenesis provides a convenient framework for modelling cancer data. Building on the two-mutation model for retinoblastoma, the model postulates that two critical rate-limiting mutations are necessary for malignant transformation. Initiated cells that have sustained the first mutation undergo a birth–death process that may result in clonal expansion of the initiated cell population. A single cancer cell formed by the occurrence of the second mutation in one of the initiated cells may then give rise to a clinically detectable cancerous tissue mass. Provision can be made in the model for the growth and development of normal tissue with age, which provides the pool of stem cells at risk.

A mathematical characterization of this two-stage model of carcinogenesis has been derived by Moolgavkar and his colleagues. An exact solution

for the hazard function for this model can be obtained by consideration of the probability generation function for the underlying stochastic process of carcinogenesis. The exact solution is recommended for use in practice rather than a commonly encountered approximation, since the hazard functions for these two versions of the model differ markedly: whereas the hazard function for the approximate version of the model increases without bound with age, the hazard function for the exact version remains bounded, approaching a finite asymptote with increasing age.

The two-stage model may be extended in different ways. As with the Armitage–Doll multistage model, more than two critical mutations may be required for malignant transformation. In such a multistage model, clonal expansion of premalignant cells at different stages of development is possible. Repair of promutagenic DNA lesions that have been fixed through cell replication may also be considered.

In the absence of complete knowledge about the mechanism of carcinogenesis in specific applications, the two-mutation model serves as a useful starting point for cancer modelling. As is the case with retinoblastoma, only two mutations may be involved in carcinogenesis. Even if more than two mutations are involved, only two of these may be rate-limiting. Allowing for the effects of tissue growth and cell kinetics, the two-stage clonal expansion model is generally sufficiently flexible to describe dose–response data derived from toxicological or epidemiological studies. In exceptional cases, such as colon cancer, where more than two mutations need to be included in the model to obtain biologically realistic estimates of mutation rates, additional parameters may be incorporated into the model.

Biologically based models of carcinogenesis are useful for several reasons. First, they provide a convenient framework within which to describe the process of carcinogenesis. Such models raise questions about the stages in carcinogenesis to be included in the model, and invite questions about their relevance to the data at hand. Second, the parameters of a biologically based model have biological meaning. With the two-stage clonal expansion model, separate parameters are used to describe the first- and second-stage mutation rates as well as the birth and death rates of initiated cells. Third, a validated biologically based model is likely to enjoy greater acceptance when used for the quantitative estimation and prediction of cancer risks. And finally, description of the temporal aspects of cancer risk is facilitated by the use of biologically based models of carcinogenesis.

Considerable experience has now accumulated in applying the two-stage clonal expansion model to toxicological and epidemiological data. Only two critical mutations are necessary to describe most data sets. The second-stage mutation rate appears to be less affected by exposure to carcinogenic stimuli than the first-stage mutation rate. This may be an artifact of fitting the model to tumour incidence or mortality data, which contain no direct information on the first- or second-stage rates, but it may also be a biological reality: agents such as radon that cause large deletions in DNA may prove lethal to the cell once a second deletion occurs, thereby preventing the second mutation.

This issue underscores the need for additional data when fitting the two-stage model. Ideally, information on the number and size of preneoplastic lesions can be used to measure cellular proliferation. Direct measures of the rates of mutation would also be useful in modelling. These data can be used to supplement rather than replace tumour-incidence or mortality data. Ideally, data on mutation and cell proliferation could be used to construct a model that could be validated using separate data on tumour incidence.

In addition to such biologically based pharmacodynamic models of carcinogenesis, biologically based pharmacokinetic models can also be used to describe the metabolism of chemical carcinogens to their reactive form. Physiologically based pharmacokinetic models envisage the body as consisting of a small number of homogeneous physiological compartments, including richly perfused tissues such m the kidney and poorly perfused tissues such as skin and fat. Because of its metabolic function, the liver is usually represented as a separate compartment. These organ and tissue compartments are interconnected by the arterial and venous blood supply.

PBPK models involve three different types of parameters. Relevant physiological parameters include tissue volumes, blood flow rates, and alveolar ventilation. Partition coefficients are used to measure the affinity of compounds in different tissue compartments. Biochemical constants are involved in the description of any metabolic process, including liver metabolism, included in the model. Estimates of all of these parameters are required to completely specify a PBPK model.

Mathematically, each compartment in a PBPK model is described as a (possibly non-linear) differential mass balance equation. Simultaneous solution of the set of equations characterizing the model permits prediction of the concentration of reactive metabolites reaching target tissues. The area under the concentration–time curve for relevant metabolites is often used as the dose metameter for carcinogenic risk assessment, although other measures such as the peak concentration in a 24-hour period may also be considered.

Because PBPK models may involve 20 or more parameters, attempts have been made to identify those parameters that contribute most to uncertainty in tissue-dose predictions. Analyses have also been conducted to identify those parameters to which predictions of tissue doses are particularly sensitive. In general, the results of such uncertainty and sensitivity analyses are compound-specific, as well as dependent on the time at which the analyses are conducted.

In addition to uncertainty and sensitivity in PBPK modelling, consideration needs to be given to interindividual variability in kinetics. The rate of metabolism can influence cancer risk, as can DNA repair rates and other factors involved in carcinogenesis that may vary substantially among individuals.

Other aspects of carcinogenesis are also candidates for biologically based model development. Receptor-mediated events such as enzyme induction, could be very early events in carcinogenesis, and may be modelled using Hill or Michaelis–Menten kinetics. The Hill equation has found recent application in the induction of the liver enzymes CYP1A1 and CYPIA2, thought to represent an early phase in the sequence of events involved in dioxin carcinogenesis.

Ideally, an integrated pharmacokinetic/pharmacodynamic model, including early biological events that may be receptor-mediated, could be constructed to obtain a complete biologically based model of carcinogenesis. Such a comprehensive biologically based model will require almost complete understanding of the biological mechanisms by which tumours are induced. The hazard functions generated by biologically based models can, in general, be used for analyses of any data sets that can be analysed using the empirical models described in Chapter 6. For proper biological interpretation of the parameters, however, much more extensive data will be required.

APPENDIX
A.I. The Armitage–Doll model

An explicit expression for $p'_n(t)$ can be obtained in one of two ways. It is not difficult to see that the Kolmogorov forward differential equations for $p_j(t)$ are:

$$p'_0(t) = -\lambda_0 p_0(t)$$

$$\cdot$$
$$\cdot$$

$$p'_k(t) = -\lambda_{k-1} p_{k-1}(t) - \lambda_k p_k(t) \qquad (A.1)$$

$$\cdot$$
$$\cdot$$

$$p'_n(t) = -\lambda_{n-1} p_{n-1}(t)$$

with initial condition $p_0(0) = 1$, $p_j(0) = 0$ for $j > 0$. These equations can be explicitly integrated. A second approach is the following. Let S_j represent the waiting time for the cell to go from stage E_j to E_{j+1}, and let $S = S_0 + S_1 + \cdots + S_{n-1}$. Then clearly, $p_n(t) = \text{Prob}\{S \le t\}$, and the problem of computing $p'_n(t)$ reduces to convolving the densities of n independent exponentially distributed random variables. If no two of the transition rates are equal (i.e. if $\lambda_i = \lambda_j \Rightarrow i = j$), then (see, e.g. Feller, 1971, p. 40):

$$p'_n(t) = \lambda_0 \lambda_1, \cdots, \lambda_{n-1} \{\Psi_{0,\,n-1} \exp(-\lambda_0 t) + \cdots + \Psi_{n-1,\,n-1} \exp(-\lambda_{n-1} t)\} \qquad (A.2)$$

where:

$$\Psi_{j,\,n-1} = [(\lambda_0 - \lambda_j)(\lambda_1 - \lambda_j) \cdots (\lambda_{j-1} - \lambda_j)(\lambda_{j+1} - \lambda_j) \\ \cdots (\lambda_{n-1} - \lambda_j)]^{-1}.$$

Now, the expression $\sum_{p=0}^{m} \Psi_{p,\,m} \exp(-\lambda_p t)$ may be expanded in a Taylor series about $t = 0$. Specifically, we have the following propositions (Moolgavkar, 1978, 1991).

Proposition 1

Let α_k be the coefficient of t^k in the power series about zero for $\sum_{p=0}^{m} \Psi_{p,\,m} \exp(-\lambda_p t)$, where the $\Psi_{p,\,m}$ are defined as above. Then:

$$\alpha_k = \begin{cases} 0 & \text{if } k < m; \\ \frac{1}{m!} & \text{if } k = m; \\ \frac{(-1)^{k-m}}{k!} \displaystyle\sum_{i1<i2<\ldots<ik-m} \lambda_{i1} \lambda_{i2} \ldots \lambda_{ik-m} & \text{if } k > m. \end{cases}$$

Proof. The proof proceeds by double induction on k and m.

Proposition 2

The coefficients α_k in the power series above are symmetric polynomials in the indeterminants $\lambda_0, \lambda_1, \cdots, \lambda_m$ and can be expressed in terms of the $m + 1$ Newton polynomials, $\sum_{i=0}^{m} \lambda_i^j$; $1 \le j \le m + 1$.

Proposition 2 says, in particular, that all the coefficients of the power series can be expressed in terms of the moments of the transition rates, i.e. in terms of the moments of the λ_i, $0 \le i \le n - 1$.

It follows immediately from Proposition 1 that the hazard function $h(t)$ can be written as:

$$h(t) \approx N p'_n(t) = \frac{N \lambda_0 \lambda_1 \cdots \lambda_{n-1}}{(n-1)!} t^{n-1} \{1 - \lambda t + f(\lambda, t)\}, \quad (A.3)$$

where λ is the mean of the transition rates, $\lambda = \frac{1}{n} \sum_{i=0}^{n-1} \lambda_i$, and $f(\lambda, t)$ involves second and higher order moments of the transition rates.

A.2 The two-mutation model
A.2.1 The hazard function

Let $Y(t)$, $Z(t)$, represent the number of intermediate and malignant cells., respectively, at time t and let

$$\Psi(y, z; t) = \sum_{j,k} P_{j,k}(t) y^j z^k$$

be the probability generating function with

$$P_{j,k}(t) = \text{Prob}[Y(t) = j, Z(t) = k \,|\, Y(0) = 0, Z(O) = 0].$$

Then $(Y(t), Z(t)$ is Markovian, and Ψ satisfies the Kolmogorov forward differential equation:

$$\Psi'(y,z;t) = \frac{\partial \Psi(y,z;t)}{\partial t} = (y-1)v(t)X(t)\Psi(y,z;t)$$

$$+ \{\mu(t)yz + \alpha(t)y^2 + \beta(t) - [\alpha(t) + \beta(t) + \mu(t)]y\}\frac{\partial \Psi}{\partial y} \qquad \text{(A.4)}$$

with initial condition Ψ $(y,z; 0) = 1$ (Moolgavkar et al., 1988). Ψ $(1, 0; t)$ is the survival function for this model, and hazard (incidence) function is given by:

$$h(t) = - \Psi'(1, 0; t) / \Psi(1, 0; t). \qquad \text{(A.5)}$$

It follows immediately from the Kolmogorov equation that:

$$\Psi'(1, 0; t) = -\mu(t)\frac{\partial \Psi}{\partial y}(1, 0; t)$$

and thus

$$h(t) = \mu(t)E[Y(t) | Z(t) = 0], \qquad \text{(A.6)}$$

where E denotes the expectation and we have used the relationship:

$$E[Y(t) | Z(t) = 0] = \frac{\partial \Psi}{\partial y}(1, 0; t)/\Psi(1, 0; t).$$

If the probability of tumour is small enough, then $E[Y(t)] \approx E[Y(t) | Z(t) = 0]$ and $h(t) \approx \mu(t)E[Y(t)]$. The differential equation, derived from the Kolmogorov equation, for $E[Y(t)]$ can be readily solved to yield:

$$h(t) \approx \mu(t) \int_0^t \left\{ v(s)X(s) \exp \int_0^t [\alpha(u) - \beta(u)]du \right\} ds \text{(A.7)}$$

This is the approximate solution that has been used for the analysis of epidemiological data. It is reasonably accurate when tumours are rare, as in epidemiological data. However, our recent experience is that it can lead to misleading results even for such data. Thus, the exact solution must be used whenever possible, and this is somewhat more complicated. Note that the approximate solution is of the proportional hazards form if only the second mutation rate is a function of the covariates of interest. Note also the similarity of equation (A.9) to equation (A.6), the exact hazard function of the Armitage–Doll model.

Two approaches can be used to obtain the exact

solution to the two-mutation model. The first involves solving the characteristic equations (see, e.g. John, 1971, pp. 6–15) associated with the Kolmogorov equation. The second approach is somewhat more general, and is not described here, but can be found in Moolgavkar & Luebeck (1990). Specifically, the characteristic equations are:

$$\frac{dy}{du} = -R(y,u) = -\{\mu(u)yz + \alpha(u)y^2 + \beta(u) - [\alpha(u) + \beta(u) + \mu(u)]y\}$$

$$\frac{dz}{du} = 0 \ (z \text{ is constant along characteristics})$$

$$\frac{dt}{du} = 1, \text{ and } \frac{d\Psi}{du} = (y-1)v(u)X(u)\Psi.$$

Now, the ordinary differential equation for Ψ may be solved along characteristics to yield:

$$\Psi(y(t),z,t) = \Psi_0 \exp \int_0^t [y(u,t)-1]v(u)X(u)du \quad \text{(A.8)}$$

where $\Psi_0 = \Psi(y(0), z, 0) = 1$ is the initial value of Ψ. We are interested in computing $\Psi(1, 0; t)$ for any t, and thus we need to find the values of Ψ along the characteristic through $(y(0), 0, 0)$, where $y(0)$ is the initial value of y and $y(t) = 1$. Now, along the characteristic, Y satisfies the differential equation $dy/du = -R(y, u)$, and this is just a Riccati equation which can be readily integrated in closed form if the parameters of the model are piecewise constant (see, e.g. Ince, 1956, p.311). To be precise, the Riccati equation for y can be solved to yield a value for $y(u)$ for any u, with initial condition $y(t) = 1$. Note that y depends on u and t.

Thus, the survival function is:

$$\Psi(1, 0; t) = \exp \int_0^t [y(u,t)-1]v(u)X(u)du \qquad \text{(A.9)}$$

where the explicit dependence of y on u and t is acknowledged. The hazard function is then given by:

$$h(t) = -\Psi'(1, 0; t) = -\int_0^t v(u)X(u)y_t(u,t)du \quad \text{(A.10)}$$

where y_t denotes the derivative of y with respect to t.

Suppose now that $0 = t_0 < t_1 \cdots < t_k = t$, and suppose that the parameters α, β and μ, are piecewise constant, i.e. on (t_{i-1}, t_i) the parameters are α_i, β_i and μ_i. Suppose further that A_i and B_i are the two roots of the polynomial $\alpha_i x^2 - [\alpha_i + \beta_i + \mu_i]x + \beta_i$.

It can be easily shown that $0 < A_i < 1 < B_i$. A closed-form expression for $y(u, t)$ can be obtained by solving the Riccati equation for y successively on each subinterval starting with (T_{k-1}, t) with initial condition $y(t_k, t_k) = 1$. The initial condition on the interval (t_{k-2}, t_{k-1}) is then the solution obtained on the interval (t_{k-1}, t_k) evaluated at t_{k-1}, i.e., $y(t_{k-1}, t)$. Thus the solution $y(u, t)$ can be inductively built up. Explicitly, for $u \in (t_{i-1}, t_i)$, $y(u, t)$ can be defined inductively by:

$$y(u, t) = \frac{B_i - A_i \frac{y(t_i, t) - B_i}{y(t_i, t) - A_i} \exp[\alpha_i(A_i - B_i)(u - t_i)]}{1 - \frac{y(t_i, t) - B_i}{y(t_i, t) - A_i} \exp[\alpha_i(A_i - B_i)(u - t_i)]} \quad (A.11)$$

with $y(t_k, t) = 1$. This is a generalization of the result in Moolgavkar & Venzon (1979).

The derivative $y_t (u, t)$ is now straightforward, albeit cumbersome, to compute using the chain rule repeatedly. The equations for $\Psi (1, 0; t)$ and $h(t)$ can be numerically integrated using the values of $y (u, t)$ and $y_t (u, t)$ computed above. If $v (u)$ is piecewise constant, too, and if, as is often the case, $X(u)$ is taken to be constant, then, in principle, these equations can be integrated in closed form. However, a numerical procedure is simpler.

Sometimes, the time-scale of interest is not the age of the animal, or time since start of treatment, but the age of *individual* intermediate clones. Then, $(Y(t), Z(t))$ is not Markovian, and the Kolmogorov differential equation does not exist. The second approach, described in Moolgavkar & Luebeck (1990), must then be used.

A.2.2 Number and size distribution of intermediate foci

The development of mathematical expressions for the number and size distribution of intermediate foci was motivated by the availability of suitable data from initiation–promotion experiments, particularly in the mouse skin system and the rodent liver system. Originally, expressions for the number and size distribution of intermediate foci were developed on the assumptions that initiated cells arose from normal cells as a non-homogeneous Poisson process, and that the clonal expansion of initiated cells gave rise to foci by way of a birth-and-death process, the waiting time distributions to cell division and cell death being exponential (Dewanji et al., 1989).

However, the latter description, which implies that mean growth of intermediate cells is exponential, is unrealistic and unduly restrictive. Hence, the model for cell division and death was extended to include Gompertz mean growth of intermediate cells, following an idea introduced by Tan (1986). This development is described in detail in Luebeck & Moolgavkar (1991). From the statistical point of view, this development leads to the introduction of one extra parameter that measures departures from exponentiality of the mean growth of initiated cells. Likelihood ratio tests can be employed to test for the significance of this extra parameter. We briefly describe the mathematical development based on the general Gompertz model.

Assume that an intermediate cell is generated at time s and thus sets off the process of (mono)clonal expansion. Now, let $N(t,s)$ be a random variable denoting the size of the intermediate cell clone at time t, given that the first cell in the clone appeared at time s. Then, the generating function, say Q, for the probabilities P_i of having $N(t, s) = i$ cells, is given (Tan, 1986) by:

$$Q(z;t,s) \equiv \sum_{i=0}^{\infty} P_i(t, s)z^i$$
$$= 1 - \frac{z - 1}{(z - 1)G(t,s) - g(t,s)} \quad (A. 12)$$

with the initial condition $P_1 (s, s) = 1$ and the definitions of the functions:

$$g(t, s) = \exp\left[\int_s^t - \delta(u, s)du\right]$$

$$\text{with } \delta(u, s) = \alpha(u, s) - \beta(u, s)$$

(the variable u denotes the age of the animal while the clone is growing) and

$$G(t, s) = \int_s^t \alpha(u, s)g(u, s)du$$

The expected number of cells in a clone which was generated at time s is then given by:

$$E[N(t, s)] = \frac{\partial Q}{\partial z}(z = 1; t, s) = [g(t, s)]^{-1}.$$

If α and β are independent of time, then the expected number of intermediate cells belonging to any one clone will grow exponentially provided that $\alpha > \beta$. On the other hand, there is a non-zero probability $P_0(t, s)$ that the clone (the initiated cell together with all its progeny) becomes extinct at time $t > s$. The number of non-extinct foci at time t will be Poisson distributed with expectation (Dewanji et al., 1989):

$$\Lambda(t) = \int_0^t X(s)v(s)[1 - P_0(t, s)]ds.$$

Since $P_0 = Q\,(z = 0) = 1 - (G + g)^{-1}$ we can also write:

$$\Lambda(t) = \int_0^t \frac{X(s)v(s)}{G(t, s) + g(t, s)}ds \qquad (A.13)$$

To derive the size distribution of non-extinct foci, let $W(t, s)$ be a random variable for the size of non-extinct foci at time t with the first initiated cell occurring at time $s < t$, i.e. $W(t,s) = [N(t,s)\,|\,N(t,s) > 0]$. Then, following Dewanji et al.(1989), we first examine the conditional probability-generating function and then derive the probability $P[W(t,s) = m]$ of observing a non-extinct clone consisting of m cells at time t given the occurrence of its progenitor cell at time s. We have:

$$E[z^{W(t,s)}] = \frac{Q(z; t, s) - Q(0; t, s)}{1 - Q(0; t, s)}$$

$$= 1 - \frac{[G(t,s) + g(t,s)](z - 1)}{(z - 1G(t,s) - g(t,s)}$$

Hence, the probability of finding a (non-extinct) clone of size $m > 0$ at time t–s after the progenitor cell was generated is:

$$P[W(t,s) = m] = \frac{1}{m!} \frac{d^m}{dz^m} E[z^W]\Big|_{z=0}$$

$$= \frac{g}{G}\left(\frac{G}{G + g}\right)^m$$

Since intermediate cells are randomly generated at all times s with $0 < s < t$, we still need to integrate over s to obtain the total probability of finding a clone of size m. However, the occurrence times of the mutations which lead to such non-extinct clones are distributed independently and identically with density function $\lambda(t, s)/\Lambda(t)$, where we have defined:

$$\lambda(t, s) = X(s)v(s)[1 - P_0(t, s)].$$

Let $p_m = P[W(t) = m]$ be the (unconditional) probability that a non-extinct clone at time t contains m cells. Then:

$$p_m(t) \equiv \frac{1}{\Lambda(t)} \int_0^t \lambda(t, s)P[W(t, s) = m]ds$$

$$= \frac{1}{\Lambda(t)} \int_0^t \lambda(t, s)\left[\frac{g}{G}\left(\frac{G}{G + g}\right)^m\right]ds \qquad (A. 14)$$

If information on tne number of foci and the size of each focus (i.e. the number of cells in each focus) were directly available, then the expression for $\Lambda(t)$ and $p_m(t)$ derived above could be immediately used for the analysis of data. However, in the rodent liver system, the available information reports the number of two-dimensional transections seen on a slide, and the size of each transection in terms of its radius. Thus, stereological considerations come into play. Details of how the expression derived above can then be used for analyses are given in recent publications (Moolgavkar et al., 1990b; Luebeck et al., 1991). Briefly, the relevant quantities are derived as follows. The expression for $\Lambda(t)$ and $p_m(t)$ given above need to be translated into expressions describing the mean number of focal transections per unit area, say $n_2(t)$, and a probability density $f_2^{\varepsilon}(y)$ for the radius of a transection, conditional on the radius being larger than a threshold ε, below which the focal transection cannot be reliably detected. In order to derive the relevant expressions we use a formula due to Wicksell (1925) that relates the distribution of radii of three-dimensional spheres to the radii of transectional disks observed in two-dimensional sections. The Wicksell formula, however, requires the three-dimensional probability density function, $f_3(r)$ as input. Hence, we need to relate three-dimensional radii to the number of (actively cycling) cells in the foci, say m. Thus, we approximate the number of cells in a focus by a smooth function of its radius r. We consider two distinct (admittedly extreme) situations.

If all cells in a spherically shaped focus are actively cycling (volume growth model), the number of cells is simply given by the ratio of clone volume to cell volume: $m(r) = r_c^3$, while if only surface cells are cycling the number of (cycling) cells is given by (surface area of clone/surface area occupied by cell) $\sim 4\pi\, r^2\,/(2r_c)^2$ (surface growth model). The cell radius r_c is assumed to be $14\mu m$, as determined by Jack et al. (1990).

Taking into account the Jacobian of the transformation $(m \to r)$, which is given by the derivative $dm(r)/dr$, the Wicksell formula reads:

$$f_2^\varepsilon(y) = \frac{y}{\mu_\varepsilon} \int_\varepsilon^\infty \frac{f_3(r)}{\sqrt{r^2 - y^2}} \, dr$$

where:

$$f_3(r) = \frac{dm(r)}{dr} \, p_{m(r)}(t),$$

with $p_{m(r)}$ given by the equation above and with the (adjusted) mean radius, μ_ε, given by:

$$\mu_\varepsilon = \int_\varepsilon^\infty \sqrt{r^2 - \varepsilon^2} f_3(r) \, dr.$$

Furthermore, the number of non-extinct transections (per unit area) is Poisson distributed with mean $n_2(t)$ and related to $\Lambda(t)$, its three-dimensional equivalent, by:

$$n_2(t) = 2\mu_\varepsilon \Lambda(t),$$

where $\Lambda(t)$ is given by the expression above. The likelihood for the experimental data is constructed as a product of the contributions that each animal makes. Each animal yields a vector of observations, with the first entry representing the number of transections observed and the remaining entries representing the radii of these transections. The likelihood contribution made by the animal is then a product of the Poisson probability of the number of transections observed and the joint density of their sizes. The likelihood is maximized with respect to the unknown model parameters.

References

Aaltonen, L.A., Peltomaki, P., Leach, F.S., Sistonen, P., Pylkkanen, L., Mecklin, J.R, Jarvinen, H., Powell, SM, Jen, J., Hamilton, SK, Peterson, GM, Kinzler, K.M., Vogelstein, B. & de la Chapelle, A. (1993) Clues to the pathogenesis of familiar colorectal cancer. Science, 260, 812-816

Adamson, R.H., Correa, P., Sieber, S.M., McIntire, KA. & Dalgard, D.W. (1976) Carcinogenicity of aflatoxin B1 in rhesus monkeys: two additional cases of primary liver cancer. J. Natl Cancer Inst., 57, 67-68

Adolph, E.F. (1949) Quantitative relations in the physiological constitutions of mammals. Science, 109, 579

Ames, B.X. & Gold, L.S. (1990) Too many rodent carcinogens: Mitogenesis increases mutagenesis. Science, 249, 970-971

Ames, B.N., Gold, L.S. & Willett, W.C. (1995) The causes and prevention of cancer. Proc. Natl Acad. Sci. USA, 92, 5258-5265

Andersen, M.E. (1981) A physiologically based toxicokinetic description of the metabolism of inhaled gases and vapors: analysis at steady state. Toxicol. Appl. Pharmacol., 60, 509-526

Andersen, M.E., Gargas, M.L. & Ramsey, J.C. (1984) Inhalation pharmacokinetics: evaluating systemic extraction, total in vivo metabolism, and the time course of enzyme induction for inhaled styrene in rats based on arterial blood: inhaled air concentration ratios. Toxicol. Appl. Pharmacol., 73, 176-187

Andersen, M.E., Clewell, H.J., III, Gargas, M.L., Smith, F.A. & Reitz, R.H. (1987) Physiologically based pharmacokinetics and the risk assessment process for methylene chloride. Toxicol. Appl. Pharmacol., 87, 185-205

Andersen, M.E., Krewski, D. & Withey, J.R. (1993) Physiologic pharmacokinetics and cancer risk assessment. Cancer Lett., 69, 1-14

Appel, K.E., Fuerstenberger, G., Hapke, H.J., Hecker, E., Hildebrandt, A.G., Koransky, W., Marks, F., Neumann, H.G., Ohnesorg, F.K. & Schulte-Hermann, R. (1990) Chemical cancerogenesis: definitions of frequently used terms. J. Cancer Res. Clin. Oncol., 116, 232-236

Armitage, P. & Doll, R. (1954) The age distribution of cancer and a multistage theory of carcinogenesis. Br. J. Cancer, 8, 1-2

Arms, A.D. & Travis, C.C. (1988) Reference Physiological Parameters in Pharmacokinetic Modelling (Final Report EPA 600/688/004), Washington, DC, US Environmental Protection Agency

Ashby, J. (1992) Use of short-term tests in determining the genotoxicity or non-genotoxicity of chemicals. In: Vainio, H., Magee, P., McGregor, D.

& McMichael A.J., eds, *Mechanisms of Carcinogenesis in Risk Identification* (IARC Scientific Publications No. 116), Lyon, International Agency for Research on Cancer, pp. 135-164

Ashby, J. & Tennant, R.W. (1988) Chemical structure, Salmonella mutagenicity and extent of carcinogenicity as indicators of genotoxic carcinogenesis among 222 chemicals tested in rodents by the US NCI/NTP. *Mutat. Res.*, **204**, 17-115

Ayesh, R., Idle, J.R., Ritchie, J.C., Crothers, M.J. & Hetzel, M.R. (1984) Metabolic oxidation phenotypes as markers for susceptibility to lung cancer. *Nature*, **312**, 169-170

Balmain, A. & Brown, K. (1988) Oncogene activation in chemical carcinogenesis. *Adv. Cancer Res.*, **51**, 147-182

Bannasch, P. (1986a) Preneoplastic lesions as end points in carcinogenicity testing. 1. Hepatic preneoplasia. *Carcinogenesis*, **7**, 689-695

Bannasch, P. (1986b) Preneoplastic lesions as end points in carcinogenicity testing. Il. Preneoplasia in various nonhepatic tissues. *Carcinogenesis*, **7**, 849-852

Bartsch, H. & Hietanen, E. (1996) The role of interindividual susceptibility in cancer burden related to environmental exposure. *Environ. Health Perspect.*, **104**, 569-577

Bartsch, H., Castegnaro, M., Rojas, M., Camus, A.M., Alexandrov, K. & Lang, M. (1992) Expression of pulmonary cytochrome P4501A1 and carcinogen adduct formation in high risk subjects for tobacco-related lung cancer. *Toxicol. Lett.*, special number 477-83, 64-65

Beland, F.A., Fullerton, N.F., Kinouchi, T. & Poirier, M.C. (1988) DNA adduct forming during continuous feeding of 2-acetylaminofluorene at multiple concentrations. In: Bartsch, H., Hemminki, K. & O'Neill, I.K., eds, *Methods for Detection of DNA Damaging Agents in Humans: Applications in Cancer Epidemiology and Prevention* (IARC Scientific Publications No. 89), Lyon, International Agency for Research on Cancer, pp. 175-180

Berenblum, I. (1941) The mechanism of cocarcinogenesis: A study of significance of cocarcinogenic action and related phenomena. *Cancer Res.*, **1**, 807-814

Berg, K. (1991) Genetic predisposition to common diseases. In: Grandjean, P., ed., *Ecogenetics*, London, Chapman and Hall, pp. 69-78

Bishop, J.M. (1991) Molecular themes in oncogenesis. *Cell*, **64**, 235-248

Blum, M., Heim, M. & Meyer, V.A. (1990) Nucleotide sequence of rabbit NAT2 encoding polymorphic liver arylamine N-acetyltransferase (NAT). *Nucleic Acids Res.*, **18**(17), 5295

Bohr, V.A., Evans, M.K., & Fornace, A.J., Jr (1989) Biology of disease: DNA repair and its pathogenetic implications. *Lab. Invest.*, **61**, 143-161

Bois, F.Y., Woodruff, T.H. & Spear, R.C. (1991) Comparison of three physiologically based pharmacokinetic models of benzene disposition. *Toxicol. Appl. Pharmacol.*, **110**, 79-88

Booth, S.C., Bosenberg, H., Garner, R.C., Hertzog, P.J. & Northop, K. (1981) The activation of aflatoxin B1 in liver slices and bacterial mutagenicity assays using livers from different species including man. *Carcinogenesis*, **2**, 1063-1068

Bos, J. (1989) *ras* oncogenes in human cancer: a review. *Cancer Res.*, **49**, 4682-4689

Boutwell, R.K. (1964) Some biological effects of skin carcinogenesis. *Prog. Exp. Tumor Res.*, **4**, 207-250

Brash, D.E., Rudolph, J.A. Simon, J.A., Lin, A., McKenna, G.J., Baden, H.P., Halperin, A.J. & Ponten, J. (1991) A role for sunlight in skin cancer: UV-induced *p53* mutations in squamous cell carcinoma. *Proc. Natl Acad. Sci. USA*, **88**, 10124-10128

Brown, C. Chu, K. (1987) Use of multistage models to infer stage affected by carcinogenic exposure; Example of lung cancer and cigarette smoking. *J. Chronic Dis.*, **40** (Suppl. 2), 171S- 179S

Burns, F.J., Vanderlaart, X.I., Snyder, E. & Albert, R.E. (1978) Induction and progression kinetics of mouse skin papillomas. In: Slaga, T.J., Boutwell, R.K. & Sivak, A., eds, *Mechanism of Tumor Promotion and Cocarcinogenesis*, New York, NY, Raven Press, pp. 91-96

Bursch, W., Lauer, B., Timmermann-Trosiener, I, Barthel, G., Schuppler, J. & Schulte-Hermann, R. (1984) Controlled cell death (apoptosis) of normal and putative preneoplastic cells in rat liver following withdrawal of tumour promoters. *Carcinogenesis*, 5, 453-458

Bursch, W., Oberhammer, F. & Schulte-Hermann, R. (1992) Cell death by apoptosis and its protective role against disease. *Trends Pharmacol. Sci.*, 13, 245-251

Campbell, H.A., Xu, Y.D., Hanigan, M.H. & Pitot, H.C. (1986) Application of quantitative stereology to the evaluation of phenotypically heterogeneous enzyme-altered foci in the rat liver. *J. Natl Cancer Inst.*, 76, 751-756

Camus, A.M., Geneste, O., Honkakoski, P., Bereziat, J.C., Henderson, C.J., Wolf, C.R., Bartsch, H. & Lang, M.A. (1993) High variability of nitrosamine metabolism among individuals: roles of cytochromes P450 2A6 and 2E1 in the dealkylation of *N*-nitrosodimethylamine and *N*-nitrosodiethylamine in mice and humans. *Mol. Carcinog.*, 7 (4), 268-275

Caporaso, N.E., Tucker, M.A., Hoover. N., Hayes, R.B., Pickle, L.W., Issaq, H.J., Muschik, G.M., Green-Gallo, L., Duivys, D. & Aisher, S., R. *et al.*(1990) Lung cancer and the debrisoquine metabolic phenotype. *J. Natl Cancer Inst.*, 85, 1264-1272

Caron de Fromentel, C. & Soussi T. (1992) *TP53* tumour suppressor gene: a model for investigating human mutagenesis. *Genes, Chromosomes Cancer*, 4, 1-15

Carter, R.L. (1984) *Precancerous States*, London, Oxford University Press

Cavanee, W.K., Dryja, T.P., Phillips, R.A., Benedict, W.F., Godbout, R., Gallie, B.D., Murphree, A.L.,

Strong, L.C. & White, R.L. (1983) Expression of recessive alleles by chromosomal mechanisms in retinoblastoma. *Nature*, 305, 779-784

Chellappan, S.P., Hiebert, S., Mudryj, M., Horowitz, J.M. & Nevins, R. (1991) The E2F transcription factor is a cellular target for the RB protein. *Cell*, 65, 1053-1061

Chen, C. & Farland, W. (1991) Incorporating cell proliferation in quantitative cancer risk assessment: Approaches, issues and uncertainties. In: *Chemically Induced Cell Proliferation: Implications for Risk Assessment*, New York, NY, Wiley-Liss, pp. 481-499

Chen, H.S.G. & Gros, J.F. (1979) Estimation of tissue-to-plasma partition coefficients used in physiological pharmacokinetic models. *J. Pharmacokin. Biopharm.*, 7, 117-125

Clarke, A.R., Purdie, C.A., Harrison, D.J., Morris, R.G., Bird, C.C., Hooper, M.L. & Wyllie, A.H. (1993) Thymocyte apoptosis induced by *p53*-dependent and independent pathways. *Nature*, 362, 849-852

Cohen, S.M. & Ellwein, L.B. (1990) Cell proliferation in carcinogenesis. *Science*, 249, 1007-1011

Cook, J.C. & Greenlee, W.F. (1989) Characterization of a specific binding protein for 2,3,7,8-tetrachlorodibenzo-*p*-dioxin in human thymic epithelial cells. *Mol. Pharmacol.*, 35, 713-719.

Craddock, V.M. (1971) Liver carcinomas induced in rats by single administration of dimethylnitrosamine after partial hepatectomy. *J. Natl Cancer Inst.*, 47, 899-907

Croy, R.G. & Wogan, G.N. (1981) Quantitative comparison of covalent aflatoxin–DNA adducts formed in rat and mouse livers and kidneys. *J. Natl Cancer Inst.*, 66, 761-768

Crump, K. & Howe, R. (1984) The multistage model with a time-dependent dose pattern: Application to carcinogenic risk assessment. *Risk Anal.*, 4, 163-176

Day, N. & Brown, C. (1980) Multistage models and primary prevention of cancer. *J. Natl Cancer Inst.*, **64**, 977-989

Denes, J., Blakey, D., Krewski, D. & Withey, J.R. (1996) Applications of receptor-binding models in toxicology. In: Fan, A.M. & Chang, L.W., eds, *Toxicology and Risk Assessment: Principles, Methods, and Applications*, New York, NY, Marcel Dekker, pp. 447-472

de Gunst, M.C.M. & Luebeck, E.G. (1994) Quantitative analysis of two-dimensional observations of premalignant clones in the presence or absence of malignant tumors. *Math. Biosci.*, **119**, 5-34

de Gunst, M.C.M. & Luebeck, E.G. (1998) A method for parametric estimation of the number and size distribution of cell clusters from observations in a section plane with an application to preneoplastic minifoci in rat liver. *Biometrics*, **54**, 100-112

Dewanji, A., Venzon, D.J. & Moolgavkar, S.H. (1989) A stochastic two-stage model for cancer risk assessment II. The number and size of premalignant clones. *Risk Anal.* **9**, 179-187

Dewanji, A., Moolgavkar, S.H., Luebeck, E.G. (1991) Two-mutation model for carcinogenesis: Joint analysis of premalignant and malignant lesions. *Math. Biosci.* **104**, 97-109

Dewanji, A., Luebeck, E.G. & Moolgavkar, S.H. (1996) A biologically based model for the analysis of premalignant foci of arbitrary shape. *Math. Biosci*, **135**, 55-68

Diller, L., Kassel, 1, Nelson, C.E., Gryka, M.A., Litwak, G., Gebhardt, M., Bressac, B., Ozturk, M., Baker, S.J., Vogelstein, B. & Friend, S.H. (1990) p53 Functions as a cell cycle control protein in osteosarcomas. *Mol. Cell Biol.*, **10**, 5772-5781

Draetta, G.F. (1994) Mammalian G cyclins. *Curr. Opin. Cell Biol.*, **6**, 842-846

Draetta, G., Luca, F., Westendorf, 1, Brizuela, L., Ruderman, J. & Beach, D. (1989) cdc2 Protein kinase is complexed with both cyclin A and B: evidence for proteolytic inaction of MPF. *Cell*, **56**, 829-838

Eacho, P.l., Lanier,, T.L. & Brodhecker, C.A. (1991) Hepatocellular DNA synthesis in rats given peroxisomal proliferating agents: comparison of Wy14,643 to clofibric acid, nafenopine and Ly 171883. *Carcinogenesis*, **12**, 1557-1561

Emery, A.E.H. (1979) *Elements of Medical Genetics*, Edinburgh, Churchill Livingstone

European Chemical Industry, Ecology and Toxicology Centre (1989) *DNA and Protein Adducts: Evaluation of their Use in Exposure Monitoring and Risk Assessment* (Monograph No. 13), Brussels

Farber, E. & Cameron, R. (1980) The sequential analysis of cancer development. *Adv. Cancer Res.*, **31**, 125-226

Farrar, D., Allen, B., Crump, K.S. & Shipp, A. (1989) Evaluation of uncertainty in input parameters to pharmacokinetic models and the resulting uncertainty in output. *Toxicol. Lett.*, **49**, 371-385

Fearon, E.R. & Vogelstein, B. (1990) A genetic model for colorectal tumorigenesis. *Cell*, **61**, 759-767

Feller, W. (1971) *An Introduction to Probability Theory and its Applications*, Vol. II, New York, NY, Wiley

Fiserova-Bergerova, V. (1983) Physiological models for pulmonary administration and elimination of inert gases. In: Fiserova-Bergerova, V., ed., *Modelling of Inhalation Exposure to Vapors: Uptake, Distribution, and Elimination*, Boca Raton, FL, CRC Press, pp. 73-100

Fiserova-Bergerova, V. & Hughes, H.C. (1983) Species differences in bioavailability of inhaled vapors and gases. In: Fiserova-Bergerova, V., ed., *Modelling of Inhalation Exposure to Vapors: Uptake, Distribution, and Elimination*, Boca Raton, FL, CRC Press, p. 97

Fisher, J.W., Whittaker, T.A., Taylor, D.H., Clewell, H.J., 111 & Andersen, M.E. (1988) Physiologically based pharmacokinetic modeling of the pregnant rat: a multiroute exposure model for trichloroethylene and its metabolite, trichloroacetic acid. *Toxicol. Appl. Pharmacol.*, 99, 395-414

Fisher, J.M., Jones, K.W & Whitlock, J.P. Jr (1989) Activation of transcription as a general mechanism of 2,3,7,8-tetrachlorodibenzo-*p*-dioxin action. *Mol. Carcinog.*, 1, 216-221.

Fitzgerald, D.J. & Yamasaki, H. (1990) Tumor promotion: models and assay systems. *Teratog. Carcinog. Mutag.*, 10, 89-102

Freedman, D.A. & Navidi, W. (1989) Multistage models for carcinogenesis. *Environ. Health Perspect.*, 81, 169-188

Fuino, T., Gottlieb, K., Manchester, D.K., Park, S.S., West, D., Gurtoo, H.L., Tarone, R.E. & Gelboin, H.V. (1984) Monoclonal antibody phenotyping of interindividual differences in cytochrome P-450-dependent reactions of single and twin human placenta. *Cancer Res.*, 44 (9), 3916-3923

Futreal, P.A. *et al.* (1994) BRCA1 mutations in primary breast cancer and ovarian carcinomas. *Science*, 266, 120-122

Gannon, J.V., Greaves, R., Iggo, R. & Lane, D.P. (1990) Activating mutations in *p53* produce a common conformational effect: a monoclonal antibody specific for the mutant form. *EMBO J.*, 9, 1595-1602

Gargas, M.L. & Andersen, M.E. (1989) Determining kinetic constants of chlorinated ethane metabolism in the rat from rates of exhalation. *Toxicol. Appl. Pharmacol.*, 99, 344-353

Gargas, M.L., Andersen, M.E. & Clewell, H.J., III (1986) A physiologically based simulation approach for determining metabolic constants from gas uptake data. *Toxicol. Appl. Pharmacol.*, 86, 341-352

Gargas, M.L., Clewell, H.J., III & Andersen, M.E. (1990) Gas uptake inhalation techniques and the rates of metabolism of chloromethanes, chloroethanes, and chloroethylenes in the rat. *Inhal. Toxicol.*, 2, 285-309

Ghering, P.J., Watanabe, P.G. & Park, C.N. (1978) Resolution of dose–response toxicity data for chemicals requiring metabolic activation: example—vinyl chloride. *Toxicol. Appl. Pharmacol.*, 44, 581-591

Gibaldi, M. & Perrier, D. (1975) *Pharmacokinetics*, New York, NY, Marcel Dekker

Godbout, R., Dryja, T.P., Squire, J., Gattie, B.L. & Phillips, R.A. (1983) Somatic inactivation of genes on chromosone 13 is a common event in retinoblastoma. *Nature*, 304, 451-453

Goerttler, K. & Loehrke, H. (1976) Improved tumour yields by means of a TPA–13MBA–TPA variation of the Berenblum–Mottram experiment on the back skin of NMR1 mice. The effect of stationary hyperplasia and without inflammation. *Exp. Pathol.*, 12, 336-341

Gold, L.S., Bernstein, L., Magaw, R. & Slone, T.H. (1989) Interspecies extrapolation in carcinogenesis prediction between rats and mice. *Environ. Health Perspect.*, 81, 211-219

Gonzalez, F.J. (1988) The molecular biology of cytochrome P450s. *Pharmacol. Rev.*, 40 (4), 243-288 [erratum, *Pharmacol. Rev.*, 1989, 41 (1), 91-92]

Goth, R. & Rajewsky, M.F. (1974) Molecular and cellular mechanisms associated with pulse-carcinogenesis in the rat nervous system by ethylnitrosourea: ethylation of nucleic acids and elimination rates of ethylated bases from DNA of different tissues. *Z. Krebsforsch.*, 82, 37-64

Gough, A.C., Miles, J.S., Spurr, N.K., Moss, J.E., Gaedigk, A., Eichelbaum, M. & Wolf, C.R. (1990) Identification of the primary gene defect at the cytochrome P450 CYP2D locus. *Nature*, 347 (6295), 773-776

Graeber, T.G., Osmanian, C., Jacks, T., Housman, D.E., Koch, C.J., Lowe, S.W & Glaccia, A.J. (1996)

Hypoxia-mediated selection of cells with diminished apoptotic potential in solid tumours. *Nature*, **379**, 88-91

Grasl-Kraupp, B., Bursch, W., Ruttka-Nedecky, B., Wagmer, A., Lauer, B. & Schulte-Hermann, R. (1994) Food restriction eliminates preneoplastic cells through apoptosis and antagonizes carcinogenesis in liver. *Proc. Natl Acad. Sci. USA*, **91**, 9995-9999

Greenblatt, M.S., Bennett, W.P., Hollstein, M. & Harris, C.C. (1994) Mutations in the *p53* tumor suppressor gene: clues to cancer etiology and molecular pathogenesis. *Cancer Res.*, **54**, 4855-4878

Guengerich, F.P. (1988) Roles of cytochrome P-450 enzymes in chemical carcinogenesis and cancer chemotherapy. *Cancer Res.*, **48**, 2946-2954

Haggard, H.W. (1924) The absorption, distribution and elimination of ethyl ether. II. Analysis of the mechanism of the absorption and elimination of such a gas or vapor as ethyl ether. *Biol. Chem.*, **59**, 753-770

Harris, C.C. (1989) Interindividual variation among humans in carcinogen metabolism, DNA adduct formation and DNA repair. *Carcinogenesis*, **10**, 1563-1566.

Harris, C.C. (1991) Chemical and physical carcinogenesis: advances and perspectives for the 1990s. *Cancer Res.*, **51** (Suppl.), 5023s-5044s

Hayashi, S., Watanabe, J. & Kawajiri, K. (1991) Genetic polymorphisms in the 5′-flanking region change transcriptional regulation of the human cytochrome *P450IIE1* gene. *J. Biochem. (Tokyo)*, **110** (4), 559-565

Heckbert, S.R., Weiss, N.S., Hornung, S.K., Eaton, D.L. & Motulsky, A.G. (1992) Glutathione S-transferase and epoxide hydrolase activity in human leukocytes in relation to risk of lung cancer and other smoking-related cancers. *J. Natl Cancer Inst.*, **84**, 414-422

Hecker, E. & Schmidt, R. (1974) Phorbol esters, the irritants and cocarcinogens of *Croton tiglium*. *Prog. Chem. Org. Nat. Prod.*, **31**, 378-467

Heidenreich, W.F. (1996) On the parameters of the clonal expansion model. *Radiat. Environ. Biophys.*, **35**, 127-129

Heidenreich, W.F., Luebeck, E.G., Moolgavkar, S.H. (1997a) Some properties of the hazard function of the two-mutation clonal expansion model. *Risk Anal.*, **17**, 391-399

Heidenreich, WY., Jacob, P. & Paretzke, H.G. (1997b) Exact solutions of the clonal expansion model and their application to the incidence of solid tumors of atomic bomb survivors. *Radiat. Environ. Biophys.*, **36**, 45-58

Hein, D.W. (1988) Genetic polymorphism and cancer susceptibility: evidence concerning acetyltransferases and cancer of the urinary bladder. *Bioessays*, **9**, 200-204

Hemminki, K. (1992) Significance of DNA and protein adducts. In: Vainio, H., Magee, P.N., McGregor, D.B. & McMichael A.J., eds, *Mechanisms of Carcinogenesis in Risk Identification* (IARC Scientific Publications No. 116), Lyon, International Agency for Research on Cancer, pp. 525-534

Hemminki, K., Reunanen, A. & Kahn, H. (1991) Use of DNA adducts in the assessment of occupational and environmental exposure to carcinogens. *Eur. J. Cancer*, **27** (3), 289-291

Hennings, H., Sjores, R., Wenk, M.L., Spangler, E.F., Tarone, R. & Yuspa, S.H. (1983) Malignant conversion of mouse skin tumours is increased by tumour initiators and unaffected by tumour promoters. *Nature*, **304**, 67-69

Herrold, K.M. (1969) Aflatoxin induced lesions in Syrian hamsters. *Br. J. Cancer*, **23**, 655-660

Herskowitz, I. (1987) Functional inactivation of genes by dominant negative mutations. *Nature*, **329**, 219-222

Hetrick, D.M., Jarabek, A.M. & Travis, C.C. (1991) Sensitivity analysis for physiologically based pharmacokinetic models. *J. Pharmacokin. Biopharm.*, **19**, 1-20

Hill, A.V. (1910) The possible effects of the aggregation of the molecules of hemoglobin on its dissociation curves. *J. Physiol.*, **40**, 4-7

Hinds, P.W., Mittnacht, S., Dulic, V., Arnold, A., Reed, S.I. & Weinberg, R.A. (1992) Regulation of retinoblastoma protein functions by ectopic expression of human cyclins. *Cell*, **70**, 993-1006

Hockenbery, D. Nuflez, G., Milliman, C., Schreiber, R.D. & Korsmeyer, S.i. (1990) Bcl2 is an inner mitochondrial membrane protein that blocks programmed cell death. *Nature*, **348**, 334-348

Holistein, M., Sidransky, D., Vogelstein, B. & Harris, C.C. (1991) *p53* Mutations in human cancers. *Science*, **253**, 49-53

Hsu, I.C., Harris, C.C., Lipsky, M.M., Snyder, S. & Trump, B.F. (1987) Cell and species differences in metabolic activation of carcinogens. *Mutat. Res.*, **177**, 1-7

Imaida, K., Tatematsu, M. Kato, T., Tsuda, H. & Ito, N. (1989) Advantages and limitations of stereological estimation of placental glutathione-S-transferase positive rat liver cell foci by computerized three-dimensional reconstruction. *Jpn J. Cancer Res.*, **80**, 326-330

Ince, E.L. (1956) *Ordinary Differential Equations*, New York, NY, Dover

Ionov, Y., Peinado, M.A., Malkhosyan, S., Shibata, D. & Perucho, M. (1993) Ubiquitous somatic mutations in simple repeated sequences reveal a new mechanism for colonic carcinogenesis. *Nature*, **363**, 558-561

Issemann, I. & Green, S. (1990) Activation of a member of the steroid hormone receptor superfamily by peroxisome proliferators. *Nature*, **347**, 645

Jack, E.M., Bentley, P., Bieri, F., Muakkassah-Kelly, S.F., Staübli, W., Suter, J., Waechter, F. & Cruz-Orive, L.M. (1990) Increase in hepatocyte and nuclear volume and decrease in the popula-tion of binucleated cells in preneoplastic foci of rat liver: A stereological study using the nucle-ator method. *Hepatology*, **11**, 286-297

Jagers, P. (1983) Stochastic models for cell kinetics. *Bull. Math. Biol.*, **45**, 507519

John, F. (1971) *Partial Differential Equations*, New York, NY, Springer-Verlag

Kagimoto, M., Heim, M., Kagimoto, K., Zeugin, T. & Meyer, U.A. (1990) Multiple mutations of the human *P450IID6* gene (CYP2D6) in poor metabolizers of debrisoquine. Study of the functional significance of individual mutations by expression of chimeric genes. *J. Biol. Chem.*, **265** (28), 17209-17214

Kai, M., Luebeck, E.G. & Moolgavkar, S.H. (1997) Analysis of solid cancer incidence among atomic bomb survivors using a two-stage model of carcinogenesis. *Radiat. Res.*, **148**, 348-358

Kamb, A., Gruis, N.A., Weaver-Feldhaus, J., Liu, Q., Harshman, K., Tavtigian, S.V., Stockert, E., Day III,. R.S., Johnson, B.E. & Scolnick, M.H. (1994) A cell cycle regulator potentially involved in genesis of many tumor types. *Science*, **264**, 436-440

Kastan, M.B., Onyekwere, 0., Sidransky, D., Vogelstein, B. & Craig, R.W. (1991) Participation of p53 protein in the cellular response to DNA damage. *Cancer Res.*, **51**, 6304-6311

Kastan, M.B., Zhan, Q, El-Deiry, W., Carrier, F., Jacks, T., Walsh, W.V., Plunkett, B.S., Vogelstein, B. & Fornace, A.J., Jr (1992) A mammalian cell cycle checkpoint pathway utilizing p53 and GADD45 is defective in ataxia telangiectasia. *Cell*, **71**, 587-597

Kawajiri, K. & Fujii-Kuriyama, Y. (1991) P450 and human cancer. *Jpn. J. Cancer Res.*, **82** (12), 1325-1335

Keiding, N., Jensen, S.T. & Ranek, L. (1972) Maximum likelihood estimation of the size distribution of liver cell nuclei from the observed distribution in a plane section. *Biometrics*, **28**, 813-829

Ketterer, B. (1988) Protective role of glutathione and glutathione transferases in mutagenesis and carcinogenesis. *Mutat. Res.*, **202** (2), 343-361

Ketterer, B., Meyer, D.J., Lalor, E., Johnson, P., Guengerich, F.P., Distlerath, L.M., Reilly, P.E., Kadlubar, F.F., Flammang, T.J., Yamazoe, Y. *et al.* (1991) A comparison of levels of glutathione transferases, cytochromes P450 and acetyltransferases in human livers. *Biochem. Pharmacol.*, **41** (4), 635-638

Kleihues, P. & Margison, G.P. (1974) Carcinogenicity of *N*-methylnitrosourea: possible role of repair of O6-methylguanine from DNA. *J. Natl Cancer Inst.*, **53**, 1839-1841

Knudson, A.G. (1971) Mutation and cancer: Statistical study of retinoblastoma. *Proc. Natl Acad. Sci.*, **68**, 820-823

Kociba, R. (1984) Evaluation of the carcinogenic and mutagenic potential of 2,3,7,8-TCDD and other chlorinated dioxins. In: Poland, A. & Kimbrough, R.D., eds, *Biological Mechanisms of Dioxin Action*, Cold Spring Harbor, NY, Cold Spring Harbor Laboratory, pp. 73-84

Kociba, R.J., D.G. Keyes, J.E. Beyer, R.M. Carreon, C.E. Wade, D.A. Dittenber, R.P. Kainins, L.E. Frauson, C.N. Park, S.D. Bernard, R.A. Hummel & C.G. Humiston (1978) Results of a two-year chronic toxicity and oncogenicity study of 2,3,7,8-tetrachlorodibenzo-*p*-dioxin in rats. *Toxicol. Appl. Pharmacol.*, **46**, 279-303

Kohn, M.C. & Portier, C2. (1993) A model of the effects of TCDD on expression of rat liver proteins. *Prog. Clin. Biol. Res.*, **387**, 211-222

Kohn, M.C., Lucier, G.W., Clark, G.C., Sewall, C., Tritschler, A.M. & Portier, C.J. (1993) A mechanistic model of the effects of dioxin on gene expression in the rat liver. *Toxicol. Appl. Pharmacol.*, **120**, 138-154

Kopp-Schneider, A. & Portier, CA. (1992) Birth and death/differentiation rates of papillomas in mouse skin. *Carcinogenesis*, **13**, 973-978

Kress, S., Sutter, C., Strickland, P.T., Mukhtar, H., Schweizer, J. & Schwarz, M. (1992) Carcinogen-specific mutational pattern in the *p53* gene in UVB-induced squamous cell carcinomas of the mouse skin. *Cancer Res.*, **52**, 6400-6403

Krewski, D., Withey, J.R., Ku, L.F. & Travis, C.C. (1991) Physiologically based pharmacokinetic models: applications in carcinogenic risk assessment. In: Rescigno, A. & Thakur, A.K., eds, *New Trends in Pharmacokinetics*, New York, NY, Plenum Press, pp. 355-390

Krewski, D., Withey, J.R., Ku, L.F. & Andersen, M.E. (1994) Applications of physiological pharmacokinetic modeling in carcinogenic risk assessment. *Environ. Health Perspect.*, **102**, Suppl.1, 37-50

Krewski, D., Wang, Y., Bartlett, S. & Krishnan, K. (1995) Uncertainty, variability, and sensitivity analysis of physiological pharmacokinetic models. *J. Biopharm. Stat.*, **5**, 245-271.

Kunz, W., Appel, K.E., Rickart, R., Schwarz, M. & Stoeckle, G. (1978) Enhancement and inhibition of carcinogenic effectiveness of nitrosamines. In: Remmer, H., Bolt, H.M., Bannasch, P. & Popper, H., eds, *Primary Liver Tumours*, Lancaster, MTP Press, pp. 261-283

Lake, B.G., Evans, J.G., Gray, T.J.B., Korosi, S.A. & North, C.A. (1989) Comparative studies on nafenopine-induced hepatic peroxisome proliferation in the rat, Syrian hamster, guinea pig, and marmoset. *Toxicol. Appl. Pharmacol.*, **99**, 148-160

Land, H., Parada, L.F. & Weinberg, R.A. (1983) Cellular oncogenes and multistep carcinogenesis. *Science*, **222**, 771-778

Lane, D.P. (1992) *p53*, guardian of the genome. *Nature*, **358**, 15-16

Leung, H.W., Paustenbach, D.J., Murray, F.J. & Andersen, M.E. (1990a) A physiological pharmacokinetic description of the tissue distribution and enzyme-inducing properties of 2,3,7,8-tetrachlorodibenzo-*o*-dioxin in the rat. *Toxicol. Appl. Pharmacol.*, **103**, 399-410

Leung, H.W., Poland, A., Paustenbach, DA, Murray, G.J. & Andersen, M.E. (1990b) Pharmacokinetics of [1251]-2-iodo-3,7,8-trichlorodibenzo-p-dioxin in mice: analysis with a physiological modeling approach. *Toxicol. Appl. Pharmacol.*, **103**, 411-419

Levine A.J., Momand J. & Finlay C.A. (1991) The *p53* tumour suppressor gene. *Nature*, **351**, 453-456

Lin, J.H., Sugiyama, Y., Awaza, S. & Hanano, M. (1982) *In vitro* and *in vivo* evaluation of the tissue-to-blood partition coefficient for physiological pharmacokinetic models. *J. Pharmacokin. Biopharm.*, **10**, 637-647

Little, M.P. (1995) Are two mutations sufficient to cause cancer? Some generalizations of the two-mutation model of carcinogenesis of Moolgavkar, Venzon and Knudson, and of the multistage model of Armitage and Doll. *Biometrics*, **51**, 1278-1291

Little, M.P. (1996) Generalizations of the two-mutation and classical multistage models of carcinogenesis fitted to the Japanese atomic bomb survivor data. *J. Radiat. Prot.*, **16**, 7-24

Little, M.P., Muirhead, C.R. & Stiller, C.A. (1996) Modelling lymphocytic leukemia incidence in England and Wales using generalizations of the two-mutation model of carcinogenesis of Moolgavkar, Venzon and Knudson. *Stat. Med.*, **15**, 1003-1002.

Livingstone, L.R., White, A., Sprouse, 1, Livanos, E., Jacks, T. & Tisty, T.A. (1992) Altered cell cycle arrest and gene amplification potential accompany loss of wild-type p53. *Cell*, **70**, 923-935

Loeb, L.A. (1989) Endogenous carcinogenesis: molecular oncology into the twenty-first century — presidential address. *Cancer Res.*, **49**, 5489-5496

Lowe, S.W., Schmitt, E.M., Smith, S.W., Osborne, B.A. & Jacks, T. (1993) p53 is required for radiation-induced apoptosis in mouse thymocytes. *Nature*, **362**, 847-849

Lubet, R.A., Nims, R.W., Ward, J.M., Rice, J.M. & Diwan, B.A. (1989) Induction of cytochrome P450b and its relationship to liver tumour promotion. *J. Am. Coll. Toxicol.*, **8**, 259-268

Lucier, G.W. (1992) Receptor mediated carcinogenesis. In: Vainio, H., Magee, P.N., McGregor, D.B. & McMichael, A.J., eds, *Mechanisms of Carcinogenesis in Risk Identification*, (IARC Scientific Publications No. 116), Lyon, International Agency for Research on Cancer, pp. 87-112

Lucier, G.W., Tritscher, A., Goldsworthy, T., Foley, 1, Clark, G., Goldstein, J. & Maronpot, R. (1991) Ovarian hormones enhance 2,3,7,8-tetrachlorodibenzo-p-dioxin-mediated increases in cell proliferation and preneoplastic foci in a two-stage model for rat hepatocarcinogenesis. *Cancer Res.*, **51**, 1391-1397

Luebeck, E.G. & Moolgavkar, S.H. (1994) Simulating the process of carcinogenesis. *Math. Biosci.*, **123**, 127-146

Luebeck, E.G., Moolgavkar, S.H., Buchmann, A. & Schwarz, M. (1991) Effects of polychlorinated biphenyls in rat liver: Quantitative analysis of enzyme altered foci. *Toxicol. Appl. Pharmacol.*, **111**, 469-484

Luebeck., E.G., Curtis, S.B., Cross, F.T. & Moolgavkar, S.H. (1996) Two-stage model of radon-induced malignant lung tumors in rats: Efrects of cell killing. *Radiat. Res.*, **145**, 163-173

Lutz, W.K. (1979) *In vivo* covalent binding of organic chemicals to DNA as a quantitative indicator in the process of chemical carcinogenesis. *Mutat. Res.*, **65**, 289-356

Lutz, W.K. (1986) Quantitative evaluation of DNA binding data for risk estimation and for classification of direct and indirect carcinogens. *J. Cancer Res. Clin. Oncol.*, **112**, 85-91

Lutz, W.K. (1990) Dose–response relationship and low-dose extrapolation in chemical carcinogenesis. *Carcinogenesis*, **11**, 1243-1247

Malkin, D., Li, F.P., Strong, L.C., Fraumeni, J.F., Jr, Nelson, C.E., Kim, D.H., Kassel, 1, Gryka, M.A., Bischoff, F.Z., Tainsky, M.A. & Friend, S.H. (1990) Germ line *p53* mutations in a familiar syndrome of breast cancer, sarcomas and other neoplasias. *Science*, **250**, 1233-1238

Marks, F., Berry, D.L., Bertsch, S., Fuerstenberger, G. & Richter, H. (1982) On the relationship between epidermal hyperproliferation and skin tumour promotion. In: Hecker, E., Fusenig, N.E., Kurtz, W., Marks, F. & Thielmann, H.W., eds, *Carcinogenesis: A Comprehensive Survey*, Vol. 7, New York, NY, Raven Press, pp. 331-346

Marshall, C.J. (1991) Tumour suppressor genes. *Cell*, **64**, 313-326

Marsman, D.S. & Popp, J.A. (1989) Importance of basophilic hepatocellular foci in the development of hepatic tumours induced by the peroxisome proliferator Wy14,643. *Proc. Am. Assoc. Cancer Res.*, **30**, 193

Marsman, D.S., Cattley, R.C., Conway, J.G. Popp, J.A. (1988) Relationship of hepatic peroxisome proliferation and replicative DNA synthesis to the hepatocarcinogenicity of the peroxisome proliferators di(2-ethylhexyl)phthalate and 4-chloro-6-(2,3-xylidino)-2-pyrimidinylthioacetic acid (Wy14,643) in rats. *Cancer Res.*, **48**, 6739-6744

Mayol, X., Perez-Tornas, R., Cullere, X., Romero, A., Estadella, M.D. & Domingo, J. (1991) Cell proliferation and tumour promotion by ethinyl estradiol in rat hepato-carcinogenesis. *Carcinogenesis*, **12**, 1133-1136

McGlynn, K.A., Rosvold, E.A., Lustbader, E.D., Hu, Y., Clapper, M.L., Zhou, T., Wild, C.P., Xia, X.L., Baffoe-Bonnie, A., Ofordi-Adei, D., Chen, QC., London, W.T. & Buetow, K.H. (1995) Susceptibility to hepatocellular carcinoma is associated with genetic variation in the enzymatic detoxification of aflatoxin B_1. *Proc. Natl Acad. Sci. USA*, **92**, 2384-2387

McGregor, D.B. (1992a) Chemicals classified by IARC: their potency in tests for carcinogenicity in rodents and their genotoxicity and acute toxicity.

In: Vainio, H., Magee, P.N., McGregor, D.B. & McMichael, A.J., eds, *Mechanisms of Carcinogenesis in Risk Identification* (IARC Scientific Publications No. 116), Lyon, International Agency for Research on Cancer, pp. 323-352

McGregor, D.B. (1992b) Chemicals classified by IARC: an investigation of some of their toxicological characteristics. *Toxicol. Lett.*, **64/65**, 637-642

McKusick, V.A. (1975) *Mendelian Inheritance in Man*, 4th ed., Baltimore, MD, Johns Hopkins University Press

McKusick, V.A. (1988) *Mendelian Inheritance in Man*, 8th ed., Baltimore, MD, Johns Hopkins University Press

Mercer, W.E., Shields, M.T., Amin, M., Sauve, G.J., Apella, E., Romano, J.W. & Ullrich, J. (1990) Negative growth control in a glioblastoma tumour cell line that conditionally expresses human wild-type *p53*. *Proc. Natl Acad. Sci. USA*, **87**, 6166-6170

Michaelis, L. & Menten, M.L. (1913) Die Kinetik der Invertinwirkung. *Biochem. Z.*, **49**, 333-369

Miller, J.A. (1970) Carcinogenesis by chemicals, an overview — G.H.A. Clowes Memorial Lecture. *Cancer Res.*, **30**, 559-576

Milner, J. & Medcalf, E.A. (1991) Cotranslation of activated mutant *p53* with wild type drives the wild-type p53 protein into the mutant conformation. *Cell*, **65**, 765-774

Mitchell & Gauthier (1992) *Advance Continuous Simulation Language*, Mitchell & Gauthier Associates (MGA) Inc.

Moles, J.P., Moyret, C., Guillot, B., Jeanteur, P., Guilhou, J.J., Theillet, C. & Basset-Seguin, N. (1993) *p53* Gene mutations in human epithelial skin cancers. *Oncogene*, **8**, 583-588

Mommsen, S., Barfold, N.M. & Aargard, J. (1985) *N*-Acetyltransferase phenotypes in the urinary bladder carcinogenesis of a low-risk population. *Carcinogenesis*, **6**, 199-201

Montesano, R., Bartsch, H., Vainio, W, Wilbourn, J. & Yamasaki, H., eds (1986) *Long-term and Short-term Assays for Carcinogens: A Critical Appraisal* (IARC Scientific Publications No.83), Lyon, International Agency for Research on Cancer, pp. 85-101

Moolgavkar, S. (1978) The multistage theory of carcinogenesis and the age distribution of cancer in man. *J. Natl Cancer Inst.*, **61**, 49-52

Moolgavkar, S. (1986) Carcinogenesis modelling: From molecular biology to epidemiology. *Ann. Rev. Public Health*, **7**, 151-169

Moolgavkar, S.H. (1991) Stochastic models of carcinogenesis. In: Rao, C.R. & Chakraborty, R., eds, *Handbook of Statistics*, Vol. 8., New York, NY, Elsevier Science, pp. 373-393

Moolgavkar, S.H. (1997) Stochastic cancer models: application to analyses of solid cancer incidence in the cohort of A-bomb survivors. *Nucl. Energy*, **36**, 447-451

Moolgavkar, S.H. & Knudson, A.G. (1981) Mutation and cancer: A model for human carcinogenesis. *J. Natl Cancer Inst.*, **66**, 1037-1052

Moolgavkar, S.H. & Luebeck, E.G. (1990) Two event model for carcinogenesis: biological, mathematical and statistical considerations. *Risk Anal.*, **10**, 323-341

Moolgavkar, S.H. & Luebeck, G. (1992a) Multistage carcinogenesis: population-based model for colon cancer. *J. Natl Cancer Inst.*, **84**, 610-618

Moolgavkar, S.H. & Luebeck, E.G. (1992b) Interpretation of labeling indices in the presence of cell death. *Carcinogenesis*, **13**, 1007-1010

Moolgavkar, S.H. & Luebeck, E.G. (1992c) Risk assessment of non-genotoxic carcinogens. *Toxicol. Lett.*, **64/65**, 631-636

Moolgavkar, S.H. & Luebeck, E.G. (1995) Incorporating cell proliferation kinetics into models for cancer risk assessment. *Toxicology*, **102**, 141-147

Moolgavkar, S.H. & Venzon, D.J. (1979) Two-event models for carcinogenesis: Incidence curves for childhood and adult tumors. *Math. Biosci.* **47**, 55-77

Moolgavkar, S.H., Dewanji, A. & Venzon, D.J. (1988) A stochastic two-stage model for cancer risk assessment. I. The hazard function and the probability tumor. *Risk. Anal.*, **8**, 383-392

Moolgavkar, S.H., Dewanji, A. & Luebeck, G. (1989) Cigarette smoking and lung cancer: Reanalysis of the British doctors' data. *J. Natl Cancer Inst.*, **81**, 415-420

Moolgavkar, S.H., Cross, F.T., Luebeck, G. & Dagle, G.E. (1990a) A two-mutation model for radonin-duced lung tumors in rats. *Radiat. Res.*, **121**, 28-37

Moolgavkar, S.H., Luebeck, G., de Gunst, M., Port, R.E. & Schwarz, M. (1990b) Quantitative analysis of enzyme altered foci in rat hepatocarcinogenesis experiments. *Carcinogenesis*, **11**, 1271-1278

Moolgavkar, S.H., Luebeck, E.G., Krewski, D. Zielinski, J.M. (1993) Radon, cigarette smoke and lung cancer: A reanalysis of the Colorado Plateau uranium miners' data. *Epidemiology*, **4**, 204-217

Moolgavkar, S.H., Luebeck, E.G., Buchmann, A., Bock & K.W. (1996) Quantitative analysis of enzyme-altered liver foci in rats initiated with diethyinitrosamine and promoted with 2,3,7,8-tetrachlorodibenzo-*p*-dioxin or 1,2,3,4,6,7,8-heptachlorodibenzo-*p*-dioxin. *Toxicol. Appl. Pharmacol.*, **138**, 31-42

Motokura, T., Bloom, T., Kim, H.G., Juppner, H., Ruderman, J.V., Kronenberg, H.M. & Arnold, A. (1991) A novel cyclin encoded by a *bcl1*-linked candidate oncogene. *Nature*, **350**, 512-515

Mulvihill, J.J. (1977) Genetic repertory of human neoplasia. In: Mulvihill, J.J., Miller, R.H. & Fraumeni, J.F., Jr, eds, *Progress in Cancer Research and Therapy*, Vol. 3, New York, NY, Raven Press, pp. 137-143

Murray, A. (1994) Cell cycle checkpoints. *Curr. Opin. Cell Biol.*, **6**, 872-876

Murray, A.W. & Kirschner, M.W. (1989) Dominoes and clocks: the union of two views of the cell cycle. *Science*, **246**, 614-621

Nair, J., Sone, H., Nagao, M., Barbin, A. & Bartsch, H. (1996) Copper-dependent formation of miscoding etheno–DNA adducts in the liver of Long Evans Cinnamon (LEC) rats developing hereditary hepatitis and hepatocellular carcinoma. *Cancer Res.*, **56**, 1267-1271

Nazar-Stewart, V., Motuisky, A.G., Eaton, D.L., White, E., Hornung, S.K., Leng, Z.T., Stapleton, P. & Weiss, N.S. (1993) The glutathione S-transferase m polymorphism as a marker for susceptibility to lung carcinoma. *Cancer Res.*, **53**, 2313-2318

Neumann, H.G. (1983) Role of extent and persistence of DNA modifications in chemical carcinogenesis by aromatic amines. *Recent Results Cancer Res.*, **84**, 77-89

Neumann, H.G. (1986) The role of DNA damage in chemical carcinogenesis of aromatic amines. *J. Cancer Res. Clin. Oncol.*, **112**, 100-106

Neyman, J. & Scott, E. (1967) Statistical aspects of the problem of carcinogenesis. In: *Fifth Berkeley Symposium on Mathematical Statistics and Probability*, Berkeley, CA, University of California Press, pp. 55-77

Nishizuka, Y. (1988) The molecular heterogeneity of protein kinase C and its implication for cellular regulation. *Nature*, **334**, 662-665

Nordling, C.O. (1953) A new theory of the cancer inducing mechanism. *Br. J. Cancer*, **7**, 68-72

Norel, R. & Agur, Z. (1990) A model for the adjustment of the mitotic clock by cyclin and MPF levels. *Science*, **251**, 1076-1078

Nurse, P. (1990) Universal control mechanism regulating onset of M-phase. *Nature*, **344**, 503-508

Nychka D., Wahba, G., Goldfarb, S. & Pugh, T. (1984) Cross validated spline methods for the estimation of three-dimensional tumor size distributions from observations on two-dimensional cross-sections. *J. Am. Stat. Assoc.*, **79**, 832-846

Oesch, F., Aulmann, W., Platt, K.L. & Doerjer, G. (1987) Individual differences in DNA repair capacities in man. *Arch. Toxicol.* (Suppl.), **10**, 172-179

O'Flaherty, E.J., Scott, W., Schreiner, C. & Belisles, R.P. (1992) A physiologically based kinetic model of rat and mouse gestation: disposition of a weak acid. *Toxicol. Appl. Pharmacol.*, **112**, 245-256

Ohgaki, H., Hard, G.C., Hirota, N., Maekawa, A., Takahashi, M. & Kleihues, P. (1992) Selective mutation of codon 204 and 213 of the *p53* gene in rat tumours induced by alkylating N-nitroso compounds. *Cancer Res.*, **52**, 2995-2998

Ohsako, S. & Deguchi, T. (1990) Cloning and expression of cDNAs for polymorphic and monomorphic arylamine N-acetyltransferases from human liver. *J. Biol. Chem.*, **265** (8), 4630-4634

Paustenbach, D.J., Clewell, H.J., III, Gargas, M.L. & Andersen, M.E. (1988) A physiologically-based pharmacokinetic model for inhaled carbon tetrachloride. *Toxicol. Appl. Pharmacol.*, **96**, 191

Pegg, A.E. & Balog, B. (1979) Formation and subsequence excision of O6-ethylguanine from DNA of rat liver following administration of diethylnitrosamine. *Cancer Res.*, **12**, 5003-5009

Pegg, A.E. & Dolan, M.E. (1987) Properties and assay of mammalian O6-alkylguanine-DNA–alkylguanine-alkyltransferase. *Pharmacol. Ther.*, **34**, 167-179

Pelekis, M.L., Krewski, D. & Krishnan, K. (1997) Physiologic-based algabraic expressions for predicting steady-state toxicokinetics of inhaled vapours. *Tox. Methods*, **7**, 207-228

Peltomaki, P., Aaltonen, L.A., Sistonen, P., Pylkkanen, L., Mecklin, J.P., Jarvinen, H., Green, J.S., Jass, J.R., Weber, J.L., Leach, F.S., Petersen, G.M., Hamilton, S.R., de la Chapelle, A. & Vogelstein, B. (1993) Genetic mapping of a locus predisposing to human colorectal cancer. *Science*, **260**, 810-812

Peraino, C., Staffeldt, E.F & Ludemann, V.A. (1981) Early appearance of altered hepatic foci and liver tumours in female rats treated once with carcinogens one day after birth. *Carcinogenesis*, **2**, 463-465

Pero, R.W., Johnson, D.B., Markowitz, M., Doyle, G., Lund-Pero, M., Seidegard, J., Halper, M. & Miller, D.G. (1989) DNA repair synthesis in individuals with and without a family history of cancer. *Carcinogenesis*, **10**, 693-697

Petruzzelli, S., Bernard, P., Paoletti, P., Rane, A., Giuntini, C. & Pacifici, G.M. (1988) Presence of epoxide hydrolase and glutathione S-transferase in human pulmonary alveolar macrophages. *Eur. J. Clin. Pharmacol.*, **34** (4), 419-421

Pitot, H.C. & Campbell, H.A. (1987) An approach to the relative potencies of chemical agents during the stages of initiation and promotion in multistage hepatocarcinogenesis in the rat. *Environ. Health Perspect.*, **76**, 49-56.

Poirier, M.C. & Beland, F.A. (1992) DNA adduct measurements and tumor incidence during chronic carcinogen exposure in animal models: implications for DNA adduct-based human cancer risk assessment. *Chem. Res. Toxicol.*, **5**, 749-755

Poland, A., Glover, E. & Kende, A.S. (1976) Stereospecific, high affinity binding of 2,3,7,8-tetrachlorodibenzo-*p*-dioxin by hepatic cytosol. Evidence that the binding species is receptor for induction of arylhydrocarbon hydroxylase. *J. Biol. Chem.*, **251**, 4936-4946

Portier, C.J. & Kaplan, N.L. (1989) Variability of safe dose estimates when using complicated models of the carcinogenic process. *Fundam. Appl. Toxicol.*, **13**, 533-544

Portier, C., Tritscher, A., Kohn, M., Sewall, C., Clark, G., Edler, L., Hoel, D.G. & Lucier, G. (1993) Ligand/receptor binding for 2,3,7,8-TCDD: implications for risk assessment. *Toxicol. Appl. Pharmacol.*, **20**, 48-56

Preston-Martin, S., Pike, M.C., Ross, R.K., Jones, P.A. & Henderson, B.E. (1990) Increased cell division as a cause of human cancer. *Cancer Res.*, **50**, 7415-7421

Quin, X.-Q., Livingston, D.M., Kaelin, W.G. & Adams, P.D. (1994) Deregulated transcription factor E2F1 expression leads to S-phase entry and p53-mediated apoptosis. *Proc. Natl Acad. Sci. USA*, **91**, 10918-10922

Ramsey, J.C. & Andersen, M.E. (1984) A physiologically based description of the inhalation pharmacokinetics of styrene in rats. *Toxicol. Appl. Pharmacol.*, **73**, 159-175

Rane, A., Wilkinson, G.R. & Shand, G. (1977) Prediction of hepatic extraction ratio from *in vitro* measurements of intrinsic clearance. *J. Pharmacol. Exp. Ther.*, **200**, 420-424

Reddy, J.K. & Lalwani, N.D. (1983) Carcinogenesis by hepatic peroxisome proliferators: evaluation of the risk of hypolipidemic drugs and industrial plasticizers to humans. *CRC Crit. Rev. Toxicol.*, **12**, 1-58

Rideout, W.M., III, Coetzee, G.A., Olumi, A.F. & Jones, P. (1990) 5-Methylcytosine as an endogenous mutagen in the human LDL receptor and *p53* genes. *Science*, **249**, 1288-1290

Robbins, P.D., Horowitz, J.M. & Mulligan, R.C. (1990) Negative regulation of human c-*fos* expression by the retinoblastoma gene product. *Nature*, **346**, 668-671

Ruediger, H.W, Schwartz, U., Serrand, E., Stief, M., Krause, T., Nowak, D., Doerjer, C. Lehnert, G. (1989) Reduced O^6-methylguanine repair in fibroblast cultures from patients with lung cancer. *Cancer Res.*, **49**, 5623-5626

Ruggeri, B., DiRado, Xl., Zhang, S.Y., Bauer, B., Goodrow, T. & Klein-Szanto, A.J.P. (1993) Benzo[*a*]pyrene-induced murine skin tumours exhibit frequent and characteristic G to T mutations in the *p53* gene. *Proc. Natl Acad. Sci. USA*, **90**, 1013-1017

Rustgi, A.K., Nicholas, D. & Bernards, R. (1991) Amino-terminal domains of c-myc and N-myc proteins mediate binding to the retinoblastoma gene product. *Nature*, **352**, 541-544

Sapienza, C. (1992) Genome imprinting and cancer genetics. *Semin. Cancer Biol.*, **3**, 151-158

Sato, A. & Nakajima, T. (1979) Partition coefficients of some aromatic hydrocarbons and ketones in water, blood and oil. *Br. J. Ind. Med.*, **36**, 231-234

Satoh, K., Hatayama, L, Tateoka, N., Tamai, K., Shimizu, T., Tatematsu, M., Ito, N. & Sato, K. (1989) Transient induction of single GST-P positive hepatocytes by DEN. *Carcinogenesis*, **10**, 2107-2111

Savitsky, K., Bar-Shira, A., Gilad, S., Rotman, G., Ziv, Y., Vanagaite, L., Tagle, D.A., Smith, S., Uziel, T., Sfez, S., *et al.* (1995) A single ataxia telangiectasia gene with a product similar to PI-3 kinase. *Science*, **268**, 1749-1753

Scherer, E., Feringa, A.W & Emmelot, P. (1984) Initiation–promotion–initiation. Induction of neoplastic foci within islands of precancerous liver cells in the rat. In: Börzsönyi, M., Laps, K., Day, N.E. & Yamasaki, H., eds, *Models, Mechanisms and Etiology of Tumour Promotion* (IARC Scientific Publications No. 56), Lyon, International Agency for Research on Cancer, pp. 57-66

Schulte-Hermann, R. (1974) Induction of liver growth by xenobiotic compounds and other stimuli. *CRC Crit. Rev. Toxicol.*, **3**, 97-158

Schulte-Hermann, R. (1985) Tumour promotion in the liver. *Arch. Toxicol.*, **57**, 147-158

Schulte-Hermann, R., Ohde, G., Schuppler, J. & Timmermann-Trosiener, I. (1981) Enhanced proliferation of putative preneoplastic cells in rat liver following treatment with the tumour promotors phenobarbital, hexachlorocyclohexane, steroid compounds and nafenopin. *Cancer Res.*, **41**, 2556-2562

Schulte-Hermann, R.. Timmermann-Trosiener, I., Barthel, G. & Bursch, W. (1990) DNA synthesis, apoptosis, and phenotypic expression as determinants of growth of altered foci in rat liver during phenobarbital promotion. *Cancer Res.*, **50**, 5127-5135

Schwarz, M., Buchmann, A., Klormann, H., Schrenk, D. & Kunz, W. (1985) Effect of phenobarbital and other liver monooxygenase modifiers on dimethylnitrosamine induced alkylation of rat liver macromolecules. *Cancer Res.*, **45**, 2020-2024

Scrable, H., Cavenee, W., Ghavimi, F., Lovell, M., Morgan, K. & Sapienza, C. (1989) A model for embryonal rhabdomyosarcorna tumorigenesis that involves genomic imprinting. *Proc. Natl Acad. Sci. USA*, **86**, 7480-7484

Seidegard, J, DePierre, J.W. & Pero, R.W. (1985) Hereditary interindividual differences in the glutathione transferase activity towards *trans*-stilbene oxide in resting human mononuclear leukocytes are due to a particular isozyme(s). *Carcinogenesis*, **6** (8), 1211-1261

Seidegard, J, Pero, R.W., Miller, D.G., & Beattie, E.J. (1986) A glutathione transferase in human leucocytes as a marker for the susceptibility to lung cancer. *Carcinogenesis*, **7**, 751-753

Seidegard, J., Pero, R.W., Markowitz, M.M., Rousch, G., Miller, D.G. & Beattie, E.J. (1990) Isoenzyme(s) of glutathione transferase (class m) as a marker for the susceptibility to lung cancer: a follow-up study. *Carcinogenesis*, **11**, 33-36

Shaw, P., Bovey, R., Tardy, S., Sahli, R., Sordat, B. & Costa, J. (1992) Induction of apoptosis by wild-type *p53* in a human colon tumor-derived cell line. *Proc. Natl Acad. Scl. USA*, **89**, 4485-4499

Shields, P.G. & Harris, C.C. (1991) Molecular epidemiology and the genetics of environmental cancer. *J. Am. Med. Assoc.*, **266**, 681-687

Silbergeld, E.K. & Gasiewicz, T.A.(1989) Dioxins and the Ah receptor. *Am. J. Ind. Med.*, **16**, 455-474.

Singer, B. & Gruenberger, D. (1983) *Molecular Biology of Mutagens and Carcinogens*, New York, NY, Plenum Press

Singer, B. & Essigmann, J.M. (1991) Site-specific mutagenesis: retrospective and prospective. *Carcinogenesis*, **12**, 949-955

Souliotis, V.L., Kaila, S., Boussiotis, V.A., Pangalis, G.A. & Kyrtopulos, S.A. (1990) Accumulation of O6-methylguenine in human blood leukocyte DNA during exposure to procarbazine and its relationships with dose and repair. *Cancer Res.*, **50** (9), 2759-2764

Souliotis, V.L., Zonga, V., Nikolopoulou, V. & Demetriadis, G.J. (1992) Measurement of O6-methylguanine-type adducts in DNA and O6-alkylguanine-DNA-alkyltransferase repair activity in normal and neoplastic human tissues. *Comp. Biochem. Physiol. [B]*, **10** (1–2), 269-275

Sozzi, G., Veronese, M.L., Negrini, M., Baffa, R., Cotticelli, M.G., Inoue, H., Tornielli, S., Pilotti, S., DeGregorio, L., Pastorino, U., Pierotti, M.A., Ohta, M., Huebner, K. & Croce, C.M. (1996) The *FHIT* gene at 3p14.2 is abnormal in lung cancer. *Cell*, **85**, 17-26

Srivastava, S., Zou, Z., Pirollo, K., Blattner, W. & Chang, E.H. (1990) Germ line transmission of a mutated *p53* gene in a cancer-prone family with Li–Fraumeni syndrome. *Nature*, **348**, 747-749

Steiner, E.C., Blau, G.E. & Agin, L.A. (1989) *Introductory Guide to Simusolv, Modeling and Simulation Software*, Midland, MI, Dow Chemical Co.

Stenbeck, F., Mori, H., Furuya, K. & Williams, G.M. (1986) Pathogenesis of dimethyl-nitrosamine-induced hepatocellular cancer in hamster liver and lack of enhancement by phe-nobarbital. *J. Natl Cancer Inst.*, **76**, 327-333

Stewart, B.W. (1992) Role of DNA repair in car-cinogenesis. In: Vainio, H., Magee, P.N., McGregor, D.B. & McMichael A.J., eds, *Mechanisms of Carcinogenesis in Risk Identification* (IARC Scientific publications No. 116), Lyon, International Agency for Research on Cancer, pp. 307-320

Stinchcombe, S., Buchmann, A., Bock, K.W. & Schwarz, M. (1995) Inhibition of apoptosis during 2,3,7,8-tetrachlorodibenzo-*p*-dioxin-mediated tumour promotion in rat liver. *Carcinogenesis*, **16**, 1271-1275.

Strasser, A., Harris, A.W. & Cory, S. (1991) *bcl-2* Transgene inhibits T cell death and perturbs thymic self-censorship. *Cell*, **67**, 889-899

Swenberg, J.A., Dyroff, M.C., Bedell, M.A., Popp, J.A., Huh, N., Kirstein, A. & Rajewsky, M.F. (1984) *O4*-Ethyldeoxythymidine, but not *O6*-ethyldeoxyguanosine accumulates in DNA of hepa-tocytes of rats exposed continuously to diethylni-trosamine. *Proc. Natl Acad. Sci. USA*, **81**, 1692-1695

Swenberg, J.A, Dietrich, D.R., McClain, R.M. & Cohen, S. (1992) Species-specific mechanisms of carcinogenesis. In: Vainio, H., Magee, P.N., McGregor, D.B. & McMichael A.A., eds, *Mechanisms of Carcinogenesis in Risk Identification* (IARC Scientific Publications No. 116), Lyon, International Agency for Research on Cancer. pp. 477-500

Takezawa, I, Miller, F.J. & 0 Neill, J.J. (1980) Single-breath diffusing capacity and lung volumes in small laboratory animals. *J. Appl. Physiol.*, **48**, 1052

Tan, W.Y. (1986) A stochastic Gompertz birth–death process. *Stat. Probab. Lett.*, **4**, 25-28

Tan, W.Y. (1991) *Stochastic Models of Carcinogenesis*. New York, NY, Marcel Dekker

Taylor, J.A., Warson, M.A., Devereux, T.R., Michels, R.Y., Saccorianno, G. & Anderson, M. (1994) *p53* mutation hotspot in radon-associated lung cancer. *Lancet*, **343**, 86-87

Thibodeau, S.N., Bren, G. & Schaid, D. (1993) Microsatellite instability in cancer of the proxi-mal colon. *Science*, **260**, 816-819

Thielmann, H.W., Popanda, 0., Edler, L. & Jung, E.G. (1991) Clinical symptoms and DNA repair characteristics of xeroderma pigmentosum patients from Germany. *Cancer Res.*, **51**, 3456-3470

Thorslund, T. & Charnley, G. (1988) Quantitative dose–response models for tumor promoting agents. In: Hart, R.W. & Hoerger, F.D., eds, *Carcinogenic Risk Assessment: New Directions in Qualitative and Quantitative Aspects*, Cold Spring Harbor, NY, Cold Spring Harbor Laboratory, pp. 245-256

Toft, D., Shyamala, G. & Gorski, J. (1967) A receptor molecule for estrogens. Studies using a cell-free system. *Proc. Natl Acad. Sci. USA*, **57**, 1740-1743

Tomatis, L., Aitio, A., Day, N.E., Heseltine, E., Kaldor, J., Miller, A.B., Parkin, D.M. & Riboli, E. (1990) *Cancer: Causes, Occurrence and Control* (IARC Scientific Publications No. 100), Lyon, International Agency for Research on Cancer

Topal, M. (1988) DNA repair, oncogenes and carcinogenesis. *Carcinogenesis*, 9, 691-696

Tritscher, A.M., Goldstein, J.A., Portier, C.J., McCoy, Z., Clark, G.C. & Lucier, G.W. (1992) Dose–response relationships for chronic exposure to 2,3,7,8-tetrachlorodibenzo-p-dioxin in a rat tumour promotion model: Quantification and immunolocalization of CYP1A2 in the liver. *Cancer Res.*, 53, 3436-3442

Trosko, J.E., Chang, C.C. & Medcalf, A. (1983) Mechanisms of tumor promotion. Potential role of intercellular communication. *Cancer Invest.*, 1, 511-526

Turtletaub, K.W., J.S. Felton, J.S. Vogel, E.G. Snyderwine, S.S. Thorgeirsson, R.H. Adamson, B.L. Gledhill & J.C. Davis (1991) Low-dose DNA dosimetry by accelerator mass spectrometry, *The Toxicologist*, 11, 131

Tyson, J.J. (1991) Modeling the cell division cycle: cdc2 and cyclin interactions. *Proc. Natl Acad. Sci. USA*, 88, 7328-7332

Uematsu, F., Kikuchi, H., Abe, T., Motomiya, M. Ohmachi, T., Sagami, I. & Watanabe, M. (1991) MspI polymorphism of the human *CYP2E* gene. *Nucleic Acids Res.*, 19 (20), 5797

US National Research Council (1990) *Health Effects of Exposure to Low Levels of Ionizing Radiation*, Washington DC, National Academy Press

US National Research Council (1993) *Issues in Risk Assessment*, Washington DC, National Academy Press

US National Toxicology Program (1982) *Bioassay of 2,3,7,8-tetrachlorodibenzo-p-dioxin for Possible Carcinogenicity (Gavage Study)* (Technical Report Series No. 102), Research Triangle Park, NC

Vähäkangas, K.H., Autrup, H. & Harris, C. (1984) Interindividual variations in carcinogen metabolism, DNA damage and DNA repair. In: Berlin, A., Draper, M., Hemminki, K. & Vainio, H., eds, *Monitoring Human Exposure to Carcinogenic and Mutagenic Agents* (IARC Scientific Publications No.59), Lyon, International Agency for Research on Cancer, pp. 85-98

Vähäkangas, K.H., Samet, J.M., Metcalf, R.A., Welsh, J.A., Bennett, W.P., Lane, D.P. & Harris, C.C. (1992) Mutations of *p53* and *ras* genes in radonassociated lung cancer from uranium miners. *Lancet*, 339, 576-580

Vainio, H., Magee, P.N., McGregor, D.B. & McMichael, A.J., eds (1992) *Mechanisms of Carcinogenesis in Risk Identification* (IARC Scientific Publications No. 116), Lyon, International Agency for Research on Cancer

van Delft, J.H., van den Ende, A.M., Keizer, H.J., Ouwerkerk, J. & Baan, R.A. (1992) Determination of N7-methylguanine in DNA of white blood cells from cancer patients treated with dacarbazine. *Carcinogenesis*, 13 (7), 1257-1259

Vesselinovitch, S.D., Rao, K.V.N. & Michailovitch, N. (1979) Neoplastic response of mouse tissues during perinatal age periods and its significance in chemical carcinogenesis. *Natl Cancer Inst. Monogr.*, 51, 239-250

Vineis, P., Caporaso, N., Tannenbaum, S.K, Skipper, P.L., Glogowski, J, Bartsch, H., Coda, M., Talaska, G. & Kadlubar, F. (1990) Acetylation phenotype, carcinogen-hemoglobin adducts, and cigarette smoking. *Cancer Res.*, 50, 3002-3004

Wang, J, Chenivesse, X., Henglein, B. & Brechot, C. (1990) Hepatitis B virus integration in a cyclin A gene in a hepatocellular carcinoma. *Nature*, 343, 555-557

Wassom, J.S., Huff, J.E. & Loprieno, N. (1977) A review of the genetic toxicology of chlorinated dibenzo-p-dioxins, *Mutat. Res.*, 47, 141-160

Wei, Q, Matanoski, G.M., Farmer, E.K., Hedayati, A. & Grossman, L. (1993) DNA repair and aging in basal cell carcinoma: a molecular epidemiology study. *Proc. Natl Acad. Sci. USA*, 90, 1614-1618

Weinberg, R.A. (1991) Tumor suppressor genes. *Science*, **254**, 1138-1146

Weinberg, R.A. (1995) The retinoblastoma protein and cell cycle control. *Cell*, **81**, 323-330

White, E. (1994) *p53*, guardian of Rb. *Nature*, **371**, 21-22

Whittemore, A.S. (1977) The age distribution of human cancer for carcinogenic exposures of varying intensity. *Am. J. Epidemiol.*, **106**, 418-432

Wicksell, D.S. (1925) The corpuscle problem, Part 1. *Biometrika*, **17**, 87-97

Wild, C.P., Hudson, G.J., Sabbioni, G., Chapot, B., Hall, A.J., Wogan, G.N., Whittle, H., Montesano, R. & Groopman, J.D. (1992) Dietary intake of aflatoxins and the level of albumin-bound aflatoxin in peripheral blood in the Gambia, West Africa. *Cancer Epidemiol. Biomarkers Prev.*, **1** (3), 229-234

Willett, W.C. (1994) Diet and health: what should we eat? *Science*, **264**, 532-537

Wogan, G.N. (1973) Aflatoxin carcinogenesis. *Methods Cancer Res.*, **7**, 309-344

Wrighton, S.A. & Stevens, J.C. (1992) The human hepatic cytochromes P450 involved in drug metabolism. *Crit. Rev. Toxicol.*, **22** (1), 1-21

Wu, X. & Levine, A.J. (1994) *p53* and E2F-1 cooperate to mediate apoptosis. *Proc. Natl Acad. Sci. USA*, **91**, 3602-3606

Yang, G.C. & Chen, C.W. (1991) A stochastic two-stage carcinogenesis model: A new approach to computing the probability of observing tumor in animal bioassays. *Math. Biosci.*, **104**, 247-258

Yin, Y., Tainsky, M.A., Bischoff, F.Z., Strong, L.C. & Wahl, G.M. (1992) Wild-type *p53* restores cell cycle control and inhibits gene amplification in cells with mutant *p53* alleles. *Cell*, **70**, 937-948

Yonish-Rouach, E., Resnitzky, D., Lotem, J., Sachs, L., Kimchi, A. & Oren, M. (1991) Wild-type *p53* induces apoptosis of myeloid leukaemic cells that is inhibited by interleukin-6. *Nature*, **352**, 345-347

Quantitative Estimation and Prediction of Human Cancer Risks
S. Moolgavkar, D. Krewski, L. Zeise, E. Cardis and H. Møller
IARC Scientific Publications No. 131
International Agency for Research on Cancer, Lyon, 1999

8: Review of Specific Examples of QEP[1]

Elisabeth Cardis, Lauren Zeise, Michael Schwarz and Suresh Moolgavkar

8.1 Introduction

The aim of this chapter is, with the help of examples, to illustrate the discussion of the problems and limitations of quantitative risk assessment in preceding chapters of this volume, not to undertake a new QEP nor to endorse any of the existing QEPs. The three agents (radon, aflatoxins and 2, 3, 7, 8-tetrachlorodibenzo-*p*-dioxin) discussed are all agents which are ubiquitous in the human environment, for which extensive data (from epidemiological studies, long-term carcinogenicity studies, molecular biology, and mechanistic studies) are available, and formal quantitative risk assessments have been carried out. A brief review of the sources of data useful for quantifying cancer risk and of the main questions of interest in QEP is presented for each, together with a summary of the assumptions made in the existing QEPs, limitations, unresolved issues and research needs.

For *radon*, available data from studies of uranium and other hard rock miners and from animal experiments provide a reasonable description of the dose–response curve for lung cancer over a wide range of exposures, including exposure levels found in some residential settings. The main questions of interest in radon risk assessment are: (1) the effect of the interaction of radon with cigarette smoking; (2) the effect of temporal patterns of exposure; and (3) the effect of lower dose-rate exposures such as are found in many residential settings. Several risk assessments have been carried out and mechanistic models have been used to infer risk as a function of pattern of exposure. Large-scale epidemiological case–control studies of residential exposures with detailed retrospective exposure reconstruction and information on tobacco smoking history are currently under way or have recently been completed. These should provide in the near future a direct test of the adequacy of current predictions of risk for residential exposure.

Naturally occurring *aflatoxins* have been found to be carcinogenic to humans (International Agency for Research on Cancer, 1993), causing primary liver cancer (PLC). Most of the existing epidemiological studies were, however, carried out in areas of relatively high aflatoxin contamination of staple foods and of high prevalence of hepatitis B virus (HBV) infection. Assessment of individual exposure to aflatoxins in most of these studies was, moreover, generally limited. As a consequence, most QEPs have been based on ecological studies. Animal experiments show large interspecies and interstrain differences in sensitivity to aflatoxin-induced liver carcinogenesis. The main questions of interest for QEP are therefore: (1) the characterization of the shape of the dose–response function, including the magnitude of the risk at the relatively low level exposures found in industrialized countries; and (2.) the possible modifying effect of HBV, hepatitis C virus (HCV) and other environmental or endogenous risk factors for PLC. Several QEPs have been carried out, using different assumptions and different data sets, resulting in markedly different risk estimates. It is known that aflatoxins are activated by cytochromes P-450 to a variety of metabolites including aflatoxin epoxide, which reacts with DNA, RNA and proteins. The level of DNA adducts of aflatoxin B_1 (AFB_1) increases roughly in linear fashion with dose in rats, mice and humans, but the level of binding to DNA varies across species and strains. Markers of recent or cumulative exposure to aflatoxin and markers of HBV infection status are being used

---

[1]   The references to this chapter are listed separately for the three substances covered, namely radon (see pp. 284–290), aflatoxin (see pp. 290–298), and 2, 3, 7, 8-tetrachlorodibenzo-p-dioxin (TCDD) (see pp. 298–304).

prospectively in epidemiological studies. Future QEPs should be based on substantial mechanistic information.

The evidence for the carcinogenicity of *TCDD* from epidemiological studies is inconclusive (International Agency for Research on Cancer, 1987), because human exposure to TCDD generally occurs in conjunction with other agents and because of the limited quantification of exposure in existing studies. Existing QEPs therefore rely mainly on data from one large animal experiment and on information on mechanisms and pharmacokinetics. The biological effects and biochemical properties of TCDD have been extensively studied. TCDD is non-DNA-reactive in standard assays and there is evidence that TCDD carcinogenesis involves receptor binding. Thus TCDD is an ideal test compound for the development of mechanistically based models for cancer prediction. Several attempts have been made to carry out such comprehensive risk assessments for this agent. At the present time, however, the relationship between the early biological events studied and cancer is not well understood, and additional information about this is needed if these data are to be of use in QEP.

8.2. Radon and lung cancer

8.2.1 Introduction

The data available currently to evaluate the carcinogenic risk associated with exposure to radon and radon progeny arise mainly from epidemiological studies of occupational exposures in underground mines and from long-term animal carcinogenicity experiments. In 1988, IARC classified radon and its progeny as human carcinogens on the basis of these data (International Agency for Research on Cancer, 1988).

Radium-226 in the earth's crust is the main source of radon-222 in the environment. Occupational exposures occur mainly in mining, particularly in uranium mines. Increases in lung cancer risk have been observed in miners even at relatively low annual exposure levels (average, 5 WLM[1] per year), comparable to exposure levels

from residential radon gas concentrations of 500–1000 Bq/m^3 (Tirmarche *et al.*, 1993). Residential radon surveys have shown that exposure to radon in homes is ubiquitous and varies widely in both magnitude and duration. As many as 5% of the houses surveyed in France and over 10% in Finland (McLaughlin, 1986) had concentrations above 200 Bq/m^3, resulting in annual exposure levels of approximately 1 WLM[2], higher than the average seen in many mines today. Thus, although residential exposure levels tend to be lower than occupational levels, radon is a public health concern in many countries.

Tobacco smoke is also a well established risk factor for human lung cancer and is responsible for a large proportion of the deaths from this disease in industrialized countries (International Agency for Research on Cancer, 1986). In view of the presence of radon gas in homes, the effects of joint exposure to radon and tobacco smoke are of interest.

The main questions of interest for radon QEP are as follows:
- What is the magnitude of the lung cancer risk associated with low cumulative doses from radon found in homes?
- How does risk vary with exposure rate?
- How does risk vary with age at exposure and sex?
- How do other environmental and endogenous exposures, in particular tobacco smoking, modify the risk of radon-induced lung cancer?

8.2.2 Sources of data

8.2.2.1 Occupational epidemiological studies

Much of the information concerning radon and lung cancer is derived from numerous mortality studies of cohorts of miners in Australia, Canada, China, Europe and the USA. Many of these were reviewed by BEIR IV (US National Academy of Sciences/National Research Council, Committee on the Biological Effects of Ionizing Radiations, 1988) and by the International Agency for Research on Cancer (1988); papers

---

[1] WLM (working level month): exposure resulting from inhalation of air with a concentration of 1 working level (WL) of radon progeny for 170h; WL: any combination of short-lived radon progeny in 1 litre of air that results in the ultimate emission of 1.3×10^5 MeV of potential α energy.

[2] Throughout this chapter, conversion from radon gas concentrations to annual exposure levels (in WLM) are made assuming a mean equilibrium factor of 0.45 and a mean residence time of 7000 h per year unless otherwise indicated.

published since then include: Morrison *et al.* (1988); Sevc *et al.* (1988); Kusiak *et al* (1991, 1993); Samet *et al.* (1991a); Woodward *et al.* (1991); Tirmarche *et al.* (1993); Tirmarche, (1995); Xuan *et al.* (1993); Fu *et al.* (1994); Lubin *et al.* (1994a, b, 1995a, b, c); Tomasek *et al.* (1994 a, b); Darby *et al.* (1995); Roscoe *et al.* (1995); Tomasek & Darby (1995) and Howe & Stager (1996). Table 8.1 shows the characteristics of the 11 large epidemiological studies of underground miners in which some measure of individual radon exposure was available.

Table 8.1 Characteristics of 11 cohort studies of underground miners

Country (Reference)	Type of mine	Number of workers	Number of lung cancer deaths	Source of information on radon	Information on other exposures
Australia (Woodward *et al.*, 1991)	Uranium	2 574	54	1954–1961: 721 measurement of radon gas	Tobacco: 1984 survey of 50% of miners
Canada, Newfoundland (Morrison *et al.*, 1988)	Fluorspar	1 772	113[a]	< 1960: none: estimation; 1960–1967: measurements of radon progeny; > 1969: daily individual levels recorded	Tobacco surveys available on 48% of miners
Canada, Ontario (Kusiak *et al.*, 1993)	Uranium	21 346	284	< 1958: none: estimation; 1958+: 1000–2000 measurements of radon gas; 1980+: radon progeny	Tobacco: survey of 1189 miners
Canada, North West Territories, Port Radium (Howe *et al.*, 1987)	Uranium	2 103	57	< 1940: none; 1945+: measurements in mines, job-exposure matrix	–
Canada, Saskatchewan, Beaverlodge (Howe *et al.*, 1986)	Uranium	8 487	65	1954–1966: air sampling of radon gas; 1967: individual progeny measurements several times a month	Tobacco: nested case–control study
China (Xuan *et al.*, 1993)	Tin	17 143	981	Work histories and WL; < 1972: radon gas measurements; > 1972: 26 000 measurements of radon and progeny; Recreation of ≤ 1972 mine conditions	Arsenic; tobacco: 1976 survey (24% missing)

Table 8.1 (Contd). Characteristics of 11 cohort studies of underground miners					
Country (Reference)	Type of mine	Number of workers	Number of lung cancer deaths	Source of information on radon	Information on other exposures
Czech Republic (Tomasek et al., 1994a)	Uranium	4 320	702	1948–1967: 39 000 measurements of radon gas in Jáchymov and Horni Slavkov; many elsewhere; > 1967: radon progeny	–
France (Tirmarche et al., 1993)	Uranium	1 735	45	< 1956: few measurements of radon gas; 1956–1985: systematic monitoring of individual exposure 1983+: individual α-dosimeters	Dust: from 1956
Sweden (Radford & St Clair Renard, 1984)	Iron	1 415	50	Measurements of radon gas Reconstruction of WL	Tobacco: > 50% of miners living in 1970 surveyed
USA, Colorado (Hornung & Meinhardt, 1987)	Uranium	3 346	256	< 1951: few measurements of radon gas; 1951–1960: 43 000 measurements of radon progeny in 2500 mines; 1969+: none (many mines closed)	Tobacco: censuses of miners between 1950 and 1969
USA, New Mexico (Samet et al., 1991b)	Uranium	3 469	68	< 1967: annual estimate per mine; 1967+: WLM estimates for individuals	Tobacco: clinic

[a] Trachea, bronchus and lung combined

In these studies, the quality of the information on the level of exposure to radon varied across cohorts and over time, from a few air measurements of radon gas and radon decay products made for control purposes in particular areas of some mines in the early years, or recreation of early mining conditions, to real-time individual exposure estimates (taking into account ventilation patterns, ore characteristics, mining methodology, weekly surveys of γ radiation, radon and dust levels, and the location and duration of work of individual miners), and even to individual estimates from personal α dosimeters in more recent years in France (Tirmarche et al., 1993).

The great majority of miners were adult men, although the Chinese study (Xuan et al., 1993) included a substantial number of women (2800) and children exposed from the age of 10 (number not specified).

Table 8.2 shows exposure characteristics and follow-up in the 11 studies. Average duration of exposure in the mines varied greatly across studies, from 1.7 years in the Beaverlodge cohort (Howe et al., 1986) to 19.5 years in the Swedish cohort (Radford & St Clair Renard, 1984). Mean cumulative exposure varied from 7.0 WLM in the Australian cohort (Woodward et al., 1991) to 430.4 WLM in the Colorado cohort (Hornung & Meinhardt, 1987) and exposure rate from approx-

Table 8.2 Characteristics of exposure, follow-up and risk estimates in 11 cohort studies

Country (Reference)	Follow-up period (years)	Average length of follow-up (years)	Mean cumulative exposure (WLM)	Mean duration (years)	Exposure rate (WLM/year)	ERR per 100 WLM[a] (95% CI)
Australia (Woodward et al., 1991)	1948–1987	19.5	7.3	1.0	7.3	5.4 (1.0–17.0)
Canada, Newfoundland (Morrison et al., 1988)	1950–1984	23.2[b]	367.315[c]	4.85[c]	76.55[c]	0.9[c] (0.6–1.2)
Canada, Ontario (Kusiak et al., 1993)	1955–1986	17.8	30.8	3.0	10.3	1.2 (0.02–2.4)
Canada, North West Territories, Port Radium (Howe et al., 1987)	1950–1980	16.5	183.3	NA[d]	NA[d]	0.3[e] (0.1–0.4)
Canada, Saskatchewan, Beaverlodge (Howe et al., 1986; Howe & Stager, 1996)	1950–1980	13.9	81.3	1.7	6.4	2.6 (1.1–5.4)[f] 3.3 (1.0–9.6)[g]
China (Xuan et al., 1993)	1976–1987	10.2	275.4	13.5	20.4	0.2[h] (0.1–0.2)
Czech Republic(Tomasek et al., 1994a)	1952–1990	24.8	219	7.9	1948: 87 1960: 17 1970: 3	0.64 (0.4–1.1)[i] 1.41 (0.7–3.3)[j]
France (Tirmarche et al., 1993)	1946–1985	25.2	70.4	14.5	4.9	0.59 (0.0–1.6)
Sweden (Radford & St Clair Renard, 1984)	1951–1976	NA[d]	93.7	19.5	4.8	2.6 (1.5–3.8) 1.4[k]
USA, Colorado(Hornung & Meinhardt, 1987)	1950–1982	NA[d]	430.4[l]	NA[d]	123.611	0.9–1.4[m] 0.6
USA, New Mexico (Samet et al., 1991b)	1943–1985	17.05	111.4	7.4	15.0	1.8[n] (0.7–5.4)

[a] Doses lagged by five years unless otherwise indicated.
[b] From Lubin et al., 1994a.
[c] Unlagged doses.
[d] NA: not available.
[e] Doses lagged by 10 years.
[f] Cohort study (Howe et al., 1986).
[g] Case-control study with revised exposure estimates (Howe & Stager, 1996).
[h] After adjustment for arsenic exposure.
[i] Whole cohort.
[j] Low exposure rate (<10 WL) subcohort.
[k] From National Academy of Sciences (1988).
[l] Median.
[m] Lag of four years and partial weighting of doses in 4–10 year period; adjusted for smoking.
[n] Unchanged by smoking adjustment.

imately 5 WLM/year in the French (Tirmarche et al., 1993) and Swedish (Radford & St Clair Renard, 1984) cohorts to over 120 WLM/year in the Colorado cohort.

In most studies, some information on tobacco use among sections of the workforce was available (Table 8.1), mostly from ad hoc single or repeated surveys carried out among active workers. The information obtained was not strictly comparable across studies because of differences in the amount of detail and method of data collection; in addition, information on smoking was lacking for substantial portions of the cohorts.

Information on histological type and localization of lung cancers was available from several studies. Review and classification methods varied. The most extensive data come from the Colorado cohort; in a study of 467 lung tumours diagnosed in uranium miners (all but 24 were in smokers) between 1947 and 1991, Saccomanno et al. (1996) found 225 squamous-cell carcinomas (48.2%), 159 small-cell carcinomas (34.0%), 72 adenocarcinomas (15.4%) and 11 large-cell carcinomas (2.4%). Among 311 lung tumours diagnosed in non-miners with the same age and calendar year of diagnosis, they found proportionally more squamous-cell carcinomas (213; 68.5%) and fewer small-cell carcinomas (40; 12.9%). The proportion of lung cancers in the central zone of the bronchial tree was significantly higher (318; 68%) among miners than non-miners (183; 58.8%). There were 10 times as many small-cell tumours in the central zone than in the middle and peripheral region among miners, and five times more among non-miners. The authors concluded that inhaled dust, radon and cigarette smoke combine to form large particulates that deposit in the central bronchial tree.

Despite differences in populations, methodology, exposure levels and exposure rates, and in the distribution of age, smoking and other factors which may modify the relation between radon exposure and risk of lung cancer, the estimates of excess relative risk (ERR) derived in these studies are within an order of magnitude of each other, ranging from 0.2 to 5.4 per WLM (Table 8.2).

8.2.2.2 Animal studies

A large number of animal experiments involving exposure to radon and its progeny, primarily through inhalation, have been carried out in the last 50 years. Several reviews of these experiments have been published (Cross, 1988; International Agency for Research on Cancer, 1988; US National Academy of Sciences/National Research Council, Committee on the Biological Effects of Ionizing Radiations, 1988). On the basis of these experiments, an IARC study group concluded that there is "sufficient" evidence for the carcinogenicity of radon and its progeny in experimental animals (International Agency for Research on Cancer, 1988).

Experiments designed to simulate the environment of underground uranium miners were carried out on SPF Wistar rats, Syrian golden hamsters and beagle dogs exposed to mixtures of radon, radon progeny, uranium ore dust, diesel engine exhaust and cigarette smoke. Experiments attempting to recreate more general environments were carried out with SPF Sprague–Dawley rats exposed to mixtures of radon, radon progeny, ambient air aerosols and cigarette smoke. Respiratory tract tumours were observed in treated animals, as well as pulmonary fibrosis, emphysema and life shortening (Cross, 1992). Most of the lung tumours were adenomas, adenocarcinomas, epidermoid carcinomas and adenosquamous carcinomas; some mesotheliomas and sarcomas were also observed.

Overall, carcinogenic risk was found to increase with increasing cumulative radon progeny exposure in the range 500–7000 WLM, as well as with unattached fraction and with cigarette smoke exposure, and to decrease with increasing exposure rate in the range 50–500 WLM/week (Cross, 1988). The estimated excess lifetime risk per million rats for lifetime exposure, based on a combined analysis of experiments performed by Pacific Northwest Laboratories, was 0.086 per $J.h.m^{-3}$ (300 per 10^6 rats per WLM) for all primary lung tumours, and 0.071 per $J.h.m^{-3}$ (250 per 10^6 rats per WLM) for carcinomas alone (Gilbert, 1989).

8.2.2.3 Residential radon studies

The lung cancer risk associated with indoor radon has been investigated directly in populations exposed residentially, primarily in numerous ecological and case–control studies.

The ecological studies carried out to date have been reviewed recently by Stidley & Samet (1993) and United Nations Scientific Committee on the Effects of Atomic Radiation (1994). Nineteen distinct studies have been carried out to date, in Canada (Létourneau et al., 1983), China (Hoffman et al., 1985, 1986), Denmark and Sweden (Gjorup & Hansen, 1987), Finland (Castren et al., 1985), Italy (Forastiere et al., 1985),

Japan (Mifune *et al.*, 1992), Norway (Stranden, 1986), Sweden (Edling *et al.*, 1982), the United Kingdom (Haynes, 1988) and the USA (Stockwell *et al.*, 1988a,b; Vonstille & Sacarello, 1990; Bean *et al.*, 1982; Hess *et al.*, 1983; Fleischer, 1986; Archer, 1987; Cohen, 1990, 1992, 1993, 1994b; Cohen & Colditz, 1994; Cohen, 1995a,b). The results of these studies are not consistent: in eight of 19 studies, there was a significant positive association between lung cancer incidence or mortality and indoor radon exposure; in one there was a positive, non-significant, association; four studies found no association and six an inverse relation.

It is difficult to interpret the results of these studies. This is due in part to the usual methodological limitations that characterize ecological studies (Piantadosi *et al.*, 1988; Greenland & Morgenstern, 1989; Greenland, 1992; see also section 4.3). Ecological regression methods are usually unsatisfactory for controlling for the effects of potential confounding variables and assessing effect modification. In addition, errors in the measurement of radon exposure as a result of using current exposure levels to infer past exposures, confounders or modifying factors can lead to biased risk estimates (Stidley & Samet, 1993). In one of the studies mentioned above, in which average radon levels in homes tested in numerous states and counties in the USA appear to be consistently negatively correlated with lung cancer mortality rates, Cohen (1990, 1993; Cohen & Colditz, 1994) used county-level information about the prevalence of smoking, indicators of a large number of socioeconomic factors, geography, altitude and weather to account for the effect of possible confounders. He concluded (Cohen, 1995a, b) that it was unlikely that smoking or other confounding factors could account for the observed negative relationship. Greenland & Morgenstern (1992) argue, however, that unexpected or biased findings may occur in ecological studies as a result of model misspecification and within-region misclassification. Stidley & Samet (1994) used simulations to examine the effects of model misspecification, inadequate control for confounding, and measurement error (related to the sampling process used to estimate radon exposure in a geographical unit) in ecological regressions of lung cancer and radon. They concluded that all of these may introduce important biases in ecological studies and compromise the results of ecological studies of radon exposure. These theoretical arguments notwithstanding, it is difficult to explain away Cohen's findings.

The association between residential radon exposure and lung cancer risk can be tested more directly using individual-level studies. Most of the studies carried out to date have used a case–control design. Exposure was estimated either using a surrogate index (e.g. type of housing) or direct radon concentration measurements in current and previous homes of the study subjects. Many of the published studies have been reviewed by Borek & Johnson (1988), International Agency for Research on Cancer (1988), Neuberger (1991) and United Nations Scientific Committee on the Effects of Atomic Radiation (1994). They include studies in Canada (Lees *et al.*, 1987, Létourneau *et al.*, 1994), China (Blot *et al.*, 1990), Finland (Auvinen *et al.*, 1996), Sweden (Axelson *et al.*, 1979, 1988; Simpson & Comstock, 1983; Edling *et al.*, 1984, 1986; Pershagen *et al.*, 1992, 1994; Svensson *et al.*, 1987, 1989; Klotz *et al.*, 1989) and the USA (Schoenberg *et al.*, 1990; Alavanja *et al.*, 1994).

Given the relatively low levels of the exposure of concern for residential exposures and the presumably small risk expected, only very large studies (including several thousands of cases (Lubin *et al.*, 1990)) and detailed individual historical exposure assessment are likely to provide useful information for the direct quantification of the effects of residential exposures. A number of such studies are currently under way in Europe and North America using similar protocols (Samet *et al.*, 1991b). Information on cigarette smoking and exposure to other potential confounding factors has been collected systematically. Together, these studies cover approximately 11 000 cases and 18 000 controls with detailed individual exposure reconstruction. The results of these studies are expected by 1998, and subsequent combined analyses are likely to provide important information about the adequacy of current extrapolations to residential settings from data on underground miners. The completed studies are described below.

The New Jersey study (Schoenberg *et al.*, 1990) covered 433 women with lung cancer and 402 controls frequency-matched for age, race and vital status. Year-long α-track measurements were made in the living areas, usually the bedrooms of dwellings, occupied for at least 10 years by the study subjects. A significant association between lung cancer risk and radon level was seen after adjustment for smoking, age and occupation. The ERR per WLM was estimated to be 3.4 per 100 WLM (0.0–8.0). The odds ratios in exposure categories 1–1.99 pCi/l (37–74 Bq/m^3), 2–3.99 pCi/l (74–148 Bq/m^3) and 4 pCi/l and above (148 Bq/m^3 and above) compared with less than 1 pCi/l were 1.1 (0.8–1.7), 1.3 (0.6–2.9) and 4.2 (1.0–17.5), respectively. The strongest association was seen among non-smokers. The study subjects generally had low exposure levels—in only 1% of homes were levels in excess of 4 pCi/l (148 Bq/m^3).

In the Shenyang study in China, α-track detectors were placed for one year in the living room and bedroom of the homes of 308 women with lung cancer and 356 age-matched population controls. No association between radon level and risk of lung cancer was found in this study, in which the median exposure level was 2.3 pCi/l (85 Bq/m^3); nearly 6% of homes had levels in excess of 8 pCi/l (296 Bq/m^3).

In the Canadian study, radon detectors were placed in current and former residences of 750 cases of lung cancer and 750 age- and sex-matched controls in Winnipeg, Manitoba. Radon concentration was determined by means of α-track detectors placed in the living areas and basement of the homes for a period of one year. No association between cumulative radon exposure and lung cancer was observed. Average concentration in living areas was 120 Bq/m^3 (resulting in annual exposures of 0.6 WLM); approximately 1% of measurements exceeded 800 Bq/m^3 (resulting in annual exposures of 4 WLM); 70% of controls were ever-smokers (Létourneau et al., 1994).

The Swedish study included 586 female and 774 male lung cancer cases, and two control groups totalling 1380 female and 1467 male controls, frequency-matched on age and calendar year. One of the control groups was also matched on vital status. Radon measurements were carried out over a period of three months in the heating season using α-track detectors in current and past dwellings of the study subjects. Relative risks (RR)

of 1.3 (95% CI 1.1–1.6) and 1.8 (1.1–2.9) were obtained, respectively, for radon concentrations of 140–400 Bq/m^3 (resulting in annual exposure levels of 0.7–2 WLM) and 400 Bq/m^3 or more (resulting in annual exposure levels of 2 WLM or more). A significant interaction with tobacco smoking was observed. The average concentration in living areas was 107 Bq/m^3 (resulting in annual exposures of 0.5 WLM) (Pershagen et al., 1994).

A population-based case–control study was also carried out among women in Missouri (USA) who were lifetime non-smokers or long-term ex-smokers (Alavanja et al., 1995). It included 618 lung cancer cases and 1402 age-matched controls. Year-long measurements of radon with α-track detectors were made in the kitchen and bedroom of residences occupied in the previous 5–30 years. A small non-significant increase in risk was found for study subjects exposed to median domestic radon concentrations—25-year time-weighted average—of 4 pCi/l (150 Bq/m^3); since only a small fraction of the population is exposed at this level, the population attributable risk was estimated to be less than 2%.

A population-based case–control study was also carried out, nested within a cohort of Finns residing in the same one-family house between 1 January 1967 and the end of 1985 (Auvinen et al., 1996). This design was chosen to maximize the validity of the estimates of long-term residential radon exposure. The study subjects were 1973 lung cancer patients (excluding cancers of the pleura) and 2885 age- and sex-matched controls drawn from the same cohort; α-track detectors were sent to the dwellings of all study subjects and the recipients were instructed to place them in the living room or bedroom for a period of 12 months. The mean radon concentration was 103 Bq/m^3 among cases and 96 Bq/m^3 among controls. A total of 517 case–control pairs were used in the matched analyses, and 1055 cases and 1544 controls in the unmatched analyses. No significant association between radon exposure and risk of lung cancer was observed. The odds ratios of lung cancer for indoor radon exposure obtained in the matched analysis was 1.01 (95% CI 0.94–1.08); for indoor concentrations of 50–99, 100–199, 200–399 400–1277 Bq/m^3, respectively, the odds ratios were 1.03 (0.8–1.3),

1.00 (0.8–1.3), 0.91 (0.6–1.4) and 1.15 (0.7–1.9) compared with those with less than 50 Bq/m^3. The unmatched analysis gave similar results.

Combined analyses of the results of lung cancer case–control studies among women from the Shenyang, New Jersey and Stockholm studies have also been carried out (Lubin et al., 1994a). They covered a total of 966 cases and 1158 controls. Close to 14% of the study subjects were estimated to have a mean time-weighted radon concentration in their homes of more than 150 Bq/m^3 in the period 5–35 years prior to the date of diagnosis. There was a non-significant trend of increasing lung cancer risk with increasing radon exposure. The overall ERR per pCi/l (i.e. per 37 Bq/m^3) was 0.00 (-0.05–0.07). The confidence interval is such that the estimate is compatible with estimates derived from studies on miners. Cigarette smoking was the predominant cause of lung cancer in the studies. Within smoking categories, the association between radon and lung cancer was inconsistent.

It is planned to combine residential radon studies. Lubin and collaborators (1994a) warn, however, that "care must be taken in combining and interpreting results from these studies because of the intrinsic limitations of studies of low levels of risk and because of the uncertainties associated with estimating cumulative residential radon levels accurately".

In a another paper, Lubin et al. (1995b) simulated a series of case–control studies and evaluated the resulting dose–response relationships. Four error distributions were assumed; for each, 10 studies of 700 cases and an equal number of controls were generated from a population with a risk of radon-induced lung cancer based on extrapolations from data on miners. When exposure was assumed to be known without error, 6/10 failed to find a significant dose–response. When errors were postulated, the situation became worse as the power was reduced. When mobility and missing measurements in homes previously occupied were incorporated in the design of the simulated studies, the power of the studies decreased, reducing the chance of detecting a statistically significant effect. On the other hand, when studies were generated on the assumption that exposure did not increase risk, up to 15% of simulated studies with 700 cases and controls resulted in an esti-

mate of the dose–response parameter in excess of that from studies on miners. This work shows that errors in exposure assessment and incomplete measurements may play a substantial role in explaining the inconsistencies of current residential studies; it also highlights the intrinsic difficulties of these studies. The authors concluded that it is unlikely that residential case–control studies alone will be able to determine precise estimates of risk from indoor radon, and that future efforts at pooling studies may not adequately address issues of risk from residential exposure.

8.2.2.4 Mechanistic studies

Radon decays with a half-life of 3.82 days into a series of short-lived isotopes (the radon progeny), including polonium-218 and polonium-214. These emit α-particles which can interact directly with DNA (Hall, 1978), most probably causing deletion-type mutations (Nakamura, 1991).

Cellular and molecular effects of α-particle irradiation have been examined in relation to radon-induced lung cancer (US National Academy of Sciences, 1988; Evans, 1990). An "inverse dose-rate effect" (i.e. an increase in carcinogenic effect per unit exposure for lower exposure rates or longer exposure times) has been observed in a number of experimental studies with high linear energy transfer (LET) radiation, neutrons and α-particles (see, for example, Hill et al., 1984, Rossi & Kellerer, 1986). This effect has been attributed to multiple traversals of a cell by α-particles (Brenner & Hall, 1992; Brenner et al., 1993; Brenner, 1994). Another explanation of this effect, based on the possible promotion of initiated cells either by radon or by the aerosol on which it is carried into the lung, has also been proposed (Moolgavkar et al., 1990, 1993; Luebeck et al., 1996). At low exposures, both postulated mechanisms predict that inverse dose-rate effects will not occur.

Recent studies have investigated the possibility that radon may induce specific mutations in the human p53 tumour-suppressor gene and the K-ras proto-oncogene in lung cancer tissues in uranium miners (Vähäkangas et al., 1992; Taylor et al., 1994; Husgafvel et al., 1995; McDonald et al., 1995). Mutations have been identified in lung tumour tissue from miners who received high exposure levels in the Colorado Plateau mines. The spectrum of mutations appears to be related to the histological type of the tumour: Taylor *et al.* (1994) reported mutations in codon 249 of the *p53* tumour-suppressor gene in 16 (31%) of 52 large- and squamous-cell tumours from the Colorado miners' cohort. McDonald *et al.* (1995) observed none among 23 adenocarcinomas studied, although they observed mutations in hotspots of the K-*ras* proto-oncogene in nine of these tumours (39%). If these mutations are indeed specific, and if they are dose-related, their detection in lung cancer cases in epidemiological studies could be of importance for characterizing the role of environmental radon in lung carcinogenesis. Studies of lung tumours among miners with lower exposures (Vähäkangas *et al.*, 1992) and among persons residentially exposed (Lo *et al.*, 1995) have so far failed to identify any mutations at codon 249 of the *p53* gene, however. Mutations in *p53* and *ras* are, moreover, common genetic defects in lung cancer: mutations in *p53* are observed in 60% of human cancers (Harris & Hollstein, 1993) and mutations in *ras* genes, mainly K-*ras*, have been observed in 20–30% of non-small-cell lung cancer cases (Bos, 1989; Minna, 1993). The interpretation of findings among uranium miners is therefore unclear at present.

8.2.2.5 Cofactors and effect modifiers

Since *tobacco smoking* is a strong lung carcinogen in humans, it may play a role in the development of lung cancer induced by radon decay products. Analyses of the joint effects of radon exposure and tobacco smoking have been carried out in most large cohort studies; they are reviewed in the BEIR IV report (US National Academy of Sciences/National Research Council, Committee on the Biological Effects of Ionizing Radiations, 1988) and in the United Nations Scientific Committee on the Effects of Atomic Radiation (UNSCEAR) report (1994). As described above, however, the data used for this purpose were limited. Most of the analyses suggest that the interaction between radon and tobacco is greater than additive, but less than multiplicative on a linear relative risk scale. The uncertainty surrounding the precise type of interaction limits the extrapolations of risk which can be made for the

general public. With a multiplicative model, exposure to radon in a population containing a large number of smokers will result in a much larger excess of lung cancer cases than in an additive model, even if the risk associated with radon exposure alone is much smaller than that associated with tobacco. The interaction between radon and tobacco smoking is also being investigated in several of the case–control studies of domestic radon exposure.

In animal experiments, the influence of cigarette smoke exposure appears to vary with the temporal pattern of the exposures: an enhanced effect was observed when cigarette exposure followed radon exposure, while no influence of tobacco smoke was seen when cigarette exposure preceded radon exposure. Results of other experiments with alternating exposures are less clear and include decreased effects of both exposures (Cross *et al.*, 1982; Cross, 1992). The observation that tumours in animals exposed to both radon progeny and cigarette smoke are larger and more invasive than in those animals exposed to radon progeny alone may be indicative of a shorter latent period in smoking-related tumours (US National Academy of Sciences, 1988).

Other *cofactors* of lung carcinogenesis may be present in mining environments, including silica, arsenic, diesel exhaust and blasting fumes. Radiogenic agents other than radon are present in uranium mines: γ-ray and prolonged ore dust exposures occur at the same time as radon exposure. Animal experiments have shown that lung tumours can be induced by radon decay products both alone and in the presence of such agents (Cross, 1988). In most of the published studies on uranium miners, no adjustment for these factors could be made since past individual exposures were not recorded systematically. Silicosis was reported in Swedish and French studies of miners (Radford & St Clair Renard, 1984; Tirmarche *et al.*, 1993). Arsenic was considered in the Czech and Chinese studies. Miners in the Czech cohort were employed in two different mines, namely Jáchymov (with average levels of arsenic in the dust of 0.5%) and Horní Slavkov (where arsenic levels were negligible) (Tomasek *et al.*, 1994a); miners who spent more than 20% of their working life in Jáchymov had an ERR of radon-induced lung cancer 1.8 times higher than those who spent less than 20% of it in that mine. In the Chinese tin miner study, many miners were also exposed to arsenic (Xuan *et al.*, 1993). Adjusting for arsenic exposure reduced the estimated ERR from 0.6 per 100 WLM to 0.2 per 100 WLM. Concomitant exposures in houses may be different from those experienced in mining environments.

The risk estimates derived from mining studies mainly concern men of working age and may not be directly applicable to women, children and older persons. Little information is available to evaluate whether age and sex modify the risk associated with radon progeny exposure. Some information comes from a small group of young tin miners (Xuan *et al.*, 1993) who did not appear to have a greatly increased risk compared with miners exposed as adults. Studies of atomic bomb survivors, who received exposures to different radiation types and in different circumstances, suggest that, for low LET radiation (predominantly γ-rays), the relative risk of solid cancers may be higher in those exposed as children (because of increased sensitivity) and in women (because of lower background rates of lung cancer) (US National Academy of Sciences/National Research Council, Committee on the Biological Effects of Ionizing Radiations, 1990).

8.2.2.6 Lung dosimetry

Lung cancer risk estimates can theoretically be derived for the general public from estimates for miners on the basis of models of the relationship between exposure and dose to target cells. Such models take account of differences in lung morphometry and levels of exertion, and depend on a large number of physical and biological factors (US National Academy of Sciences/National Research Council, Committee on the Biological Effects of Ionizing Radiations, 1988, 1991):

- Age
- Sex
- Aerosol size distribution
- Unattached fraction of radon progeny
- Breathing rate and route (oral versus nasal)
- Pattern and efficiency of deposition of radon progeny
- Solubility of radon progeny in mucus
- Influence of smoking on aerosol characteristics and lung morphometry.

The US National Academy of Sciences Panel on Dosimetric Assumptions Affecting the Application of Radon Risk Estimates (US National Academy of Sciences, 1991) has attempted a comprehensive comparison of exposure–dose relations for mining and home environments using a dosimetric model. Calculations indicated that doses of α energy per unit exposure delivered to target cells in the respiratory tract tend to be generally a little lower, and never higher, in the home environment compared with the mining environment. This reduction is of the order of 30% for adults of both sexes and less than 20% for infants and children; such estimations are, however, subject to considerable uncertainty (US National Academy of Sciences, 1991).

8.2.3 Empirical approach to QEP

The data sets of many of the epidemiological studies of miners have been combined and analysed by different investigators and international groups, using different risk models (US National Academy of Sciences, 1980; US National Council on Radiation Protection and Measurements, 1984; Thomas *et al.*, 1985; International Commission on Radiation Protection, 1987; US National Academy of Sciences/National Research Council, Committee on the Biological Effects of Ionizing Radiations, 1988; Lubin *et al.*, 1994b, 1995a). Early analyses by the US National Council on Radiation Protection and Measurements (1984) and the BEIR III committee (US National Academy of Sciences/National Research Council, Committee on the Biological Effects of Ionizing Radiations, 1980) were based on a constant absolute risk model; the International Commission on Radiation Protection (1987) favoured a constant relative risk model.

8.2.3.1 BEIR IV

The report of the US National Academy of Sciences/National Research Council, Committee on the Biological Effects of Ionizing Radiation (1988) (BEIR IV) was based on a joint analysis of data from four cohorts of miners: uranium miners from Ontario (Kusiak *et al.*, 1991), Saskatchewan (Howe *et al.*, 1986), and the Colorado plateau (Hornung & Meinhardt, 1987) and Swedish metal miners (Radford & St Clair Renard, 1984). In these analyses, the Colorado cohort was restricted to miners with cumulative exposure below 2000 WLM. Both internal comparisons by level of risk and comparisons with external reference populations were carried out. The Committee fitted families of time-dependent relative risk models to the data on miners, using Poisson regression and taking into account cumulative exposure, duration of exposure, attained age, age at first exposure, time since cessation of exposure as well as exposure in different time intervals. The final model chosen was a time-dependent relative risk model in which ERR varies with time since exposure and depends on attained age, but does not take into account either exposure rate or smoking. The model is written as follows:

$$r(a) = r_0(a) \left[1 + 0.025 \ c(a) \ (W_1 + 0.5 \ W_2) \right]$$

where:

$r(a)$ is the age-specific lung cancer mortality rate in a given calendar period for attained age a;

$r_0(a)$ is the age-specific background lung-cancer mortality rate (assumed to include the effect of smoking);

$c(a)$ is 1.2 for age a less than 55 years, 1.0 for age a between 55 and 64 years, 0.4 for age a greater than or equal to 65;

W_1 is the cumulative dose in WLM incurred between five and 15 years in the past; and

W_2 is the cumulative dose in WLM incurred 15 years or more in the past.

In this model, radon exposures distant in time have less impact on the age-specific ERR than more recent exposures. In these analyses, information on tobacco smoking used to examine the interaction between radon and tobacco on the risk of lung cancer came primarily from the Colorado miners' cohort. Although a sub-multiplicative model provided the best fit, the Committee chose the more parsimonious multiplicative model for use in risk projection. This implies that the coefficients in the model are averaged over the smoking patterns of the four cohorts and may not be directly applicable to other populations (the risk estimates may be biased because no adjustment for tobacco smoking was possible,).

The BEIR IV Committee used this model to predict risks to residentially exposed populations, assuming that the above risk estimates could be extended over the entire life span, that cigarette smoke and radon exposure interact multiplicatively on the age-specific relative risk, that exposure to radon progeny increases the risk of lung cancer in proportion to the age and sex-specific baseline risk of lung cancer associated with other causes, and that a WLM results in approximately the same dose to the bronchial epithelium in both occupational and residential settings (US National Academy of Sciences, 1988). Mortality rates for smokers and non-smokers in the USA over the period 1980–1984 for men and women were used, assuming a steady-state pattern of tobacco consumption (with approximately 48% of men and 36% of women smoking), a uniform age at beginning of smoking of 18, and RRs of lung cancer for smokers versus non-smokers of 12 and 10, respectively, for men and women. The age-specific lung cancer rates for non-smokers r_n (a) were calculated from population rates, $r_0(a)$ as follows:

$$r_n \ (a) = r_0(a) \ / \ (P + RR(1 - P))$$

where P is the proportion of non-smokers and RR is the relative risk of lung cancer for smokers versus non-smokers.

As a result, the Committee estimated that a lifetime exposure to 1 WLM per year would increase the number of deaths due to lung cancer by a factor of about 1.5 over the background rate for both men and women in populations with the same prevalence rate of tobacco smoking. In the American population, this correspond to 506 extra deaths per 100 000 men and to 186 extra deaths per 100 000 women. Most of these additional deaths would be in smokers, for whom the radon-related risk would be approximately 10 times greater than that in non-smokers (US National Academy of Sciences, 1988).

8.2.3.2 Joint analyses of 11 studies on miners

A joint analysis of data from the 11 cohorts of miners listed in Table 8.1 has recently been carried out (Lubin *et al.*, 1994b) with the aim of evaluating further the exposure–response relationship and, in particular, of assessing the effects of attained age, exposure rate, age at first exposure, time since exposure and tobacco smoking on estimates of excess relative risk per WLM (ERR/WLM). The analyses covered data on 68 000 miners, 2700 lung cancer deaths and 1.2×10^6 person–years of observation. Linear relative risk models were fitted, using Poisson regression, stratifying for cohort, attained age and, when available, other occupational exposures and ethnicity, and modelling the effects of the variables listed above for the BEIR IV model. The analyses were not stratified on calendar time, although the study periods covered several decades during which lung cancer rates, tobacco consumption and radon exposure have changed.

The results showed that the ERR of lung cancer mortality was consistently linearly related to cumulative exposure to radon progeny within the range of miner exposures, and strongly modified by attained age, time since exposure and time since cessation of exposure to radon progeny, but was not associated with age at first exposure. The ERR/WLM decreased with attained age, time since exposure and time since cessation of exposure to radon progeny. Over a broad range of cumulative exposures, a higher lung cancer risk was associated with underground exposures received at low rates, suggesting an inverse-dose-rate effect. The data were too sparse, however, to determine whether this inverse-dose-rate effect applied to ranges of exposure found in most homes, although there were indications of a decreased effect of exposure rate at low cumulative exposures (Lubin *et al.*, 1994b).

Two different models were selected as best representing the joint miners' data, namely:

1. The time since exposure, age, intensity model:

$$RR = 1 + \beta \times (w_{5-14} + \theta_2 w_{15-24} + \theta_3 w_{25+}) \times \phi_{age} \times \gamma_{WL},$$

where $\beta = 0.0611$, $\theta_2 = 0.81$, $\theta_3 = 0.40$, and ϕ_{age} and γ_{WL} have the following values:

$$\phi_{age} \begin{cases} 1.0 \text{ for age} < 55 \\ 0.65 \text{ for age } 55 \leq \text{age} < 65 \\ 0.38 \text{ for age } 65 \leq \text{age} < 75 \\ 0.22 \text{ for age } 75 \leq \text{age} \end{cases}$$

$$\gamma_{WL} \begin{cases} 1.0 \text{ for WL} < 0.5 \\ 0.51 \text{ for } 0.5 \leq \text{WL} < 1.0 \\ 0.32 \text{ for } 1.0 \leq \text{WL} < 3.0 \\ 0.27 \text{ for } 3.0 \leq \text{WL} < 5.0 \\ 0.13 \text{ for } 5.0 \leq \text{WL} < 15.0 \\ 0.10 \text{ for } 15.0 \leq \text{WL} \end{cases}$$

In this model, β denotes the ERR per WLM in the time period 5–14 years after exposure, θ_2 and θ_3 the relative effects of exposure in the 15–24 and 25+ years time since exposure windows, w_{5-14}, w_{15-24} and w_{25+} represent respectively the cumulative exposure in WLM received in the periods 5–14, 15–24 and 25 or more years previously, ϕ_{age} is the modifying effect of attained age and γ_{WL} is the modifying effect of exposure rate.

2. The time since exposure, age, duration (dur) model:

$$RR = 1 + \beta \times (w_{5-14} + \theta_2 w_{15-24} + \theta_3 w_{25+}) \times \phi_{age} \times \gamma_{dur}$$

where $\beta = 0.0039$, $\theta_2 = 0.76$, $\theta_3 = 0.31$, and ϕ_{age} and γ_{WL} have the following values:

$$\phi_{age} \begin{cases} 1.0 \text{ for age} < 55 \\ 0.57 \text{ for } 55 \leq \text{age} < 65 \\ 0.34 \text{ for } 65 \leq \text{age} < 75 \\ 0.28 \text{ for } 75 \leq \text{age} \end{cases}$$

$$\gamma_{WL} \begin{cases} 1.0 \text{ for dur} < 5 \text{ years} \\ 3.17 \text{ for } 5 \leq \text{dur} < 15 \text{ years} \\ 5.27 \text{ for } 15 \leq \text{dur} < 24 \text{ years} \\ 9.27 \text{ for } 25 \leq \text{dur} < 35 \text{ years} \\ 13.6 \text{ for } 35 \text{ years} \leq \text{dur} \end{cases}$$

The role of smoking was investigated separately in the six cohorts where some information was available. For joint exposure, the data were consistent with a relative risk that was greater than additive but less than multiplicative. A separate analysis of data on non-smokers (based on 64 cases and 50 000 person–years) indicated that non-smokers had a threefold higher risk (measured in ERR per WLM) of lung cancer induced by radon progeny than smokers.

Based on these models, it was estimated that, for miners, 39% of lung cancer deaths among smokers and 73% of the lung cancer deaths among never-smokers may have been due to radon progeny exposure.

Findings were extrapolated to indoor settings (Lubin *et al.*, 1994b, 1995a) and showed that, among residents of single-family dwellings in the USA, 11% of lung cancer deaths in smokers and 30% among non-smokers may be attributable to indoor exposure to radon. These estimates were obtained using 1985–1989 American population mortality rates and are similar to those based on the BEIR IV risk model. For the year 1993, they correspond to about 15 000 lung cancer deaths—approximately 10 000 among smokers and 5000 among never-smokers—attributable to indoor radon in the USA.

8.2.4 Mechanistic modelling

Although important insights into the effects of radon and tobacco smoke have been derived from the study of cohorts of uranium miners, questions remain about how the pattern of exposure may affect risk. As seen above, such questions are difficult to address using conventional statistical methods for the analysis of epidemiological studies. Additional difficulties arise when studying joint exposure patterns to two or more agents. In contrast, as discussed in Chapter 7, the incorporation of age-related exposure patterns is relatively straightforward in biologically based models of carcinogenesis. Furthermore, the parameters of such models are directly interpretable in biological terms, and may thus afford some insight into the mechanisms of action of the agents under study.

Among the cohort studies that have contributed to understanding of the aetiology of lung cancer, two are of particular importance. The British doctors' study (Doll & Peto, 1978), undertaken to investigate the adverse health effects of tobacco smoking, is noted for completeness of follow-up. The Colorado Plateau uranium miners' study has provided insights into the interaction between radon and cigarette smoke in the induction of lung cancer (Lundin *et al.*, 1971; Whittemore & McMillan, 1983; Hornung & Meinhardt, 1987; Krewski *et al.*, 1989; Roscoe *et al.*, 1989). A simultaneous analysis of the Colorado Plateau miners' data and the British doctors' data within the framework of the two-mutation clonal expansion model of carcinogenesis (Moolgavkar & Knudson, 1981; Moolgavkar & Luebeck, 1990) was recently carried out by Moolgavkar *et al.* (1993)

The biological basis of the two-mutation model has been extensively discussed in previous publications (Moolgavkar & Knudson, 1981; Moolgavkar & Luebeck, 1990) and is presented in Chapter 7. Briefly, the model is based on the following fundamental biological assumptions:

1 In any tissue, there is a pool of cells susceptible to malignant transformation. This pool is generally identified with the stem-cell pool in the tissue of interest.

2 Malignant tumours are clonal, arising from a single transformed progenitor cell.

3 Malignant transformation of a susceptible cell is the result of two specific, rate-limiting, hereditary (at the level of the cell) and irreversible events. In chemical carcinogenesis, the first rate-limiting event is identified with initiation, and the second rate-limiting event with malignant conversion. Clonal expansion of intermediate cells is associated with promotion. Once a malignant cell is generated, it is assumed to give rise to a histologically detectable tumour after a constant lag time.

For the mathematical development, $X(t)$ is the number of susceptible cells at age t, and $n(d_r, d_s)$ is the rate of the first mutation as a function of the exposure rate of radon, d_r, measured in WLM/month (WLM/m), and the exposure rate of cigarette smoke, d_s, measured in numbers of cigarettes per day. Specifically, intermediate or initiated cells are generated from normal ones as a non-homogeneous Poisson process with intensity nX. The intermediate cells divide with rate α, die or differentiate with rate ß, and divide into one intermediate and one malignant cell with rate m. Each of these rates may be influenced by exposure to radon or cigarette smoke. The manner in which rates of mutation and cell proliferation depend on exposure to these two agents is discussed below.

The objectives of the analysis were to estimate the parameters of the two-mutation model as functions of the exposure rates of radon and cigarette smoke, to use the fitted model to make inferences about the risk of lung cancer associated with exposure to radon and tobacco smoke, and to characterize the interaction between radon and tobacco smoke with concurrent exposure to both agents. Estimates of the model parameters were obtained using the method of maximum likelihood. Details of the likelihood construction and fitting are provided in the original publication.

The likelihood was parameterized as a function of nX, μ, $a-b$, and b/a. Throughout this analysis, X was taken to be a constant equal to 10^7.

The Colorado miners' data and the British doctors' data were first analysed separately. However, an analysis assuming that the effects of tobacco on the mutation rates were equal in the two data sets produced a likelihood that was virtually identical to that resulting from the separate analyses. Thus the data were consistent with the hypothesis that the spontaneous and tobacco-related mutation rates are identical in the two cohorts. Explicitly, the following dose–response functions were used for each of the parameters:

$$n(d_s,d_r) = a_0 + a_s d_s + a_r d_r,$$
$$\mu(d_s,d_r) = b_0 + b_s d_s + b_r d_r$$

and

$$(a-b)(d_s,d_r) = c_0 + c_{s1}(1 - \exp[-c_{s2}\,d_s]) + c_{r1}$$
$$(1 - \exp[-c_{r2}d_r])$$

in the Colorado miners' data, and

$$(a-b)(d_s) = e_0 + e_{s1}(1 - \exp[-e_{s2}d_r])$$

in the British doctors' data. In both data sets, the ratio b/a was taken to be constant and independent of the level of exposure to radon or tobacco.

In this model, referred to as model A, 15 parameters were estimated from the data. Estimates of the spontaneous mutation rates a_0 and b_0 were almost equal, and the second mutation rate m appeared to be unaffected by either radon or cigarette smoke. The likelihood was little changed by setting $a_0 = b_0$ and $b_s = b_r = 0$. Hence, a reduced form of model A was considered in which only 12 parameters were estimated. In model B, all model parameters common to the Colorado miners' and British doctors' cohorts are equal. Thus, in this model $c_0 = e_0$, $c_{s1} = e_{s1}$, and $c_{s2} = e_{s2}$, and 9 parameters were estimated.

The fitted models were used to predict the number of lung cancer deaths in different exposure categories (Figure 8.1). In addition to the total number of deaths in each category, the temporal pattern of deaths is also important. This pattern is well described by the model. The reader is referred to the original paper for details.

The analysis indicated an inverse-exposure-rate effect (Figure 8.2), i.e. for the same cumulative exposure, protraction of the exposure increased the lifetime probability of a tumour.

The analysis indicated that both radon and cigarette smoking affect the first mutation rate and the kinetics of intermediate cell division. The second mutation rate appeared to be independent of radon and cigarette smoke. Similar conclusions regarding the role of radon daughters were drawn from analyses of experimental data (Moolgavkar et al., 1990; Luebeck et al., 1996). An earlier analysis of the British doctors' data, on the other hand, had suggested that cigarette smoke was not a promoting agent (Moolgavkar et al., 1989). This analysis was based on the approximate solution of the two-mutation model, and the possibility of saturation of the dose–response function for the promotional effect was not considered. The current analysis, based on the exact solution to the two-mutation model, is to be preferred.

Figure 8.3 shows the probability of lung cancer at age 70 as a function of age at start of exposure. From this figure it is clear that, for the exposure scenario considered, the probability of tumour at age 70 is more or less constant for ages at start of exposure between 20 and 30, and declines rapidly thereafter with increasing age at first exposure. The hazard function at age 70, on the other hand, increases with increasing age at first exposure, as reported by Hornung & Meinhardt (1987). Thus, the effect of age at first exposure depends upon whether one is studying the probability of tumour or the hazard function. Furthermore, the conclusions will also depend on the age at which observations are made and on the pattern of exposure considered.

As described above, there is interest in the question whether joint exposure to radon and cigarette smoke is synergistic (US National Academy of Sciences/National Research Council, Committee on the Biological Effects of Ionizing Radiations, 1988). The answer to this question depends upon the definition of synergy adopted, and some attempts have been made to define

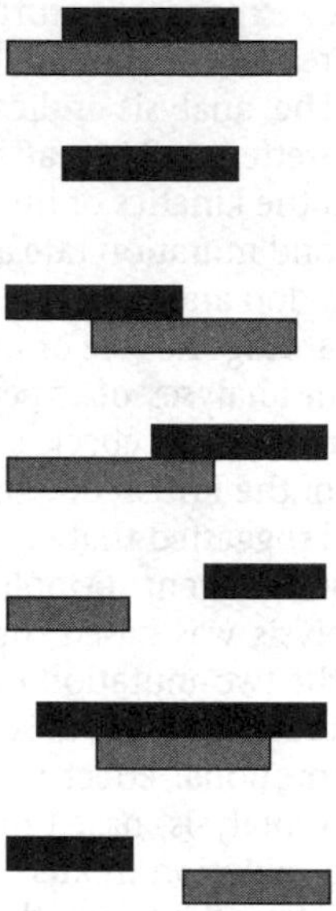

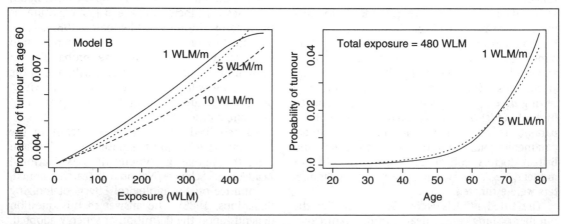

Group	Exposure profile	No. of miners	No. of lung cancer deaths		
			Observed	Model A	Model B
I. No exposure		8	0	0.0084	0.0046
II. Radon Tobacco smoke		2224	235	237.1	234.4
III. Radon Tobacco smoke		477	13	16.04	12.03
IV. Radon Tobacco smoke		116	15	15.25	16.02
V. Radon Tobacco smoke		118	20	14.18	12.72
VI. Radon Tobacco smoke		159	8	8.17	6.10
VII. Radon Tobacco smoke		19	3	0.71	0.68
VIII. Radon Tobacco smoke		11	0	0.53	0.40
Total		3132	294	292.0	282.4

Figure 8.1. Schematic representation of patterns of exposure. Length of bars does not represent actual duration of exposure. In each category, the number of miners, the observed number of lung cancer deaths and the expected numbers generated by models A and B are shown

Figure 8.2. Effect of fractionation of exposure. Curves generated by model B; model A yields similar results. Probability of tumour at age 60 plotted against total exposure to radon for different exposure rates

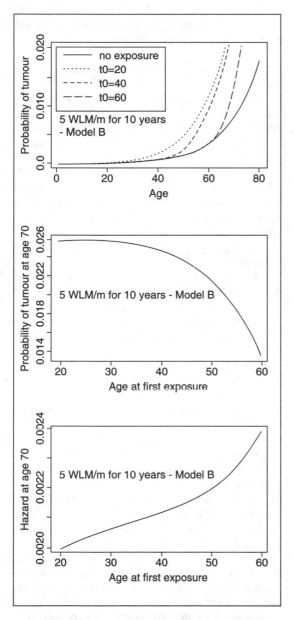

Figure 8.3. Effect of age at first exposure to radon on risk of lung cancer. Curves generated using model B: model A yields similar results. Upper panel: the probability of tumour at age 70 plotted against age at first exposure for an exposure regimen of 5 WLM/m for 10 years. Note that, for exposures starting very early, the curve is horizontal, indicating that the probability of tumour is independent of age at first exposure if exposure starts early enough, but that, with later ages at first exposure, probability of tumour is inversely related to age at exposure. The lower panel shows that the hazard (incidence) function at age 70 increases with age at first exposure

independence and synergy on the basis of the relationship of those risks of joint exposure to those of independent exposure to the two agents. In view of the complicated biology that may intervene between the exposure and the ultimate risk of cancer, such an undertaking would appear to be of dubious validity. Thus, there is no suggestion of any interaction between radon and cigarette smoke on the cellular level, i.e. there is no indication that interaction terms need to be considered when describing the dose–response functions for any of the parameters of the model. Nevertheless, the relative risk of joint exposure is somewhere between additive and multiplicative.

An interesting phenomenon has been reported with exposure to high LET radiation, e.g. from radon daughters, namely the inverse-exposure-rate effect, discussed above and described both in experimental (Moolgavkar *et al.*, 1990) and epidemiological (Hornung & Meinhardt, 1987; Darby & Doll, 1990) data: for a given total exposure, fractionation of exposure increases the lifetime probability of tumour. As Figure 8.2 shows, this analysis confirmed the inverse-exposure-rate effect in the Colorado miners' cohort. This effect can be attributed to the promotional effect of radon (see Moolgavkar *et al.*, 1993, for details). An earlier analysis of radon-induced malignant lung tumours in rats had arrived at the same conclusion (Moolgavkar *et al.*, 1990). A later analysis of an extended data set (Luebeck *et al.*, 1996) took explicit account of cell killing by radon and concluded that the promotion of intermediate lesions may be attributable to the uranium ore dust used as the carrier aerosol in the experiments. One conclusion of this analysis is that the inverse-exposure-rate effect would not be seen in the absence of an irritant (see also Chapter 7).

If an average annual exposure to the American population of 0.2 WLM from birth is assumed (US National Council on Radiation Protection and Measurements, 1984), model B predicted approximately two extra lung cancer deaths per 10 000 non-smoking individuals by age 70, compared with approximately 18 among 10 000 individuals smoking 20 cigarettes per day from age 20. The corresponding ERRs are 0.026 and 0.02, respectively, among non-smokers and smokers, which are smaller than those reported by Lubin *et al.*, (1994b). Note that, because of the high risk of lung cancer among smokers, the ERR associated with radon is higher among non-smokers than smokers, although the excess risk is much higher among smokers.

8.2.5 Comparison of QEP results

If we consider the questions of interest for radon QEP listed in section 8.2.1 above, we can conclude that, although the results of the QEP may differ, both empirical and mechanistic approaches provide an answer to the first question, namely the magnitude of the lung cancer risk associated with low cumulative doses from radon in a population under study.

As predictions of risks may imply extrapolations to populations with different patterns of exposure to radon (exposure rate, exposure duration, age at beginning and ending of exposure), to tobacco and to other agents, answers to the other three questions are also essential. Empirical approaches to QEP may provide answers to these questions: the effect of age at exposure and the interaction between radon and tobacco exposures have been studied by Thomas *et al.* (1985), the BEIR IV Committee (US National Academy of Sciences/National Research Council, Committee on the Biological Effects of Ionizing Radiations, 1988), Steenland (1994), Lubin *et al.* (1994a) and Hornung *et al.* (1995). Dose-rate effects have also been studied in detail by Lubin *et al.* (1995c).

These questions are, however, difficult to address and to interpret using conventional, statistical approaches because a number of *a priori* hypotheses must be made for the modelling of such effects. In contrast, the incorporation of temporal patterns of exposure and of multiple exposures is normal in biologically based models of carcinogenesis (Moolgavkar *et al.*, 1993). Indeed, of the various approaches described in the preceding section, only the analyses of Moolgavkar and collaborators (1993) have provided biologically interpretable hypotheses concerning the effects of dose rate, age at exposure and tobacco on the risk of radon-induced lung cancer. It must, however, be emphasized that many of these conclusions probably depend on the model used, and thus must be considered as hypotheses to be tested. Additional information (biological as well as epidemiological) would, however, be needed to characterize the effect of

sex and other endogenous and environmental, factors when using this model.

8.2.6 Remaining uncertainties, needs for the future

Most of the information used for the quantification of risk in the QEPs described above was obtained from epidemiological studies of men exposed as adults in the mining environment. Although the results of such studies carried out in several countries are generally consistent within a factor of 10 (despite differences in exposure rates, smoking patterns and age distribution), there is little direct evidence to test the adequacy of extrapolations from these studies to the risk to the general population following indoor air exposures.

The use of these data for predicting risks due to domestic exposures to radon and its progeny entails a number of uncertainties, as follows:

- Random statistical variability in miners' data and biases and uncertainties in mine dosimetry.
- Models for projecting risk over time.
- Models for extrapolating from mine settings to the home environment, in particular for describing the interaction with tobacco smoke.
- Assumptions about exposure-rate effects.
- Models for extrapolating to specific subgroups of the population: children, women, pregnant women, never-smokers, former smokers, etc.

While efforts need to be made to quantify these uncertainties, it is important to note that, unlike the risks associated with many other environmental pollutants, radon risk assessment does not require extrapolation from animal studies, and extrapolations are not carried out over a particularly large range of exposures. Additional studies of exposure-rate effects in joint analyses of miners cohorts with different exposure patterns, combined with the results of recently published and ongoing case–control studies of residential exposures and with continued experimental work to determine the biological bases for exposure-rate effects, should provide, in the near future, a useful test of current estimates of risk and of the validity of the models used for extrapolating risks from mining to residential environments.

8.3 Aflatoxins and Liver Cancer

8.3.1 Introduction

The aflatoxin-producing *Aspergillus* species, and consequently aflatoxin contamination, are ubiquitous in areas of the world with hot, humid climates. Exposure arises mainly from contamination of food staples, and levels are particularly high in parts of sub-Saharan Africa, South-east Asia and Central America. Widespread low-level contamination of, for example, corn and peanuts, occurs in industrialized countries. Occupational exposure can result from farming and milling operations. The relative proportions of the different aflatoxins, e.g. G_1, G_2, B_1 and B_2, depend on the species of *Aspergillus* present. AFB_1 is the type most frequently present in contaminated samples.

Aflatoxins have been recognized as liver carcinogens in both humans and in experimental animals (International Agency for Research on Cancer, 1993). The incidence of liver cancer varies widely across the world (Parkin *et al.*, 1992). In China and Thailand, it is one of the most prevalent types of cancers (Parkin *et al.*, 1992), causing at least 100 000 deaths annually (Qian *et al.*, 1994), and 250 000 deaths worldwide (Scholl *et al.*, 1995). Aflatoxin clearly plays a role in the induction of liver cancers in these countries (International Agency for Research on Cancer, 1993), and reduction of dietary aflatoxin may be an important preventive measure. Another important risk factor for primary liver cancer is infection with the hepatitis B virus (HBV) (International Agency for Research on Cancer, 1994). Mechanistic data provide further evidence of liver cancer causation by both hepatitis B and aflatoxin.

Despite the considerable information from epidemiological studies and animal bioassays, risks from specific exposures to aflatoxins are difficult to estimate and predict. There are questions regarding the extent to which hepatitis B infection and other factors modify the effect of aflatoxin, the applicability of findings from countries with high liver cancer rates and high prevalence of HBV to those with low rates and vice versa, the shape of the dose–response relationship over the ranges of aflatoxin exposure found worldwide, and the wide variability in susceptibility observed in animal bioassays. The results of mechanistic studies provide some insight on these issues, and in this section, the extent to which such information may improve confidence in risk predictions for aflatoxin is explored. Although mechanistic data cannot be formally and explicitly integrated into QEP for aflatoxin, they are critical in interpreting the findings and guiding the development of empirical approaches.

The discussion of aflatoxin QEP begins with a review of the available epidemiological and experimental bioassay data, and the risk assessments derived from them. It then considers these assessments in the light of recently published mechanistic studies, and concludes with a list of research initiatives that, if undertaken, would improve the epidemiological database for QEP, as well as the confidence in selecting modelling procedures for low-dose predictions.

8.3.2 Epidemiological studies

A large number of epidemiological studies have been carried out, particularly in African and Asian countries where high incidence and mortality from liver cancer have been reported. These studies (reviewed in International Agency for Research on Cancer, (1993)) fall into three categories, namely, correlation, case–control and cohort studies.

8.3.2.1 Correlation studies

Table 8.3 lists the characteristics and results of the correlation studies in which liver cancer rates (incidence or mortality) were studied in relation to estimated levels of aflatoxin intake in different regions. Highly positive correlations were observed in all but three studies (Stoloff, 1983; Campbell *et al.*, 1990; Srivatanakul *et al.*, 1991a,), providing strong evidence of an association. Outcome assessment was, of necessity, ecological in these studies, which therefore provided limited information for use in quantification of the risk of liver cancer in relation to level of aflatoxin exposure, even though exposures were measured in some studies by detection of urinary metabolites or DNA adducts of aflatoxins in large numbers of subjects (Autrup *et al.*, 1987; Campbell *et al.*, 1990; Srivatanakul *et al.*, 1991a). In addition, as all studies but one (Stoloff, 1983) were based on populations living in areas of high prevalence of HBV, they provide limited information on the magni-

Table 8.3 Correlation studies[a]

Region/country (reference)	No. of areas	Liver cancer rate (per 100 000 per annum except where otherwise indicated)		Aflatoxin (AF) exposure			Correlation	Information on hepatitis B virus (HBV) (prevalence)
		Type of measurement	Range	Type of measurement	No. of samples	Range		
Africa								
Kenya (Peers & Linsell, 1973)	3	Incidence (≥=16 years)	3.11–12.92 (M) 0.0–5.44 (F)	Same as Peers et al. (1976)	2431	4.88–14.81 (M) 3.46–10.03 (F)	0.87 (M+F)	-
Kenya (Autrup et al., 1987)	9	Crude incidence	0.24–2.69 (M) 0.24–0.88 (F)	Proportion with urinary AF adduct	983	11.8–41.7 (M) 5.0–22.1 (F)	0.75 (M+F)	sAg, cAb
Mozambique, (van Rensburg et al., 1985)	8	Age-adjusted incidence	9.1–60.7 (M) 2.2–13.0 (F)	Average intake from prepared meals (ng/kg per day)	2183	18.9–189.1 (all types)	0.64 (M) 0.71 (F)	-
	17[b]	Crude incidence	1.2–17.7	-		3.5–183.7(B_1)	0.88	-
South Africa, Transkei (van Rensburg et al., 1990)	4	Age-adjusted incidence	3.2–10.3	Same as Autrup et al. (1987)	623	5.14–23.21	0.80	-
Swaziland (Keen & Martin, 1971)	3	Crude incidence	2.2–9.7	Proportion positive in groundnuts	NA	20–60%	+	-
Swaziland (Peers et al., 1976)	4	Incidence (≥=15 years)	7.0–26.65 (M) 0.0–5.62 (F)	Average intake from prepared meals and beer (ng/kg per day)	1056	8.34–53.34 (M) 5.11–43.14 (F)	0.988 (M) 0.957 (F)	-
Swaziland (Peers et al., 1987)	10	Incidence (M:15–64)	2.9–24.85	Average intake from four kinds of foods and beer (µg per day)	2583	1.4–20.8 (all types) 0.8–11.1 (B_1)	$p < 0.01$	sAg, sAb, cAb
Uganda (Alpert et al., 1971)	7	Crude incidence	1.4–15.0	Proportion positive in food samples	NA	10.3–43.8	+	-

Table 8.3 (Contd). Correlation studies[a]

Region/country (reference)	No. of areas	Liver cancer rate (per 100 000 per annum except where otherwise indicated)		Aflatoxin (AF) exposure			Correlation	Information on hepatitis B virus (HBV) (prevalence)
		Type of measurement	Range	Type of measurement	No of samples	Range		
Asia								
China, Guangxi (Yu, 1992; Yu, 1995)	10	Crude mortality	1.06–125	AFB_1 intake; AFM_1 urinary excretion	81	-	$p<0.001$ (intake) $p>0.05$ AFM_1 urinary excretion	-
China (Yaobin et al., 1983)	29	Crude mortality	NA	Proportion positive (grain and oil)	20 000	NA	0.653 (M) 0.438 (F)	sAg
China (Campbell et al., 1990)	48	Cumulative mortality per 1000 in men aged 0–64 years	2.46–96.33	Urinary AF metabolites (ng/kg per 4h)	1200	0–611	-0.17	sAg
				Average corn intake (g per day)	NA	0–624	-0.20	
				% mouldy peanuts consumed	NA	0–87	0.17	
China (Yeh et al., 1986)	2	Age-adjusted mortality	25.9–49.1	Average intake from cooked staple foods (ng/kg per day)	395	35–55	+	-
China (Armstrong, 1980)	7	Crude mortality	8.3–25.6	Relative proportion positive food samples (lowest = 1.0)	NA	1.0–4.4	+	-
Taiwan, China (Hatch et al., 1993)	8	Age-adjusted	18.9–60.0 (M) 5.5–22.7 (F)	Mean urinary AF metabolites (pg/ml)	250	31.6–107.7 (M) 20.3–61.9 (F)	$p = 0.001$	sAg
Thailand (Shank et al., 1972a,b)	2	Crude incidence	2.0–6.0	Same as Autrup et al. (1987)	7591	6.5–61.0 (all types) 5.5–39.5 (B_1)	+	-

Region/Country (reference)	No. of areas	Liver cancer rate (per 100 000 per annum except where otherwise indicated)		Aflatoxin (AF) exposure			Correlation	Information on hepatitis B virus (HBV) (prevalence)
		Type of measurement	Range	Type of measurement	No of samples	Range		
Thailand (Srivatanakul et al., 1991a)	5	Standardized proportional mortality ratio (all deaths)	0.66–0.92 (HCC) 0.32–3.34 (CC)	Proportion with serum albumin-bound	351	2.0–13.9	-0.75 (HCC) -0.03 (CC)	sAg, sAb, cAb
				Proportiont with urinary AF and adduct	241	6.5–23.4	-0.64 (HCC) 0.17 (CC)	
Americas								
USA (Stoloff, 1983)	2	Standardized proportional mortality ratio (all deaths)	235–259	Average intake from cooked cornmeals and roasted peanut products (ng/kg per day)	NA	0.25–105	No	-

Table 8.3 (Contd). Correlation studies[a]

[a] NA: not available; HCC: heptocellular carcinoma; CC:cholangiocarcinoma.
[b] Combined analyses including data from previous studies in other areas.

tude of the association between aflatoxin exposure and liver cancer in the absence of HBV infection. This limits their usefulness for QEP for populations living in areas with low HBV prevalence.

8.3.2.2 Case–control studies

Table 8.4 shows the characteristics and results of the case–control studies. Five such studies of the impact of aflatoxin exposure on hepatocellular carcinoma (HCC) were carried out in Asian countries. In the earliest study, in the Philippines (Bulatao-Jayme et al., 1982), aflatoxin intake was estimated based on a food frequency questionnaire, the measurement of aflatoxin levels in food samples, and the measurement of AFB_1 and AFM_1 in 24-h urine samples. Information was requested in the questionnaire, inter alia, on the frequency of consumption and usual amount consumed of specific food items for each period of a subject's residential history. Of urine samples taken, 51% from cases versus 35% from controls were positive for AFB_1 and/or AFM_1 ($p<0.05$). No information on HBV infection status was available in this study. The relative risks of primary liver cancer increased with estimates of daily aflatoxin exposure intake.

In a case–control study in Thailand (Srivatanakul et al., 1991b), aflatoxin intake was determined by measurement of total serum aflatoxin–albumin adducts, and by the frequency of intake of several major sources of aflatoxins. Statistically significant associations were not observed between liver cancer risk and either aflatoxin–albumin adducts or aflatoxin intake in these studies. The prevalence of individuals with detectable levels of serum aflatoxin–albumin adducts was approximately 16% in these studies (Srivatanakul et al., 1991a). In a study in Hong-Kong (Lam et al., 1982), no significant association was observed between liver cancer risk and frequency of intake of corn and beans, the chief sources of aflatoxin. Associations were not observed in a case–control study in Guangxi, China (Zhang, 1992) where exposures to both cases and controls were observed to be high. In the only study conducted in Africa (Olubuyide et al., 1993), significant increases were reported in HCC with AFB_1 albumin-adduct levels.

8.3.2.3 Cohort studies

The cohort studies, also presented in Table 8.4, can be divided into two groups: general popula-

Table 8.4 Case–control and cohort studies[a]

Country or territory (reference)	Study subjects and number of deaths	Aflatoxin (AF) exposure	Results	Covariates considered
Case–control studies				
Philippines (Bulatao-Jayme et al., 1982)	90 PLC cases; 90 hospital controls	Estimated intake based on food frequency questionnaire (µg per day)	RR vs 0–3µg per day: 13.9 for 4–6µg per day 17.0 for 7+µg per day	Ethanol (g per day)
		Detection of urinary AF(B_1+M_1)	Cases: 51%; Controls: 35% ($p<0.05$)	
Hong Kong (Lam et al., 1982)	107 PLC cases; 107 hospital controls	Frequency of intake of seven AF–containing foods	No association	HBsAg, salted fish, blood transfusion, alcohol, smoking
Thailand (Srivatanakul et al., 1991b)	65 HCC cases; 65 hospital controls	Serum AF–albumin adducts (pg/mg albumin)	RR 1.0 (0.4–2.4) ≥ 3pg vs < 3pg	HBsAg, fresh vegetables, drinking,
		Frequency of intakes of major food sources of AF	1.9 (NS)	Regular consumption of betel nut
Thailand (Parkin et al., 1991)	103 CC cases;103 hospital controls	Serum AF–albumin adducts (pg/mg albumin)	RR 1.0 (0.1–16.0) ≥ 3pg vs <3	Anti-OV, HBsAg, betal-nut, sticky rice
		Frequency of intakes of major sources of AF	1.4 (NS) Regular consumption 1.4 (NS) Total food group	
Taiwan, China (Wang et al., 1996a)	56 HCC cases; 220 controls	Albumin adducts	OR among HBsAg+: 2.8 (0.9–9.1) detectable albumin adducts;	HBsAg, alcohol, cigarette smoking
		Urinary AF metabolites	5.5 (1.3-23.4) high vs low urinary metabolite levels	
Nigeria (Olubuyide et al., 1993)	22 HCC cases; 22 matched controls	Serum albumin adducts	$p<0.005$	-
China, Guangxi (Zhang, 1992)	99 PLC cases; 99 matched controls	Serum albumin adducts	Association with aflatoxin not significant (p>0.05)	HBV infection, drinking pond/ditch water, family PLC history, alcohol
Cohort studies				
China (Yeh et al., 1985)	551 HBsAg-positive and 551 HBsAg-negative	Living in village with light (avg. 0.65 mg per year) or heavy (6.02 mg per year) contamination	Mortality rate from HCC per 100 000 cases HBsAg-positive: heavy AF contamination 649.35; light AF contamination 65.92	HBsAg
	16 HCC deaths		HBsAG–negative: heavy AF contamination 98.57;	

Table 8.4 (Contd). Case–control and cohort studies[a]

Country or territory (reference)	Study subjects and number of deaths	Aflatoxin (AF) exposure	Results	Covariates considered
			light AF contamination 0.00	
			RR: 9.58 heavy vs light (HBsAg–positive)	
China (Yeh et al., 1989)	7917 men aged 25–64 years	Estimated intake from raw staple food samples in four districts; range: 0.3–51.8 mg per year	Age-adjusted mortality rate per 100 000: 175.4–613.5	HBsAg
	149 PLC deaths		Pearson r = 1.00	
China (Ross et al., 1992)	18 244 men aged 45–64 years	Presence of urinary AF or DNA adducts	RR 3.8 (1.2–12.2) 1.9 (0.5–7.5) HBsAg-negative 60.1 (6.4–561.8) HBsAg-positive	HBsAg, smoking, alcohol,education
	22 PLC cases; 140 matched controls			
China (Qian et al., 1994)	Same as Ross et al. 55 cases 267 controls	In-person questionnaire and market samples; Urinary AF metabolites for 50 cases	No association RR: 3.4 (1.1–10) AF positive/HBsAg-negative 7.3 (2.2–24.4) AF negative/HBsAg-negative 59 (16.6-212) AF positive/HBsAg-positive	Cigarette smoking
China, Haimen City (London et al., 1995)	60 984 men aged 30–64 years	Questionnaire on staple food consumption by decade (1960s, 1970s, 1980s and 1990s)	Corn consumption – p = 0.003 (1970s) p > 0.05 (other decades)	HBsAg
	183 HCC deaths; 5 matched controls per case			
Taiwan, China, Penghu Islands (Chen et al., 1996a)	6847 aged 30–65 years; 20 HCC cases; 86 controls	Serum AFB$_1$–albumin adducts	OR; 5.5 (1.2–24.5) for detected albumin adducts	HBsAg; anti-HCV, family history of HCC or cirrhosis
Taiwan, China (Chen et al., 1996b)	4841 HBsAg carriers; 32 HCC; 73 matched controls	AFB$_1$–albumin adducts collected at time of recruitment; GST M1 and T1 phenotypes characterized	ORs null GST M1 genotype: 4.1 (low AF; p<0.05); 12.4 (high AF; p<0.01) ORs null GST T1: 1.8 (low AF; NS); 10.4 (high AF; p<0.05)	Cigarette smoke, alcohol drinking

Table 8.4 (Contd). Case–control and cohort studies[a]

Country or territory (reference)	Study subjects and number of deaths	Aflatoxin (AF) exposure	Results	Covariates considered
Sweden (Alavanja et al., 1987)	2649 grain millers; 10 PLC	NA	SIR 238 ($p<0.05$)	-
Denmark (Olsen et al., 1988)	Male workers at livestock feed processing companies	Estimated from AF content in crops and concentration of organic dust (170 ng per day)	SPIR - 246 (108–486) HCC 298 (109–659) CC for processing companies (≥10 years before)	None

[a] PLC: primary liver cancer; HCC: hepatocellular carcinoma; NS: not significant; Anti-OV: titre of antibody to *Opisthorchis viverrini*; SIR: standard incidence ratio; SPIR: standardized proportional incidence ratio; CC: cholangiocarcinoma; HBsAg: hepatitis B virus surface antigen; HCV hepatitis C virus.

tion studies, carried out in China (Yeh *et al.*, 1985, 1989; Ross *et al.*, 1992; Qian *et al.*, 1994); and occupational cohort studies, carried out in Northern Europe (Alavanja *et al.*, 1987; Olsen *et al.*, 1988).

A significant increase in liver cancer incidence was seen among 2649 Swedish grain millers (Alavanja *et al.*, 1987) and significant increases in both hepatocellular and cholangiocarcinoma incidence in employees of Danish livestock feed processing companies (Olsen *et al.*, 1988). Although these studies suggest aflatoxin effects in areas of low prevalence of HBV infection, only fairly crude estimates of aflatoxin exposure level were available, so that they are of limited use for QEP.

The first Chinese cohort study (Yeh *et al.*, 1985) included 551 HBsAg-positive and an equal number of HBsAg-negative inhabitants of Fusui County, China, who were identified between 1974 and 1977 and followed up to 1982. Subjects were classified according to whether they lived in an area of heavy or light aflatoxin exposure. Regardless of HBsAg status, the mortality from liver cancer was higher in "heavily exposed" (estimated average intake, 6.02 mg per year) than in "lightly exposed" (0.64 mg per year) subjects; the relative risk among those found to be HBsAg-positive was 8.58. A multiplicative effect was observed between aflatoxin exposure and HBsAg

status but, as noted by the International Agency for research on Cancer (1993), misclassification of HBsAg status could have affected that finding.

In southern Guangxi, China, 7917 men aged 25–64, resident in one of five communities, were identified in 1982–1983 and followed up to 1986 (Yeh *et al.*, 1989). Mean aflatoxin intake per year was estimated in four of the five communities based on the mean aflatoxin content of raw food samples and on the average yearly consumption of these foods; they ranged from 0.3 to 51.8 mg per person per year. Study subjects were judged to be free of liver cancer at the time of enrolment by physical examination and negative serum α-foetoprotein test. HBsAg positivity was tested for all liver cancer deaths and for a 25% stratified random sample of the cohort. A strong positive correlation ($p = 0.004$) was found between primary liver cancer risk and estimated mean aflatoxin intake. Of the 76 liver cancer deaths, 69 were HBsAg-positive and seven HBsAg-negative at the time of enrolment. As noted by Wu-Williams *et al.* (1992), this study is better than the earlier studies for QEP because of improvements in the assessment of exposure, outcome and confounding variables: (1) although calculated on a population basis, staple foods were sampled twice yearly over several years to estimate aflatoxin dose; (2) the ascertainment of HCC rates was based on active follow-up; and (3) the assessment of the hepatitis B infection rate was based on extensive testing of the cohort (25%) and all cases.

A cohort of 18 244 men living in Shanghai, aged 45–64, was identified between 1986 and 1989 and followed up to 1990 (Ross *et al.*, 1992). A nested case–control study was carried out, based on the 22 cases of primary liver cancer observed and 140 controls matched on age and residence. Aflatoxin exposure of the cases and controls was determined as the presence of (AF) B_1, P_1 or M_1 or of AFB_1–N7-guanine adducts in the urine. The relative risk of primary liver cancer for detectable urinary aflatoxins or aflatoxin–guanine adducts, adjusted for HBsAg status, cigarette smoking and alcohol intake, was 3.8 (95% CI, 1.2–12.2). Relative risk from aflatoxin was dependent on HBsAg status: it was 1.9 (95% CI, 0.5–7.5) among HBsAg-negative and 60.1 (95% CI, 6.4–561.8) among HBsAg-positive subjects, although this estimate is based on only seven cases and two controls. No information was provided on individual exposure levels, limiting the usefulness of this study for QEP. A follow-up study (Qian *et al.*, 1994) similarly found that the presence of urinary aflatoxin and HBsAg was positively associated with HCC, greatest risk being observed in those positive for both markers (Table 8.4). The relative risk for AFB_1–guanine adducts in the urine, in HBsAg-negative subjects (adjusted for cigarette smoking), was found to be 3.4 (95% CI, 1.1–10.0), while no association was found between liver cancer risk and dietary aflatoxin level as determined from surveys of market foods. The adducts were measured prior to the observation of tumours, precluding the possibility that elevated adduct levels were due to the modulation of metabolism resulting from liver carcinogenesis. Among the HBsAg-positive subjects, the relative risk was 7.3 (2.2–24.4) for those without detected urinary aflatoxin biomarkers, and 59.4 (16.6–212.0) for those in whom biomarkers were present. Thus a strong interaction between the two factors and HCC risk was again observed. This study should be useful for QEP evaluations of the potential magnitude of the interaction between HBV and aflatoxin.

A total of 25 616 individuals from seven townships in Taiwan, China were enrolled in a cohort from 1990 to 1992. A total of 56 cases of HCC were diagnosed and individually matched with 220 healthy controls from within the cohort. Blood samples were analysed for aflatoxin–albumin adducts and tested for HBV, while urine was tested for aflatoxin metabolites. There appeared to be a synergism between aflatoxin exposure and chronic HBV infection in this study. In male HBsAg-positive individuals there were increased odds ratios of 2.8 (95% CI, 0.9–9.1) and 5.5 (95% CI, 1.3–23.4) for detectable compared with non-detectable aflatoxin–albumin adducts and high versus low urinary aflatoxin, respectively. Two further cohorts in Taiwan, China, in which AFB_1–albumin adducts were used as a marker also found an association between aflatoxin exposure and HCC risk (Table 8.4; Chen *et al.*, 1996a, b).

8.3.3 Experimental data
8.3.3.1 Animal bioassay

Aflatoxin carcinogenicity studies have been reviewed by the International Agency for Research on Cancer (1993). The susceptibility to aflatoxin carcinogenicity varies markedly between animal species (see Busby & Wogan, 1984). The Fischer rat is extremely sensitive to aflatoxin, a significant increase in hepatocellular carcinoma being seen at dietary AFB_1 levels of 4 ppb while the adult mouse is refractory to 1000 ppb AFB_1 in the diet. Hamsters and guinea-pigs and other rat strains are of intermediate sensitivity, although carcinogenicity data are less comprehensive than for the mouse and Fischer rat.

8.3.3.2 Pharmacokinetics

The interspecies variation in susceptibility has been at least partially explained by the expression of specific isoenzymes of glutathione-S-transferases (GST). The mouse constitutively expresses a hepatic alpha class GST, Yc, which has a 50-fold higher activity in conjugating AFB_1-8,9-epoxide to glutathione than the constitutive rat protein, Yc1 (Buetler *et al.*, 1992). These differences in expression result in markedly lower AFB_1-DNA adduct levels in mouse liver than in rat (Ramsdell & Eaton 1990). An alpha class GST subunit, Yc2, which has a high AFB_1-8,9-epoxide conjugating activity, is not constitutively expressed in the adult male rat but is induced in this animal by various antioxidants, such as ethoxyquin, butylated hydroxyanisole and oltipraz (Hayes *et al.*, 1994). This induction confers resistance in the rat to AFB_1 induced DNA adduct formation, preneoplastic lesions and HCC (Hayes *et al.*, 1991). Yc2 is also constitutively expressed in female rat liver, which could explain the greater sensitivity of male rats to AFB_1 (Hayes *et al.*, 1993). It is noteworthy that the rat and mouse have similar capacities to activate AFB_1 to the DNA-binding metabolite AFB_1-8,9-epoxide; however, recently two forms of epoxide, the *exo* and *endo* AFB_1-8,9-epoxide, have been described (Raney *et al.*, 1992a,b), and the relative proportions of each metabolite could be species-dependent.

In humans, GSTs appear to be relatively ineffective at detoxifying AFB_1 (Raney *et al.*, 1992a; Kirby *et al.*, 1993), and this is consistent with the difference in amino acid sequence compared with the Yc and rat Yc2 which are active in the AFB_1-8,9-epoxide conjugation (Raney *et al.*, 1992a). In addition to the GST enzymes determining interspecies susceptibility, an inducible aldehyde-reductase has been identified in rat liver, and this enzyme is induced by phenolic antioxidants (Hayes *et al.*, 1993). It will be of interest to determine whether this enzyme is constitutively expressed in different species, including humans. Other routes of detoxification, such as hydroxylation to AFQ_1, may be important in humans (Raney *et al.*, 1992c). Some studies have been conducted in human populations to assess the possible impact of polymorphisms in carcinogen metabolizing enzymes on induction of AFB_1–serum albumin adducts and HCC risk. In a population with high aflatoxin exposure, lack of GST M1, due to a deletion in the gene coding for this protein, was not associated with higher aflatoxin–albumin adducts (Wild *et al.*, 1993b), while in a lower-exposure population adducts were more frequently found in individuals with the GST M1 null genotype (McGlynn *et al.*,, 1995). In addition, in the latter study, a polymorphism in the microsomal epoxide hydrolase (EPXH) gene, resulting in an enzyme with a lower activity, was associated with a higher prevalence of aflatoxin–albumin adducts in Ghana (McGlynn *et al.*, 1995). The association of lower EPXH activity with a higher prevalence of aflatoxin–albumin adducts requires further

study because, in principle, this protein adduct could result not only from the direct binding of AFB_1-8,9-epoxide but also indirectly via the binding of the AFB_1-dihydrodiol formed by the action of the EPXH, i.e. it could also be postualated that the lower EPXH activity reduces the albumin adduct levels. The impact of these polymorphisms on HCC risk has been examined in a few studies and this is discussed below, but further case–control and cross-sectional studies in populations at different levels of aflatoxin exposure should help to resolve some of these outstanding questions with respect to the importance of the above polymorphisms in determining human HCC risk.

As far as the modulating effects of HBV infection on aflatoxin metabolism are concerned, one study reported that a small group of healthy HBsAg carriers had higher antipyrine and cortisol metabolism, two markers of cytochrome P–450 activity, compared with a group of controls (Geubel *et al.*, 1987). De Flora *et al.* (1985) studied 129 human liver biopsies pooled according to liver pathology, and a significant enhancement of AFB_1 activation was seen in mild chronic active, but not severe, hepatitis. In the woodchuck model, animals infected with woodchuck hepatitis virus had a tendency to a higher activation of promutagens, including AFB_1 (De Flora *et al.*, 1989). Aflatoxin metabolism has also been studied in a HBV transgenic mouse strain in which synergy for hepatocarcinogenesis between HBV and AFB_1 was observed (Kirby *et al.*, 1994). An increase in the level of some cytochrome P-450 isoenzymes was observed, notably cytochrome P-450 2a-5, which is partly responsible for AFB_1 metabolism in the mouse.

8.3.3.3 DNA-adducts

Data from experimental studies to date describe a linear dose–response relationship between AFB_1 exposure and liver AFB_1–DNA adducts, urinary nucleic acid adducts and peripheral blood albumin adducts. AFB_1–DNA adducts in rat liver are linearly related to AFB_1 dose following single exposures as low as 1 ng/kg, i.e. within the range of reported human dietary exposures; no threshold response was reported. Similarly, repeated-dose experiments revealed a linear dose–response model for AFB_1 ingestion and steady-state AFB_1–DNA adducts in rat liver (for a review, see California Department of Health Services, 1991; Choy, 1993). Experiments in other species performed at higher doses have given the same result, although the data are far less extensive. Linear relationships between urinary excretion of the major AFB_1-nucleic acid adduct, AFB_1–N7-guanine, and both dose of AFB_1 and hepatic AFB_1–DNA adduct level were reported in rats (Groopman et al., 1993). In addition, in the same species, a linear dose–response relation between AFB_1 and AFB_1–albumin adducts after single and multiple exposures was observed (Wild et al., 1986).

Several aflatoxin metabolites and nucleic acid adducts have also been measured in human urine. Some urinary metabolites, particularly AFM_1 and AFB_1–N7-guanine, show an excellent linear correlation with recent intake of AFB_1 at the individual level. In contrast, other metabolites, e.g., AFP_1, or the parent compound AFB_1, do not correlate with dietary aflatoxin intake (for review, see Groopman, 1993). Aflatoxin bound covalently to peripheral blood albumin, which is formed following activation of aflatoxin in the liver, shows a linear correlation with aflatoxin intake and with urinary excretion of AFB_1–N7-guanine adduct (Gan et al., 1988; Wild et al., 1992; Groopman, 1993).

In general, the level of AFB_1–DNA adducts formed for a given dose is increased in sensitive (e.g. rat) as compared to resistant (e.g. mouse) species (see Choy, 1993). However, the strains of animals used, dose levels and routes of exposure have often not been comparable between the carcinogenicity and DNA-adduct studies, and data for chronic dosing are available only for few species. Species comparisons of the level of aflatoxin–albumin adducts also casts light on species differences in susceptibility due to pharmacokinetics. Data from chronic dosing studies are available for three strains of rat, hamsters, guinea-pigs and mice (Wild et al., 1996). Comparisons of urinary AFB_1–N7-guanine and peripheral blood aflatoxin–albumin adducts suggest that, for a given exposure, the level of adduct formed is similar in rats (sensitive to aflatoxin carcinogenesis) and humans (Gan et al., 1988; Groopman,1993; Wild et al., 1996).

8.3.3.4 Target gene

A striking difference in the position and type of mutations in specific genes has been observed in liver tumours from different parts of the world. A specific mutation in the third nucleotide of codon 249 (AGG to AGT transversion) in the p53-tumour-suppressor gene has been observed at a high frequency (up to 50%) in HCC from countries such as Mozambique and in southern China. Individuals in these countries are expected to have a high aflatoxin exposure, and it has been hypothesized that this carcinogen is responsible for the induction of the mutation. This is consistent with the observation that the same mutation is rare in European countries and in Japan, where aflatoxin exposure would be expected to be low. Similarly, other researchers have observed low frequencies of this mutation in HCC from areas or groups with high HBV prevalence but low aflatoxin exposure (Hong Kong Chinese (Ng et al., 1994), Beijing (Fujimoto et al., 1994), Shanghai (Li et al., 1993)). Finally, there continue to be case series reports of high occurrence of the mutation in HCC from areas of high aflatoxin exposure (Senegal (Coursaget et al., 1993), Qidong, China (Li et al., 1993; Fujimoto et al., 1994)), and low occurrence from areas of low exposure (e.g., Britain (Challen et al., 1992); France and Italy (Debuire et al., 1993)). The type of mutation observed, a G to T transversion, is what would be expected to result from the AFB_1–N7-guanine adduct, and the third nucleotide of codon 249 is a target for AFB_1 in in vitro assays (Puisieux et al., 1991).

There are, however, questions outstanding with regard to the above hypothesis. For example, the data on aflatoxin exposure in the different countries is weakly documented and the studies have been limited to case series. Thus the possibility remains that this remarkable specificity in mutation spectra in different geographical areas is related to environmental exposures other than AFB_1.

Nevertheless, while it is not clear whether HBV infection is required for the specific p53 mutation which has been associated with aflatoxin to occur, a small number of liver tumours in those negative for HBV in heavily aflatoxin-exposed populations have contained the mutation. In addition, HBV carriage does not appear to be sufficient to explain the mutation spectra, given the infrequent occurrence of AGG to AGT mutations in codon 249 in HBV-positive HCC from low aflatoxin-exposure countries. In experiments conducted with the human hepatocyte-like cell line, Hep G2, Aguilar and colleagues (1993) showed that this same nucleotide is mutated more frequently by AFB_1 than are nucleotides in the adjacent codons 248 and 250. Furthermore, Aguilar *et al.*, (1994) examined mutations in hepatocytes from parts of the liver free from tumours, and showed that HCC patients from a high-aflatoxin exposure region (Qidong, China) had a higher frequency of G to T transversions at the third nucleotide of codon 249 than HCC patients from low-aflatoxin exposure areas (Thailand, USA).

To date, *p53* mutations have not been observed in AFB_1-induced HCC in experimental animals including rats, mice, ducks and monkeys. For the first three of these species, the DNA sequence corresponding to codon 249 in humans is different, and therefore the sequence specificity of AFB_1 binding would not be expected to be the same. In monkeys, the sequence is the same but only four HCC have been examined (Fujimoto *et al.*, 1992). In addition, *p53* mutations in experimentally induced tumours are generally rare in contrast to humans, where some 50% of tumours have a mutation in this gene (Hollstein *et al.*, 1991). The genes important in the carcinogenic process may therefore differ across species, thus complicating cross-species extrapolations.

8.3.3.5 Animal models of aflatoxin and HBV interaction

Experimental models of HBV infection, including HBV transgenic mice, woodchucks and ducks, have been used in tests for interactions with aflatoxin. In ducks, relatively minor liver damage is associated with duck HBV infection and few tumours have been reported in the absence of other treatment. There is no evidence of a synergistic effect with aflatoxin in terms of HCC induction (Uchida *et al.;* 1988, Cova *et al.;* 1990, Cullen *et al.;* 1990). In woodchucks, synergism was reported between woodchuck hepatitis virus (WHV) and aflatoxin B_1 (Bannasch *et al.*, 1995). In this experiment there was an earlier appearance of hepatocellular neoplasms and a higher incidence of hepatocellular carcinomas in WHV-

infected woodchucks treated with AFB_1 compared with those not receiving the carcinogen. In HBV transgenic mice, which also develop HCC in the absence of carcinogen treatment, there was also an earlier onset of HCC in those animals also treated with AFB_1 (Sell *et al.*, 1991). In tree shrews, combined exposure to HBV and aflatoxin produced roughly a 4.5-fold increase in HCC above that produced by either factor alone (Yan *et al.*, 1996)

In general, animal models of HBV in which there is an associated liver injury (woodchucks, tree shrews and HBV transgenic mice) have supported the notion of a synergistic interaction with AFB_1. The mechanism underlying the observed synergism is unknown, but a number of hypotheses have been put forward including an altered carcinogen metabolism in association with HBV-related liver injury (Kirby *et al.*, 1994; Izzotti *et al.*, 1995; Chemin *et al.*, 1996), and this is discussed below.

AFB_1 is immunosuppressive in various animal species, acting on both circulating and humoral immune systems (see Richard, 1991). An effect on HBV replication or the development of chronic HBV infection has been postulated (Lutwick, 1979) but not examined to date.

8.3.4. Review of risk assessments

Typically, in deriving dose–response relationships to assess the dietary risks from aflatoxin, the various human and animal data sets are analysed, frequently with different mathematical models, and comparisons are made between the predicted incidence of liver cancer and general population values. In this way, the assessments attempt to address issues such as the varying susceptibility across species, extrapolations from epidemiological studies with relatively high background liver cancer rates, and the influence of HBV on aflatoxin-induced liver cancer. Various cancer potency estimates for aflatoxin have been made from animal bioassay data (Cornfield, 1977; US Food and Drug Administration, 1978; Carlborg, 1979; Dichter, 1984; California Department of Health Services, 1990, 1991). Results depend on the choice of the mathematical model used for estimating potency and the test species and strain (see e.g. Table 8.5, and Carlborg, 1979). There are clearly species differences in susceptibility to

Table 8.5 Measures of carcinogenic activity derived from bioassay data[a]			
Test animal	Cancer potency[b] (mg/kg per day)	TD_{50} (mg/kg per day)	Reference
Rat			
Buffalo	1530	< 0.00675	Angsubhakorn *et al.* (1981a)
	517	0.00573	Angsubhakorn *et al.* (1981b)
Charles River CD	1170	0.00419	Newberne & Rogers (1973)
Fischer 344	89[c]	0.148	Ward *et al.* (1975)
	2700	0.00093	Wogan *et al.* (1974)
	26000		Cullen *et al.* (1987)
	1000		Butler & Hempsell (1981)
	2100	0.00134	Nixon *et al.* (1981)
MRC	880 (M)		Butler *et al.* (1969)
	1200 (F)		
Wistar	680		Epstein *et al.* (1969)
	80[d]	0.0366	Merkow *et al.* (1973)
Mouse			
A/J	> 64[e]		Stoner *et al.* (1986)
C57BL (ip)	380		Vesselinovitch *et al.* (1972)
C57BL/BV1 (ip)	3500 (F)[f]	0.00402	Griciute (1980)[g]
A/He (ip)	700[e]		Wieder *et al.* (1968)
Hamster			
Syrian golden	36		Moore *et al.* (1982)
Tree shrew	60	0.027	Reddy *et al.* (1976)
Monkey			
Cynomolgus		0.107	Adamson & Sieber (1983)
Rhesus		0.071	Adamson & Sieber (1983)
Rhesus/ cynomolgus[h]	100		Sieber *et al.* (1979)

[a] Data from California Department of Health Services (1990) or derived by means of the procedure described in Hoover *et al.* (1995).

[b] Derived from dose–response data for hepatocellular neoplasia, except for [c] colon, [d] kidney, [e] lung or [f] lymphoreticular system. Results are for the male of the species unless otherwise indicated (male, M; female, F).

[g] Reported by the authors as a negative study. Gold & Zeiger (1997) indicate a statistically significant trend ($p<0.007$).

[h] Combined data from male and female cynomolgus and rhesus monkeys.

induction of liver cancer by aflatoxin (Busby & Wogan, 1984; International Agency for Research on Cancer, 1993). For the Fischer rat, a significant increase in HCC is seen at dietary AFB_1 levels as low as 4 ppb, while the adult mouse is refractory to 1000 ppb AFB_1 in the diet. Predictions made from rat data using standard assumptions are inconsistent with observations of human liver cancer rates in the USA (Stoloff, 1983; California Department of Health Services, 1991), and it is not clear which animal species is the best surrogate for defining aflatoxin carcinogenesis in humans. Although the observed interspecies dif-

ferences can be partially explained by the pharmacokinetic and other mechanistic data, they have not been quantitatively reconciled.

As outlined below, the first-generation risk assessments relied on correlational epidemiological studies. Despite crude estimates for intake and incidence, the results of analyses of studies in several locations with high liver cancer incidence and HBV prevalence have been fairly consistent. Given the clear association between HBV and liver cancer, the application of these assessments to areas with much lower HBV prevalence has been questioned. The cohort study of Yeh *et al.*

(1989), with its careful ascertainment of HBsAg status and extended intake assessment, initiated the next generation of analyses. Dose–response analyses by various researchers found a roughly 10-fold increase in aflatoxin potency associated with HBV infection. Questions remain regarding the appropriateness of different models used for low-dose risk prediction. Since the development of these assessments, the generation of epidemiological data, with refined evaluations of markers for exposure and other pertinent factors in aflatoxin carcinogenesis has continued apace and in parallel with experimental work on aflatoxin metabolism, target genes, and interactions with HBV. Subsequent sections address further research needs and the possibility of improved predictions.

8.3.4.1 Assessments based on the correlation studies

African and Asian studies Perhaps the most widely quoted assessment is that of Peers & Linsell (1977), who analysed the combined data sets from their studies of aflatoxin exposure and liver cancer in the Murang'a district of Kenya (Peers & Linsell, 1973) and in Swaziland (Peers *et al.*, 1976). They compared crude annual incidence rates of liver cancer with the logarithm of daily aflatoxin intake (*x*), and noted that "it almost invariably has been found that a semi-logarithm relationship gave a higher correlation coefficient than either a simple regression line or a log-log relation." In an expanded analysis of all studies for which dose–response data were available at the time (Table 8.6), they found that the following simple linear relationship provided a better fit:

Annual cases per 100 000 = 0.106 daily aflatoxin intake (ng/kg) + 2.2.

The alternative semi-log relationship that they derived was unrealistic in that it implied that liver cancer incidence in the absence of aflatoxin exposure was zero. They remarked that the background rates of liver cancer in Caucasian populations in North America and Western Europe are similar to the value of 2.2 per 100 000 in their simple linear relationship. The linear relationship has been widely reported, and used either to

estimate excess risks from aflatoxin exposures in the USA, or to provide a basis for comparing other estimates (Dichter, 1984; US Food and Drug Administration, 1978; Bruce, 1990; California Department of Health Services, 1990, 1991). The US Food and Drug Administration (1978) relied on this analysis for assessing cancer risks from aflatoxin in peanuts both at the regulatory level in use at the time, and at alternative levels considered for regulation. Other researchers have performed similar analyses on various selected correlation studies from Africa and Asia with results comparable (within a factor of 4) to the initial findings of Peers & Linsell (See Table 8.6).

American studies Stoloff (1983) estimated aflatoxin exposures in south-eastern states of the USA, and used them in the log-linear relationship of Peers *et al.* (1976) to predict liver cancer incidence in white males in the region. He found the predictions to be inordinately high, and concluded that the correlations between aflatoxin intake and liver cancer observed in Asia and Africa should not be used for making predictions in the USA. He calculated that the excess mortality from primary liver cancer in rural white males was 10% higher in the South-east compared with the northern and western USA. Bruce (1990) used Stoloff's estimates of intake and excess liver cancer rates to derive a cancer potency estimate lower by roughly a factor of 30 than the value that he, as well as others, found from the Asian and African data (see Table 8.6). Others have questioned the aflatoxin intake estimates serving as the basis for the potency estimate because of possible bias in the sampling (Wild & Montesano, 1991) and the lack of confirmation of the high levels of aflatoxin contamination assumed (Wood, 1989). In addition, other major factors associated with liver cancer may vary in the USA by geographical region (Sandler et al. 1983), and these differences were not taken into account in the analyses of data from the USA by Stoloff (1983) and Bruce (1990).

8.3.4.2 Analyses based on the Guangxi, China cohort data

The prospective cohort study of Yeh *et al.* (1989), described above, provided the opportunity to explicitly address the relative contributions to liver cancer of hepatitis B and aflatoxin in

Table 8.6 Cancer potency estimates derived from correlation studies

Data sets analysed	Annual risk per 100 000 population for average daily consumption of ng/kg body weight aflatoxin[a]	Cancer potency slope (in lifetime risk per μg/kg body weight per day aflatoxin)
Peers & Linsell (1977): Mozambique (van Rensburg et al.,1974); Thailand (Shank et al., 1972a,b); Kenya (Peers & Linsell, 1973); Swaziland (Peers et al.,1976)	0.106	74.2[b]
Carlborg (1979): Thailand (Shank et al., 1972a,b); Kenya (Peers & Linsell, 1973); Swaziland (Peers et al., 1976)	0.21[b]	96 (145: 70-year life)
Bruce (1990): Mozambique (van Rensburg et al., 1985); Thailand (Shank et al., 1972a,b); Kenya (Peers et al., 1976); Swaziland (Peers et al., 1976, 1987)	0.0951	47.6 (50-year life) 66[c] (70-year life)
United States (Stoloff, 1983)	0.0031	
Croy & Crouch (1991): Swaziland (Peers et al., 1987)	0.153 (0.09 – 0.23)	107 (63 – 161)
California Department of Health Services (1990): Swaziland (Peers et al., 1976)	0.375 (0.154 – 0.599)	263 (107 – 419)
Swaziland (Peers et al., 1987)	0.168 (UCL[c]: 0.365)	118 (UCL[c]: 256)
Mozambique (van Rensburg et al., 1985)	0.135 (0.103 – 0.169)	94 (72 – 118)

[a] Confidence limits given in parentheses.
[b] Derived from values given in Croy & Crouch (1991).
[c] Upper 95% confidence limit.

dose–response and risk evaluations. HBsAg status was made available for liver cancer deaths and a 25% stratified random sample of the total cohort at the time of enrolment. In addition, liver cancer mortality rates were ascertained by active follow-up of the cohort, thus addressing the problem of underreporting plaguing several of the other studies. Aflatoxin intake was determined through biannual sampling of raw foods collected from study areas over a six year period. Each of the four subareas in Guangxi could be characterized in terms of mean daily intake of aflatoxin, age-adjusted liver cancer mortality rates, prevalence of HBsAg positivity, and "age-adjusted" person–years of follow-up among HBsAg-positive

and HBsAg-negative subjects (Croy & Crouch, 1991; California Department of Health Services, 1990, 1991; Wu-Williams et al. 1992).

Separate estimates of aflatoxin cancer potency for hepatitis-B-negative and positive individuals (Croy & Crouch, 1991; California Department of Health Services, 1990, 1991; Wu-Williams et al. 1992) have been derived from this study. Croy & Crouch (1991) assumed a linear relationship between aflatoxin exposure and age-adjusted mortality rate for liver cancer, with the expected number of cases r seen during N person–years of observation for exposure at dose rate d given by:

$$r = N(a + bd).$$

Table 8.7 Cancer potency estimates as a function of hepatitis status[a]

Type of analysis (reference)	Cancer potency (units per mg/kg body weight per day) by HBsAg status[b]		
	Negative	Positive	Average for population
Linear regression (Croy & Crouch, 1991)	25 (55)	350 (540)	–
Linear regression (California Department of Health Services, 1990)	50	469	–
Multiplicative relative risk model (California Department of Health Services, 1991; Wu-Williams et al., 1992)	2.6 (4.4)	66 (130)	3.2 (5.6)
Interactive model (excess risk form) (California Department of Health Services, 1991; Wu-Williams et al., 1992)	22 (42)	301 (447)	24 (46)
Two-stage clonal expansion model (Bowers et al. 1993)	9	230	10
Exponential relative risk model (Hosenyi, 1992)	(2.2)[c]	(56)[c]	1.6 (2.8)

[a] Derived from the data of Yeh et al. (1989), as reanalysed by Bowers et al. (1993).
[b] Figures in parentheses are the upper 95% confidence bounds, except where otherwise indicated.
[c] Upper confidence bounds.

The number of cases was assumed to be Poisson distributed, and estimates of a and the "cancer potency" b, obtained separately for HBsAg-positive and -negative subjects, were derived by maximum likelihood techniques. Significantly different estimates were derived for the two populations, aflatoxin being far more potent in those who were HBsAg-positive than in those who were negative; a similar analysis was performed by the California Department of Health Services (1990), with comparable results (Table 8.7).

Prediction of risk in the general population using the above approach was criticized because of the small number of liver cancer cases (7) among those with negative HBsAg status (Thomas, 1990). Following the suggestions of Thomas (1990), analyses to evaluate the combined effects of aflatoxin and hepatitis B were undertaken (Wu-Williams et al., 1992; Hosenyi, 1990, 1992; California Department of Health Services, 1991).

Wu-Williams et al. (1992) fitted a number of models, which are presented in Table 8.8. The relative and absolute risk forms tried were mathematically equivalent (i.e. they were reparametrizations of one another) and could not be distinguished on the basis of fits to the Chinese data, yet when they were used to make risk predictions in the USA, on the assumption that background incidence was known, the relative and absolute different risk forms produced substantially different risk predictions because the background liver cancer incidence in the Chinese cohort is much greater than that in the USA.

Hoseyni (1990, 1992) also applied relative and absolute risk models to the data set of Yeh et al. (1989), and found the best fit to be the relative risk model of the form $a \exp(b_1 d_1 + b_2 d_2)$, where d_1 is the daily intake of aflatoxin, and d_2 is an indicator for hepatitis B status. Bowers et al., (1993), however, found an absolute risk model $(a + b_1 d_1 + b_2 d_2 + b_3 d_1 d_2)$

Table 8.8 Model fits to annual liver cancer incidence (y) versus aflatoxin (d) and HBV infection (h) for the Guangxi, China (Yeh *et al.*, 1989) data[a]

Combined HBV–aflatoxin effect	Risk models[b,c]	
	Excess risk form	Relative risk form[d]
Additive model	$y = a+b_1h+b_2d$	$y = a(1+b_1{'}h+b_2{'}d)$
Parameter estimates:		
a: Background incidence (per year)	$2.87{\times}10^{-5}$ ($7.55{\times}10^{-5}$–$2.25{\times}10^{-4}$)	$2.87{\times}10^{-5}$ ($7.55{\times}10^{-5}$–$2.25{\times}10^{-4}$)[e]
b_1: HBV effect (annual increase in incidence due to HBV	0.0055 (0.0045-0.0067)	191 a (NC)[c]
		14520 a (NC)[c]
b_2: Aflatoxin effect (annual incidence per mg/kg per day)	0.42 (0.072-1.76)	
Goodness of fit: $\chi^2 = 17.27$ (5df)[f]		
Interactive model	$y = a+b_1h+b_2d+b_3hd$	$y = a(1+b_1{'}h+b_2{'}d+b_3{'}hd)$
Parameter estimates:		
a: Background incidence (per year)	$6.17{\times}10{-5}$ (0-$2.25{\times}10^{-4}$)	$6.17{\times}10^{-5}$ ($7.55{\times}10^{-5}$–$2.2{\times}10^{-4}$)
b_1: HBV effect (annual increase in incidence due to HBV)	0.0035 (0.002-0.0046)	56.04 a (NC)[c]
b_2: Aflatoxin effect (annual incidence per mg/kg per day)	0.29 (0.069-0.55)	4690 a (NC)[c]
b_3: Aflatoxin–HBV interaction (annual incidence per mg/kg-day)	3.72 (2.20-5.41)	60380 a (NC)[c]
Goodness-of-fit: $\chi^2 = 6.11$ (4df)[f]		
Multiplicative in relative risk model		$y = a(1+b_1{'}h)(1+b_2{'}d)$
Parameter estimates:		
a: Background (per year)		$1.35{\times}10^{-4}$ ($7.55{\times}10^{-5}$–$2.25{\times}10^{-4}$)
b_1: HBV effect (annual increase in incidence due to HBV)		25.10 (15.57–43.64)
b_2: Aflatoxin effect (annual incidence per mg/kg per day)		1242 a (666a–2150a)
Goodness-of-fit: $\chi^2 = 6.68$ (5df)[f]		

[a] Source: Wu-Williams *et al.* (1992).
[b] HBV negative: $h = 0$; HBV positive: $h = 1$.
[c] Table gives maximum likelihood estimates, with likelihood-based upper and lower 95% confidence bounds given in parentheses; NC, confidence limit(s) were infinite.
[d] Parameter estimates for relative risk model are expressed in terms of corresponding excess risk model by multplying by the parameter a.
[e] Confidence limits calculated using asymptotic Wald limits because likelihood-based estimates did not converge.
[f] df: Degrees of freedom.

that fitted the data of Yeh *et al.* (1989) better than the relative-risk model selected by Hoseyni and noted that "one of the better fitting relative risk models was being compared to one of the poorer fitting absolute risk models." Bowers goes on to point out that an alternative to a purely absolute or relative-risk model may be appropriate in this case. He suggests a model of the form $(a + \exp(b_1d_1))$

(exp (b_2d_2)) for the data of Yeh *et al.*, indicating that the risk due to aflatoxin exposure is additive for the model with respect to background in the absence of HBV. In the presence of hepatitis infection, additional risk is proportional to the sum of background and aflatoxin-related risk.

Finally, Bowers and colleagues (1993) reanalysed the data of Yeh *et al.* (1989), using the two-stage clonal expansion model (see Chapter 7) in the form proposed by Thorslund *et al.* (1987). In applying that model, they assumed that aflatoxin is an initiator of primary liver cancer independently of HBV infection, and that HBV promotes liver cancer in the absence of aflatoxin exposure and further that it multiplicatively interacts with aflatoxin to promote liver cancer. They modelled incidence by the function $(a_0 + a_1 d_1)$ [$\exp(b_0 + b_2 d_2 + b_3 d_1 d_2) - 1$]/$(b_0 + b_2 d_2 + b_3 d_1 d_2)$, with d_1 the intake of aflatoxin, and d_2 indicating hepatitis B status. Assuming that background mutation alone (i.e. a_0) accounts for the eight-fold difference between China and the USA in background liver cancer in the absence of HBV and aflatoxin exposure, they estimated the cancer potency for aflatoxin for HBsAg-negative and -positive populations (Table 8.7).

8.3.5 Discussion

The empirical approaches described above to predict aflatoxin risk from epidemiological data did not formally take into account mechanistic information in the assessment. Much research, however, has been undertaken in an attempt to gain an understanding of aflatoxin carcinogenesis, as well as to identify sensitive and specific markers of individual exposure levels for use in epidemiological studies. The results of these efforts, described in section 8.3.2, provide guidance during QEP for selecting models and considering alternative empirical approaches.

8.3.5.1 Reliability of exposure estimates in epidemiological studies

At the population level, dose–response analyses of the correlation studies from different geographical areas of high HBV prevalence, and of the cohort study of Yeh *et al.* have given fairly consistent results. The epidemiological studies relied on surveys of staple foods in the relevant geographical areas and on detailed dietary intake questionnaires; some misclassification of individual exposure levels is thus inevitable. The sampling and analytical difficulties and complexities of accurately measuring aflatoxins in bulk food commodities are well recognized (Campbell *et al.*, 1986; Whitaker & Park 1994) but have generally not been taken into account. In addition, classical epidemiological methods of dietary measurement at the individual level are difficult to apply in the

types of communities where aflatoxin exposures occur, and may not take into account all sources of aflatoxin exposure (Hall & Wild, 1994).

Observations of aflatoxin bound covalently to peripheral blood albumin (Gan *et al.*, 1988; Wild *et al.*, 1993b) provide information on the pattern of exposure at different ages and the variation of aflatoxin exposures among individuals. Several populations have been studied using the aflatoxin–in–albumin marker and have shown that exposure in parts of Africa begins in the perinatal period, continues throughout life, and can vary both geographically and seasonally for a given population (see Wild *et al.*, 1993b; Wang *et al.*, 1996b); considerable day-to-day variation has also been observed (Groopman *et al.*, 1992). The range of interindividual variation in adduct level within a defined population is marked, being greater than two orders of magnitude even in individuals from the same villages and the same ethnic groups, and sampled at the same time of the year.

Use of current exposures as a surrogate for past exposures in dose–response analyses has become a more important issue for QEP, as measures are taken in areas with high aflatoxin levels to reduce them.

8.3.5.2 Impact of hepatitis B virus on aflatoxin risk

The degree to which the observed quantitative relationships between aflatoxin exposure and risk apply to areas with a low prevalence of hepatitis B infection is an important question for aflatoxin QEP. Interactions between HBV and aflatoxin are evident in the dose–response analyses of the data of Yeh *et al.* (1989), with about an order of magnitude difference in the risk of aflatoxin at a given exposure between those of positive and negative HBsAg status These findings are consistent with the more recent epidemiological studies addressing this issue using urinary aflatoxin metabolites or albumin adducts as biomarkers of exposure (Ross *et al.*, 1992; Qian *et al.*, 1994; Wang *et al.*, 1996a), as well as with the mechanistic evidence from studies of *p53* mutation spectra and animal models of hepatitis B infection and aflatoxin.

To predict risks in areas of low aflatoxin exposure and low HBV prevalence, a better understanding of the nature of their interaction is needed; the hypotheses in this regard are consistent with a variety of dose–response models giving different predictions of risk at low exposure levels. Both HBV and aflatoxin are genotoxic and can induce liver injury, and interactions. There are several possible mechanisms of interaction, including modulation of AFB_1 metabolism by viral infection, HBV-induced cell proliferation, and altered viral replication due to the immunosuppressive actions of AFB_1.

Two types of studies indicate the modulation of aflatoxin metabolism by HBV infection:

(1) those which have examined either *in vitro* or *in vivo* the metabolism of carcinogens, or marker drugs, in relation to HBV infection status; and
(2) those which have measured *in vivo* the level of aflatoxin bound to cellular macromolecules in HBV-infected or non-infected subjects as a marker of the biologically effective dose of aflatoxin.

In the second type of study, differences in aflatoxin metabolism have been observed in children. In one study of 323 subjects in the Gambia, a significantly higher mean aflatoxin–albumin adduct level was observed in HBsAg-seropositive individuals compared with those negative for this marker (Allen *et al.*, 1992). In another study in the Gambia, a moderately higher adduct level was also observed in HBsAg carriers (Wild *et al.*, 1993a). In this case, a positive correlation was observed between the levels of serum transaminases and aflatoxin–albumin adduct, independently of HBV infection. These data are consistent with the hypothesis that liver injury caused by HBV and/or other factors may alter aflatoxin metabolism and hence the level of binding of aflatoxin to cellular macromolecules. However, similar differences have not been observed in adults. In China, a study of 120 adults (approximately 60 of whom were HBsAg-positive and the same number negative) failed to find any difference in aflatoxin–albumin adduct levels with respect to HBV infection status (Wang *et al.*, 1996b). A similar result has recently been obtained in a study of 180 chronic HBV carriers and a similar number of controls in the Gambia (Wild *et al.*, unpublished data). The reason for the differences between adults and children is unclear but merits further investigation.

8.3.5.3 Genetically determined differences in human susceptibility

An important factor in the assessment of aflatoxin risk, which has until recently been over-looked, is the variation in human susceptibility due to individual differences in human metabolism. Enzymes implicated in aflatoxin metabolism are being identified, and cytochrome P-450s (CYP) important in the bioactivation of aflatoxin include CYP1A2 and 3A4 (Gallagher *et al.*, 1994). In terms of aflatoxin detoxification, the situation is less clear. Glutathione-S-transferases (GSTs) may play a role (Liu *et al.*, 1991; Raney *et al.*, 1992b), but activities in human liver are generally low compared with those in the mouse and hamster (Kirby *et al.*, 1993). A proportion of the human population have deletions in the *GST M1* and/or *GST T1* genes resulting in the absence of functional protein and it is hypothesized that these individuals would be at an increased HCC risk for a given exposure to aflatoxin. Epoxide hydrolase is also of potential importance in aflatoxin detoxification by converting the AFB_1-8,9-epoxide to dihydrodiol. There are also polymorphisms in this gene which appear to alter enzyme activity and therefore potentially affect individual susceptibility.

Case–control studies have been performed in a search for an association between people homozygous for deletions in the *GST M1* and *T1* genes (null genotype) and HCC risk. In the first study, in Shanghai, China, a study of 52 cases and 116 controls revealed a slightly increased risk of HCC among *GST M1* null individuals (OR (95% CI) = 1.9 (0.94–3.63); $p = 0.06$) (McGlynn *et al.*, 1995). This study also revealed a significant increase in risk (OR (95% CI) = 3.3 (1.2–9.2); $p = 0.01$) associated with the presence of at least one mutant "low-activity" epoxide hydrolase allele. There was also a greater increase in risk in the "low-activity" allele group in association with chronic HBV infection. This may reflect the HBV–aflatoxin interaction observed in the prospective cohort studies in mainland China and Taiwan, China (Qian *et al.*, 1994; Wang *et al.*, 1996a). A nested case–control study in Taiwan, China, among a cohort of HBsAg carriers gave results consistent with those obtained in Shanghai (Chen *et al.*, 1996b). There was a significant increase in risk of HCC among HBsAg carriers with increasing aflatoxin exposure. When this trend was examined in relation to the *GST M1* and *T1* genotypes, it was found that the increased risk with increasing aflatoxin exposure was significant only in the subjects who were null for either *M1* or *T1*.

The importance of the above-mentioned polymorphisms for HCC risk associated with aflatoxin exposure is only beginning to be understood. It is still not clear whether the impact of the genotype is dependent on the level of aflatoxin exposure. In this context, it is of interest that the prevalence of the null genotype for $GST M1$ is less than 20% in some populations in West Africa but 100% in parts of Micronesia and Polynesia (Wild $et\ al.$, 1993a; Board $et\ al.$, 1990).

8.3.5.4 Shape of the dose–response curve
Models used to predict risks from low-level exposure to aflatoxins in the diet have usually assumed that risks increase linearly either with dose or the logarithm of dose. Data from studies of DNA adducts are consistent with the assumption of linearity for aflatoxin pharmacokinetic processes. Such data, however, do not provide information about later steps in aflatoxin carcinogenesis. For example, one can question whether the adducts observed are a good surrogate measure of mutation and whether the dose–response for mutation increases linearly with adduct exposures. None the less, linearity in the aflatoxin dose-response relationship has been observed in epidemiological studies in areas of high HBV prevalence and aflatoxin exposure, and the extent to which this is true for other regions awaits clarification, perhaps through studies of biomarkers and target gene prevalence in populations with low levels of exposure.

8.3.5.5 Impact of background exposures
A number of other risk factors besides HBV and aflatoxin have been identified for HCC, including cigarette smoking, alcohol consumption and age (Sandler $et\ al.$, 1983; Yu $et\ al.$ 1996) and some of these factors may also interact with aflatoxin (Yu $et\ al.$, 1996). Furthermore, prediction of risk in one geographical region using results from another involves at least implicit assumptions regarding the prevalence of risk factors and their interaction with aflatoxin.

8.3.6 Research needs
A number of broad areas of research could provide valuable data to strengthen the risk assessment process for aflatoxin, namely:

(i) improved evaluation of the properties of biomarkers of aflatoxin exposure and susceptibility;
(ii) improved understanding of the mechanisms of carcinogenesis involving aflatoxin and other factors including HBV, and HCV; and
(iii) prospective epidemiological studies using appropriate biomarkers in individuals.

The risk assessments for aflatoxin are based on epidemiological studies in which aflatoxin exposure is measured at the population level. The use of sensitive and specific markers of individual exposure levels in epidemiological studies may therefore improve the basis of QEP in the future. Significant progress has been made in methods of detecting and quantifying human exposure, but the following questions have yet to be answered:

• What are the quantitative relationships between the biomarkers in blood and urine and external exposures?

• What is the relationship between the biomarkers in blood and urine, and the AFB_1–DNA adduct levels in hepatocytes (the target cell)? If AFB_1 adducts in blood and urine are to be used for characterizing the relationship between aflatoxin exposure and liver cancer risk, they must be predictive of the presumed important lesion induced by aflatoxin in the target cell.

• What is the relationship between aflatoxin exposure and the high frequency of mutation in the third nucleotide of codon 249 of the $p53$ gene? This requires more rigorous study to exclude the possibility that the mutation is not a result of aflatoxin exposure. If a specific association is established, and if this mutation is the only mechanism whereby aflatoxin induces liver cancer, this may permit the identification of those cases of HCC in which aflatoxin has played a role within a population, and thus a refinement of risk assessment.

• What is the temporal behaviour of aflatoxin–albumin or aflatoxin–DNA adducts in an individual? How representative of long-term exposure are these biomarkers for a given individual? Does this vary across individuals?

• What are the factors (aflatoxin metabolism, DNA repair) influencing interindividual variation in aflatoxin–adduct levels? Does the expression of aflatoxin–metabolizing enzymes (e.g. GST isoenzymes) alter individual risk in the same way as interspecies susceptibility is influenced by this parameter? Are some individuals or populations at higher risk because of polymorphisms in these and/or other enzymes?

The mechanism of aflatoxin hepatocarcinogenesis is not known; it may be that aflatoxin induces cancer because of its mutagenicity, its mitogenicity, its immunosuppressive activities, or some combination of these. The relationship between aflatoxin exposure and liver cancer will differ, depending on the actual carcinogenic mechanism. The mechanism of interaction with HBV is also not known. These issues are an important area for further research, since QEP generally involves extrapolation of risks across populations exposed to combinations (and often different levels) of risk factors. Specific questions of interest include the following:

• Are the available biomarkers of aflatoxin exposure, namely aflatoxin adducts, involved in the aetiopathogenesis of liver cancer or not?
• How important are the mitogenic activities of aflatoxin and chronic HBV infection in determining risk?
• Does the immunosuppressive action of aflatoxin modify the risk of chronic infection with HBV?
• To what extent is aflatoxin metabolism altered by viral hepatitis and liver injury?
• At what stage of the hepatocarcinogenic process does aflatoxin act, and consequently at what point in the life span of an individual should the measurement of exposure be made upon which risk assessments could be based? How important is the temporal pattern of aflatoxin exposure in determining risk (chronic versus intermittent exposure)?

8.4 2,3,7,8-Tetrachlorodibenzo-para-dioxin (TCDD)

8.4.1 Introduction

Both radon and aflatoxin, discussed earlier in this chapter, are associated with cancer in humans at specific sites, namely radon with cancer of the lung and aflatoxin with cancer of the liver. There is, moreover, concordance of tumour sites in epidemiological and toxicological studies of these two agents. By contrast, TCDD may be associated with cancer at multiple sites, and there appears to be little concordance between the sites affected in toxicological studies and those for which elevated risks have been reported in epidemiological studies.

TCDD is ubiquitous in the environment. It occurs as a toxic by-product in many industrial processes, most notably during the synthesis of many halogenated aromatic compounds, such as the phenoxy herbicides and the trichlorophenols. Experiments in animals show that, on a molar basis, it is one of the most toxic chemicals known to man. Thus, there is legitimate concern regarding allowable levels of human exposure. At the same time, TCDD is one of the most extensively studied chemicals, and we have considerable knowledge of its biological effects. Many epidemiological studies on human populations exposed to TCDD-contaminated chemicals are available as well.

The evidence that TCDD is non-DNA-reactive in standard assays and that the biological effects of TCDD involve receptor binding holds out the possibility that the dose–response curve for carcinogenesis has a threshold below which cancer and the induction of other toxic effects will not occur. The biological effects and biochemical properties, such as TCDD receptor binding, have been extensively studied. Thus, TCDD was seen as an ideal test compound for which to attempt to develop mechanistically based models for cancer prediction.

Many issues have been faced, and some have been resolved, in the effort to develop mechanistic and mathematical models of TCDD carcinogenesis. This section will describe some attempts to address these issues. For example, as discussed below, although TCDD is, on the whole, negative in the standard short-term assays, some studies are at least suggestive of genotoxicity, and theoretically there is the possibility of indirect activity, e.g. via TCDD induction of metabolism in other xenobiotics and endogenous compounds to DNA-reactive forms. Modelling the development of liver foci has provided some support for this hypothesis. Much of the modelling and experimental work has been on the liver, yet non-hepatic tumours have been the primary tumours in some bioassays. There are also the general issues of the extent to which such tumours should be taken into account in predictive modelling for humans, and whether the animal models used so far can reasonably be expected to be predictive of human responses.

8.4.2 Experimental data

8.4.2.1 Animal bioassay

TCDD-induced carcinogenesis has been observed by multiple routes of administration in long-term bioassays in mice, rats and hamsters (as reviewed by US Environmental Protection Agency, 1985; California Department of Health Services, 1986; International Agency for Research on Cancer, 1987a; Huff *et al.*, 1991; Kociba 1991). The studies serving as the basis for dose–response evaluations in risk assessments were oral bioassays in rats by Kociba *et al.* (1978) and in mice and rats by the US National Toxicology Program (1982a). Both commonly and uncommonly occurring tumours were observed in these studies, as discussed in greater detail below. Other bioassays confirm the need to consider multiple target sites in assessing risks of TCDD to humans. In a skin painting study in mice, fibrosarcomas were induced (US National Toxicology Program, 1982b). B6C3 mice developed thymic lymphoma after intraperitoneal exposure; B6C3 mice of each sex developed liver neoplasms after gavage or intraperitoneal exposure (Della Porta *et al.*, 1987). Liver tumours were also induced in Swiss/H/Riop mice exposed *via* gavage (Toth *et al.*, 1979). After receiving six injections either intraperitoneally or subcutaneously of 100 mg/kg TCDD, Syrian Golden hamsters developed squamous-cell carcinomas of the facial skin (distant from the site of administration) (Rao *et al.*, 1988). In ovariectomized rats, TCDD promoted lung tumours but was not observed to induce liver tumours (Clark *et al.*, 1991). Initiation–promotion studies are discussed below.

The early definitive carcinogenesis study was that of Kociba *et al.* (1978, 1979) in which male and female Sprague–Dawley rats were fed TCDD-contaminated diets resulting in doses of approximately 0.001, 0.01 or 0.1 mg/kg body weight per day. Kociba *et al.* observed dose-related increases in squamous-cell carcinoma of the nasal turbinates or hard palate in both sexes, of the tongue in male rats and of the lung in female rats. These tumours are not commonly seen in control animals of this strain. An independent assessment of pathology by Squire (as reported by US Environmental Protection Agency, 1985) confirmed these findings, although the numbers of animals with tumours in particular dose groups varied slightly in the two evaluations. The most widely noted finding in this study is of hepatocellular carcinomas and neoplastic nodules in female rats. The dose–response data for this lesion serve as the basis of levels used by several agencies to regulate exposures to dioxin. Squire

also assessed the pathology of the liver lesions and found several more liver neoplasms in females in the control and lowest dose groups than did Kociba *et al.*, but the overall statistical significance of the findings remained high. More recently, another histopathological re-evaluation of the liver tumours has been undertaken by a group chaired by Sauer (1990), using the diagnostic criteria for liver tumours described in Maronpot *et al.* (1986), which provides counts of animals with liver adenomas instead of neoplastic nodules. In the re-evaluation, the numbers of animals with neoplasms in the mid- and high-dose groups were substantially lower than those noted by Kociba *et al.* and Squire (Brown, 1991; Huff *et al.*, 1991). Nevertheless, the Sauer re-evaluation of these groups still indicates significant increases above controls for liver adenomas and, in the high-dose group, for liver carcinomas.

The US National Toxicology Program (1982a,b) conducted bioassays in a different strain, the Osborne Mendel rat, administering for two years to both sexes weekly doses of vehicle only, or 0.01, 0.05 or 0.5 mg/kg body weight TCDD in two administrations. Averaging the weekly amount results in daily doses similar to those in the Kociba *et al.* study. In male rats, the Program found thyroid follicular-cell tumours significantly elevated in the three treatment groups, in contrast to the results for this sex obtained by Kociba *et al.*; neoplastic nodules in the liver, uncommon in males of this strain, were elevated in the highest-dose group. In female rats, the incidence of liver tumours was elevated in the highest-dose group only; adenomas of the adrenal cortex and fibrosarcomas of the subcutaneous tissue were also elevated in a dose-dependent manner.

The US National Toxicology Program (1982b) gavage studies in B6C3F1 mice were similarly designed, with low-, mid- and high-dose groups of males receiving the same levels as the rats, and the respective female groups receiving four times those levels. The liver was again a target for TCDD carcinogenesis, with malignant hepatocellular tumours seen in both sexes. Fibrosarcomas of the subcutaneous tissue and lymphomas were elevated in high-dose female mice. A dose-related trend in alveolar/bronchiolar tumours, which may have been caused by TCDD treatment, was observed in male mice.

8.4.2.2. Pharmacokinetic data

Pharmacokinetic data are typically used in risk assessments to account for species and dose-dependent differences in absorption, distribution, metabolism and elimination. As outlined below, dose-dependent and interspecies differences in these processes have been observed for TCDD, and have been attributed to protein regulation by TCDD (e.g. disproportionately high clearance at high doses due to TCDD induction of clearance enzymes) (for review, see Byard, 1987; Zeise et al., 1990; Neubert et al., 1991). Thus, additional data on pharmacodynamic parameters such as enzyme induction have been developed and used in coupled "pharmacokinetic/pharmacodynamic" models which quantitatively describe the relationship between TCDD intake and tissue and cellular concentrations of free and bound TCDD (Andersen et al., 1993).

Approximately 50–90% TCDD administered orally to laboratory animals is absorbed. At low doses, percentage absorption may increase as the dose level decreases, and varies with dosing vehicle (Abraham et al., 1988). The extent of percutaneous absorption also increases with decreasing dose (Brewster et al., 1989).

TCDD is widely distributed but accumulates in liver and fat depots. Although accumulation in the liver has been reported to be more pronounced in rodents than in monkeys (Byard, 1987), most studies in rodents were conducted at doses capable of inducing binding proteins. In humans, the predominant deposition site for TCDD at the usual levels of human exposure is adipose tissue, whereas in rats exposed to considerably higher levels, it is the liver (Schlatter, 1991). For example, Schlatter (1991) calculates that, under typical conditions, 60% of total TCDD body burden is present in rat liver, in contrast to 2.5% in human liver, with a 12-fold greater concentration in rat liver. In rodents, the ratio of liver to fat concentrations decreased with decreasing dose (Kociba et al., 1978; Abraham et al., 1988, 1989). Much of this dose dependence has been attributed to binding to CYP1A2 (Andersen et al., 1993), one of the hepatic proteins induced by TCDD which has a high affinity for the compound (Poland et al., 1989; Voorman & Aust, 1989). The concentrations of this protein are increased in induced rats by eight- to 10-fold (Kedderis et al., 1991).

In experimental studies, elimination of TCDD primarily occurs via the excretion of metabolites in the bile and urine and, to a lesser extent, via passive diffusion through the gut wall. Greenlee et al., (1991) report that passive faecal elimination in humans may occur to a greater extent than previously thought, but that this requires study. Relative to life span, the biological half-life measured in humans (six to seven years; Poiger & Schlatter, 1986; Schlatter, 1991) and non-human primates (rhesus: 56 weeks, Bowman et al., 1988; marmoset: 10 weeks, Neubert et al., 1990) is longer than that measured in rodents (31 days in rats, 11 days in mice and hamsters; Byard, 1987). For example, measured TCDD half-life as a function of life span is twice as long for humans as for rats. This has been attributed to dose-dependent differences in elimination due to enzyme induction at the relatively high doses of TCDD used in rodent studies (Abraham et al., 1988). As reviewed by Neubert et al. (1991), the elimination kinetics of TCDD have been observed to be significantly altered in pregnant mice (Krowke, 1986), much lower liver concentrations being observed in the pregnant animal. This was not seen for marmosets (Krowke, 1986; Hagenmaier et al., 1990).

In modelling TCDD pharmacokinetics/dynamics for quantitative risk assessment, several observations pertaining to TCDD protein regulation are being considered. These include TCDD-induced increases in the concentration of the Ah receptor (Poland & Knutson, 1982; Sloop & Lucier, 1987); induction of transforming growth factor-alpha (TGF-alpha) (Choi et al., 1991); modulation of the epidermal growth factor (EGF) receptor (Clark et al., 1991; Lin et al., 1991); and induction of cytochrome P-450 (Tritscher et al., 1992; Portier et al., 1993).

8.4.2.3 Initiation–promotion studies

Several initiation–promotion studies have been performed with 2,3,7,8-TCDD in the mouse skin (Berry et al., 1978; US National Toxicology Program, 1982a,b; Poland et al., 1982), mouse liver (Beebe et al., 1995) and rat liver (Pitot et al., 1980, 1987; Flodström et al., 1991; Lucier et al., 1991; Waern et al., 1991; Dragan et al., 1992; Tritscher et al., 1992; Buchmann et al., 1994; Stinchcombe et al., 1995). On the skin, TCDD is ineffective as a promoter in the classical two-stage initiation–promotion assay in CD-1 and Swiss-Webster mice (Berry et al., 1978; US National Toxicology Program, 1982b); however, chronic administration of the toxicant to HRS/J (hr/hr) mice subsequent to an initiating dose of N-methyl-N'-nitrosoguanidine (MNNG) elicits strong promoting effects at a dose as low as 35.7 ng/kg body weight per day (Poland et al., 1982). This latter strain of mice bears the recessive trait hairless and responds to topical TCDD administration with epidermal hyperplasia and hyperkeratosis. Mice that are wild-type or heterozygous at this locus do not show these morphological alterations (Knutson & Poland, 1982), indicating that there exists some correlation between promotion of papilloma formation and hyperplastic response in mouse skin (Poland et al., 1982).

Pitot and co-workers studied the promoting effects of chronic administration of TCDD on the evolution of enzyme-altered foci in livers of female F344 rats that were administered intragastrically a single dose of N-nitrosodiethylamine combined with a partial hepatectomy (Pitot et al., 1980, 1987; Dragan et al., 1992). The number and liver volume fraction of altered hepatic foci (AHF), characterized by multiple marker enzyme changes, were determined at various doses of TCDD. Strong enhancement of AHF volume fraction and numbers was seen at a dose equivalent to 100 ng/kg body weight per day, while no statistically significant increases were obtained at doses below 10 ng/kg body weight per day. Pitot et al. (1987) proposed a definition of a promotion index, and calculated that TCDD had a promotion index of 106 compared with an index of 6.0 for the classical liver tumour promoter phenobarbital. On a molar basis, TCDD is therefore the most powerful tumour promoter known in rat liver. Promotion by TCDD is primarily seen in female rats and is much less pronounced in males. This is presumably due to synergistic effects mediated by oestrogens, since ovariectomy of rats leads to strongly decreased preneoplastic responses when compared with the effects obtained with TCDD in the intact female animals (Lucier et al., 1991).

8.4.2.4 Short-term tests
TCDD is generally considered to be non-DNA-reactive because of the large body of evidence for its activity via the receptor-binding mechanism (Whitlock, 1990; also see below), and because

TCDD does not appear to form DNA adducts and on the whole is negative in short-term tests for genotoxicity (Wassom et al., 1977; International Agency for Research on Cancer, 1987b; Shu et al. 1987; Greenlee et al., 1991; Lucier, 1992; Lucier et al., 1993). The molecular structure of TCDD does not have apparent electrophilic sites (Ashby & Tennant, 1988). TCDD may damage DNA by indirect mechanisms, e.g. by elevating the production of DNA-reactive metabolites of both xenobiotic and endogenous compounds, as noted by Lucier et al. (1993), Lucier (1992) and US Environmental Protection Agency (1988), and TCDD-mediated elevation of CYP1A1 may be associated with oxidative DNA damage (Park et al., 1996). TCDD treatment of rats resulted in increased in vitro induction of sister chromatid exchanges by alpha-naphthoflavone (Lundgren et al., 1986); indirect induction of sister chromatid exchanges and chromosomal aberrations has also been reported (Lundgren et al., 1988). Interestingly, TCDD induced neoplastic transformation in immortalized human keratinocytes (Yang et al., 1992), and the results of mathematical modelling of liver foci are reported to be consistent with the hypothesis that TCDD acts as an initiator (Moolgavkar et al., 1996; Portier et al., 1996). Thus, the issue of whether (and how) to account for the possibility of TCDD genotoxicity in mathematical modelling to estimate TCDD risks has not been resolved.

8.4.2.5 Mechanistic aspects of TCDD action
Many of the effects induced by TCDD are mediated by an intracellular receptor, the Ah (aromatic aryl hydrocarbon) receptor, to which TCDD binds with high affinity (Poland & Knutson, 1982; Safe, 1986; Whitlock, 1990). The Ah receptor consists of two subunits: the Ah receptor ligand-binding subunit (ALBS) (Burbach et al., 1992), and two 90 kDa heat-shock proteins (hsp90) (Cuthill et al., 1987; Poland et al., 1991). Binding of TCDD to ALBS leads to dissociation of hsp90 from the complex. Ligand-bound ALBS then associates with another protein, the aryl hydrocarbon receptor nuclear translocator (ARNT) (Reyes et al., 1992). The dioxin/Ah receptor complex binds with high affinity to specific sequences in DNA, called dioxin-responsive elements (DREs) (Denison et al., 1988; Hapgood et al., 1989; Neuhold et al., 1989). DRE sequences have been detected in the enhancer

domains of a number of genes (Rushmore *et al.*, 1990); NADP(H) quinone reductase (Favreau & Pickett *et al.*, 1991) and cytochrome P1-450 (CYP1A1) (Gonzales & Nebert, 1985; Fujisawa-Sehara *et al.*, 1987; Nebert & Jones, 1989). The enhancer of the mouse CYP1A1 gene contains four DREs (Fisher *et al.*, 1990) and the enhancer of the human gene probably contains six (Wu & Whitlock, 1993). DRE-binding of the TCDD-activated Ah receptor is assumed to lead to bending of the DNA (Elferink & Whitlock, 1990), resulting in activation of the promoter by other constitutively expressed transcription factors (Wu & Whitlock, 1993).

Differences in sensitivity to TCDD with regard to biochemical changes and toxic effects have been demonstrated in congenic mouse strains expressing low or high affinity forms of the Ah receptor (Poland & Knutson, 1982). Thus, congenic mice expressing the lower-affinity form of the receptor require higher doses of TCDD to elicit the effects than strains expressing the higher-affinity forms. A similar difference in sensitivity to polychlorodibenzodioxins (PCDDs) has also been demonstrated in tumour-promotion studies in skin of congenic mouse strains (Knutson & Poland, 1982). In these studies, PCDDs showed the same rank order of potency in Ah receptor binding *in vitro* and tumour induction *in vivo*. The requirement for a functional Ah receptor has been demonstrated during TCDD-induced tumour promotion in mouse liver (Beebe *et al.*, 1995). Taken together, these data strongly support a receptor-mediated mechanism for TCDD-induced carcinogenesis.

Although most of the biochemical effects of TCDD are believed to be mediated via receptor binding, some researchers have suggested that some responses may not require the receptor–ligand complex to act as a transcription factor (Bombick *et al.*, 1988; Beebe *et al.*, 1990; Matsumura *et al.*, 1984; Enan & Matsumura, 1996).

TCDD is a powerful inducer of cytochrome P-450 (Poland & Knutson, 1982). Several studies on a wide range of chemically quite diverse xenobiotics indicate that induction of cytochrome P-450 in liver by these agents correlates well with their promoting efficiency in this organ. Similar species differences in promoting effects and

enzyme induction by barbiturates and related compounds have been demonstrated (Lubet *et al.*, 1989), and structure-activity differences in both parameters correlated well within a series of barbiturates (Nims *et al.*, 1987), polyhalogenated biphenyls (Buchmann *et al.*, 1991) and certain polychlorinated dibenzofuran and dibenzo-*p*-dioxin congeners (Waern *et al.*, 1991); similar dose–response characteristics of 2,4,8-trichlorodibenzofuran and cytochrome P-450 induction have been described (Deml *et al.*, 1989). Induction of cytochrome P-450 may therefore serve as a sensitive early marker for the promoting activity of TCDD in liver. Lucier and colleagues recently established dose–response relationships for the induction of two cytochrome P-450 isoenzymes, CYP1A1 and CYP1A2, respectively, in liver of rats chronically exposed to TCDD (Tritscher *et al.*, 1992). Female Sprague–Dawley rats were administered *N*-nitrosodiethylamine as initiator and were subsequently treated chronically with four different doses of TCDD (equivalent to 3.5, 10.7, 35.7 and 125 ng/kg body weight per day) for 30 weeks; additional groups of rats were given TCDD alone. Liver concentrations of TCDD were determined for each individual rat. CYP1A1 and CYP1A2 were quantitated by radioimmunoassay and immunolocalized within frozen liver sections by means of specific antibodies.

TCDD-mediated increases in CYP1A1 and CYP1A2 have been mathematically modelled (Kohn *et al.*, 1993; Portier *et al.*, 1993). The best fitting model is consistent with linearity of response at low doses. However, a model implying a threshold at low doses is also consistent with the data. Other biochemical end-points, such as EGF-receptor binding, were also investigated in these studies. The issues are complex, and we refer the reader to the relevant publications for further details.

Although there is a good correlation between enzyme induction and promotion by TCDD, as pointed out above, this correlation is by no means perfect. Thus, while TCDD is ineffective as a promoter in ovariectomized rats and does not stimulate liver cell proliferation in these animals, it is still capable of inducing cytochrome P-450 (CYP1A2) in roughly the same magnitude as in the intact female rats (Lucier *et al.*, 1991). Both haired (hr/+) and hairless (hr/hr) HRS/J mice respond to TCDD with epidermal aryl hydrocarbon hydroxylase induction, but the proliferative response and promotion of papilloma formation can be stimulated only in the hr/hr mice (Knutson & Poland, 1982; Poland et al., 1982). Enzymes controlling DNA synthesis and cell proliferation are likely to be regulated in a much more complex manner than enzymes of the liver mono-oxygenase system, including cytochromes P-450; while the latter are constitutively expressed in liver cells (even though at low levels in the case of some isoenzymes), cell cycle-regulating genes are not.

Chronic treatment of rats with high doses of TCDD leads to sustained proliferation of normal appearing hepatocytes (Lucier et al., 1991). Less is known about hepatocyte proliferation kinetics at lower TCDD doses and, in particular, about the induction of proliferation of initiated hepatocytes in TCDD-treated animals. Recent results suggest that TCDD has only minor effects on the proliferation of enzyme-altered hepatocytes in rat liver (Buchmann et al., 1994). Since many other liver tumour promoters inhibit apoptosis in both normal and preneoplastic liver cells (Schulte-Hermann, 1985), TCDD might be expected to elicit similar effects. A recent study (Stinchcombe et al., 1995) indicates that TCDD inhibits apoptosis in enzyme-altered hepatocytes. TCDD might therefore increase cell death at high doses, where cytotoxicity plays a major role, while it might decrease cell death by inhibition of apoptosis at low doses, where cytotoxicity is of minor importance. Future studies should therefore address the question of changes in the rates of proliferation and of apoptosis of initiated hepatocytes at different doses of TCDD, in particular very low ones. Analyses should be performed at different time points during chronic exposure in order to allow temporal changes in the patterns of proliferation and apoptosis to be detected.

8.4.3 Epidemiological studies

Because TCDD occurs as an unwanted contaminant during various chemical processes, humans are exposed to it only in combination with other, possibly toxic, chemicals. Thus, the biggest problem in epidemiological studies is that of isolating the effects of TCDD from those of other chemicals with which it is associated. Epidemiological studies have, by and large, focused on populations exposed to the phenoxy herbicides and trichlorophenols, either during the manufacture of these chemicals or during their use.

Early case reports suggested associations between exposure to phenoxy herbicides or to the chlorophenols and the subsequent development of malignant lymphomas and soft-tissue sarcomas (STS). These reports have subsequently been investigated by case–control studies. The early work in this area by Swedish investigators reported significant associations between exposure to these compounds and the risk of malignant lymphomas (Hardell, 1981; Hardell et al., 1981) and STS (Hardell & Sandström, 1979). A recent review article by Johnson (1992) states that, at the time of writing, 10 case–control studies on the association between these chemicals and malignant lymphomas, and 15 case–control studies of STS and phenoxy herbicide and chlorophenol exposure, were being conducted.

Most of the case–control studies of malignant lymphoma failed to find any association of this group of diseases with exposure to TCDD. Cohort studies, which are discussed below, likewise do not support any association between exposure to TCDD and malignant lymphoma.

Johnson (1992) pointed out that, of the 15 case–control studies of STS, 13 have provided information on the possible effect of dioxin exposure. Of these, four showed a statistically significant association of exposure to the phenoxy herbicides or the trichlorophenols and STS. In three of the remaining studies, significant associations were found in some subgroups of the study population. By far the highest risks were found by the Swedish investigators, whose studies, however, have been severely criticized on the grounds, inter alia, of inappropriate choice of controls, recall bias, interviewer bias and inappropriate use of statistical methodology. For reviews of the case–control studies see the papers by Lilienfeld & Gallo (1989) and Johnson (1992). The case–control studies raise some concerns about the role of TCDD in STS, but do not provide a definite answer.

In the early 1990s, four cohort studies (Zober et al., 1990; Fingerhut et al., 1991; Manz et al., 1991; Saracci et al., 1991) explored the association between exposure to TCDD-contaminated chemicals, such as the phenoxy herbicides and the trichlorophenols, and the subsequent development of cancer. These are important studies because they contain sizeable subpopulations with substantial exposures to TCDD, documented by workplace measurements, the occurrence of chloracne and, in some instances, measurements in blood or adipose tissue. It must be emphasized, however, that tissue measurements were available only on subsets of exposed individuals not necessarily representative of the groups as a whole.

The tumours of *a priori* interest are malignant lymphomas and STS. None of the cohort studies report an increased risk of lymphomas in the exposed groups. With STS, the picture is mixed. No increase is reported in the studies of Zober *et al.* (1990) and Manz *et al.* (1991). These are, however, the smallest of the cohort studies, and STS are rare tumours. The study of Fingerhut *et al.* (1991) reports a standardized mortality ratio (SMR) of 922, with a wide confidence interval in the subgroup of workers who presumably received the highest exposure to TCDD-contaminated chemicals. The estimate of risk is based on a small number (four) of cases. Further, as pointed out by Collins *et al.* (1993), all cases of STS in the Fingerhut cohort occurred in individuals who had also been exposed to a potent human bladder carcinogen, 4-aminobiphenyl. The study of Saracci *et al.* (1991) is the largest of the cohort studies, and is a multinational study conducted on 20 study groups in 10 countries. In this study, a statistically non-significant SMR of 196 based on four cases was reported. However, "the excess does not seem to be specifically associated with those herbicides probably contaminated by TCDD". Subsequently, Peto (1991) pointed out that there was no significant trend in risk with either duration of exposure or time since first exposure to the phenoxy herbicides and trichlorophenols. Moreover, two of the four cases of STS had occurred in individuals who had been exposed for less than one year. The cohort studies taken together, therefore, raise some concern about the role of TCDD in STS, but the evidence at the present time is inadequate to conclude that it has a causal role in STS.

All four cohort studies found an elevation in the risk of respiratory cancer in some subgroup of the exposed cohort. However, there is no apparent dose–response relationship, and, importantly,

little smoking information is available. One would expect a high prevalence of smoking in industrial cohorts. With the exception of the Saracci cohort, there is also some indication of an increase in total cancer mortality in these cohorts. Again, no dose–response relationship is evident.

Bertazzi *et al.* (1993) have reported on an industrial accident that occured in 1976 near Seveso in Italy, which exposed the local population to TCDD. Three areas, A, B and R, with decreasing TCDD contamination were identified, and the populations of these areas, together with a reference population, were followed between 1977 and 1986 for cancer occurrence. The population of area A was small and there were only 14 cancer cases. STS were elevated in zone R, but not in zone B. There was also an increase in zone B of hepatobiliary neoplasms in both men and women. The increase was statistically significant among women. In addition, some lymphoid and haematological malignancies were increased in both men and women in zone B.

A report on a fifth cohort study of TCDD has recently been published (Becher *et al.*, 1996). This study of over 2000 workers in four phenoxy herbicide production plants in Germany reported a statistically significant increased mortality from all cancers, respiratory cancers and Hodgkin's lymphoma. The largest group of workers in this study is from the same plant as that investigated in the study conducted by Manz *et al.*, (1991)

Overall, the strongest evidence for the human carcinogenicity of TCDD is for all cancers combined, rather than for those at any specific site. Smoking and ionizing radiation are the only other agents associated with cancers at many different sites. Even for these carcinogens, however, there are clearly elevated risks for certain specific sites. The lack of precedent for a general multisite carcinogen suggests circumspection in the interpretation of the epidemiological data on TCDD.

Although the epidemiological data provide some (weak) support for the hypothesis that TCDD is a human carcinogen, the absence of any dose–response relationship makes these data unsuitable for QEP, which must, therefore, be based on animal data.

8.4.4 Risk assessment

The levels of dioxin considered to be safe by regulatory agencies and other institutions vary by three orders of magnitude, as indicated by several authors (Leung *et al.*, 1988; Zeise *et al.*, 1990; Kociba, 1991). Canada, the German Federal Environmental Agency, the Netherlands Institute of National Health and the New York State Department of Health all apply a safety factor to an assumed no-observed-adverse-effect level (NOAEL) derived from the study by Kociba *et al.* to specify maximal allowable daily intake levels of 1–10 pg/kg per day. The differences are attributable to the safety factor applied to the NOAEL, although the selection of the NOAEL can be questioned. In the USA, Federal agencies (the Environmental Protection Agency (EPA), the Centers for Disease Control (CDC) and the Food and Drug Administration (FDA)) fit the linearized multistage model to dose–response data from the Kociba bioassay in female rats to derive cancer potency estimates. The doses associated with an increase in lifetime risk of 10^{-6} (referred to by some as "virtually safe doses") by these agencies vary from 0.006 to 0.057 fg/kg body weight per day. The differences in these values are the result of differences in the choice of dose measures in model fitting (administered dose [US EPA, US FDA] or liver concentration [US CDC]), the assumption that dose measure is equivalent across species (amount per surface area [US EPA]; amount per body weight [US FDA]; rat liver concentration [US CDC]), differences in tumour counts (pathology of Squire [US CDC] or Kociba [US FDA] or both [US EPA]), the use of crude adjustments for early mortality in the Kociba study (US EPA only), and differences in the target site selected (liver only [US CDC, US FDA]; those causally related to TCDD exposure [liver, lung, hard palate/turbinates; US EPA]). The California Department of Health Services (1986) derived a cancer potency value slightly different from that of the US EPA (within 10%) from the dose–response data for liver tumours in male mice (US National Toxicology Program, 1982a).

Assessments following the multistage approach used by regulatory agencies in the USA have included: time-dependent analyses to account better for the high mortality in the study by Kociba *et al.* (Portier *et al.*, 1984; Sielken, 1987); fitting the models to the latest pathology evaluation by Sauer (1990) of female rat liver tumours (California Department of Health Services, 1990; Paustenbach *et al.*, 1991); fitting models to additional target sites and experiments (Portier *et al.*, 1984; US Environmental Protection Agency, 1985; California Department of Health Services, 1990) and analyses accounting for interdose differences in pharmacokinetics (CDC [Kimborough, 1984]; Portier *et al.*, 1984).

The US EPA (1985) adjusted for early mortality in the study by Kociba *et al.* by eliminating from the analysis animals that died during the first year (before the first tumour appeared). In the time-dependent re-evaluations, an approximate form of the hazard function of the multistage model was used. This procedure led to higher estimates of potency, with the highest potency estimated when the tumours were assumed to be rapidly lethal.

Use of the pathology re-evaluation of Sauer results in a two-fold decrease in the potency estimate derived from liver tumours in the female rat using the standard procedures of US EPA (California Department of Health Services, 1990). Paustenbach *et al.* (1991) reported that fitting the linearized multistage model to "survival adjusted tumour incidence data" from the re-evaluation results in an estimate of potency about a half to a third that derived from data of the original Kociba histopathology evaluation. They also reported that fitting the approximate form (see Chapter 7) of a stochastic two-stage model (Moolgavkar & Luebeck, 1990) to individual animal data (i.e. Sauer-diagnosed tumour status and time of death) results in a decrease in potency of two orders of magnitude for liver carcinomas and by a factor of eight for all liver tumours.

Consideration of estimates derived from the other US NTP and Kociba experiments (Portier *et al.*, 1984; US Environmental Protection Agency, 1985; see Zeise *et al.*, 1990 for compilation) indicate that exclusion or re-evaluation of a particular experimental result is not expected to change the cancer potency by more than a factor of two or three if estimated using standard approaches. The cancer potency estimated by US EPA in 1985 (156 000 (mg/kg per day)$^{-1}$) is the geometric mean of two values, one derived from the Squire histopathology evaluation for female rat tumours, the other from that of Kociba.

Excluding the high-dose group due to lack of fit results in a higher estimate (425 000 (mg/kg per day)$^{-1}$). The next highest potency value is derived from thyroid tumour data from the US NTP male rat experiment (222 000 (mg/kg per day)$^{-1}$), followed by that for data on liver tumours in the male mouse US NTP experiment (130 000 (mg/kg per day)$^{-1}$). Potencies lower than the current US EPA value by a factor of three or more are derived from dose–response data in the remaining experiments (squamous-cell tumours of the nasal and oral cavity in the male rat [Kociba]: 15 000–40 000 [mg/kg per day]$^{-1}$); liver tumours in the female rat [NTP]: 33 000 [mg/kg per day]$^{-1}$; sites causally related to TCDD treatment in the female [NTP] mouse [subcutaneous fibroma, lymphoma, leukaemia or liver tumours]: 46 000 [mg/kg per day]$^{-1}$).

The US EPA has undertaken a re-evaluation of its 1985 risk assessment for TCDD, at least partly in the hope that mechanistic considerations would inform the prediction of the dose–response curve in the low-dose region. At the time of writing, the new US EPA report has not been officially released. Draft chapters have been available, however, and it is clear from these that the EPA has attempted to incorporate mechanistic information in this re-evaluation. The analyses presented include a physiologically based pharmacokinetic (PBPK) model to describe the uptake and metabolism of TCDD, as well as receptor-binding models to describe early biological events along the pathway to carcinogenesis. Analyses of altered hepatic foci using the methods described in Chapter 7 have also been undertaken. Because of critical knowledge gaps, however, an integrated biologically based QEP does not appear feasible at the present time. It seems likely that, despite all the effort put into the re-evaluation, the US EPA will fall back on the Kociba study for the estimation of the potency of TCDD.

8.4.5 Conclusions

Epidemiological evidence of human carcinogenicity of TCDD is limited. It causes tumours at multiple sites in toxicological studies, depending upon the species and the sex of the animals used. The estimates of unit risk (potency) vary widely, depending upon the species, sex and site used to derive the estimate. The issue of whether or not there is a threshold for the carcinogenicity of TCDD remains unresolved. The dose–response curve for enzyme induction by TCDD is consistent both with linearity and with the existence of a threshold. Because the sequence of steps between enzyme induction and biological effects relevant to malignancy, e.g. induction of cell division or inhibition of apoptosis, is not known, the dose–response curve for enzyme induction cannot be used to infer dose–response relationships for these biological effects. Prediction of human cancer risk from toxicological studies is further complicated by the absence of information on which specific species, sex, and tumour type are most relevant to human carcinogenesis.

References – radon

Alavanja, M.C., Brownson, R.C., Lubin, J. H., Berger, E., Chang, J. & Boice, J.D., Jr (1994) Residental radon exposure and lung cancer among nonsmoking women. *J. Natl Cancer Inst.*, **86**, 1829-1837

Archer, V.E. (1987) Association of lung cancer mortality with precambrian granite. *Arch. Environ. Health*, **42**, 87-91

Auvinen, A., Makelainen, I., Hakama, M., Castren, O., Pukkala, E., Reisbacka, H. & Rytomaa, T. (1996) Indoor radon exposure and risk of lung cancer: a nested case–control study in Finland. *J. Natl Cancer Inst.*, **88**, 966-972

Axelson, O., Andersson, K., Desai, G., Fagerlund, I., Jansson, B., Karlsson, C. & Wingren, G. (1988) Indoor radon exposure and active and passive smoking in relation to the occurrence of lung cancer. *Scand. J. Work Environ. Health*, **14**, 286-292

Axelson, O., Edling, C. & Kling, H. (1979) Lung cancer and residency—a case–referent study on the possible impact of of exposure to radon and its daughters in dwellings. *Scand. J. Work Environ. Health*, **5**, 10-15

Bean, J.A., Isacson, P., Hahne, R.M.A. & Kohler, J. (1982) Drinking water and cancer incidence in Iowa. II. Radioactivity in drinking water. *Am. J. Epidemiol.*, **116**, 924-932

Blot, W.J., Xu, Z.Y., Boice, J.D., Jr., Zhao, D.Z., Stone, B.J., Sun, J., Jing, L.B. & Fraumeni, J.F. (1990) Indoor radon and lung cancer in China. *J. Natl Cancer Inst.*, **82**, 1025-1030

Borek, T.D. & Johnson, J.A. (1988) *Estimating the Risk of Lung Cancer from Inhalation of Radon Daughters Indoors: Review and Evaluation* (EPA 600/6-88/008), Las Vegas, NV, US Environmental Protection Agency

Bos, J.L. (1989) *ras* oncogenes in human cancer: a review. *Cancer Res.*, **49**, 4682-4689

Brenner, D.J. (1994) The significance of dose rate in assessing the hazards of domestic radon exposure. *Health Phys.* **67**, 76-79

Brenner, D.J. & Hall, E.J. (1990) The inverse dose–rate effect for oncogenic transformation by neutrons and charged particles: a plausible interpretation consistent with published data. *Int. J. Radiat. Biol.*, **58**(5), 745-758

Brenner, D.J., Hall, E.J., Randers-Pehrson, G. & Miller, R.C. (1993) Mechanistic considerations on the dose-rate/LET dependence of oncogenic transformation by analyzing radiation. *Radiat. Res.*,**133**, 365-369

Castren, O., Voutilainen, A., Winqvist, K. & Makelainen, I. (1985) Studies of high indoor radon areas in Finland. *Sci. Total. Environ.*, **45**, 311-318

Cohen, B.L.(1990) A test of the linear–no threshold theory of radiation carcinogenesis. *Environ. Res.*, **53**, 193-220

Cohen, B.L. (1992) Problems in ecological studies [letter; comment]. *Int. J. Epidemiol.*, **21**, 422-425

Cohen, B.L. (1993) Relationship between exposure to radon and various types of cancer. *Health Phys.*, **65**, 529-31

Cohen, B.L. (1994) Dose–response relationship for radiation carcinogenesis in the low-dose region. . *Int. Arch. Occup. Environ. Health*, **66**, 71-75

Cohen, B.L. (1995a) Test of the linear–no threshold theory of radiation carcinogenesis for inhaled radon decay products. *Health Phys.*, **68**, 157-174

Cohen, B.L. (1995b) How dangerous is low level radiation? *Risk. Anal.*, **15**, 645-653

Cohen, B.L. & Colditz, G.A. (1994) Tests of the linear-no threshold theory for lung cancer induced by exposure to radon. *Environ. Res.*, **64**, 65-89

Cross, F.T. (1988) *Radon Inhalation Studies in Animals* (DOE/ER-0396), Springfield, VA, National Technical Information Service

Cross, F.T. (1992) Experimental statistical and biological models of radon carcinogenesis. *Radiat. Prot. Dosimetry*, **45**, 629-633

Cross, F.T., Palmer, R.F., Filipy, R.E., Dayle, G.E. & Stuart, B.O. (1982) Carcinogenic effects of radon daughters, uranium ore dust and cigarette smoke in beagle dogs. *Health Phys.*, **42**, 33-52

Damber, L.A. & Larsson, L.G. (1987) Lung cancer in males and type of dwelling. An epidemiologic pilot study. *Acta Oncol.*, **26**, 211-215

Darby, S.C. & Doll, R (1990) Radiation and exposure rate. *Nature*, **344**, 824

Darby, S.C., Whitley, E., Howe, G.R., Hutchings, S.J., Kusiak, R.A., Lubin, J.H., Morrison, H.I., Tirmarche, M., Tomasek, L., Radford, E.P. *et al.*, (1995) Radon and cancers other than lung cancer in underground miners: a collaborative analysis of 11 studies. *J. Natl Cancer Inst.* **87**, 378-384

Doll, R. & Peto, R. (1978) Cigarette smoking and bronchial carcinoma: dose and time relationships among regular smokers and life-long non-smokers. *J. Epidemiol. Community Health*, **32**, 303-313

Edling, C., Comba, P., Axelson, O. & Flodin, U. (1982) Effects of low-dose radiation—a correlation study. *Scand. J. Work Environ. Health*, **8**, Suppl. 1, 59-64

Edling, C., Kling, H. & Axelson, O. (1984) Radon in homes—a possible cause of lung cancer. *Scand. J. Work Environ. Health*, **10**, 25-34

Edling, C., Wingren, G. & Axelson, O. (1986) Quantification of the lung cancer risk from radon daughter exposure in dwellings—an epidemiological approach. *Environ. Int.,* **12**, 55-60

Evans, H.H. (1992) Relationship of the cellular and molecular effects of alpha-particle irradiation to radon-induced lung cancer. In: Cross, F.T. ed., *Proceedings of the 29th Hanford Symposium on Health and the Environment, Richland, Washington,* Richland, WA, Battelle Press, pp. 537-554

Fleischer, R.L. (1986) A possible association between lung cancer and a geological outcrop. *Health Phys.,* **50**, 823-827

Forastiere, F., Valesini, S., Arca, M., Maglioia, M.E., Michelozzi, P. & Tasco, C. (1985) Lung cancer and natural radiation in an Italian province. *Sci. Total Environ.,* **45**, 519-526

Fu, H., Gu, X., Jin, X., Yu, S., Wu, K. & Guidotti, T.L. (1994) Lung cancer among tin miners in southeast China: silica exposure, silicosis, and cigarette smoking. . *Am. J. Ind. Med.* **26**, 373-381

Gilbert, E.S. (1989) Lung cancer risk models from experimental animals. In: *Proceedings of the 24th Annual Meeting of the National Council on Radiation Protection and Measurements (NCRP),* Bethesda, MD, National Council on Radiation Protection and Measurements , pp. 141-145

Gjorup, H.L. & Hansen, H.J. (1985) Lifetime loss through lung cancer in Denmark and Sweden. *Nord. Med.,* **100**(4), 100-103

Greenland, S. (1992) Divergent biases in ecologic and individual level studies. *Stat. Med.,* **11**, 1209-1223

Greenland, S. & Morgenstern, H. (1989) Ecological bias, confounding, and effect modification. *Int. J. Epidemiol.,* **18**, 269-274

Greenland, S. & Morgenstern, H. (1992) Problems in ecological studies. Letter to the editor. *Int. J. Epidemiol.,* **21**, 424-425

Hall, E.J. (1978) *Radiobiology for the Radiologist,* Philadelphia, PA, Harper and Row

Harris, C.C. & Hollstein (1993) Clinical implications of the *p53* tumor-suppressor gene. *New Engl. J. Med.,* 1318-1327

Haynes, R.M. (1988) The distribution of domestic radon concentrations and lung cancer mortality in England and Wales. *Radiat. Prot. Dosimetry,* **25**, 93-96

Hess, C.T., Weiffenbach, C.V. & Norton, S.A. (1983) Environmental radon and cancer correlations in Maine. . *Health Phys.,* **45**, 339-348

Hill, C.K., Han, A. & Elkind, M.M. (1984) Fission spectrum neutrons at a low dose rate enhance neoplastic transformation in the linear dose region (0–10 cGy). *Int. J. Radiat. Biol.,* **46**, 11-15

Hofmann, W., Katz, R. & Zhang, C. (1985) Lung cancer incidence in a Chinese high background area—epidemiological results and theoretical interpretation. *Sci. Total Environ.,* **45**, 527-534

Hofmann, W., Katz, R. & Zhang, C. (1986) Lung cancer risk at low doses of alpha particles. *Health Phys.,* **51**, 457-468

Hollstein, M., Sidransky, D., Vogelstein, B. & Harris, C.C. (1991) *p53* mutations in human cancers. *Science,* **253**(5015), 49-53.

Hornung, R.W. & Meinhardt, T.J. (1987) Quantitative risk assessment of lung cancer in U.S. uranium miners. *Health Phys.,* **52**, 417-430

Hornung, R.W., Deddens, J. & Roscoe, R. (1995) Modifiers of exposure response estimates for lung cancer among miners exposed to radon progeny. *Environ. Health Perspect.* **103**, 49-53

Howe, G.R. & Stager, R.H. (1996) Risk of lung cancer mortality after exposure to radon decay products in the Beaverlodge cohort based on revised exposure estimates. *Radiat. Res.,* **146**, 37-42

Howe, G.R., Nair, R.C., Newcombe, H.B., Miller, A.B. & Abbat, J.D. (1986) Lung cancer mortality (1950–1980) in relation to radon daughter exposure in a cohort of workers at the Eldorado Beaverlodge radium uranium mine. *J. Natl Cancer Inst.,* **77**, 357-362

Howe, G.R., Nair, R.C., Newcombe, H.B., Miller, A.B., Burch, J. D. & Abbatt, J.D. (1987) Lung cancer mortality (1950–80) in relation to radon daughter exposure in a cohort of workers at the Eldorado Port Radium Uranium Mine: Possible modification of risk by exposure rate. *J. Natl Cancer Inst.*, **79**, 1255-1260

Husgafvel Pursiainen, K., Ridanpaa, M., Anttila, S. & Vainio, H. (1995) *p53* and *ras* gene mutations in lung cancer: implications for smoking and occupational exposures. *J. Occup. Environ. Med.* **37**, 69-76

International Agency for Research on Cancer (1986) *Tobacco: A Major International Health Hazard* (IARC Scientific Publications No. 74), Lyon

International Agency for Research on Cancer (1988) *IARC Monographs on the Evaluation of Carcinogenic Risks to Humans*, Vol. 43, *Man-made Mineral Fibres and Radon*, Lyon

International Commission on Radiological Protection (1987) *Lung Cancer Risk from Indoor Exposures to Radon Daughters* (ICRP-Publication 50), Oxford, Pergamon Press

Klotz, J.B., Petix, J.R. & Zagraniski, R.T. (1989) Mortality of a residential cohort exposed to radon from industrially contaminated soil. . *Am. J. Epidemiol.*, **129**, 1179-1186

Krewski, D., Miller, T., Eaton, R.S., Meyerhof, D.P. & Létourneau, E.G. (1989) Managing environmental radon risk: a Canadian perspective. In: Freij, L., ed., *Management of Risk from Genotoxic Substances in the Environment*, Stockholm, Swedish National Chemicals Inspectorate

Kusiak, R.A., Springer, J., Ritchie, A.C. & Muller, J. (1991) Carcinoma of the lung in Ontario gold miners: possible aetiological factors. *Br. J. Ind. Med.*, **48**, 808-817

Kusiak, R.A., Ritchie, A.C., Muller, J. & Springer, J. (1993) Mortality from lung cancer in Ontario uranium miners. *Br. J. Ind. Med.*, **50**, 920-928

Lees, R.E., Steele, R. & Roberts, J.H. (1987) A case–control study of lung cancer relative to domestic radon exposure. *Int. J. Epidemiol.*, **16**, 7-12

Létourneau, E.G., Krewski, D., Choi, N.W., Goddard, M.J., McGregor, R.G., Zielinski, J.M. & Du, J. (1994) Case–control study of residential radon and lung cancer in Winnipeg, Manitoba, Canada. *Am. J. Epidemiol.*, **140**, 310-322

Lo, Y.M., Darby, S., Noakes, L., Whitley, E., Silcocks, P.B., Fleming, K.A. & Bell, J.I. (1995) Screening for codon 249 *p53* mutation in lung cancer associated with domestic radon exposure [letter]. *Lancet*, **345**, 60

Lubin, J.H. & Gail, M.H. (1990) On power and sample size for studying features of the relative odds of disease. *Am. J. Epidemiol.*, **131**, 552-566

Lubin, J.H., Samet, J.M. & Weinberg, C. (1990) Design issues in epidemiologic studies of indoor exposure to Rn and risk of lung cancer. *Health Phys.*, **59**, 807-817

Lubin, J.H., Liang, Z., Hrubec, Z., Pershagen, G., Schoenberg, J.B., Blot, W.J., Klotz, J.B., Xu, Z.Y. & Boice, J.D. (1994a) Radon exposure in residences and lung cancer among women: combined analysis of three studies. *Cancer Causes Control*, **5**, 114-128

Lubin, J.H, Boice, J.D., Jr, Hornung, R.W., Edling, C., Howe, G., Kunz, E., Kusiak, R.A., Morrison, H.I., Radford, E.P., Samet, J.M., Tirmarche, M., Woodward, A., Xiang, Y.S. & Pierce, D.A. (1994b) *Lung Cancer and Radon: A Joint Analysis of 11 Underground Miners Studies* (NIH Publication No 94-3644), Washington, DC, US Department of Health and Human Services

Lubin, J.H., Boice, J.D., Jr., Edling, C., Hornung, R.W., Howe, G.R., Kunz, E., Kusiak, R.A., Morrison, H.I., Radford, E.P., Samet, J.M. et al., (1995a) Lung cancer in radon-exposed miners and estimation of risk from indoor exposure. *J. Natl Cancer Inst.*, **87**, 817-827

Lubin, J.H., Boice, J.D., Jr & Samet, J.M. (1995b) Errors in exposure assessment, statistical power and the interpretation of residential radon studies. *Radiat. Res.*,**144**, 329-341

Lubin, J.H., Boice, J.D., Jr., Edling, C., Hornung, R.W., Howe, G., Kunz, E., Kusiak, R.A., Morrison, H.I., Radford, E.P., Samet, J.M. & et al., (1995c) Radon-exposed underground miners and inverse dose-rate (protraction enhancement) effects. *Health Phys.*, **69**, 494-500

Luebeck, E.G., Curtis, S.B., Cross, F.T. & Moolgavkar, S.H. (1996) Two-stage model of radon-induced malignant tumors in rats: Effects of cell killing. *Radiat. Res.*, **145**,163-173

Lundin, F.E., Wagoner, J.K. & Archer, V.E. (1971) *Radon Daughter Exposure and Respiratory Cancer: Quantitative and Temporal Aspects* (Joint Monograph 1), Springfield, VA, National Institute of Occupational Safety and Health and National Institute of Environmental Health Science

McDonald, J.W., Taylor, J.A., Watson, M.A., Saccomanno, G. & Devereux, T.R. (1995) *p53* and K-*ras* in radon-associated lung adenocarcinoma. *Cancer Epidemiol. Biomarkers Prev.*, **4**, 791-793

McLaughlin, J.P. (1986) *Exposure to Natural Radiation in Dwellings of the European Communities (EURATOM Treaty)*, Brussels, Commission of the European Communities

Mifune, M., Sobue, T., Arimoto, H., Komoto, Y., Kondo, S. & Tanooka, H. (1992) Cancer mortality survey in a spa area (Misasa, Japan) with a high radon background. *Jpn. J. Cancer Res.*, **83**, 1-5

Minna, J.D. (1993) The molecular biology of lung cancer pathogenesis. *Chest,* **103**, 449-456

Moolgavkar, S.H. & Knudson, A.G. (1981) Mutation and cancer: a model for human carcinogenesis. *J. Natl Cancer Inst.*, **66**, 1037-1052

Moolgavkar, S.H. & Luebeck, E.G. (1990) Two-event model for carcinogenesis: biological, mathematical and statistical considerations. *Risk Anal.*, **10**, 323-341

Moolgavkar, S.H., Dewanji, A. & Luebeck, G. (1989) Cigarette smoking and lung cancer: reanalysis of the British Doctors' Data. *J. Natl Cancer Inst.*, **81**, 415-420

Moolgavkar, S.H., Cross, F.T., Luebeck, G. & Dayle, G.E. (1990) A two-mutation model for radon-induced lung tumours in rats. *Radiat. Res.*, **131**, 28-37

Moolgavkar, S.H., Luebeck, E.G., Krewski, D. & Zielinski, J.M. (1993) Radon, cigarette smoke and lung cancer: a reanalysis of the Colorado plateau uranium miners' data. *Epidemiology*, **4**, 204-217

Morrison, H.I., Semenciv, R.M., Mao, Y. & Wigle, D.T. (1988) Cancer mortality among a group of fluorspar miners exposed to radon progeny. *Am. J. Epidemiol.*, **128**, 1266-1275

National Council on Radiation Protection and Measurements (1984) *Evaluation of Occupational and Environmental Exposures to Radon and Radon Daughters in the United States* (NCRP-Report No. 78), Washington, DC

Neuberger, J.S. (1991) Residential radon exposure and lung cancer: an overview of published studies. *Cancer Detect. Prev.*, **15**, 435-443

Pershagen, G., Akerblom G., Axelson, O., Clavensjo, B., Damber, L., Desai, G., Enflo, A., Lagarde, F., Mellander, H., Svartengren, M. *et al.*, (1994) Residential radon exposure and lung cancer in Sweden. *New Engl. J. Med.*, **330**, 159-164

Pershagen, G., Liang, Z.H., Hrubec, Z., Svensson, C. & Boice, J.D. (1992) Residential radon exposure and lung cancer in Swedish women. *Health Phys.*, **63**, 179-186

Piantadosi, S., Byar, D. & Green, S. (1988) The ecological fallacy. *Am. J. Epidemiol.*, **127**, 893-904

Radford, E.P. & St Clair Renard, K.G. (1984) Lung cancer in Swedish miners exposed to low doses of radon daughters. *New Engl. J. Med.*, **310**, 1485-1994

Roscoe, R.J., Steenland, K., Halperin, W.E., Beaumont, J.J. & Waxweiler, R.J. (1989) Lung cancer mortality among nonsmoking uranium miners exposed to radon daughters. *J. Am. Med. Assoc.*, **262**, 629-633

Roscoe, R.J., Deddens, J.A., Salvan, A. & Schnorr, T.M. (1995) Mortality among Navajo uranium miners. *Am. J. Public Health*, **85**, 535-540

Rossi, H.H. & Kellerer, A.M. (1986) The dose rate dependence of oncogenic transformation by neutrons may be due to variation in response during the cell cycle. *Int. J. Radiat. Biol.*, **50**, 353-361

Saccomanno, G., Auerbach, O., Kuschner, M., Harley, N.H., Michels, R.Y., Anderson, M.W. & Bechtel, J.J. (1996) A comparison between the localization of lung tumors in uranium miners and in nonminers from 1947 to 1991. *Cancer*, **77**, 1278-1283

Samet, J.M., Pathak, D.R., Morgan, M.V., Key, C.R., Valdivia, A.A. & Lubin, J.H. (1991a) Lung cancer mortality and exposure to Rn progeny in a cohort of New Mexico underground U miners. *Health Phys.*, **61**, 745-752

Samet, J.M., Stolwijk, J. & Rose, S.L. (1991b) Summary: International Workshop on residential Rn epidemiology. *Health Phys.*, **60**, 223-227

Schoenberg, J.B, Klotz, J.B., Wilcox, H.B, Nicholls, G.P., Gil-del-Real, M.T., Stemhagen, A. & Mason, T.J. (1990) Case–control study of residential radon and lung cancer among New Jersey women. *Cancer Res.*, **50**, 6250-6254

Sevc , J., Kunz, E., Tomasek, L., Plack, V. & Horacek, J. (1988) Cancer in man after exposure to Rn daughters. *Health Phys.*, **54**, 27-46

Simpson, S.G. & Comstock, G.W. (1983) Lung cancer and housing characteristics. *Arch. Environ. Health*, **38**, 248-251

Steenland, K. (1994) Age specific interactions between smoking and radon among United States uranium miners. *Occup. Environ. Med.*, **51**, 192-194

Stidley, C.A. & Samet, J.M. (1993) A review of ecologic studies of lung cancer and indoor radon. *Health Phys.*, **65**, 234-251

Stidley, C.A. & Samet, J.M. (1994) Assessment of ecologic regression in the study of lung cancer and indoor radon. *Am. J. Epidemiol.*, **139**, 312-322

Stockwell, H.G., Lyman, G.H., Waltz, J. & Peters, J.T. (1988) Lung cancer in Florida. Risks associated with residence in the central Florida phosphate mining region. *Am. J. Epidemiol.*, **128**, 78-84

Stranden, E. (1986) Radon in Norwegian dwellings and the feasibility of epidemiological studies. *Radiat. Environ. Biophys.*, **25**, 37-42

Svensson, C., Eklund, G. & Pershagen, G. (1987) Indoor exposure to radon from the ground and bronchial cancer in women. *Int. Arch. Occup. Environ. Health*, **59**, 123-131

Svensson, C., Pershagen, G. & Klominek, J. (1989) Lung cancer in women and type of dwelling in relation to radon exposure. . *Cancer Res.* **49**, 1861-1865

Taylor, J.A., Watson, M.A., Devereux, T.R., Michels, R.Y., Saccomanno, G. & Anderson, M. (1994) *p53* mutation hotspot in radon-associated lung cancer. *Lancet*, **343**, 86-87

Thomas, D.C., McNeil, K.G. & Dougherty, C. (1985) Estimates of lifetime lung cancer risks resulting from Rn progeny exposures. *Health Phys.*, **49**, 825-846

Tirmarche, M. (1995) Radon and cancer risk: epidemiological studies after occupational or domestic exposure. *Rev. Epidemiol. Santé Publique*, **43**, 451-60

Tirmarche, M., Raphalen, A., Allin, F., Chameaud, J. & Bredon, P. (1993) Mortality of a cohort of French uranium miners exposed to relatively low radon concentrations. *Br. J. Cancer*, **67**, 1090-1097

Tomasek, L. & Darby, S.C. (1995) Recent results from the study of West Bohemian uranium miners exposed to radon and its progeny. *Environ. Health Perspect.*, **103**, Suppl. 2, 55-57

Tomasek, L., Darby, S.C., Fearn, T., Swerdlow, A.J., Placek, V. & Kunz, E. (1994a) Patterns of lung cancer mortality among uranium miners in West Bohemia with varying rates of exposure to radon and its progeny. *Radiat. Res.*, **137**, 251-261

Tomasek, L., Swerdlow, A.J., Darby, S.C., Placek, V. & Kunz, E. (1994b) Mortality in uranium miners in west Bohemia: a long-term cohort study. *Occup. Environ. Med.*, **51**, 308-315

United Nations Scientific Committee on the Effects of Atomic Radiation (1994) *Sources and Effects of Ionizing Radiation*, New York, NY, United Nations

US National Academy of Sciences (1991) *US NAS Panel on Dosimetric Assumptions Affecting the Application of Radon Risk Estimates*, Washington, DC, National Research Council

US National Academy of Sciences/National Research Council, Committee on the Biological Effects of Ionizing Radiations (1980) *The Effects on Populations of Exposure to Low Levels of Ionizing Radiation*, BEIR III, Washington, DC, National Academy Press

US National Academy of Sciences/National Research Council, Committee on the Biological Effects of Ionizing Radiations (1988) *Health Risks of Radon and Other Internally Deposited Alpha-Emitters*, BEIR IV, Washington, DC, National Academy Press

US National Academy of Sciences/National Research Council, Committee on the Biological Effects of Ionizing Radiations (1990) *Health Effects of Exposure to Low Levels of Ionizing Radiation*, BEIR V, Washington, DC, National Academy Press

US National Council on Radiation Protection and Measurements (1984) *Evaluation of Occupational and Environmental Exposures to Radon and Radon Daughters in the United States* (NCRP Report 78), Washington, DC

Vähäkangas, K.H., Samet, J.M., Metcalf, R.A., Welsh, J.A., Bennett, W.P., Lane, D.P. & Harris, C.C. (1992) Mutations of *p53* and *ras* genes in radon-associated lung cancer from uranium miners. *Lancet*, **339**, 576-580

Vonstille, W.T. & Sacarello, H.L.A. (1990) Radon and cancer. *J. Environ. Health*, **53**, 25-28

Whittemore, A.S. & McMillan, A. (1983) Lung cancer mortality among US uranium miners: a reappraisal. *J. Natl Cancer Inst.*, **71**, 489-499

Woodward, A., Roder, D., McMichael, A.J., Crouch, P. & Mylvaganam, A. (1991) Radon daughter exposures at the radium H:11 uranium mine and lung cancer rates among former workers, 1952–87. *Cancer Causes Control*, **2**, 213-220

Xuan, X.Z., Lubin, J.H., Li, J.Y., Young, L.F.L, Luo, Q.S., Yang, L., Wang, J.Z. & Blot, W.J. (1993) A cohort study in southern China of workers exposed to radon and radon decay products. *Health Phys.*, **64**, 120-131

References—aflatoxin

Adamson, R.H. & Sieber, S.M. (1983) Carcinogenesis studies in nohuman primates. In: Langenback, R. & Nesnow, S., eds, *Organ and Species Specificity in Chemical Carcinogenesis*, New York, NY, Plenum Press, pp. 129-156

Aguilar, F., Hussain, S.P. & Cerutti, P. (1993) Aflatoxin B1 induces the transversion of G→T in codon 249 of the *p53* tumor suppressor gene in human hepatocytes. *Proc. Natl Acad. Sci. USA*, **90**, 8586-8590

Aguilar, F., Harris, C.C., Sun, T., Hollstein, M. & Cerutti, P. (1994) Geographic variation of *p53* mutational profile in nonmalignant human liver. *Science*, **264**, 1317-1319

Alavanja, M.C.R., Malker, H. & Hayes, R.B. (1987) Occupational cancer risk associated with the storage and bulk handling of agricultural foodstuff. *J. Toxicol. Environ. Health*, **22**, 247-254

Allen, S.J., Wild, C.P., Wheeler, J.G., Riley, E.M., Montesano, R., Bennett, S., Whittle, H.C., Hall,

A.J. & Greenwood, B.M. (1992) Aflatoxin exposure, malaria, and hepatitis B infection in rural Gambian children. *Trans. R. Soc. Trop. Med. Hyg.*, **86**, 426-430

Alpert, M.E., Hutt, M.S.R., Wogan, G.N. & Davidson, C.S. (1971) Association between aflatoxin content of food and hepatoma frequency in Uganda. *Cancer*, **28**, 253-260

Angsubhakorn, S., Bharmarapravati, N., Romruen, K., Sahaphong, S., Thanmavit, W. & Miyamoto, M. (1981a) Further study of alpha benzene hexachloride inhibition of aflatoxin B1 hepatocarcinogenesis in rats. *Br. J. Cancer*, **43**, 881-883

Angsubhakorn, S., Bharmarapravati, N., Romruen, K. & Sahaphong, S. (1981b) Enhancing effects of dimethylnitrosamine on aflatoxin B1 hepatocarcinogenesis in rats. *Int. J. Cancer*, **28**, 621-626

Armstrong, B. (1980) The epidemiology of cancer in the People's Republic of China. *Int. J. Epidemiol.*, **9**, 305-315

Autrup, H., Seremet, T., Wakhisi, J. & Wasunna, A. (1987) Aflatoxin exposure measured by urinary excretion of aflatoxin B1–guanine adduct and hepatitis B virus infection in areas with different liver cancer incidence in Kenya. *Cancer Res.*, **47**, 3430-3433

Bannasch, P., Khoshkhou, N.I., Hacker, H.J., Radaeva, S., Mrozek, M., Zillmann, U., Kopp Schneider, A., Haberkorn, U., Elgas, M., Tolle, T., *et al.* (1995) Synergistic hepatocarcinogenic effect of hepadnaviral infection and dietary aflatoxin B1 in woodchucks. *Cancer Res.*, **55**, 3318-3330

Board, P., Coggan, M., Johnston, P., Ross, V., Suzuki, T. & Webb, G. (1990) Genetic heterogeneity of the human glutathione transferases: a complex of gene families. *Pharmacol. Ther.*, **48**, 357-369

Bowers, J., Brown, B., Springer, J., Tollefson, L., Lorentzen, R. & Henry, S. (1993). Risk assessment for aflatoxin: an evaluation based on the multistage model. *Risk Anal.*, **13**, 637-642

Bruce, R.D. (1990) Risk assessment for aflatoxin: II. Implications of human epidemiology data. *Risk Anal.*, **10**, 561-569

Buetler, T.M., Slone, D. & Eaton, D.L. (1992) Comparison of the aflatoxin B1–8,9 epoxide conjugating activities of two bacterially expressed alpha class glutathione S-transferase isoenzymes from mouse and rat. *Biochem. Biophys. Res. Commun.*, **188**, 597-603

Bulatao-Jayme, J., Almero, E.M., Castro, M.C.A., Jardeleza, M.T.R. & Salamat, L.A. (1982) A case–control dietary study of primary liver cancer risk from aflatoxin exposure. *Int. J. Epidemiol.*, **11**, 112-119

Busby, W.F. & Wogan, G.N. (1984) Aflatoxins. In: Searle, C.D., ed., *Chemical Carcinogens* (ACS Monograph No. 182), Washington, DC, American Chemical Society, pp. 945-1136

Butler, W.H. & Hempsall, V. (1981) Histochemical studies of hepatocellular carcinomas in the rat induced by aflatoxin. *J. Pathol.*, **134**, 157-170

Butler, W.H., Greenblut, M. & Lijinsky, W. (1969) Carcinogenesis in rats by aflatoxins B_1, G_1 and B_2. *Cancer Res.*, **29**, 2206-2211

California Department of Health Services (1990) *DRAFT Risk Specific Intake Levels for Aflatoxin (March) Presented to the Proposition 65 Scientific Advisory Panel*, Sacramento, CA, University of California at Davis

California Department of Health Services (1991) *Risk Specific Intake Levels for Aflatoxin*, Berkeley, CA, CDHS Reproductive and Cancer Hazard Assessment Section

Campbell, T.C., Chen, J., Liu, C., Li, J. & Parpia, B. (1990) Nonassociation of aflatoxin with primary liver cancer in a cross-sectional ecological survey in the People's Republic of China. *Cancer Res.*, **50**, 6882-6893

Campbell, A.D., Whitaker, T.D., Pohland, A.E., Dickens, J.W. & Park, D.L. (1986) Sampling, sample preparation, and sampling plans for foodstuffs for mycotoxin analysis. *Pure Appl. Chem.*, **58**, 305-314

Carlborg, F.W. (1979) Cancer, mathematical models, and aflatoxin. *Food Cosmet. Toxicol.*, **17**, 169-166

Challen, C., Lunec, J., Warren, W., Collier, J. & Bassendine, M.F. (1992) Analysis of the *p53* tumor suppressor gene in hepatocellular carcinomas from Britain. *Hepatology*, **16**, 1362-1366

Chemin, I., Takahashi, S., Belloc, C., Lang, M.A., Ando, K., Guidotti, L.G., Chisari, F. & Wild, C.P. (1996) Differential induction of carcinogen metabolising enzymes in a transgenic mouse model of fulminant hepatitis. *Hepatology*, **24**, 649-656

Chen, C.J.,Wang, L.Y., Lu, S.N., Wu, M.H., You, S.L., Zhang, Y.J., Wang, L.W. & Santella R.M. (1996a) Elevated aflatoxin exposure and increased risk of hepatocellular carcinoma. *Hepatology*, **24**, 38-42

Chen, C.J., Yu, M.W., Liaw, Y.F., Wang, L.W., Chiamprasert, S., Matin, F., Hirvonen, A., Bell, D.A. & Santella, R.M. (1996b) Chronic hepatitis B carriers with null genotypes of glutathione S-transferase M1 and T1 polymorphisms who are exposed to aflatoxin are at increased risk of hepatocellular carcinoma. *Am. J. Hum. Genet.*, **59**, 128-134

Choy, W.N. (1993) A review of the dose–response induction of DNA adducts by aflatoxin B1 and its implications to quantitative cancer-risk assessment. *Mutat. Res.*, **296**, 181-198

Cornfield, J. (1977) Carcinogenic risk assessment, *Science*, **198**, 693

Coursaget, P., Depril, N., Chabaud, M., Nandi, R., Mayelo, V., Lecann, P. & Yvonnet, B. (1993) High prevalence of mutations at codon 249 of the *p53* gene in hepatocellular carcinomas from Senegal. *Br. J. Cancer*, **67**, 1395-1397

Cova, L., Wild, C.P., Mehrotra, R., Turusov, V., Shirai, T., Lambert, V., Jacquet, C., Tomatis, L., Trepo, C. & Montesano, R. (1990) Contribution of aflatoxin B1 and hepatitis B virus infection in the induction of liver tumours in ducks. *Cancer Res.*, **50**, 2156-2163

Croy, R.G. & Crouch, E.A.C. (1991) Interaction of aflatoxin and hepatitis B virus as carcinogens in human populations. In: Bray, G.A. & Ryan, D.H., eds, *Mycotoxins, Cancer and Health* (Pennington Nutrition Series Vol. 1), Baton Rouge, LA, Louisiana State University Press, pp. 87-100

Cullen, J.M., Ruebner, B.H., Hsieh, L.S., Hyde, D.M. & Hsieh, D.P. (1987) Carcinogenicity of dietary aflatoxin M_1 in male Fischer rats compared to aflatoxin B_1. *Cancer Res.*, **47**, 1913-1917

Cullen, J.M., Marion, P.L., Sherman, G.J., Hong, X. & Newbold, J.E. (1990) Hepatic neoplasms in aflatoxin B1–treated, congenital duck hepatitis B virus-infected, and virus-free Pekin ducks. *Cancer Res.*, **50**, 4072-4080

Debuire, B., Paterlini, P., Pontisso, P., Basso, G. & May, E. (1993) Analysis of the *p53* gene in European hepatocellular carcinomas and hepatoblastomas. *Oncogene*, **8**, 2303-2306

De Flora, S., Romano, M., Basso, C., Serra, D., Astengo, M. & Picciotto, A. (1985) Metabolic activation of hepatocarcinogens in chronic hepatitis B. *Mutat. Res.*, **144**, 213-219

De Flora, S., Hietanen, E., Bartsch, H., Camoirano, A., Izzotti, A., Bagnasco, M. & Millman, I. (1989) Enhanced metabolic activation of chemical hepatocarcinogens in woodchucks infected with hepatitis B virus. *Carcinogenesis*, **10**, 1099-1106

Dichter, C,R, (1984) Risk estimates of liver cancer due to aflatoxin exposure from peanuts and peanut products. *Food Chem. Toxicol.*, **22**, 431-437

Epstein, S.M., Bartus, B. & Farber, E. (1969) Renal epithelial neoplasms induced in male Wistar rats by oral aflatoxin B^1. *Cancer Res.*, **29**, 1045-1050

Fujimoto, Y., Hampton, L.L., Luo, L.D., Wirth, P.J., & Thorgeirsson, S.S. (1992) Low frequency of *p53* gene mutation in tumors induced by aflatoxin B1 in nonhuman primates. *Cancer Res.* **52**, 1044-1046

Fujimoto, Y., Hampton, L.L., Wirth, P.J., Wang,N.J., Xie, J.P. & Thorgeirsson, S.S. (1994)

Alterations of tumor suppressor genes and allelic losses in human hepatocellular carcinomas in China. *Cancer Res.*, **54**, 281-285

Gallagher. E.P., Wienkers, L.C., Stapleton, P.L. & Eaton, D.L. (1994) Role of human microsomal and human complementary DNA-expressed cytochromes P4501A2 and P4503A4 in the bioactivation of aflatoxin B1. *Cancer Res.*, **54**, 101-108

Gan, L.S., Skipper, P.L., Peng, X., Groopman, J.D., Chen, J.-S., Wogan, G.N. & Tannenbaum, S.R. (1988) Serum albumin adducts in the molecular epidemiology of aflatoxin carcinogenesis: correlation with aflatoxin B1 intake and urinary excretion of aflatoxin M1. *Carcinogenesis*, **9**, 1323-1325

Geubel, A.P., Pauwels, S., Buchet, J.P., Dumont, E. & Dive, C. (1987) Increased cyt P-450 dependent function in healthy HBsAg carriers. *Pharmacol. Ther.*, **33**, 193-196

Gold, L.S. & Zeiger, E., eds (1997) *Handbook of Carcinogenic Potency and Genotoxicity Databases*, Boca Raton, FL, CRC Press

Griciute, L. (1980) Investigation on the combined action of N-nitrosodiethylamine with other carcinogens. In: Walker, E.A., Griciute, L., Castegnaro, M. & Börzsönyi, M., eds, N-*Nitroso Compounds: Analysis, Formation and Occurrence* (IARC Scientific Publications No. 31), Lyon, International Agency for Research on Cancer, pp. 813-822

Groopman, J.D., Zhu, J., Donahue, P.R., Pikul, A., Zhang, L., Chen, J.S. & Wogan, G.N. (1992) Molecular dosimetry of urinary aflatoxin–DNA adducts in people living in Guangxi Autonomous Region, People's Republic of China. *Cancer Res.*, **52**, 45-52

Groopman, J.D., Wild, C.P., Hasler, J., Chen, J., Wogan, G.N. & Kensler, T.W. (1993) Molecular epidemiology of aflatoxin exposures: validation of aflatoxin-N7-guanine levels in urine as a biomarker in experimental rat models and humans. *Environ. Health Perspect.*, **99**, 107-13

Hall, A.J. & Wild, C.P. (1994) The epidemiology of aflatoxin related disease. In: Eaton, D.L. & Groopman, J.D., eds, *The Toxicology of Aflatoxins:*

Human Health, Veterinary and Agricultural Significance, San Diego, CA, J.D. Academic Press, pp. 233-258

Hatch, M.C., Chen, C.J., Levin, B.T., Yang, G.Y., Hsu, S.W., Wang, L.W., Hsieh, L.L. & Santella, R.M. (1993) Urinary aflatoxin levels, hepatitis-B virus infection and hepatocellular carcinoma in Taiwan. *Int. J. Cancer*, **54**, 931-934

Hayes, J.D., Judah, D.J., McLellan, L.I., Kerr, L.A., Peacock, S.D. & Neal, G.E. (1991) Ethoxyquin-induced resistance to aflatoxin B1 in the rat is associated with the expression of a novel alpha-class glutathione S-transferase sub-unit, Yc2, which possesses high catalytic activity for aflatoxin B_1-8,9-epoxide. *Biochem. J.*, **279**, 385-398

Hayes, J.D., Judah, D.J. & Neal, G.E. (1993) Resistance to aflatoxin B1 associated with the expression of a novel aldo-keto reductase which has catalytic activity towards a cytotoxic aldehyde-containing metobolite of the toxin. *Cancer Res.*, **53**, 3887-3894

Hayes, J.D., Nguyen, T., Judah, D.J., Petersson, D.G. & Neal, G.E. (1994) Cloning of cDNAs from fetal rat liver encoding glutathione S-transferase Yc polypeptides. The Yc2 subunit is expressed in adult rat liver resistant to the hepatocarcinogen aflatoxin B1. *J. Bio. Chem.*, **269**, 20707-20717

Hollstein, M.C., Sidransky, D., Vogelstein, B. & Harris, C.C. (1991) *p53* Mutations in human cancers. *Science*, **253**, 49-53

Hoover, S.M., Zeise, L., Pease, W.S., Lee, L.E., Henning, M.P. Weiss, L.B. & Cranor, C. (1995) Improving the regulation of carcinogens by expediting cancer potency estimation. *Risk Anal.*, **15**, 267-280

Hoseyni, M.S. (1990) *Aflatoxin Risk Assessment. Attachment in Comment on the California Department of Health Services Draft Aflatoxins Document. Submitted by the Aflatoxins Task Force of the Proposition 65 Committee*, Washington, DC, International Life Sciences Institute–Nutrition Foundation

Hoseyni, M.S. (1992) Risk assessment for aflatoxin: III. Modeling the relative risk of hepatocellular carcinoma. *Risk Anal.*, **12**, 123-126

International Agency for Research on Cancer (1993) *IARC Monographs on the Evaluation of Carcinogenic Risks to Humans*, Vol. 56, *Some Naturally Occurring Substances: Food Items and Constituents, Heterocyclic Aromatic Amines and Mycotoxins*, Lyon

International Agency for Research on Cancer (1994) *IARC Monographs on the Evaluation of Carcinogenic Risks to Humans*, Vol. 59, *Hepatitis Viruses*, Lyon

Izzotti, A., Scatolini, L., Lewtas, J., Walsh, D. & De Flora, S. (1995) Enhanced levels of DNA adducts in the liver of woodchucks infected with hepatitis virus. *Chem. Biol. Inter.*, **97**, 273-285

Keen, P. & Martin, P. (1971) Is aflatoxin carcinogen in man? The evidence in Swaziland. *Trop. Geogr. Med.*, **23**, 44-53

Kirby, G.M., Wolf, C.R., Neal, G.E., Judah, D.J., Henderson, C.J., Srivaranakul, P. & Wild, C.P. (1993) *In vitro* metabolism of aflatoxin Ba by normal and tumorous liver tissue from Thailand. *Carcinogenesis*, **14**, 2613-2620

Kirby, G.M., Chemin, I., Montesano, R., Chisari, F.V., Lang, M.A. & Wild, C.P. (1994) Induction of specific cytochrome P450s involved in aflatoxin B1 metabolism in hepatitis B virus transgenic mice. *Mol. Carcinog.*, **11**, 74-80

Lam, K.C., Yu, M.C., Leung, J.W.C. & Henderson B.E. (1982) Hepatitis B virus and cigarette smoking: risk factors for hepatocellular carcinoma in Hong Kong. *Cancer Res.*, **42**, 5246-5248

Li, J., Lin, B., Li, G., *et al.* (1979) *Atlas of Cancer Mortality in the People's Republic of China*, Shanghai, China Map Press, pp. 39-46

Li, D., Cao, Y., He, L., Wang, N.J. & Gu, J.R. (1993) Aberrations of *p53* gene in human hepatocellular carcinoma from China. *Carcinogenesis*, **14**, 169-173

Liu, Y.H., Taylor, J., Linko, P., Lucier, G.W. & Thompson, C.L. (1991) Glutathione S-transferase mu in human lymphocyte and liver: role in modulating formation of carcinogen-derived DNA adducts. *Carcinogenesis*, **12**, 2269-2275

London, W.T., Evans, A.A., McGlynn, K., Buetow, K., An, P., Gao, L.L., Lustbader, E., Ross, E., Chen, G.C. & Shen, F.M. (1995). Viral, host and environmental risk factors for hepatocellular carcinoma: A prospective study in Haimen City, China. *Intervirology*, **38**, 155-161

Lutwick, L.I. (1979) Relation between aflatoxin, hepatitis-B virus, and hepatocellular carcinoma. *Lancet*, **1**, 755-757

McGlynn, K.A., Rosvold, E.A., Lustbader. E.D., Hu, Y., Clapper, M.L., Zhou, T., Wild C.P., Xia, X.L., Baffoe Bonnie, A., Ofori Adjei, D., *et al.* (1995) Susceptibility to hepatocellular carcinoma is associated with genetic variation in the enzymatic detoxification of aflatoxin B1. *Proc. Natl Acad. Sci. USA*, **92**, 2384-2387

Merkow, L.P., Epstein, S.M., Slifkin, M. & Pardo, M. (1973) The ultrastructure of renal neoplasms induced by aflatoxin B1. *Cancer Res.*, **33**, 1608-1614

Moore, M.R., Pitot, H.C., Miller, E.C. & Miller, J.A. (1982) Cholangiocellular carcinoma incidence in Syrian hamsters administered aflatoxin B1 in large doses. *J. Natl Cancer Inst.*, **68**, 271-278

Newberne, P.M. & Rogers, A.W. (1973) Rat colon carcinomas associated with aflatoxin and marginal vitamin A. *J. Natl Cancer Inst.*, **50**, 439-444

Ng, I.O.L., Chung, L.P., Tsang, S.W.Y., Lam, C.L., Lai, E.C.S., Fan, S.T. & Ng, M. (1994) *p53* gene mutation spectrum in hepatocellular carcinomas in Hong Kong Chinese. *Oncogene*, **9**, 985-990

Nixon, J.E., Hendricks, J.D., Pawlowski, N.E., Loveland, P.M. & Sinnhuber, R.O. (1981) Carcinogenicity of aflatoxin in Fischer 344 rats. *J. Natl Cancer Inst.*, **66**, 1159-1163

Olsen, J.H., Dragsted, L. & Autrup, H. (1988) Cancer risk and occupational exposure to aflatoxins in Denmark. *Br. J. Cancer*, **58**, 392-396

Olubuyide, I.O., Maxwell, S.M., Hood, H., Neal, G.E. & Hendrickse R.G. (1993) HBsAg, aflatoxin and primary hepatocellular carcinoma. *Afr. J. Med. Med. Sci.*, **22**, 89-91

Parkin, D.M., Srivatanakul, P., Khlat, M., Chenvidhya, D., Choticoan, P., Insiripong, S., L'Abbe, K.A. & Wild, C.P. (1991) A case–control study of cholangiocarcinoma. *Int. J. Cancer*, **48**, 323-326

Parkin, D.M., Muir, C.S., Whelan, S.L., Gao, T.-T., Ferlay, J. & Powell, J., eds (1992) *Cancer Incidence in Five Continents*, Vol. VI (IARC Scientific Publications No. 120), Lyon, International Agency for Research on Cancer

Peers, F.G. & Linsell, C.A. (1973) Dietary aflatoxins and liver cancer—a population based study in Kenya. *Br. J. Cancer*, **27**, 473-484

Peers, F.G. & Linsell, C.A. (1977) Dietary aflatoxins and human primary liver cancer. *Ann. Nutr. Aliment.* **31**, 1005-1018

Peers, F.G., Gilman, G.A. & Linsell C.A. (1976) Dietary aflatoxins and human liver cancer. A study in Swaziland. *Int. J. Cancer*, **17**, 167-176

Peers, F., Bosch, X., Kaldor, J., Linsell, A. & Pluijmen, M. (1987) Aflatoxin exposure, hepatitis B virus infection and liver cancer in Swaziland. *Int. J. Cancer*, **39**, 545-553

Puisieux, A., Lim, S., Groopman, J. & Ozturk, M. (1991) Selective targeting of *p53* mutational hotspots in human cancers by etiologically defined carcinogens. *Cancer Res.*, **51**, 6185-6189

Qian, G.S., Ross, R.K., Yu, M.C., Yuan, J.M., Gao, Y.T., Henderson, B.E. Wogen, G.N. & Groopman, J.D. (1994) A follow-up study of urinary markers of aflatoxin exposure and liver cancer risk in Shanghai, People's Republic of China. *Cancer Epidemiol. Biomarkers Prev.*, **3**, 3-10

Ramsdell, H.S. & Eaton, D.L. (1990) Mouse liver glutathione S-transferase isoenzyme activity toward aflatoxin B1-8,9-epoxide and benzo[*a*]pyrene-7,8-dihydrodiol-9,10-epoxide. *Toxicol. Appl. Pharmacol.*, **105**, 216-225

Raney, K.D., Meyer, D.J., Ketterer, B., Harris, T.M. & Guengerich, F.P. (1992a) Glutathione conjugation of aflatoxin B1 exo- and endo-epoxides by rat and human glutathione S-transferases. *Chem. Res. Toxicol.*, **5**, 470-478

Raney, K.D., Coles, R., Guengerich, F.P. & Harris, T.P. (1992b) The endo-8 9-epoxide of aflatoxin B-1. A new metabolite. *Chem. Res. Toxicol.*, **5**, 333-335

Reddy, J.K., Svoboda, D.J. & Rao, M.S. (1976) Induction of liver tumours by aflatoxin B1 in the tree shrew (*Tupaia glis*), a nonhuman primate. *Cancer Res.*, **36**, 151-160

Richard, J.L. (1991) Mycotoxins as immunomodulators in animal systems. In: Bray, G.A. & Ryan, D., eds, *Mycotoxins, Cancer and Health*, Baton Rouge, LA, Louisiana State University Press, pp. 197-220

Ross, R.K., Yuan, J.-M., Yu, M.C., Wogan, G.N., Qian, G.-S., Tu, J.-T., Groopman, J.D., Gao, Y.-T. & Henderson, B.E. (1992) Urinary aflatoxin biomarkers and risk of hepatocellular carcinoma. *Lancet*, **339**, 943-946

Sandler, D.P., Sandler, R.S. & Horney, L.F. (1983). Primary liver cancer mortality in the United States. *J. Chronic Dis.*, **36**, 227-236

Scholl, P., Musser, S.M., Kensler T.W. & Groopman J.D. (1995) Molecular biomarkers for aflatoxins and their application to human liver cancer. *Pharmacogenetics*, **5**, S171-S176

Sell, S., Hunt, J.M., Dunsford, H.A. & Chisari, F.V. (1991) Synergy between hepatitis B virus expression and chemical hepatocarcinogenesis in transgenic mice. *Cancer Res.*, **51**, 1278-1285

Shank, R.C., Gordon, J.E., Wogan, G.N., Nondasuta, A. & Subhamani, B. (1972a) Dietary aflatoxins and human liver cancer. III. Field survey of rural Thai families for ingested aflatoxins. *Food Cosmet. Toxicol.*, **10**, 71-84

Shank, R.C., Bhamarapravati, N., Gordon, J.E. & Wogan, G.N. (1972b) Dietary aflatoxins and human liver cancer. IV. Incidence of primary liver cancer in two municipal populations of Thailand. *Food Cosmet. Toxicol.*, **10**, 171-179

Sieber, S.M., Correa, P., Dalgard, D.W. & Adamson, R.H. (1979) Induction of osteogenic sarcomas and tumours of the hepatobiliary system in human primates with aflatoxin B_1. *Cancer Res.*, **39**, 4545-4554

Srivatanakul, P., Parkin, D.M., Jiang, Y.-Z., Khlat, M., Kao-Ian, U.-T., Sontipong, S. & Wild, C. (1991a) The role of infection by *Opisthorchis viverrini*, hepatitis B virus, and aflatoxin exposure in the etiology of liver cancer in Thailand. A correlation study. *Cancer*, **68**, 2411-2417

Srivatanakul, P., Parkin, D.M., Khlat, M., Chenvidhya, D., Chotiwan, P., Insiripong, S., L'Abbé, K.A. & Wild, C.P. (1991b) Liver cancer in Thailand. II. A case–control study of hepatocellular carcinoma. *Int. J. Cancer*, **48**, 329-332

Stoloff, L. (1983) Aflatoxin as a cause of primary liver-cell cancer in the United States: a probability study. *Nutr. Cancer*, **5**, 165-186

Stoner, G.D., Conran, P.B., Greisiger, E.A., Stober, J., Morgan, M. & Pereira, M.A. (1986) Comparison of two routes of chemical administration on the lung adenoma response in strain A/J mice. *Toxicol. Appl. Pharmacol.*, **82**, 19-31

Tennant, B.C., Hornbuckle, W.E., Yeager, A.E., Baldwin, B.H., Sherman, W.K., Anderson, W.I., Steinberg, H., Cote, P.J., Korba, B.E. & Gerin, J.L. (1991) Effects of aflatoxin B1 on experimental woodchuck hepatitis virus infection and hepatocellular carcinoma. In: Hollinger, F.B., Lemon, S.M. & Margolis, H., eds, *Viral Hepatitis and Liver Disease*, Baltimore, MD, Williams & Wilkins, pp. 599-600

Thomas, D. (1990) Discussion of risk assessments: aflatoxin. In: *Proceedings of the Meeting of the Safe*

Drinking Water and Toxic Enforcement Act of 1986 Scientific Advisory Panel (Capitol Reports), Sacramento, CA, University of California at Davis

Thorslund, T.W., Brown, C.C. & Charnley, G. (1987). Biologically motivated cancer risk models. *Risk Anal.*, **7**, 109-119

Uchida, T., Suzuki, K., Esumi, M., Arii, M. & Shikata T. (1988) Influence of aflatoxin B1 intoxication on duck livers with duck hepatitis B virus infection. *Cancer Res.*, **48**, 1559-1565

US Food and Drug Administration (1978) *Assessment of Estimated Risk Resulting from Aflatoxins in Consumer Peanut Products and Other Food Commodities*, Washington, DC, Bureau of Foods

van Egmond, H.P., ed. (1989) *Mycotoxins in Dairy Products*, Amsterdam, Elsevier

van Rensburg, S.J., van der Watt, J.J., Purchase, I.F.H, Pereira Coutinho, L. & Markham, R. (1974) *S. Afr. Med. J.*, **48**, 2508a-2508d

van Rensburg, S.J., Cook-Mozaffari, P., van Schalkwyk, D.J., van der Watt, J.J., Vincent, T.J. & Purchase, I.F. (1985) Hepatocellular carcinoma and dietary aflatoxin in Mozambique and Transkei. *Br. J. Cancer*, **51**, 713-726

van Rensburg, S.J., van Schalkwyk, G.C. & van Schalkwyk, D.J. (1990) Primary liver cancer and aflatoxin intake in Transkei. *J. Environ. Pathol. Toxicol. Oncol.*, **10**, 11-16

Vesselinovitch, S.D., Mihailovich, N., Wogan, G.N., Lombard, L.S. & Rao, K.V.N. (1972) Aflatoxin B1, a hepatocarcinogen in the infant mouse. *Cancer Res.*, **32**, 2289-2291

Wang, L.Y., Hatch, M., Chen, C.J., Levin, B., You, S.L., Lu, S.N.,Wu, M.H., Wu, W.P., Wang, L.W., Wang, Q., Huang, G.T., Yang, P.M., Lee, H.S. & Santella, R.M. (1996a) Aflatoxin exposure and risk of hepatocellular carcinoma in Taiwan. *Int. J. Cancer*, **67**, 620-625

Wang, J.S., Qian, G.S., Zarba, A., He, A., Zhu, Y.R., Zhang, B.C. Jacobson, L,. Grange, S.J., Munoz, A.,

Kensler, T.W. & Groopman, J.D. (1996b) Temporal patterns of aflatoxin–albumin adducts in hepatitis B surface antigen-positive and antigen-negative residents of Daxin, Qidong County, People's Republic of China. *Cancer Epidemiol. Biomarkers. Prev.*, **5**, 253-261

Ward, J.M., Sontag, J.M., Weisburger, E.K. & Brown, C.A. (1975) Effect of lifetime exposure to aflatoxin B1 in rats. *J. Natl Cancer Inst.*, **55**, 107-110

Whitaker, T.B. & Park, D.L. (1994) Problems associated with accurately measuring aflatoxin in food and feeds: errors associated with sampling, sample preparation and analysis. In: Eaton, D.A. & Groopman, J.D., eds, *The Toxicology of Aflatoxins: Human Health, Veterinary and Agricultural Significance*, San Diego, CA, Academic Press, pp. 433-450

Wieder, R., Wogan, G.N. & Shimkin, M.A. (1968) Pulmonary tumours in strain A mice given injections of aflatoxin B1. *J. Natl Cancer Inst.*, **40**, 1195-1197

Wild, C.P. & Montesano, R. (1991) Detection of alkylated DNA adducts in human tissues. In: Groopman, J.D. & Skipper, P.L. eds., *Molecular Dosimetry and Human Cancer: Analytical, Epidemiological and Social Considerations*, Boca Raton, FL, CRC Press, pp. 263-280

Wild, C.P., Hudson, G.J., Sabbioni, G., Chapot, B., Hall, A.J., Wogan, G.N., Whittle, H., Montesano, R. & Groopman, J.D. (1992) Dietary intake of aflatoxins and the level of albumin-bound aflatoxin in peripheral blood in The Gambia, West Africa. *Cancer Epidemiol. Biomarkers Prev.*, **1**, 229-34

Wild, C.P., Fortuin, M., Donato, F., Whittle, H.C., Hall, A.J., Wolf, C.R. & Montesano, R. (1993a) Aflatoxin, liver enzymes and hepatitis B virus infection in Gambian children. *Cancer Epidemiol. Biomarkers Prev.*, **2**, 555-61

Wild, C.P., Jansen, L.M., Cova, L. & Montesano, R. (1993b) Molecular dosimetry of aflatoxin exposure: contribution to understanding the multifactorial aetiopathogenesis of primary hepatocellular carcinoma (PHC) with particular reference to hepatitis B virus. *Environ. Health Perspect.*, **99**, 115-122

Wild, C.P., Hasegawa, R., Barraud, L., Chutimataewin, S., Chapot, B., Ito, N. & Montesano, R. (1996) Aflatoxin–albumin adducts: a basis for comparative carcinogenesis between animals and humans. *Cancer Epidemiol. Biomarkers. Prev.*, **5**, 179-189

Wogan, G.N., Palianlunga, S. & Newberne, P.M. (1974) Carcinogenic effects of low dietary levels of aflatoxin B1 in rats. *Food Cosmet. Toxicol.*, **12**, 681-685

Wood, W.E. (1989) Aflatoxins in domestic and imported foods and feeds. *J. Assoc. Off. Anal. Chem.*, **72**, 543-548

Wu-Williams, A.H., Zeise, L. & Thomas, D. (1992) Risk assessment for aflatoxin B_1: a modeling approach. *Risk Anal.*, **12**, 559-567

Yan, R.Q., Su, J.J., Huang, D.R., Gan, Y.C., Yang, C. & Huang, G.H. (1996). Human hepatitis B virus and hepatocellular carcinoma. II. Experimental induction of hepatocellular carcinoma in tree shrews exposed to hepatitis B virus and aflatoxin B1. *J. Can. Res. Clin. Oncol.*, **122**(5), 289-295

Yaobin, W., Lizun, L., Benfa, Y., Yaochu, X., Yunyuan, L. & Wenguang, L. (1983) Relation between geographical distribution of liver cancer and climate–aflatoxin B1 in China. *Sci. Sin. (B)*, **26**, 1166-1175

Yeh, F.-S., Mo, C.-C. & Yen, R.-C. (1985) Risk factors for hepatocellular carcinoma in Guangxi, People's Republic of China. *Natl Cancer Inst. Monogr.*, **69**, 47-48

Yeh, F.-S., Yu, M.C., Mo, C.-C., Luo, S., Tong, M.J. & Henderson B.E. (1989) Hepatitis B virus, aflatoxins, and hepatocellular carcinoma in southern Guangxi, China. *Cancer Res.*, **49**, 2506-2509

Yu, S.Z. (1992) Aflatoxins and liver cancer in Guangxi, China. *Chin. J. Prev. Med.*, **26**(3), 162-164

Yu, S-Z. (1995) Primary prevention of hepatocellular carcinoma. *J. Gastroenterol. Hepatol.*, **10**, 674-682

Yu, M.W., Lien, J.P., Liaw, Y.F., Chen, C.J. (1996) Effects of multiple risk factors for hepatocellular carcinoma on formation of aflatoxin B1–DNA adducts. *Cancer Epidemiol. Biomarkers Prev.*, **5**, 613-619

Zhang, M.D. (1992) Aflatoxins and primary liver cancer—a population based case–control study. *Chin. J. Prev. Med.*, **26**(6), 331-333

References—TCDD

Abraham, K., Krowke, R. & Neubert, D. (1988) Pharmacokinetics and biological activity of 2,3,7,8-tetrachlorodibenzo-*p*-dioxin. *Arch. Toxicol.*, **62**, 359-368

Abraham, K., Wiesmuller, T., Brunner, H., Krowke, R., Hagenmeier, H. & Neubert, D. (1989) Absorption and tissue distribution of various polychlorinated dibenzo-*p*-dioxins and dibenzofurans (PCDDs and PCDFs) in the rat. *Arch. Toxicol.*, **63**, 193-202

Andersen, E.L. & the US Environmental Protection Agency Carcinogen Assessment Group (1983) Quantitative approaches in use to assess cancer risk. *Risk Anal.*, **3**, 277-295

Anderson, M.E., Mills, J.J., Gargas, M.L., Kedderis, L., Birnbaum, L.S., Neubert, D. & Greenlee, W.F. (1993) Modeling receptor-mediated processes with dioxin: implications for pharmacokinetics and risk assessment. *Risk Anal.*, **13**, 25-35

Ashby. J. & Tennant, R.W. (1988) Chemical structure, Salmonella mutagenicity and extent of carcinogenicity as indicators of genotoxic carcinogenesis among 222 chemicals tested in rodents by the US NCI/ NTP. *Mutat. Res.*, **204**, 17-115

Becher, H., Flesch-Janys, D., Kauppinen, T., Kogevinas, M., Steindorf, K., Manz, A. & Wahrendorf, J. (1996) Cancer mortality in German male workers exposed to phenoxy herbicides and dioxins. *Cancer Causes Control*, **7**, 312-321

Beebe, L., Park, S.S. & Anderson, L.M. (1990) Differential enzyme induction of mouse liver and lung following a single low or high dose of 2,3,7,8-tetrachlordibenzo-*p*-dioxin (TCDD). *J. Biochem. Toxicol.*, **5**, 211-219

Beebe, L.E., Fornwald, L.W., Diwan, B.A., Anver, M.R., Anderson, L.M. (1995) Promotion of *N*-nitrosodiethylamine-initiated hepatocellular tumors and hepatoblastomas by 2,3,7,8-tetrachlorodibenzo-*p*-dioxin or Aroclor 1254 in C57BL/6, DBA/2, and B6D2F1 mice. *Cancer Res.*, **55**, 4875-4880

Berry, D.L., DiGiovanni, J., Juchau, M.R., Bracken, W.M., Gleason, G.L. & Slaga, T.J. (1978) Lack of tumour-promoting ability of certain environmental chemicals in a two-stage mouse skin tumorigenesis assay. *Res. Commun. Chem. Pathol. Pharmacol.*, **20**, 101-107

Bertazzi, P. A., Pesatori, A.C., Consonni, D., Tironi, A., Landi, M.T., & Zoccheti, C. (1993) Cancer incidence in a population accidentally exposed to 2,3,7,8-tetrachlorodibenzo-*para*-dioxin. *Epidemiology*, **4**, 398-406.

Bombick, D.W., Jankun, J., Tullis, K. & Matsumara, F. (1988) 2,3,7,8-Tetrachlordibenzo-*p*-dioxin causes increases in expression of c-*erb*-A and levels of protein–tyrosine kinases in selected tissues of responsive mouse strains. *Proc. Natl Acad. Sci. USA*, **85**, 4128-4132

Bowman, R.E., Schantz, S.L., Werasinghe, N.C.A., Gross, M.L. & Barsoti, D.A. (1988) Chronic dietary intake of 2,3,7,8-tetra-chlorodibenzo-*p*-dioxin (TCDD) at 5 or 25 parts per trillion in the monkey: TCDD kinetics and dose effect estimate of reproductive toxicity. *Chemosphere*, **18**, 243-252

Brewster, D.W., Banks, Y.B., Clark, A.M. & Birnbaum, L.S. (1989) Comparative polychlorinated dibenzofurans. *Toxicol. Appl. Pharmacol.*, **97**, 156-166

Brown, W.R. (1991) Implications of the reexamination of the liver sections from the TCDD chronic rat bioassay. In: Gallo, M.A., Scheuplein, R.J. & van der Heijden, C.A., eds, *Biological Basis for Risk Assessment of Dioxins and Related Compounds* (Banbury Report 35), Cold Spring Harbor, NY, CSH Press, pp. 13-26

Buchmann, A., Ziegler, S., Wolf, A., Robertson, L.W., Durham, S.K. & Schwarz, M. (1991) Effects of polyhalogenated biphenyls in rat liver: correlation between primary subcellular effects and promoting activity. *Toxicol. Appl. Pharmacol.*, **111**, 454-468

Buchmann, A., Stinchcombe, S., Koerner, W., Hagenmaier, H.P., & Bock, K.W. (1994) Effects of 2,3,7,8-tetrachloro- and 1,2,3,4,6,7,8-heptachlorodibenzo-*p*-dioxin on the proliferation of preneoplastic liver cells in the rat. *Carcinogenesis*, **15**, 1143-1150.

Burbach, K.M., Poland, A. & Bradfield, C.A. (1992) Cloning of the Ah-receptor reveals a distinctive ligand-activated transcription factor. *Proc. Natl Acad. Sci. USA*, **89**, 8185- 8189

Byard, J.L. (1987) The toxicological significance of 2,3,7,8-tetrachlorodibenzo-*p*-dioxin and related compounds in human adipose tissue. *J. Toxicol. Environ. Health*, **22**, 61-83

California Department of Health Services (1986) *Health Effects of Chlorinated Dioxins and Dibenzofurans*, Berkeley, CA

Choi, E.J. Toscano, J.A. Tyan, N., Riedel, W.A. & Toscano, W.A. (1991) Dioxin induces transforming growth factor-alpha in human keratinocytes. *J. Biol. Chem.*, **266**, 9591-9597

Clark, G., Tritscher, A., Maronpot, R., Foley, J. & Lucier, G. (1991) Tumour promotion by TCDD in female rats. In: Gallo, M.A., Scheuplein, R.J. & van der Heijden, C.A., eds, *Biological Basis for Risk Assessment of Dioxins and Related Compounds* (Banbury Report 35), Cold Spring Harbor, NY, CSH Press, pp. 389-404

Collins, J.J., Strauss, M.E., Levinskas, G.J., & Conner, P.R. (1993) The mortality experience of workers exposed to 2,3,7,8-tetrachlorodibenzo-*p*-dioxin in a trichlorophenol process accident. *Epidemiology*, **4**, 8-13

Cuthill, S., Poellinger, L. & Gustafsson, J.-A. (1987) The receptor for 2,3,7,8-tetrachlordibenzo-*p*-dioxin in the mouse hepatoma cell line Hepa 1c1c7. A comparison with the glucocorticoid receptor and the mouse and rat hepatic dioxin receptors. *J. Biol. Chem.*, **262**, 3477-3481

Della Porta, G., Dragani, T.A. & Sozzi, G. (1987) Carcinogenic effects of infantile and long term 2,3,7,8-tetrachlorodibenzo-*p*-dioxin treatment in the mouse. *Tumori*, **73**, 99-107

Deml, E., Wiebel, F.J. & Oesterle, D. (1989) Biological activity of 2,4,8-trichlorodibenzofuran: promotion of rat liver foci and induction of cytochrome P-450-dependent monooxygenases. *Toxicology*, **59**, 229-238

Denison, M.S., Fischer, J.M., Whitlock, J.P. (1988) The DNA recognition site for the dioxin-Ah receptor complex: nucleotide sequence and functional analysis. *J.Biol.Chem.*, **263**, 17221-17224

Dragan, Y.P., Xu, X., Goldsworthy, T.L., Campbell, H.A., Maronpot, R.R. & Pitot, H.C. (1992) Characterisation of the promotion of altered hepatic foci by 2,3,7,8-tetrachlorodibenzo-*p*-dioxin in the female rat. *Carcinogenesis*, **13**, 1389-1395

Elferink, C.J. & Whitlock, J.P., Jr (1990) 2,3,7,8-Tetrachlordibenzo-*p*-dioxin-inducible, Ah receptor-mediated bending of enhancer DNA. *J. Biol. Chem.*, **265**, 5718-5721

Enan, E., & Matsumura, F.(1996) Identification of c-Src as the integral component of the cytosolic Ah receptor complex, transducing the signal of 2,3,7,8-tetrachlordibenzo-*p*-dioxin (TCDD) through the protein phosphorylation pathway. *Biochem. Pharmacol.*, **52**, 1599-1612.

Favreau, L.V. & Pickett, C.B. (1991) Transcriptional regulation of the rat NAD(P)H:quinone reductase gene. Identification of regulatory elements controlling basal level expression and inducible expression by planar aromatic compounds and phenolic antioxidants. *J. Biol. Chem.*, **266**, 4556-4561

Fingerhut, M.A., Halperin, W.E., Marlow, D.A., Piacitelli, L.A., Honchar, P.A., Sweeney, M.H., Greife, A.L., Dill, P.A., Steenland, K. & Suruda, A.J.

(1991) Cancer mortality in workers exposed to 2,3,7,8-tetrachlorodibenzo-*p*-dioxin. *New Engl. J. Med.*, **324**, 212-218

Fisher, J.M., Wu, L., Denison, M.S. & Whitlock, J.P., Jr (1990) Organization and function of a dioxin-responsive enhancer. *J. Biol. Chem.*, **265**, 9676-9681

Flodström, S.L. & Ahlborg, U.G. (1989) Tumour promoting effects of 2,3,7,8-tetrachlorodibenzo-*p*-dioxin (TCDD)—effects of exposure duration, administration schedule and type of diet. *Chemosphere*, **19**, 779-783

Flodström, S.L., Busk, L., Kronevi & Ahlborg, U.G. (1991) Modulation of 2,3,7,8-tetrachlorodibenzo-*p*-dioxin and phenobarbital-induced promotion of hepatocarcinogenesis in rats by the type of diet and vitamin A deficiency. *Fundam. Appl. Toxicol.*, **16**, 375-391

Fujisawa-Sehara, A., Sogawa, K., Yamane, M. & Fujii-Kuriyama, Y. (1987) Characterisation of xenobiotic responsive elements upstream from the drug-metabolising cytochrome P-450c gene: a similarity to glucocorticoid regulatory elements. *Nucleic Acids Res.*, **15**, 4179-4191

Gonzalez, F.J. & Nebert, D.W. (1985) Autoregulation plus upstream positive and negative control regions associated with transcriptional activation of the mouse cytochrome P1-450 gene. *Nucleic Acids Res.*, **13**, 7269-7288

Greenlee, W.F., Anderson, M.E. & Lucier, G.W. (1991) A perspective on biologically based approaches to dioxin risk assessment. *Risk Anal.*, **11**, 565-568

Hagenmaier, H., Wiesmuller, T., Golor, G., Krowke, R., Helge, H. & Neubert, D. (1990) Transfer of various polychlorinated dibenzo-*p*-dioxins and dibenzofurans (PCDDs and PCKFs) via placenta and through milk in a marmoset monkey. *Arch. Toxicol.*, **64**, 601-615

Hapgood, J., Cuthill, S., Denis, M., Poellinger, L. & Gustafsson, J.-A. (1989) Specific protein-DNA interactions at a xenobiotic-responsive element: copurification of dioxin receptor and DNA-binding activity. *Proc. Natl Acad. Sci. USA*, **86**, 60-64

Hardell, L. (1981) Relation of soft-tissue sarcoma, malignant lymphoma and colon cancer to phenoxy acids, chlorophenols and other agents. *Scand. J. Work Environ. Health*, **7**, 119-130

Hardell, L. & Sandström, A. (1979) Case–control study: soft-tissue sarcomas and exposure to phenoxyacetic acids or chlorophenols. *Br. J. Cancer*, **39**(6), 711-717

Hardell, L., Eriksson, M., Lenner, P. & Lundgren, E. (1981) Malignant lymphoma and exposure to chemicals, especially organic solvents, chlorophenols and phenoxy acids: a case–control study. *Br. J. Cancer*, **269**, 169-176

Huff, J.E., Salmon, A.G., Hooper, N.K. & Zeise, L. (1991) Long-term carcinogenesis studies on 2,3,7,8-tetrachlorodibenzo-*p*-dioxin and hexachlorodibenzo-*p*-dioxins. *Cell Biol. Toxicol.*, **7**, 67-94

International Agency for Research on Cancer (1987a) *IARC Monographs on the Evaluation of Carcinogenic Risks to Humans*, Suppl. 7, *Overall Evaluations of Carcinogenicity: An Updating of IARC Monographs Volumes 1 to 42*, Lyon, pp. 350-354

International Agency for Research on Cancer (1987b) *IARC Monographs on the Evaluation of Carcinogenic Risks to Humans*, Suppl. 6, *Genetic and Related Effects: An Updating of Selected IARC Monographs from Volumes 1 to 42*, Lyon, pp. 508-510

Johnson, E.S. (1992) Human exposure to 2,3,7,8-TCDD and risk of cancer. *Crit. Rev. Toxicol.*, **21**, 451-463

Kedderis, L., Diliberto, J., Linko, P., Goldstein, J. & Birnbaum, L. (1991) Disposition of 2,3,7,8-tetrabromodibenzo-*p*-dioxin and 2,3,7,8-tetrachlorodibenzo-*p*-dioxin in the rat: biliary excretion and induction of cytochromes CYP1A1 and CYP1A2. *Toxicol. Appl. Pharmacol.*, **11**, 163-172

Kimborough, R.D. (1984) The epidemiology and toxicology of TCDD. *Bull. Environ. Contam. Toxicol.*, **33**, 636-647

Knutson, J.C. & Poland, A. (1982) Response of murine epidermis to 2,3,7,8-tetrachlorodibenzo-p-dioxin: interaction of the Ah and hr locus. *Cell*, 30, 225-234

Kociba, R. (1991) Rodent bioassays for assessing chronic toxicity and carcinogenic potential of TCDD. In: Gallo, M.A., Scheuplein, R.J. & van der Heijden, C.A., eds, *Biological Basis for Risk Assessment of Dioxins and Related Compounds* (Banbury Report 35), Cold Spring Harbor, NY, CSH Press, pp. 3-11

Kociba, R.J., Keyes, D.G., Beyer, J.E., Carreon, R.M., Wade, D.A., Dittenberger, D.A., Kalnins, R.P., Frauson, L.E., Park, C.N., Bernard, S.D., Hummel, R.A. & Humiston, C.G. (1978) Results of a two-year chronic toxicity and oncogenicity study of 2,3,7,8-tetrachlorodibenzo-p-dioxin in rats. *Toxicol. Appl. Pharmacol.*, 46, 279-303

Kociba, R.J., Keyes, D..G., Beyer, J.E. & Carreon, R.M. (1979) Toxicologic studies of 2,3,7,8- tetrachlorodibenzo-p-dioxin in rats. In: Deichman, W.B., ed., *Toxicology and Occupational Medicine*, New York, NY, Elsevier, pp. 281-287

Kohn, M., Lucier, G., Clark, G., Sewall, C., Tritscher, A. & Portier, C. (1993) A mechanistic model of the effects of dioxin on gene expression in rat liver. *Toxicol. Appl. Pharmacol.*, 120, 138-154

Krowke, R. (1986) Studies on distribution and embyrotoxicity of different PCDD and PCDF in mice and marmosets. *Chemosphere*, 15, 2011-2022

Leung, H.W., Murray, F.J. & Paustenbach, D.J. (1988) A proposed occupational exposure limit for 2,3,7,8-tetrachlorodibenzo-p-dioxin. *Am. Ind. Hyg. Assoc. J.*, 49, 466-474

Lilienfeld, D. & Gallo, M.A. (1989) 2,4-D, 2,4,5-T, and 2,3,7,8-TCDD: an overview. *Epidemiol. Rev.*, 11, 28-58

Lin, F.H., Birnbaum, L.S., Lucier, G.W. & Goldstein, J.A. (1991) Influence of the Ah locus on the effects of 2,3,7,8-tetrachlorodibenzo-p-dioxin on the hepatic epidermal growth factor receptor. *Mol. Pharmacol.*, 39, 307-313

Lubet, R.A., Nims, R.W., Ward, J.M., Rice, J.M. & Diwan, B.A. (1989) Induction of cytochrome P450b and its relationship to liver tumour promotion. *J. Am. Coll. Toxicol.*, 8, 259-268

Lucier, G.W. (1992) Receptor-mediated carcinogenesis. In: Vainio, H., Magee, P.N., McGregor, D.B. & McMichael, A.J., eds, *Mechanisms of Carcinogenesis in Risk Identification* (IARC Scientific Publications No. 116), Lyon, International Agency for Research on Cancer, pp. 87-112

Lucier, G.W., Tritscher, A., Goldsworthy, T., Foley, J., Clark, G., Goldstein, J. & Maronpot, R. (1991) Ovarian hormones enhance 2,3,7,8-tetrachlorodibenzo-p-dioxin-mediated increases in cell proliferation and preneoplastic foci in a two-stage model for rat hepatocarcinogenesis. *Cancer Res.*, 51, 1391-1397

Lucier, G.W., Portier, C.J. & Gallo, M.A. (1993) Receptor mechanisms and dose response models for the effects of dioxins. *Environ. Health Perspect.*, 101, 36-44

Lundgren, K., Andries, M., Thompson, C. & Lucier, G.W. (1986) Dioxin treatment of rats results in increased *in vitro* induction of sister chromatid exchanges by alpha-naphthoflavone: an animal model for exposure to halogenated aromatics. *Toxicol. Appl. Pharmacol.*, 85, 189-195

Lundgren, K., Collman, G.W., Wu-Wang, S., Tiernan, T., Taylor, M., Thompson, C.L. & Lucier, G.W. (1988) Cytogenetic and chemical detection of human exposure to polyhalogenated aromatic hydrocarbons. *Environ. Mol. Mutag.*, 11, 1-11

Manz, A., Berger, J., Dwyer, J.H., Flesch-Janys, D., Nagel, S. & Waltsgott, H. (1991) Cancer mortality among workers in chemical plant contaminated with dioxin. *Lancet*, 338, 959-964

Maronpot, R.R., Montgomery, C.A., Boorman, G.A. & McConnell, E.E. (1986) National Toxicology Program nomenclature for hepatoproliferative lesions of rats. *Toxicol. Pathol.*, 14, 263-273

Matsumura, F., Brewster, D.W., Madhukar, B.V. & Bombick, D.W. (1984) Alteration of rat hepatic plasma membrane functions by 2,3,7,8-tetrachlordibenzo-*p*-dioxin (TCDD). *Arch. Environ. Contam. Toxicol.*, **13**, 509-515

Moolgavkar, S. & Luebeck, G. (1990) Two event model for carcinogenesis: biological, mathematical, and statistical considerations. *Risk Anal.*, **10**, 323-341

Moolgavkar, S.H., Luebeck, E.G., Buchmann, A. & Bock, K.W. (1996) Quantitative analysis of enzyme-altered liver foci in rats initiated with diethylnitrosamine and promoted with 2,3,7,8-tetrachlorodibenzo-*p*-dioxin or 1,2,3,4,6,7,8-heptachlorodibenzo-*p*-dioxin. *Toxicol. Appl. Pharmacol.*, **138**, 509-515

Nebert, D.W. & Jones, J.E. (1989) Regulation of the mammalian cytochrome P1450 (CYP1A1) gene. *Int. J. Biochem.*, **21**, 243-252

Neubert, R., Wiesmuller, T., Abraham, K., Krowke, R. & Hagenmaier, H. (1990) Persistence of various polychlorinated dibenzo-*p*-dioxins and dibenzofurans (PCDDs and PCDFs) in hepatic and adipose tissue of marmoset monkeys. *Arch. Toxicol.*, **64**, 431-442

Neubert, D., Abraham, K., Golor, G., Krowke, R., Kruger, N., Nagao, T., Neubert, R., Schulz-Schalge, T., Stahlmann, R., Wiesmuller, T. & Hagenmaier, H. (1991) Comparison of the effects of PCDDs and PCDFs on different species taking kinetic variables into account. In: Gallo, M.A., Scheuplein, R.J. & van der Heijden, C.A., eds, *Biological Basis for Risk Assessment of Dioxins and Related Compounds* (Banbury Report 35), Cold Spring Harbor, NY, CSH Press, pp. 27-49

Neuhold, L.A., Shirayoshi, Y., Ozato, K., Jones, J.E. & Nebert, D.W. (1989) Regulation of mouse CYP1A1 gene expression by dioxin: requirement of two cis-acting elements during induction. *Mol. Cell. Biol.*, **9**, 2378-2386

Nims, R.W., Devor, D.E., Hennemann, J.R. & Lubet, R.A. (1987) Induction of alkoxyresorufin O-dealkylases, epoxide hydrolase, and liver weight gain: correlation with liver tumour promoting potential in a series of barbiturates. *Carcinogenesis*, **8**, 67-71

Park, J.Y., Shigenaga, M.K. & Ames, B.N. (1996) Induction of cytochrome P4501A1 by 2,3,7,8-tetrachlorodibenzo-*p*-dioxin or indolo(3,2-b) carbazole is associated with oxidative DNA damage. *Proc. Natl Acad. Sci. USA*, **93**, 2322-2327

Paustenbach, D.J., Layard, M.W., Wenning, R.J. & Keenan, R.E. (1991) Risk assessment of 2,3,7,8-TCDD using a biologically based cancer model: a reevaluation of the Kociba *et al.* bioassay using 1978 and 1990 histopathology criteria. *J. Toxicol. Environ. Health*, **34**, 11-26

Peto, R. (1991) Occupational exposure to chlorophenoxy herbicides and chlorophenols. *Lancet*, **388**, 1392.

Pitot, H.C., Goldsworthy, T., Campbell, H.A & Poland, A. (1980) Quantitative evaluation of the promotion by 2,3,7,8-tetrachlorodibenzo-*p*-dioxin of hepatocarcinogenesis by diethylnitrosamine. *Cancer Res.*, **40**, 3616-3620

Pitot, H.C., Goldsworthy, T.L., Moran, S., Kennan, W., Glauert, H.P., Maronpot, R.R. & Campbell, H.A. (1987). A method to quantitate the relative initiating and promoting potencies of hepatocarcinogenic agents in their dose–response relationships to altered hepatic foci. *Carcinogenesis*, **8**, 1491-1499

Poiger, H. & Schlatter, C. (1986) Pharmacokinetics of 2,3,7,8-TCDD in man. *Chemosphere*, **15**, 1489-1494

Poland, A. & Knutson, J. (1982) 2,3,7,8-Tetrachlordibenzo-*p*-dioxin and related halogenated aromatic hydrocarbons: examination of the mechanism of toxicity. *Ann. Rev. Pharmacol. Toxicol.*, **22**, 517-554

Poland, A., Palen, D. & Glover, E. (1982) Tumour promotion by TCDD in skin of HRS/J hairless mice. *Nature*, **300**, 271-273 oland, A., Teitelbaum, P. & Glover, E. (1989) 125Ia2-Iodo-3,7,8-trichlorodibenzo-p-dioxin binding species in mouse liver induced by agonists for the Ah receptor: characterisation and identification. *Mol. Pharmacol.*, **36**, 113-120

Poland, A., Glover, E. & Bradfield, C.A. (1991) Characterisation of polyclonal antibodies to the Ah receptor prepared by immunization with a synthetic peptide hapten. *Mol. Pharmacol.*, **39**, 20-26

Portier, C.J., Hoel, D.G. & Van Ryzin, J. (1984) Statistical analysis of the carcinogenesis bioassay data relating to the risks from exposure to 2,3,7,8-tetrachlorodibenzo-p-dioxin. In: Lowrence, W.W., ed., *Public Health Risks of the Dioxins*, Los Altos, CA, William Kaufmann, pp. 99-119

Portier, C.J., Tritscher, A., Kohn, M., Sewell, C., Clark, G., Edler, L., Hoel, D. & Lucier, G. (1993) Ligand/receptor binding for 2,3,7,8-TCDD: implications for risk assessment. *Fundam. Appl. Toxicol.*, **20**, 48-56

Portier, C.J, Sherman, C., Kohn, M., Edler, L., Kopp-Schneider, A., Maronpot, R.M. & Lucier, G. (1996) Modeling the number and size of hepatic focal lesions following exposure to 2,3,7,8-TCDD. *Toxicol. Appl. Pharmacol.*, **138**, 20-30

Rao, M.S., Subbarao, V., Prasad, J.D. & Scarpelli, D.G. (1988) Carcinogenicity of 2,3,7,8-tetrachlorodibenzo-p-dioxin in the Syrian golden hamster. *Carcinogenesis*, **9**, 1677-1679

Reyes, H., Reisz-Porszasz, S. & Hankinson, O. (1992) Identification of the Ah receptor nuclear translocation protein (Arnt) as a component of the DNA binding form of the Ah receptor. *Science*, **256**, 1193-1195

Rushmore, T.H., King, R.G., Paulson, K.E. & Pickett, C.B. (1990) Regulation of glutathione S-transferase Ya sub-unit gene expression: identification of a unique xenobiotic-responsive element controlling inducible expression by planar aromatic compounds. *Proc. Natl Acad. Sci. USA*, **87**, 3826-3830

Safe, S.H. (1986) Comparative toxicology and mechanism of action of polychlorinated dibenzo-p-dioxins and dibenzofurans. *Ann. Rev. Pharmacol. Toxicol.*, **26**, 371-399

Saracci, R., Kogenivas, M., Bertazzi, P.A., Bueno-de-Mesquita, B.H., Coggon, D., Green, L.M., Kauppinen, T., L'Abbe, K.A., Littorin, M., Lynge, E. *et al.* (1991) Cancer mortality in workers exposed to chlorophenoxy herbicides and chlorophenols. *Lancet,* **338**(8774), 1027-1032

Sauer, R.M. (1990) *Pathology Working Group. 2,3,7,8,-Tetracholorodibenzo-p-dioxin in Sprague Dawley Rats*, Ivansville, MD, Pathco, Inc.

Schlatter, C. (1991) Data on kinetics of PCDDs and PCDFs as a prerequisite for human risk assessment. In: Gallo, M.A., Scheuplein, R.J. & van der Heijden, C.A., eds, *Biological Basis for Risk Assessment of Dioxins and Related Compounds* (Banbury Report 35), Cold Spring Harbor, NY, CSH Press, pp. 215-226

Schulte-Hermann, R. (1985) Tumour promotion in the liver. *Arch. Toxicol.*, **57**, 147-158

Shu, H.P., Paustenbach, D.J. & Murray, F.J. (1987) A critical evaluation of the use of mutagenesis, carcinogenesis and tumour promotion data in a cancer risk assessment of 2,3,7,8-tetrachlorodibenzo-p-dioxin. *Reg. Toxicol. Pharmacol.*, **7**, 57-58

Sielken, R.L. (1987) Quantitative cancer risk assessments for 2,3,7,8-tetrachlorodibenzo-p-dioxin (TCDD). *Food Chem. Toxicol.*, **25**, 257-267

Sloop, T.C. & Lucier, G.W. (1987) Dose dependent elevation of Ah receptor binding by TCDD in rat liver. *Toxicol. Appl. Pharmacol.*, **8**, 329-337

Stinchcombe, S., Buchmann, A., Bock, K.W. & Schwarz, M. (1995) Inhibition of apoptosis during 2,3,7,8-tetrachlorodibenzo-p-dioxin-mediated tumour promotion in rat liver. *Carcinogenesis*, **16**, 1271-1275.

Tanaka, N., Nettesheim, P., Gray, T., Nelson, K. & Barrett, J.C. (1989) 2,3,7,8-tetrachlorodibenzo-p-dioxin enhancement of N-methyl-N'-nitro-N nitrosoguanidine-induced transformation of rat tracheal epithelical cells in culture. *Cancer Res.*, **49**, 2703-2708

Toth, K. Somfai-relle, S., Sugar, J. & Bence, J. (1979) Carcinogenicity testing of herbicide 2,4,5-trichlorophenoxyethanol containing dioxin and of pure dioxin in Swiss mice. *Nature*, **278**, 548-549

Tritscher, A.M., Goldstein, J.A., Portier, C.J., McCoy, Z., Clark, G.C. & Lucier, G.W. (1992) Dose–response relationships for chronic exposure to 2,3,7,8-tetrachlorodibenzo-*p*-dioxin in a rat tumour promotion model: quantification and immunolocalization of CYP1A1 and CYP1A2 in the liver. *Cancer Res.*, **52**, 3436-3442

US Environmental Protection Agency (1985) *Health Assessment Document for Polychlorinated Dibenzo-*p-*dioxins* (EPA 600/8-84-014F), Washington, DC, Office of Health and Environmental Assessment

US Environmental Protection Agency (1988) *A Cancer Risk-Specific Dose Estimate for 2,3,7,8-TCDD (Review Draft)*, Washington, DC

US National Toxicology Program (1982a) *Bioassay of 2,3,7,8-Tetrachlorodibenzo-*p-*dioxin for Possible Carcinogencity (Gavage Study)* (Technical Report Series No. 209), Research Triangle Park, NC

US National Toxicology Program (1982b) *Bioassay of 2,3,7,8-Tetrachlorodibenzo-*p-*dioxin for Possible Carcinogenicity (Dermal Study)* (Technical Report Series No. 201; NTP 80-32; NIH Publ. No. 82-1757), Research Triangle Park, NC

Voorman, R. & Aust, S.D. (1989) TCDD (2,3,7,8 tetrachlorodibenzo-*p*-dioxin) is a tight binding inhibitor of cytochrome P450d. *J. Biochem. Toxicol.*, **4**, 105-109

Waern, F., Flodström, S., Busk, L., Kronevi, T., Nordgren, I. & Ahlborg, U.G. (1991) Relative liver tumour promoting activity and toxicity of some polychlorinated dibenzo-*p*-dioxin- and dibenzofuran congeners in female Sprague–Dawley rats. *Pharmacol. Toxicol.*, **69**, 450-458

Wassom, J.S., Huff, J.E. & Loprieno, N. (1977) A review of the genetic toxicology of chlorinated dibenzo-*p*-dioxins. *Mutat. Res.*, **47**, 141-160

Whitlock, J.P., Jr (1990) Genetic and molecular aspects of 2,3,7,8-tetrachlordibenzo-*p*-dioxin action. *Ann. Rev. Pharmacol. Toxicol.*, **30**, 251-277

Wu, L. & Whitlock, J.P., Jr (1993) Mechanism of dioxin action: receptor–enhancer interactions in intact cells. *Nucleic Acids Res.*, **21**, 119-125

Yang, J.-H., Thraves, P., Dritschilo, A. & Rhim, J.S. (1992) Neoplastic transformation of immortalised human keratinocytes by 2,3,7,8-tetrachlordibenzo-*p*-dioxin. *Cancer Res.*, **52**, 3478-3482

Zeise, L., Huff, J.E., Salmon, A.G. & Hooper, N.K. (1990) Human risks from 2,3,7,8-tetrachlorodibenzo-*p*-dioxin and hexachlorodibenzo-*p*-dioxins. *Adv. Mod. Environ. Toxicol.*, **17**, 293-342

Zober, A., Messerer, P. & Huber, P. (1990) Thirty-four-year mortality follow-up of BASF employees exposed to 2,3,7,8-TCDD after the 1953 accident. *Int. Arch. Occup. Environ. Health.* **62**(2), 139-157

Quantitative Estimation and Prediction of Human Cancer Risks
S. Moolgavkar, D. Krewski, L. Zeise, E. Cardis and H. Møller
IARC Scientific Publications No. 131
International Agency for Research on Cancer, Lyon, 1999

9: Future Perspectives, Unresolved Issues and Research Needs

Suresh Moolgavkar, Alistair Woodward, Dan Krewski, Elisabeth Cardis and Lauren Zeise

9.1 Introduction

In this volume, we have reviewed the scientific bases and the state of the art of quantitative estimation and prediction (QEP) of cancer risk. Improvements in the future will depend on improvements in the design of epidemiological and experimental studies, on the quality and detail of information collected in these studies, and on increased understanding of the biological mechanisms of carcinogenesis. In this chapter, we discuss some unresolved issues and research needs in cancer QEP.

Ideally, as we have discussed elsewhere, QEP should be based on appropriate epidemiological data. Because such data are rarely available, however, the risk of cancer in populations exposed to low levels of putative carcinogenic agents must often be inferred from experiments in which animals, usually rodents, are exposed to high concentrations of the agent of interest. The attendant problems of interspecies and low-dose extrapolation are among the most contentious scientific issues of the day. Even when epidemiological data are available, the problem of low-dose extrapolation often remains because, typically, these data are available on occupationally exposed cohorts which have been exposed to relatively high concentrations of the agent under investigation. Currently available approaches for addressing these issues have been discussed in detail in this volume. There is a growing consensus that, when mechanistic information is available, models that take it into account are preferable to empirical statistical models for use in prediction.

9.2 An example: the case of dioxin (TCDD)

The QEP for dioxin was discussed in some detail in Chapter 8. Dioxin is not typical of the compounds for which QEPs are required. More is known about the uptake, distribution in tissues, and biological mechanism of action of dioxin than about most other chemical agents for which QEP must be carried out. Epidemiological studies, both case–control and cohort, are available as well. The US Environmental Protection Agency is currently conducting a new QEP for dioxin in order to accommodate the new epidemiological and mechanistic information now available.

The early epidemiological data suggested a possible association between exposure to dioxin and soft-tissue sarcomas and lung cancer (see Chapter 8). There are serious problems, however, with the selection of controls in the case–control studies of the soft-tissue sarcomas; exposure assessment is a problem in both cohort and case–control studies, and there is no information on cigarette smoking in the cohort studies suggesting an increased risk of lung cancer. Little exposure–response information is available. In a recent monograph, the International Agency for Cancer Research (1997) concluded that the epidemiological data showed a stronger association between exposure to TCDD and all cancers than for cancer at any specific site. It also noted that such a finding was highly unusual for a carcinogen. Although the Agency classified TCDD as a category 1 carcinogen (i.e. TCDD is carcinogenic to humans), this classification was not based solely on epidemiological evidence, which was judged to be limited, but also on considerations of carcinogenicity in animals and biological mechanisms. The committee responsible for the monograph concerned did not conduct a QEP.

Experiments in rodents have consistently shown an increase in tumours of various sites, most notably the liver, in animals exposed to dioxin (Chapter 8). The old QEP (US Environmental Protection Agency, 1985) for dioxin was based on a study of rodent liver tumours conducted in 1978 (Kociba *et al.*, 1978). In a more recent re-examination of the pathology, the majority of tumours in this study were classified as liver nodules (Sauer, 1990), which are believed to be premalignant lesions. These tumours were treated as malignant in the original analysis (US Environmental Protection Agency, 1985). There is no information in the Kociba study (Kociba *et al.*, 1978) on the number and size distribution of intermediate foci, or on measures of cell proliferation.

More recently, quantitative analyses of early biological events in response to dioxin exposure have been undertaken. The dose–response curves for receptor binding and for induction of the cytochrome P-450 enzymes are consistent with linearity at low doses (Kohn *et al.*, 1993; Portier *et al.*, 1993). Unfortunately, there is no information on how these early events are related to fundamental cellular processes, such as cell proliferation, relevant to carcinogenesis. In the absence of any information on how the early dioxin-induced events are related to carcinogenesis, it is not clear how the quantitation of these events can be used in risk assessment. Thus, even with epidemiological studies and much information on the biological mechanism by which dioxin acts, there are crucial data gaps that preclude the use of these data in QEP. It is depressing to note that the current re-evaluation of dioxin QEP by the US Environmental Protection Agency will probably have to be substantially based on the old Kociba study. What kind of information is required to rectify this situation?

9.3 Future perspectives and research needs in epidemiology

We know now that the burden of cancer falls unequally on different populations and on different subgroups within the same population, and that genetic, environmental, and lifestyle factors are all important in determining risk. The central challenge of cancer epidemiology in the forseeable future is to quantify the contributions made by each of these factors to the burden of cancer in a population. Meeting this challenge will require progress in the design of studies to incorporate both genetic and environmental factors in epidemiological investigations; improvements in analytical techniques to address the problems posed by errors in measurement of exposure; and the development of biological markers of exposure to the agent of interest and of surrogate endpoints for the cancer under investigation.

9.3.1 Genetic and environmental factors in cancer epidemiology

Although it has been appreciated for some time, from both epidemiological and experimental studies, that genetics and environment interact in carcinogenesis (see, e.g. the discussions in Chapters 7 and 8 and below), the central focus of epidemiological investigations has not, until recently, been on this interaction. Conventional epidemiology was instead focused on the discovery of environmental and lifestyle factors involved in carcinogenesis. Genetic factors, if they were considered at all, were thrown in almost as an afterthought by way of a few questions regarding family history. Geneticists, on the other hand, developed the powerful statistical techniques of segregation and linkage analyses for the identification of major genes involved in disease. Environmental factors were not considered in these analyses. It appears clear now that, although the major cancer genes, such as the retinoblastoma gene and the gene for familial adenomatous polyposis, confer a huge risk on individuals who are unfortunate enough to inherit them (Moolgavkar & Luebeck, 1992a; Strong & Amos, 1996), these genes occur with low frequency and may therefore not contribute substantially to the burden of cancer in populations. Subtle gene–environment interactions, such as those engendered by polymorphisms in enzymes involved in metabolizing environmental carcinogens, are likely to be of greater importance in populations. Examples of such polymorphisms are discussed in Chapters 7 and 8 and below.

An example of great contemporary interest is provided by radiation-induced thyroid cancer, which illustrates nicely that both host (age at exposure, sex, genetic predisposition) and environmental factors play important roles in determining the risk of cancer following exposure to an environmental agent. Studies of atomic bomb survivors indicate that the risk of radiation, as measured by the excess relative risk (ERR), varies nearly 100-fold by age at exposure: ERR per Sv is 0.1 for those exposed as adults (above the age of

20) and 10.3 for those exposed as children (below the age of 10) (Thompson *et al.*, 1994). While this this difference in risk may be due to increased susceptibility of young tissue to radiation, a recent analysis (Kai *et al.*, 1997) of the incidence of three solid cancers (lung, stomach and colon) in the same cohort using the two-mutation clonal expansion model shows that increased susceptibility of young tissue need not be invoked to explain the high ERRs in those exposed as children. Comparison of risk estimates across populations of children exposed in different countries show great variability (Ron *et al.*, 1995), with the highest risk estimates in the population of Israeli children exposed for treatment of tinea capitis (Ron *et al.*, 1989). A study in the USA also indicates that children of Jewish origin have a higher risk of radiation-induced thyroid cancer than non-Jewish children (Perkel *et al.*, 1988).

The risk may be even higher than previously estimated for very young children: a very early and large increase in the incidence of thyroid cancer in children and young adults in Belarus, and later in the Ukraine and Russia (Kazakov *et al.*, 1992; Tronko *et al.*, 1994; Tsyb *et al.*, 1994; Stsjazhko *et al.*, 1995) has been reported following the Chernobyl accident. While, based on data from other exposed populations, an increase in thyroid cancer was anticipated in this population, the magnitude of the increase is striking, particularly in the Gomel region of Belarus, where the number of cases in children is more than 10 times higher than predicted (Cardis *et al.*, 1996). This discrepancy may, at least partly, be due to errors in dose estimates; it may also reflect an exceptional sensitivity of those who were very young at the time of the accident or a genetic predisposition, possibly related to ethnic background. Modifying effects of iodine deficiency in the affected area must also be considered. The identification of the combination of factors responsible for the high risk is the key to the accurate prediction of the future risk of thyroid cancer in other populations exposed to radiation.

It is clear that, in the future, epidemiological studies will need to cover both genetics and environmental epidemiology. Study designs for such investigations that involve combining population-based case–control studies and family studies have been proposed (Zhao & LeMarchand, 1992;

Whittemore & Gong, 1994; Liang & Pulver, 1996). Since the majority of families may not carry the disease gene, one concern is that these designs may be inefficient. In order to address this concern, multiphase sampling designs have been proposed (Whittemore, 1995; Whittemore & Halpern, 1997; Zhao *et al.*, 1997). A number of technical issues remain to be resolved, however (Zhao *et al.*, 1997).

9.3.2 Exposure/dose assessment

As discussed in detail in Chapter 4, errors in measurement of exposure and outcome can have substantial effects on the direction and shape of dose–response relationships. Measurement error can be minimized by careful selection and design of measurement instruments, and strict quality control in their use and in the processing and analysis of the measurement results. If not prevented, it can be controlled to some degree by the use of multiple measures of exposure and outcome, the adjustment of dose–response relationships for the effects of measurement error, and the control of covariates related to such error. While in some cases the application of these procedures may make the effects of measurement error negligible in QEP, this is probably rarely the case.

Statistical techniques have been developed to adjust for errors in measurement during analyses of epidemiological studies (Armstrong *et al.*, 1992; Carroll *et al.*, 1995). In epidemiological studies, both the "classical" and the "Berkson" error structure can occur. For example, exposure to radiation in a cohort of nuclear workers may be measured on an individual basis by means of film badges. The error structure in this case is most conveniently represented by the "classical" model or extensions of it. Explicitly, let X be the true value of the exposure of interest and W be the exposure measured with error (by the film badge). Then the simplest classical error model postulates that $W = X + U$. The classical model can be extended to include dependence of W on other covariates of interest. In particular, the error term U may depend upon the true value of the exposure (X), in which case the model is called an error calibration model (Carroll *et al.*, 1995).

In other situations, the Berkson error model may be more appropriate. For example, Constantino *et al.* (1995) describe a cohort of steel workers who were exposed to emissions from coke ovens. Average concentrations of the emissions were measured for topside, part-time topside and side oven work, and each worker was assigned an exposure based on the length of time worked in each job. In this case, the Berkson error structure is appropriate: $X = W + U$, with notation as above. In other situations, when exposures are reconstructed from complex job exposure matrices, the error structure may be neither classical nor Berksonian (Gilks & Richardson, 1992).

Whatever the error structure, if the likelihood of the data can be written down, it can be maximized, at least in theory, to yield estimates of the parameters. Unfortunately, it is seldom possible to maximize the likelihood directly because of formidable computational difficulties. Computer-intensive methods, such as Markov Chain Monte Carlo (MCMC) methods, are currently being intensively investigated to address this problem (see, e.g. the recent monograph edited by Gilks *et al.*, 1996).

9.3.3 Biomarkers of exposure and surrogate end-points

Complementary to the development of better statistical methods for addressing errors in measurement of exposure is that of methods for the direct measurement of internal dose (e.g. polychlorinated biphenyls in serum and adipose tissue, and salivary cotinine from tobacco smoke), and of better measurements of biologically relevant dose (e.g. DNA or protein adducts) and early markers of biological response (which may also be thought of as markers of cumulative exposure, e.g. specific locus mutations). Examples of protein adducts that have been looked at in human studies are haemoglobin adducts of ethylene oxide, 4-aminobiphenyl and *N*-nitroso compounds. Studies have shown that smokers have significantly higher levels of 4-amino-biphenyl–haemoglobin adducts than non-smokers. Measurable levels of these adducts have also been reported in non-smokers, however, possibly as a result of exposure to environmental tobacco smoke (Bryant *et al.*, 1987; Perera *et al.*, 1987). DNA adducts of aflatoxin have been detected in human urine (Groopman *et al.*, 1985), and DNA adducts have also been used as markers of exposure to aromatic compounds (Hemminki *et al.*,

1990). Specific mutations at the hypoxanthine guanine phosphoribosyl transferase (HPRT) and the glycophorin A loci have been looked at in human populations exposed to chemotherapeutic agents and radiation (Perera & Santella, 1993). Interpretation of studies using biological markers of exposure is complicated by the large intra- and interindividual variability that is observed. Additionally, the use of DNA or protein adducts is limited by the short exposure period that these adducts cover, and that of specific locus mutations by the fact that these can give essentially no information about dose rate or pattern of exposure. To evaluate these problems and their significance, it would be desirable to incorporate in large cohort studies the periodic collection of biological samples for recurrent measurement of exposure so as to obtain information on dose rate, pattern of exposure and, ultimately, cumulative exposure over some period of time. Other markers of exposure have been developed as well, and the field of molecular epidemiology is growing rapidly, offering the hope of eventually yielding accurate measures of exposure and of early biological response. The reader is referred to recent monographs (Hulka *et al.*, 1990; Schulte & Perera, 1993; Perera, 1996) for further details.

Because of the dual problems of the cancer latency period and the difficulty in detecting small increments in cancer risk associated with low exposures, increasing attention is being paid to the use of surrogate end-points. Since, by definition, these occur earlier than clinical cancer, and since they also (tend to) occur at higher frequency than the eventual cancer, their use as end-points affords a potential increase in both study efficiency and statistical power. Where early examples might have included preclinical macroscopic lesions (e.g. polyps of the large bowel or dysplastic naevi on the skin), there is now the opportunity to use specific (combinations of) mutations from among the rapidly increasing repertoire of mutations positively associated with human cancers. These mutations—particularly of tumour-suppressor genes and of proto-oncogenes—may accrue sequentially, as has been suggested for the mutations associated with colon cancer (Fearon & Vogelstein, 1990). Nevertheless, there is a general dearth of information about the prospective link between the occurrence of such mutations in non-neoplastic (or at least premalignant) tissue and the subsequent occurrence of tumours. Therefore, it is not yet possible to know the predictive significance of such mutations, whether measured in tissue from the target organ of interest or in other tissue (e.g. white blood cell DNA). Moreover, for valid statistical inferences, a potential surrogate end-point must satisfy certain fairly stringent criteria (Prentice, 1989).

Important information has recently been obtained on the activated *ras* oncogene, expressed as the elevated concentration of gene product in serum, measured in initially cancer-free pneumoconiosis patients, and followed subsequently to the development of lung cancer in some of these patients (Brandt-Rauf *et al.*, 1992). Also, there is an opportunity to obtain data from studies of cancer patients treated with cytotoxic drugs, by measuring mutations (and adducts and other cytogenetic events) induced by therapy, and then observing their predictive relationship to subsequent second primary cancers. An ongoing Nordic cohort study provides a further example: the follow-up of approximately 2000 occupationally exposed workers in whom cytogenetic abnormalities were documented at recruitment and then related to cancer incidence (Brogger *et al.*, 1990). This approach is being applied in Australia to a cohort of underground uranium miners (Woodward *et al.*, 1991), in whom the glycophorin-A and HPRT somatic mutations in peripheral blood cells have been measured, and who are now being followed to observe rates of cancer occurrence.

Both the potential and the limitations of this approach are illustrated by recent work on ultraviolet radiation (UVR)-related mutations in skin, and their relationship to skin cancer. Over the past 15 years, a number of epidemiological studies have been conducted around the world and have shown that exposure to sunlight (and, presumably, specifically to UVR) entails increased risks for the three main types of skin cancer (Armstrong & English, 1996; Scotto *et al.*, 1996). Nevertheless, the dose–response relationship has not been readily derivable from these (mostly case–control) studies. Furthermore, it seems likely that the situation is complex—the temporal pattern of exposure, age at first substantive exposure, and peak versus average exposure may all have

important influences on the extent of the increase in risk, particularly for malignant melanoma. The existing dose–response information has largely been derived from ecological data, based on UVR levels and skin cancer rates in geographically disparate populations. Those data, however, are almost certainly biased by local behavioural factors that modify the typical dose of UVR received in each population, and by variations in average host susceptibility (e.g. due to differences in skin pigmentation between populations).

It now seems possible that new information about the dose–response relationship—particularly within the relatively narrow dose range that represents the likely shift in UVR exposure due to stratospheric ozone depletion over the coming several decades—could rapidly be obtained with a sensitive and highly specific cancer-predictive mutation in skin cells (e.g. Brash *et al.*, 1991). Some recent evidence suggests that such a mutation may exist; namely the formation of pyrimidine dimers (entailing CC→TT transversion) within the *p53* gene (Nakazawa *et al.*, 1994). Nevertheless, until there are prospective data confirming the predictive significance of this mutation in humans, it cannot be used as a surrogate end-point for UVR-induced skin cancer.

9.3.4 Interindividual variation in susceptibility to carcinogen exposure

Improved measures of exposure to carcinogens will lead to more precise estimates of dose, and hence reduce the variability associated with calculated cancer risks. However, there is considerable variability between individuals in susceptibility to a given exposure. Depending on the needs of public health science and policy-making, the quantitation of cancer risk may need to take account, at some level, of this interindividual variation.

The factors responsible for such variability may act at any point in a pathway extending from absorption or uptake of carcinogen to the critical cellular step that marks the progression of a preneoplastic lesion to a new cancer. There are four broadly defined types of determinant of individual susceptibility to cancer, of which three refer to endogenous characteristics: variations in the metabolic handling of procarcinogens or carcinogens, variations in DNA repair capacity, and germline genetic mutations that predispose to cancer. The fourth is an acquired type, and refers, prototypically, to conjoint exposures such as cigarette smoking and dietary deficiencies of antioxidant micronutrients.

A variety of interindividual variations in metabolic phenotype influence the metabolism of carcinogens, and therefore influence the individual's risk of cancer. This metabolic characterization can be effected either with biochemical tests (especially the excretion of urinary metabolites) or, increasingly, with molecular genetic assays. Some examples have been discussed in Chapters 7 and 8.

Because the cytochrome P-450 system is involved in the metabolic activation and detoxification of carcinogens, it is not surprising that polymorphisms in the enzymes of this system are associated with cancer risk. The CYP2D6 enzyme, which is part of this system, has been well studied as an inherited metabolic characteristic. The rate of 4-hydroxylation of debrisoquine varies several thousand-fold between the extensive and poor "debrisoquine metabolizer" phenotypes (Harris, 1989, 1991). Two studies have shown an approximately five-fold increase in lung cancer in individuals who are "extensive" metabolizers (Ayesh et al., 1984; Caporaso et al., 1990).

The "acetylator phenotype" is a genetically inherited metabolic trait that determines the rate at which aromatic amines are metabolized. It has a bimodal distribution within populations, and the proportions of fast and slow acetylators vary by racial group; around 90% of Oriental peoples, 40–50% of Caucasians, and 20–30% of Israelis and Egyptians are fast acetylators (Evans, 1984). Slow acetylators are at increased risk for bladder cancer (Mommsen & Aagard, 1986). This is probably because, in slow acetylators, an alternative (non-acetylation) hepatic pathway is used for the metabolism of aromatic amines, which increases the level of promutagenic glucuronide metabolites in urine. On the other hand, fast acetylators appear to be predisposed to colon cancer, although the results of studies have not been fully consistent (Minchin et al., 1993). Much similar research is now under way in relation to variations in cancer risk as a function of other sources of metabolic phenotypic heterogeneity.

Variations in DNA repair capacity constitute a second type of innate susceptibility. Over 20 years ago, persons with xeroderma pigmentosum, an autosomal recessive condition, were shown to be defective in the repair of UV-induced damage of DNA in skin cells (Cleaver & Kraemer, 1995). Other heritable conditions such as Bloom's syndrome, ataxia telangiectasia and Fanconi's anaemia also entail defective DNA repair and increased susceptibility to cancer (Stewart, 1992; Strong & Amos, 1996). These conditions are rare, and so, presumably, they would be treated as special cases within a clinical context, rather than as a subpopulation for the formal quantitation of cancer risks.

Certain inherited genetic mutations pose a more direct risk of cancer. The classic example (Knudson, 1971) is the (occasional) inheritance of the mutated retinoblastoma tumour-suppressor gene (RB1), which renders the individual liable to (bilateral) retinoblastoma in early life. In Li–Fraumeni syndrome, patients with inherited mutations in the p53 gene are at greatly enhanced risk for cancers at multiple sites (Li, 1996; Strong & Amos, 1996). More recently, higher-prevalence genes predisposing to cancers of the colon, breast and to malignant melanoma have been reported (Li, 1996; Strong & Amos, 1996). The gene(s) for hereditary non-polyposis colon cancer have been briefly discussed in Chapter 7.

As previously mentioned, the fourth type of individual susceptibility is of the acquired variety. Cigarette smoking, for example, is one such characteristic that appears to amplify the cancer risks induced by exposures to other factors, such as asbestos fibres and ionizing radiation (α particles) from radon decay products.

The purpose in studying individual susceptibility differs, depending on whether the issue is examined from the point of view of public health, biomedical science, or clinical medicine. Public health aims to find efficient means of protecting populations from ill-health due to cancer. Better information about individual susceptibility may lead to greater efficiency in public health programmes (by concentrating screening programmes or primary prevention on high-risk categories of the population). However, such gains will be made only if research leads to acceptable and affordable interventions at the population level. Clinical medicine is concerned with the identification and management of increased susceptibility at the individual level, and again the emphasis must be placed on detecting determinants of susceptibility that are modifiable. Biomedical science has a focus that is narrower still than the clinical view, and essentially seeks knowledge about variations in individual susceptibility in order to improve understanding of the mechanisms of cancer.

Knowledge of the causes of individual susceptibility has grown enormously in the last five years. Examples of significant recent findings have been mentioned above. The immediate questions calling for future research include identifying: (i) the range and components of interindividual susceptibility to common carcinogens; (ii) variables that reduce susceptibility to carcinogens (such as possibly protective dietary factors); and (iii) genetic mutations that predispose to common cancers (advancing the work already reported on breast and colon cancer).

A central procedural question for QEP is: How much account should be taken of the differing risks experienced by identifiable subgroups within the population? This question poses a dilemma that did not previously press upon us. Populations of laboratory animals are genetically identical, so that the question of stratifying the calculation of their tumour risk does not arise. In the absence of biochemical and molecular measurements, populations of humans, studied epidemiologically, have necessarily been treated in unstratified fashion; average risks have been calculated at specified exposure levels. Now, there is the emerging possibility of multifactorial stratification of human subjects, in relation to a rapidly expanding repertoire of biological measures of host characteristics.

9.4 Future perspectives and research needs in toxicological studies

Because experimental studies are generally conducted on inbred strains of animals, the problems of heterogeneity, which must be addressed in epidemiological studies, do not arise in toxicological studies. Likewise, exposures can be precisely measured and disease outcomes carefully determined by necropsy so that the problems of mismeasured exposure and misclassification of

outcome need not be considered. There are other issues, however, of fundamental importance that arise in toxicological studies. These have to do with the *relevance* of the findings to QEP. A well designed and carefully conducted experimental study may add to our knowledge regarding mechanisms of carcinogenesis, but unless care has been taken to collect the appropriate quantitative data, the study may not be useful for QEP. We briefly discuss the ideal toxicological experiment for QEP below. A more fundamental problem arises if the agent under investigation causes cancer in the experimental model by a mechanism that does not exist in humans. For example, certain critical activating (or detoxifying) enzymes present in one species might be absent in another. Thus, when using toxicological data for QEP, careful consideration should be given to the relevance of any findings to human cancer.

9.4.1 Intermediate lesions

A critical issue is the relationship of intermediate lesions to the malignant tumour. A better understanding of the temporal course of the development of intermediate lesions, such as enzyme-altered foci in the rodent liver, and of the events involved in converting intermediate lesions into malignant tumours is required. Only a small fraction of enzyme-altered foci (or papillomas) develop into malignant tumours. This is an inevitable consequence of the stochastic nature of the events leading to malignant transformation. There is a second possibility, however, which is of great practical importance: not all intermediate lesions may have the potential to develop into malignant tumours. It would be very useful to have a marker (or markers) for intermediate lesions that do have the potential for malignant transformation. Essentially, such a marker would distinguish a lesion consisting of initiated cells from intermediate lesions that share a number of properties (such as enzyme alterations) with initiated lesions, but do not have the capacity to progress to fully malignant lesions.

9.4.2 Cell proliferation kinetics

It is now widely appreciated that cell proliferation kinetics play an important role in the carcinogenic process (Cohen & Ellwein, 1990). Furthermore, both cell division kinetics and the kinetics of differentiation and apoptosis are important. Indeed, some oncogenes block apoptosis and some promoters are presumed to act by decreasing the rate of apoptosis of initiated cells. Mathematically, it is important to consider cell division and apoptosis explicitly: it is not sufficient to consider only the net rate of cell division, i.e. the difference between the rates of cell division and apoptosis. Thus, ideally, one should have data on the dose–response curves for cell division rates and rates of apoptosis in both normal and initiated cells. Some attempts to obtain these data in the rodent liver have already been made.

Some comments on the methods used for estimating these rates are in order. For cell division, several different methods are now available, including flow cytometric methods for measurement of DNA content. If, however, proliferation rates on both normal and focal tissue are to be estimated, then *in vivo* pulse or continuous labelling with DNA precursors, such as tritiated thymidine or 2-bromo-2'-deoxyuridine (BrdU), are used. The interpretation of the labelling index and the estimation of division rates from pulse labelling experiments are difficult because the length of time that cells are exposed to label is not known with any precision. The interpretation of continuous labelling indices and their translation into division rates are easier. It should be emphasized, however, that estimation of cell division rates from labelling indices depends implicitly upon an assumed underlying model for cell division. When intermitotic times are assumed to be exponentially distributed, a likelihood-based approach has recently been advocated for estimating the parameter of this exponential distribution, which can be interpreted as the division rate (Moolgavkar & Luebeck, 1992b). With archived tissue, the fraction of cells in the S phase of the cell cycle can be estimated by immunohistochemical techniques for the detection of proliferation-associated antigens, such as PCNA or Ki67. As in the case of pulse labelling, it is not clear how this estimate can be converted into an estimate of the cell division rate.

Although the use of DNA precursor labelling is very convenient, a potential disadvantage of this method is that it is a measure, not of cell division, but of DNA synthesis. Under conditions where DNA synthesis is elevated by processes such as polyploidization or massive induction of DNA repair, this technique may be misleading. A more specific, although labour-intensive, measure of cell proliferation is the mitotic index. It is, however, not possible to convert this index into a rate for cell division without knowledge of the fraction of time that actual mitosis occupies in the cell cycle. For quantitative estimation of risk, therefore, the best procedure at present appears to be the measurement of a continuous labelling index, which can be used to estimate the rate of cell division (Moolgavkar & Luebeck, 1992b).

Rates of apoptosis are even more difficult to estimate directly than rates of cell division. Although markers for cells undergoing apoptosis are being developed (Stinchcombe et al., 1995), it is still too early to tell whether their use gives results in good agreement with those obtained with the more traditional approach, which depends on recognizing anatomical features of apoptotic cells under the microscope. Whether markers of apoptosis or more traditional methods are used, there are fundamental difficulties in converting counts of apoptotic bodies, which is how the data are presented, into rates of apoptosis. The difficulties arise from the fact that the number of visible apoptotic bodies depends upon two quantities: the rate at which cells enter apoptosis (which is the rate that we need to estimate) and the time that apoptotic bodies remain visible after cells have entered apoptosis. Estimates of the latter quantity are available, but are unlikely to be precise. To make matters even more complicated, the time to disappearance of apoptotic bodies will certainly depend upon the tissue and possibly also on the agent under investigation.

9.4.3 Statistical considerations

Finally, better statistical methods are required for analyses of toxicological data with serial sacrifices. Because the time to appearance of tumour is rarely known, statistical analyses of time-to-tumour data, whether empirical or biologically based, depend upon simplifying assumptions. In order to construct the likelihood, tumours have to be classified as being either incidental or fatal. Such a classification is usually made by the pathologist at necropsy. For incidental tumours, it is assumed that the tumour appeared at some time during the entire period that the animal was under observation, and that death or sacrifice of the animal was completely independent of the tumour. For fatal tumours, it is assumed that the tumour was instantaneously fatal. These are strong assumptions and unlikely to hold in practice. Even if a tumour is classified as being incidental, it may well hasten death from other causes. A tumour that is classified as being fatal may well have been present for a considerable period of time before causing death. Thus, such simplifying assumptions, without which likelihood analysis is currently not feasible, certainly lead to some bias in the estimates of parameters. More general methods for addressing these problems of interval-censored data need to be developed. Frequent serial sacrifices have been suggested to estimate the incidence of tumours (McKnight & Crowley, 1984). An alternative approach based on estimation of an extra "lethality" parameter has been proposed by Dewanji et al. (1993).

The analysis of intermediate lesions, such as altered hepatic foci or skin papillomas, in toxicological experiments has not received adequate statistical attention. As discussed in Chapter 7, methods based on the two-mutation clonal expansion model have been developed for analyses of altered hepatic foci. Until the recent development of these methods based on mechanistic considerations, the quantitative information in these data remained largely unexploited. Stereological considerations play an important role in the analyses of altered hepatic foci because observations made in two dimensions (histological examination under a microscope) have to be translated into information in three dimensions. The classical methods employed by experimentalists use a "binning" procedure introduced by Saltykov (see, e.g. Campbell et al., 1986) to estimate the number of three-dimensional spheres in certain predetermined size classes from information on two-dimensional discs. This procedure has the unpleasant property that the number of foci in some of the bins might be estimated to be negative. Nychka and colleagues (1984) have used statistical smoothing techniques to estimate the size distribution of foci from that of two-dimensional sections of foci. The latter method requires considerably more data than are available in the typical experiment. Both approaches require the

assumption of perfectly spherical foci and make crucial use of results due to Wicksell (1925). There is clear evidence, however, that the foci are not spherical. Preliminary attempts (Imaida et al., 1989) have been made to investigate the bias in the Saltykov procedure that may be introduced by departures from sphericity; no systematic study has been undertaken, however. In a recent paper, Dewanji et al. (1996) relaxed the assumption of spherical foci when analyses are conducted using the two-mutation clonal expansion model. Their proposed method presents difficult computational challenges, however.

The approaches briefly discussed above cannot be applied to very small foci consisting of a single cell or a very small number of cells. Recently, the placental form of glutathione-S-transferase (GST-P) has been used as a marker to detect foci consisting of a single cell or a few altered cells in liver transections (Satoh et al., 1989). These small lesions afford the opportunity to study early events in carcinogenesis, provided that the appropriate stereological techniques can be developed. Work has recently been started on this problem (de Gunst & Luebeck, 1998).

9.5 Future perspectives and research needs for biologically based models of carcinogenesis

In this volume, we have given many examples of the use of biologically based models for the estimation of effects, and for the construction of dose–response curves. When extrapolating outside the range of the data, however, there are no guarantees that these models will do any better than the traditional method of linear extrapolation. It must be remembered that these biologically based models were not developed originally for QEP of cancer risk but rather to provide explanations of phenomena that had been observed, either in the epidemiology of human cancer or in experimental carcinogenesis. Thus, biologically based cancer models have two very different functions. First, from the scientific point of view, a model provides a framework within which the process of carcinogenesis can be viewed and questions about it asked. A good model must provide explanations for observations and insights into data, and suggest experiments or epidemiological studies. Second, when used for the analysis of a data set, the parameters of the model should provide useful summary information. In short, from the scientific point of view, a biologically based model is good if it is useful, but it is widely understood that no model provides an absolutely "true" picture of the world. All scientific explanations are provisional, based on the knowledge that is available at the time.

Quantitative cancer risk assessment, on the other hand, is less forgiving of error. Policy-makers typically seek certainty rather than provisional assessment. Non-scientists often expect that the biological formulation of the model will accurately reflect reality, and therefore that the translation of this model into mathematical terms must be correctly specified. Obviously, we are very far from developing such a model. Nonetheless, biologically based models could prove to be very useful in QEP by focusing attention on data needs, and by breaking up a large and complex problem into smaller and more manageable pieces. Although quantitative extrapolations of risk to low doses based on such models cannot be demonstrated to be more "accurate" than those based on empirical procedures, some information on the shape of the dose–response curve may be obtained.

As illustrated elsewhere in this volume, biologically based models have a useful role to play in data analysis. When studying dose–response, some of the most important questions are concerned with the effect of pattern of exposure on risk. Thus, for example, there is some evidence that fractionation of a given exposure to high linear energy transfer (LET) radiation leads to an increased lifetime risk of malignancy. Another question of interest is how ages at first and last exposure influence subsequent risk of cancer. Such questions may be difficult to study using traditional statistical techniques, particularly when joint exposure to two agents, such as radon and cigarette smoke, are of interest. On the other hand, such analyses are relatively straightforward using hazard functions generated by cancer models. Problems can also arise when both premalignant and malignant lesions are discovered in a bioassay. For example, in some rodent hepatocarcinogenesis studies, altered hepatic foci, many of which are thought to be premalignant lesions, or adenomas are scored in addition to frank malig-

nancies. Currently, there are no good procedures for handling such data. Often, the premalignant and malignant lesions are combined in the analysis, a procedure that is clearly inappropriate because it gives equal weight to the two types of lesion. Sometimes, the premalignant lesions are omitted from the analysis, but this is equally inappropriate because valuable information is then discarded. Carcinogenesis models offer a way out of this dilemma by providing the potential for analyses that can simultaneously handle premalignant and malignant lesions (Dewanji *et al.*, 1991).

Because biologically based models seek to describe the fundamental biological events involved in carcinogenesis, the parameters of such models have direct biological interpretation. How meaningful these interpretations are will depend upon how faithfully the model reflects underlying biological processes. The two-stage clonal expansion model discussed in detail in Chapter 7, for example, includes parameters that explicitly represent the rates of occurrence of certain genetic lesions, and the birth and death rates of cells that have sustained the first genetic alteration. To some extent, the validity of parameter estimates can be gauged by determining whether they are of reasonable biological plausibility.

Ideally, the use of biologically based models of carcinogenesis should be "technology-forcing" in the sense that lack of fit may lead to revisions of the model, including a possible rethinking of the sequence of events involved in neoplastic transformation. For example, Moolgavkar & Luebeck (1992a) analysed human colon cancer data and concluded that more than two rate-limiting events were involved in colon carcinogenesis. Similarly, Kopp-Schneider & Portier (1992) analysed data from a mouse skin initiation–promotion experiment, and concluded that more than two rate-limiting events were required to describe the process of neoplastic transformation. The process of model fitting, evaluation, and updating need not be limited to pharmacodynamic models used to describe cellular events involved in carcinogenesis. Early work on the development of physiological pharmacokinetic models often failed to produce satisfactory results, leading to biologically motivated model refinements and corresponding improvements in fit.

The example of dioxin shows that even detailed biological information may not be be very useful in risk assessment because of crucial gaps in knowledge. While it is true that a detailed understanding of mechanism is likely to translate into better risk assessment, the data needs for rational risk assessment overlap, but are not identical with, those for detailed mechanistic understanding. The example of dioxin again illustrates this point. A detailed mechanistic understanding of dioxin-induced cell proliferation would entail knowledge of all the steps, after the early biological responses to dioxin such as receptor binding and enzyme induction, that ultimately lead to cell proliferation. For QEP, it would appear to be sufficient to know the dose–response curves for cell division and apoptosis. In fact, direct measurement of cell division and apoptosis in response to dioxin is preferable to detailed knowledge of mechanism, particularly if the mechanism is complex, as is likely.

One of the fundamental problems in carcinogenesis modelling is that, although carcinogenesis is a multistage process, little or no information is generally available on the intermediate stages to malignancy except in a few experimental systems. Most often, particularly in epidemiological studies, only incidence or prevalence data are available, and estimates of parameters associated with intermediate stages are obtained from these data. This procedure, which is akin to deconvolving a distribution into the sum of two distributions, can yield misleading results. For example, in the analyses of the epidemiological and experimental data on radon-induced lung tumours in Chapter 8, the two-mutation clonal expansion model was used. Information was available only on the malignant tumours; the intermediate stage was essentially hypothesized but unobserved. Even if the model used for the analysis is correct, much more precise information would be obtained if direct observations could be made on the intermediate stage. Some recent simulation results have shown that end-point, i.e. tumour-incidence, data have little power to discriminate among mechanisms. This is one of the reasons why the rodent liver system is an attractive model system for quantitative risk assessment. As described earlier, this system is characterized by the appearance of early altered lesions, at least

some of which are believed to be premalignant. The technology for counting these lesions and for measuring their sizes is now fairly well developed. Information on premalignant (papillomas) and malignant (carcinomas) lesions is available also in the mouse skin system, which is probably the oldest animal model system under study. The quantitative information, particularly on the size distribution of papillomas, is not as precise as in the liver system, however. Although a formal analysis in which both premalignant and malignant lesions are simultaneously considered has not hitherto been carried out, such an analysis would offer the maximum power to discriminate between mechanisms and the most precise estimates of parameters. Methods for simultaneous analyses of premalignant and malignant lesions are currently being investigated. At the same time, better experimental methods need to be developed to identify and quantify the foci within foci in the rodent liver. These are often considered to be the first signs of malignancy in the premalignant focus. Development of markers for intermediate lesions on the pathway to malignancy, and of methods for the quantitation of these intermediate lesions in animal model systems other than the rodent liver and mouse skin, would be most useful for QEP. Some work along these lines is being done with the rodent pancreas.

When mechanistic models are used for data analysis, another problem arises from the fact that most tumours are occult until they reach a certain size. Thus, most carcinogenesis models explicitly consider only the time to appearance of the first malignant cell in the tissue, whereas the data consist of observations on whether or not a malignant tumour is present at a given time. One, rather ad hoc, approach that has been used is to assume a constant lag time between the appearance of the first malignant cell and the detection of a malignant tumour. This assumption is clearly a gross oversimplification of biological reality. For one thing, even malignant cells undergo differentiation and may die. Thus, the first malignant cell in a tissue may not give rise to a malignant tumour, and even if the first malignant cell did do so, there is clearly a time-to-tumour distribution. The impact of such considerations on the estimates of parameters of the two-mutation model has been investigated by simulation (Luebeck & Moolgavkar, 1994), although much work remains to be done. Models that consider explicitly the proliferation kinetics of malignant cells have also been developed (Dewanji *et al.*, 1991; Yang & Chen, 1991), although statistical methods for applying these models to the analyses of data are not yet available. Another problem, which has been briefly discussed above, is that likelihood analyses of incidence data require assumptions regarding tumour lethality.

Implicit in current attempts to incorporate cell proliferation kinetics into carcinogenesis models are the assumptions that cells in a tissue divide, die and mutate independently, and that the waiting time distributions of these events are exponential. These assumptions are convenient because they simplify the mathematics, but they are certainly not true. Whole volumes have been published on mathematical models of the cell cycle, and it is well known that intermitotic times are not exponentially distributed. Thus, it is necessary to develop the mathematical tools required to incorporate more realistic models of the cell cycle into carcinogenesis models. At the same time, the application of these more realistic models will require collection of the appropriate data.

We have given examples of the application of biologically based models to analyses of epidemiological data in Chapter 7 of this volume. Heretofore, these models have been used almost exclusively for analyses of cohort data. Few attempts have been made to analyse case–control data. Although the likelihood for case–control data can easily be constructed (Moolgavkar, 1995) based on ideas put forward by Prentice & Breslow (1978) and Prentice (1986), estimation of parameters appears to require ancillary information on background cancer rates. This is because the hazard functions derived from mechanistic models are not, in general, of the proportional hazards form, and therefore the background hazards cannot be eliminated from the expression for the likelihood. Methods for fitting these models to case–control data need to be developed.

As a consideration of biologically based models of carcinogenesis makes clear, what is required for a rational approach to QEP is fundamental biological information. Some information that would be useful has been discussed above, but

other fundamental issues also need to be addressed, as follows. Is there a subset of cells in tissues susceptible to malignant transformation? It is generally believed that only the stem cells in a tissue are susceptible, but there does not appear to be strong evidence in support of this view. How does the size of this susceptible subpopulation change with age? Can this susceptible subpopulation be identified, and rates of cell division and apoptosis measured? In experimental systems, clonogenic subpopulations of cells susceptible to malignant transformation have been identified (Clifton, 1990).

Although the foregoing discussion has focused on pharmacodynamic models used to characterize biological interactions between the proximate carcinogen and the target tissue, the development and application of biologically based pharmacokinetic models to describe the metabolism of xenobiotics have also received considerable attention in recent years, as discussed in Chapter 7. Physiologically based pharmacokinetic (PBPK) models which view the body as consisting of a small number of relatively homogeneous physiologically relevant compartments are now commonplace. Such multiparametric PBPK models are of particular biological relevance since all of the parameters have clear biological interpretation; consequently, estimates of the values of allometric and other PBPK model parameters can easily be evaluated for biological plausibility.

Inhaled carcinogens pose an additional challenge. Not only are PBPK models required to describe the uptake and disposition of inhaled toxicants, but the dynamics of air flow respiration also play an essential role in determining dose to various parts of the respiratory system. Recent work on modelling air flow in the respiratory passages holds out the promise of precise estimates of dose of inhaled toxicants to various parts of the respiratory tree (Kimbell *et al.*, 1993).

Many carcinogens, of which dioxin is one example, are thought to act through receptor-mediated mechanisms (Lucier, 1992). Although models to describe receptor binding are available (Chapter 7), the nature of the biological receptors and the formation of the receptor–ligand complexes are less well understood than other pharmacokinetic processes. The Hill and Michaelis–Menten equations (see Chapter 7) are useful tools, but may not represent adequately the fundamental processes governing the complex ligand–receptor interactions involved in carcinogenesis. None the less, the importance of receptor-mediated events in neoplastic transformation warrants further work in the identification of critical cellular receptors and in developing better models of the binding of ligands to the receptors.

If a series of models (PBPK, receptor-binding, pharmacodynamic) can be developed to describe distinct aspects of the overall biological process occurring between exposure to an environmental agent and subsequent malignant transformation, consideration may be given to combining these models to arrive at an integrated biologically based model of the entire process of carcinogenesis following exposure to a carcinogen (Connolly & Andersen, 1991). The construction of such integrated models may be thought of as the holy grail of carcinogenesis modelling, and will be possible only when sufficient data on each aspect of the carcinogenic process are available.

9.6 The bioassay

From the discussion above, it is clear that the current bioassay does not provide the information that is required for a QEP based on mechanistic considerations. Because the rodent liver model system is so well characterized, we describe here an "ideal" bioassay in rodents with liver lesions as the end-points of interest. First, although practical considerations always dictate the size of an experiment, the number of animals studied should be as large as possible. Second, as many dose groups as possible should be included in the study. It may be useful to undertake a "range-finding" study first in order to obtain some information on necessary sample sizes, particularly at low doses. Finally, serial sacrifices should always be planned so that important information on the time to tumour development can be obtained.

At each sacrifice, the animals should be necropsied and the liver carefully examined for the presence or absence of malignant tumours. The sizes of these tumours (if any are present) should be measured, if possible. In addition, two to three sections from each lobe of the liver should be stained and examined for altered foci.

It is advisable to use two markers, one positive such as the induction of GST-P, the other negative, such as the absence of ATPase. The area of each section should be measured carefully and the number of transections (through altered foci) in each section of the liver should be counted, after which the area of each transection should be measured. If possible, foci within foci should be counted and sized, although the quantitative technology for converting these data into three-dimensional information on the number and size distribution of foci within foci does not exist at present. If possible, the average size of the cells in the normal liver and in the foci should be determined. The concentration of the active metabolite should be measured in the liver, and, if relevant and possible, DNA adducts should be measured as functions of the dose of the agent under study. Similarly, continuous (two-to-three-day) labelling indices should be measured in normal and focal tissue as functions of the dose of the agents. Ideally, labelling indices should be measured in the same sections as those used for quantifying foci. This can be accomplished by using double stains, e.g. by combining immunohistochemical demonstration of the induction of GST-P and the incorporation of BrdU. Rates of apoptosis should be measured as well, if possible.

9.7 Conclusions

Improvements in the future will depend on the quality and detail of information collected in epidemiological and experimental studies, on increased understanding of the biological mechanisms of carcinogenesis, and on improvements of cancer risk models. Results of QEPs in the future are unlikely to be single numbers: our current understanding of carcinogenesis indicates that an individual's risk of developing cancer from a given agent will depend on a number of host factors—including age at exposure, sex, genetic make-up—and exposure to other environmental agents. It is essential, therefore, in order for predictions to be applicable, that proper account be taken of possible modifying factors in the quantitative estimation process and that estimates be derived, where appropriate, for different levels of these factors (e.g. risk in children, adolescents and adults, in smokers and in non-smokers, etc.).

While we have focused our attention in this volume on the scientific aspects of QEP, it must be remembered that assessments of risk are often conducted in a politically charged environment. The result is a "fusion of facts and values in the masquerade of politics as science contradicts the prevailing notion that risk assessment for toxic substances is (or should be) entirely objective or scientific" (Whittemore, 1996). Risk assessments of the future should be more explicit regarding the sources of uncertainty and should explicitly acknowledge the assumptions made to bridge existing data gaps. There are consequently important questions for research that include quantitative and qualitative elements. What is the plausible range (which is not the same as the statistical confidence interval) of risks ? What are the best means of expressing uncertainty in QEP? Where are the critical decision points? What are the consequences of applying different strategies in research and analysis? What values do scientists apply in choosing between these strategies?

As discussed above, there is a growing consensus that, when mechanistic information is available, models that take it into account are preferable to purely empirical models for predictions. Not surprisingly, therefore, a scientific approach to QEP requires information on fundamental biological quantities. It is unlikely, however, that, even with this information, we shall be able to solve the problems of interspecies and low-dose extrapolation. We should, however, obtain some insights into reasons for species differences in response to carcinogenic agents, and into the shape of the dose–response curve. Anything more will probably remain beyond the ken of Science.

References

Armstrong, B.K. & English, D.R. (1996) Cutaneous malignant melanoma. In: Schottenfeld, D. & Fraumeni, J.F., eds, *Cancer Epidemiology and Prevention, 2nd ed.*, New York, NY, Oxford University Press, pp. 1282-1312

Armstrong, B.K., White E. & Saracci R. (1992) *Principles of Exposure Measurement Error in Epidemiology* (Monographs in Epidemiology and Biostatistics, Vol. 21), New York, NY, Oxford University Press

Ayesh, R., Idle, J., Richie, J., Crothers, M. & Hetzel, M. (1984) Metabolic oxidation phenotypes as markers for susceptibility to lung cancer. *Nature*, 312, 169-170

Brandt-Rauf, P.W., Smith, S., Hemminki, K., Vainio, H. & Ford, J. (1992) Serum oncoproteins and growth factors in asbestosis and silicosis patients. *Int. J. Cancer*, 50, 881-885

Brash, D.E., Rudolph, J.A., Simon, J.A., Lin, A., McKenna, G.J., Baden, H.P., Halperin, A.J. & Ponten, A. (1991) A role for sunlight in skin cancer: UV-induced *p53* mutations in squamous cell carcinoma. *Proc. Natl Acad. Sci. USA*, 88, 10124-10128

Brogger, A., Hagmar, L, Hansteen, I.L., Heim, S., Hogstedt, B., Knudsen, L., Lambert, B., Linnainmaa, K., Mitelman, F., Nordenson, I., Reuterwall, C., Salomaa, S., Skerfving, S. & Sorsa, M. (1990) An inter-Nordic prospective study on cytogenetic endpoints and cancer risk. *Cancer Genet. Cytogenet.*, 45, 1264-1272

Bryant, M.S., Skipper, P.L., Tannenbaum, S.R. & Niure, M. (1987) Hemoglobin adducts of 4-aminobiphenyl in smokers and nonsmokers. *Cancer Res.*, 47, 612-618

Campbell, H.A., Xu, Y.D., Hanigan, M.H. & Pitot, H.C. (1986) Application of quantitative stereology to the evaluation of phenotypically heterogeneous enzyme-altered foci in the rat liver. *J. Natl Cancer Inst.*, 76, 751-756

Caporaso, N.E., Tucker, M.A., Hoover, R.N., Hayes, R.B., Pickle, L.W., Issaq, H.J. & Muschik, G.M. (1990) Lung cancer and the debrisoquine metabolic phenotype. *J. Natl Cancer Inst.*, 82, 1264-1272

Cardis, E., Okeanov, A.E., Anspaugh, L., Mabuchi, K., Likhtarev, I., Ivanov, V.K. & Prisyazhniuk, A.E. (1996) Estimated long-term health effects of the Chernobyl accident. In: *One Decade After Chernobyl. Summing up the Consequences of the Accident. Proceedings of an International Conference*, Vienna, International Atomic Energy Agency

Carroll, R.J., Ruppert, D. & Stefanski, L.A. (1995) *Measurement Error in Nonlinear Models* (Monographs on Statistics and Applied Probability, Vol. 63), London, Chapman and Hall

Cleaver, J.E. & Kraemer, K.H. (1995) Xeroderma pigmentosum and Cockayne syndrome. In: Scriver, C.R., Beaudet, A.L., Sly, W.S. & Valle, D., eds, *The Metabolic and Molecular Basis of Inherited Disease*, New York, NY, McGraw-Hill, pp. 4393-4419

Clifton, K.H. (1990). The clonogenic cells of the rat mammary and thyroid glands: their biology, frequency of initiation, and promotion/progression to cancer. In: Moolgavkar, S.H., ed., *Scientific Issues in Quantitative Cancer Risk Assessment*, Boston, MA, Birkhäuser, pp. 1-21

Cohen, S.M. & Ellwein, L.B. (1990) Cell proliferation in carcinogenesis. *Science*, 249, 1007-1011

Connolly, R.B. & Andersen, M.E. (1991) Biologically based pharmacodynamic models: Tools for toxicological research and risk assessment. *Ann. Rev. Pharmacol. Toxicol.*, 31, 503-523

Costantino, J.P., Redmond, C.K. & Bearden, A. (1995) Occupationally related cancer risk among coke oven workers: 30 years of follow-up. *J. Occup. Environ. Med.*, 37, 597-604.

de Gunst, M.C.M. & Luebeck, E.G. (1998) A method for parametric estimation of the number and size distribution of cell clusters from observations in a section plane. *Biometrics*, 54, 100-112

Dewanji, A., Luebeck, E.G. & Moolgavkar, S.H. (1991) Two-mutation model for carcinogenesis: Joint analysis of premalignant and malignant lesions. *Math. Biosci.*, 104, 97-109

Dewanji, A., Krewski, D. & Goddard, M.J. (1993) A Weibull model for estimation of tumorigenic potency. *Biometrics*, 49, 367-377

Dewanji, A., Moolgavkar, S.H. & Luebeck, E.G. (1996) A biologically based model for the analysis of premalignant foci of arbitrary shape. *Math. Biosci.*, 135, 55-68

Evans, D.A.P. (1984) Survey of the human acetylator polymorphism in spontaneous disorders. *J. Med. Genet.*, 21, 243-253

Fearon, E.R. & Vogelstein, B. (1990) A genetic model for colorectal tumorigenesis. *Cell*, 61, 759-767

Gilks, W.R. & Richardson, S. (1992) Analysis of disease risks using ancillary risk factors, with application to job exposure matrices. *Stat. Med.*, 11, 1443-1463

Gilks, W.R., Richardson, S. & Spiegelhalter, D.J., eds (1996) *Markov Chain Monte Carlo in Practice*, London, Chapman & Hall

Groopman, J.D., Donahue, P.R., Zhu, J., Chen, J. & Wogan, G.N. (1985) Aflatoxin metabolism and nucleic acid adducts in urine by affinity chromatography. *Proc. Natl Acad. Sci. USA*, 82, 6492-6496

Harris, C.C. (1989) Interindividual variation among humans in carcinogen metabolism, DNA adduct formation and DNA repair. *Carcinogenesis*, 10, 1563-1566

Harris, C. (1991) Chemical and physical carcinogenesis: Advances and perspectives for the 1990s. *Cancer Res.*, Suppl, 51, 50235-50445

Hulka, B.S., Wilcosky, T.C. & Griffith, J.D. (1990) *Biological Markers in Epidemiology*, New York, NY, Oxford University Press

Hemminki, K., Grzybowska, E., Chorazi, M., Twardowska-Sau-Cha, K., Sroczynski, J.W., Putman, K.L., Randerath, K., Phillips, D.H., Hewer, A., Santella, R.M., Young, T.L. & Perera, F.P. (1990) DNA adducts in humans environmentally exposed to aromatic compounds in an industrial area of Poland. *Carcinogensis*, 11, 1229-1231

Imaida, K., Tatematsu, M., Kato, T., Tsuda, H. & Ito, N. (1989) Advantages and limitations of stereological estimation of placental glutathione-S-transferase-positive rat liver cell foci by computerized three-dimensional reconstruction. *Jpn J. Cancer Res.*, 80, 326-330

International Agency for Research on Cancer (1997) *IARC Monographs on the Evaluation of Carcinogenic Risk to Humans*, Vol 69, *Polychlorinated Dibenzo-para-dioxins and Polychlorinated Dibenzofurans*, Lyon

Kai, M., Luebeck, E.G. & Moolgavkar, S.H. (1997) Analysis of the incidence of solid cancer among atomic bomb survivors using a two-stage model of carcinogenesis. *Radiat Res.*, **148**, 348-358

Kazakov, V.S., Demidchik, E.P. & Astakhova, L.N. (1992) Thyroid cancer after Chernobyl. *Nature*, **359**, 21

Kimbell, J.S., Gross, E.A., Joyner, D.R., Godo, M.N. & Morgan, K.T. (1993) Application of computation fluid dynamics to regional dosimetry of inhaled chemicals in the upper respiratory tract of the rat. *Toxicol. Appl. Pharmacol.*, **121**, 253-263

Knudson, A.G. (1971) Mutation and cancer: Statistical study of retinoblastoma. *Proc. Natl Acad. Sci. USA*, **68**, 820-823

Kohn, M.C., Lucier, G.W., Clark, G.C., Sewall, C., Tritscher, A.M. & Portier, C.J. (1993) A mechanistic model of effects of dioxin on gene expression in the rat liver. *Toxicol. Appl. Pharmacol.*, **120**, 138-154

Kociba, R.J., Keyes, D.G., Beyer, J.E., Carreon, R.M., Wade, C.E., Dittenber, D.A., Kainins, R.P., Frauson, L.E., Park, C.N., Bernard, S.D., Hummel, R.A. & Humiston, C.G. (1978) Results of a two-year chronic toxicity and oncogenicity study of 2,3,7,8-tetrachlorodibenzo-*p*-dioxin in rats. *Toxicol. Appl. Pharmacol.*, **46**, 279-303

Kopp-Schneider, A. & Portier, C.J. (1992) Birth and death/differentiation rates of papillomas in mouse skin. *Carcinogenesis*, **13**, 973-978

Li, F.P. (1996) Familial aggregation. In: Schottenfeld, D. & Fraumeni, J.F., eds, *Cancer Epidemiology and Prevention*, 2nd ed., New York, NY, Oxford University Press, pp. 546-558

Liang, K.Y. & Pulver, A.E. (1996) Analysis of case–control/family sampling design. *Genet. Epidemiol.*, **13**, 253-270

Lucier, G.W. (1992) Receptor-mediated carcinogenesis. In: *Mechanisms of Carcinogenesis in Risk Identification* (IARC Scientific Publications No. 116), Lyon, International Agency for Research on Cancer, pp. 87-112

Luebeck, E.G. & Moolgavkar, S.H. (1994) Simulating the process of malignant transformation. *Math. Biosci.*, **123**, 127-146

McKnight, B. & Crowley, J. (1984) Tests for differences in tumor incidence based on animal carcinogenesis experiments. *J. Am. Stat. Assoc.*, **79**, 639-648

Minchin, R.F., Kadlubar, F.F. & Ilett, K.F. (1993) Role of acetylation in colorectal cancer. *Mutat. Res.*, **290**, 35-42

Mommsen, S. & Aagaard, J. (1986) Susceptibility in urinary bladder cancer: Acetyltransferase phenotypes and related risk factors. *Cancer Lett.*, **32**, 199-205

Moolgavkar, S.H. (1995) When and how to combine results from multiple epidemiological studies in risk assessment. In: Graham, J.D., ed., *The Role of Epidemiology in Regulatory Risk Assessment*, Amsterdam, Elsevier Science, pp. 77-90

Moolgavkar, S.H. & Luebeck, G. (1992a) Multistage carcinogenesis: population-based model for colon cancer. *J. Natl Cancer Inst.*, **84**, 610-618

Moolgavkar, S.H. & Luebeck, G. (1992b) Interpretation of labeling indices in the presence of cell death. *Carcinogenesis*, **13**, 1007-1010

Nakazawa, H., English, D., Randell, P.L., Nakazawa, K., Martel, N., Armstrong, B.K. & Yamasaki, H. (1994) UV and skin cancer: specific *p53* gene mutation in normal skin as a biologically relevant exposure measurement. *Proc. Natl Acad. Sci. USA*, **91**, 360-364.

Nychka, D., Wahba, G., Goldfarb, S. & Pugh, T. (1984) Cross validated spline methods for the estimation of three-dimensional tumor size distributions from observations on two-dimensional cross-sections. *J. Am. Stat. Assoc.*, **79**, 832-846

Perera, F.P. (1996) Molecular epidemiology in cancer prevention. In: Schottenfeld, D. & Fraumeni, J.F., eds, *Cancer Epidemiology and Prevention,* 2nd ed., New York, NY, Oxford University Press, pp. 101-115

Perera, F.P. & Santella, R. (1993) Carcinogenesis. In: Schulte, P.A. & Perera, F.P., eds, *Molecular Epidemiology: Principles and Practices,* San Diego, CA, Academic Press, pp. 277-300

Perera, F.P., Santella, R.M., Brenner, D., Poirier, M.C., Munshi, A.A., Fischman, H.K. & van Ryzin, J. (1987) DNA adducts, protein adducts and sister chromatid exchange in cigarette smokers and non-smokers. *J. Natl Cancer Inst.,* 79, 449-456

Perkel, V.S., Gail, M.H., Lubin, J., Pee, D.Y., Weinstein, R., Shore-Freedman, E. & Schneider, A.B. (1988) Radiation-induced thyroid neoplasms: evidence for familial susceptibility factors. *J. Clin. Endocrinol. Metab.,* 66, 1316-1322

Portier, C., Tritscher, A., Kohn, M., Sewall, C., Clark, G., Edler, L., Hoel, D. & Lucier, G. (1993) Ligand/receptor binding for 2,3,7,8-TCDD: Implications for risk assessment. *Fundam. Appl. Toxicol.,* 20, 48-56

Prentice, R.L. (1986) A case–cohort design for epidemiologic cohort studies and disease prevention trials. *Biometrika,* 73, 1-11

Prentice, R.L., (1989) Surrogate endpoints in clinical trials: definition and operational criteria. *Stat. Med.,* 8, 431-440

Prentice R.L., & Breslow, N.E. (1978) Retrospective studies and failure time models. *Biometrika,* 65, 153-158

Ron, E., Modan, B., Preston, D.L., Alfandary, E., Stovall, M. & Boice, J.D., Jr (1989) Thyroid neoplasia following low-dose radiation in childhood. *Radiat. Res.,* 20, 516-531

Ron, E., Lubin, J., Shore, R.E., Mabuchi, K., Modan, B., Pottern, L.M., Schneider, A.B., Tucker, M.A. & Boice, J.D., Jr (1995) Thyroid cancer after exposure to external radiation: a pooled analysis of seven studies. *Radiat. Res.,* 141, 259-277

Satoh, K., Hatayama, I., Tateoka, N., Tamai, K., Shimizu, T., Tatematsu, M., Ito, N. & Sato, K. (1989) Transient induction of single GST-P positive hepatocytes by DEN. *Carcinogenesis,* 10, 2107-2111

Sauer, R.M. (1990) *Pathology Working Group. 2,3,7,8-Tetrachlorodibenzo-p-dioxin in Sprague–Dawley Rats,* Ivansville, MD, Pathco, Inc.

Schulte, P.A. & Perera, F.P., eds (1993) *Molecular Epidemiology: Principles and Practices,* San Diego, CA, Academic Press

Scotto, J., Fears, T.R., Kraemer, K.H. & Fraumeni, J.F., Jr (1996) Nonmelanoma skin cancer. In: Schottenfeld, D. & Fraumeni, J.F., eds, *Cancer Epidemiology and Prevention,* 2nd ed., New York, NY, Oxford University Press, pp. 1313-1330

Stewart, B.W. (1992) Role of DNA repair in carcinogenesis. In: *Mechanisms of Carcinogenesis in Risk Identification,* (IARC Scientific Publications No. 116), Lyon, International Agency for Research on Cancer, pp. 307-320

Stinchcombe, S., Buchmann, A., Bock, K.W. & Schwarz, M. (1995) Inhibition of apoptosis during 2,3,7,8-tetrachlorodibenzo-*p*-dioxin-mediated tumour promotion in rat liver. *Carcinogenesis,* 16, 1271-1275

Strong, L.C. & Amos, C.I. (1996) Inherited susceptibility. In: Schottenfeld, D. & Fraumeni, J.F., eds, *Cancer Epidemiology and Prevention,* 2nd ed., New York, NY, Oxford University Press, pp. 559-586

Stsjazhko, V.A., Tsyb, A.F., Tronko, N.D., Souchkevitch, G. & Baverstock, K.F. (1995) Letter to the editor. *Br. Med. J.,* 310, 801

Thompson, D.E., Mabuchi, K., Ron, E., Soda, M., Tokunaga, M., Ochikubo, S., Sugimoto, S., Ikeda, T., Terasaki, M., Izumi, S. & Preston, D.L. (1994) Cancer incidence in atomic bomb survivors. Part II: Solid tumors, 1958–87. *J. Radiat. Res.,* 137, S17-S67

Tronko, N.D., Epstein, Y., Oleinik, V., Bogdanova, T., Likhtarev, I., Gulko, G., Kairo, I. & Sobolev, B. (1994) Thyroid gland in children after the Chernobyl accident (yesterday and today). In: Nagataki, S., ed., *Nagasaki Symposium on Chernobyl: Update and Future*, Amsterdam, Elsevier Science, pp. 31-46

Tsyb, A.F., Parshkov, E.M., Ivanov, V.K., Stepanenko, V.F., Matveenko, E.G. & Skoropad, Y.D. (1994) Disease indices of thyroid and their dose dependence in children and adolescents affected as a result of the Chernobyl accident. In: Nagataki, S., ed., *Nagasaki Symposium on Chernobyl: Update and Future*, Amsterdam, Elsevier Science, pp. 9-19

US Environmental Protection Agency (1985) *Health assessment document for polychlorinated dibenzo-p-dioxins* (Document EPA/600/8-84-014F), Cincinnati, OH, Office of Health and Environmental Assessment

Whittemore, A.S. (1995) Multiphase sampling designs and estimating equations. *J. R. Stat. Soc., Series B*, **59**, 589-602

Whittemore, A.S. (1996) Quantitative risk assessment. In: Schottenfeld, D. & Fraumeni, J.F., eds, *Cancer Epidemiology and Prevention*, 2nd ed., New York, NY, Oxford University Press, pp. 116-126

Whittemore, A.S. & Gong, G. (1994) Segregation analysis of case–control data using generalized estimating equations. *Biometrics*, **50**, 1073-1087

Whittemore, A.S. & Halpern, J. (1997) Multiphase sampling designs in genetic epidemiology. *Stat. Med.*, **16**, 153-167

Wicksell, D.S. (1925) The corpuscle problem, Part I. *Biometrika*, **17**, 87-97

Woodward, A., Roder, D., McMichael, A.J., Crouch, P. & Mylvaganam, A. (1991) Radon daughter exposures at the Radium Hill Uranium Mine and lung cancer rates among former workers. *Cancer Causes Control*, **2**, 213-220

Yang, G.C. & Chen, C.W. (1991) A stochastic two-stage carcinogenesis model: A new approach to computing the probability of observing tumor in animal bioassays. *Math. Biosci.*, **104**, 247-258

Zhao, L.P. & LeMarchand, L. (1992) An analytical method for assessing patterns of familial aggregation in case–control studies. *Genet. Epidemiol.*, **9**, 141-154

Zhao, L.P., Hsu, L., Davidov, O., Potter, J., Elston, R.C. & Prentice, R.L. (1997) Population-based family study designs: An interdisciplinary research framework for genetic epidemiology. *Genet Epidemiol.*, **14**, 365-388

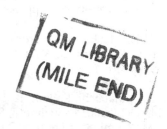
Achevé d'imprimer sur rotative par l'Imprimerie Darantiere à Dijon-Quetigny en mai 1999
Dépôt légal : 2e trimestre 1999 - N° d'impression : 99-0435